Measuring Outcomes in Speech-Language Pathology

Measuring Outcomes in Speech-Language Pathology

EDITED BY

Carol M. Frattali

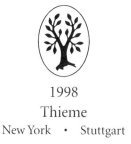

1998

Thieme

New York • Stuttgart

Thieme New York
333 Seventh Ave.
New York, NY 10001

Measuring Outcomes in Speech-Language Pathology
Carol M. Frattali, Ph.D.

RC423
.M39
1997

Library of Congress Cataloging-in-Publication Data

Measuring outcomes in speech-language pathology / edited by Carol M.
  Frattali.
      p.   cm.
    Includes bibliographical references and index.
    ISBN 0-86577-718-7 (TMP).—ISBN 3-13-109731-0 (GTV)
    1. Speech therapy—Evaluation.   2. Outcome assessment (Medical
care) I. Frattali, Carol.
    [DNLM: 1. Speech Disorders—therapy.   2. Treatment Outcome.
3. Language Disorders—therapy.   4. Speech-Language Pathology.   WL
340.2 M484   1997]
RC423.M39   1997
616.85'506—dc21
DNLM/DLC   97-26377
for Library of Congress   CIP

Important note: Medical knowledge is ever-changing. As new research and clinical experience broaden our knowledge, changes in treatment and drug therapy may be required. The authors and editors of the material herein have consulted sources believed to be reliable in their efforts to provide information that is complete and in accord with the standards accepted at the time of publication. However, in view of the possibility of human error by the authors, editors, or publishers of the work herein, or changes in medical knowledge, neither the authors, editors, publisher, nor any other party who has been involved in the preparation of this work, warrants that the information contained herein is in every respect accurate or complete, and they are not responsible for any errors or omissions or for the results obtained from use of such information. Readers are encouraged to confirm the information contained herein with other sources. For example, readers are advised to check the product information sheet included in the package of each drug they plan to administer to be certain that the information contained in this publication is accurate and that changes have not been made in the recommended dose or in the contraindications for administration. This recommendation is of particular importance in connection with new or infrequently used drugs.

Some of the product names, patents, and registered designs referred to in this book are in fact registered trademarks or proprietary names even though specific reference to this fact is not always made in the text. Therefore, the appearance of a name without designation as proprietary is not to be construed as a representation by the publisher that it is in the public domain.

Printed in the United States of America

5 4 3   2   1

TNY ISBN 0-86577-718-7
GTV ISBN 3-13-109731-0

Contents

Foreword   xi
Rosemary Lubinski

Preface   xiii
Acknowledgments   xv
Contributors   xvii

Section I.   OVERVIEW

Chapter 1. Outcomes Measurement: Definitions,
Dimensions, and Perspectives   1
Carol M. Frattali

Chapter 2. Outcomes Measurement Requirements   28
Patricia Larkins Hicks

Section II.   MEASURES

Chapter 3. Measuring Modality-Specific Behaviors,
Functional Abilities, and Quality of Life   55
Carol M. Frattali

Chapter 4. Measuring Consumer Satisfaction   89
*Paul R. Rao,
Jean Blosser, and
Nancy P. Huffman*

Chapter 5. Collecting, Analyzing, and Reporting
Financial Outcomes Data   113
*Michael I. Rolnick and
Richard M. Merson*

Section III.   METHODS

Chapter 6. Treatment Efficacy Research   134
Lesley B. Olswang

Chapter 7. Program Evaluation   151
Deborah L. Wilkerson

v

Chapter 8. Quality Improvement 172
Carol M. Frattali

Chapter 9. Designing Automated Outcomes Management Systems 186
Mary Ann Keatley,
Thomas I. Miller, and
Alex F. Johnson

Chapter 10. Overcoming Barriers to Outcomes Measurement 209
Reg Warren

Section IV. OUTCOMES MEASUREMENT IN SPECIAL POPULATIONS

Chapter 11. Outcomes Measurement in Culturally and Linguistically Diverse Populations 225
Hortencia Kayser

Chapter 12. Outcomes Measurement in Aphasia 245
Audrey L. Holland and
Cynthia K. Thompson

Chapter 13. Outcomes Measurement in Cognitive Communication Disorders 267
Section 1. Traumatic Brain Injury 268
Brenda L. B. Adamovich
Section 2. Right Hemisphere Brain Damage 281
Connie A. Tompkins and Margaret T. Lehman
Section 3. Dementia 292
Michelle Bourgeois

Chapter 14. Efficacy, Outcomes, and Cost Effectiveness in Dysphagia 321
Jeri A. Logemann

Chapter 15. Outcomes Measurement in Motor Speech Disorders 334
David R. Beukelman,
Pamela Mathy, and
Kathryn Yorkston

Chapter 16. Outcomes Measurement in Voice Disorders 354
Katherine Verdolini,
Lorraine Ramig, and
Barbara Jacobson

Chapter 17. Outcomes Measurement Issues in Fluency Disorders   387
Gordon W. Blood and
Edward G. Conture

Chapter 18. Outcomes Measurement in Child Language
and Phonological Disorders   406
Howard Goldstein and
Judith Gierut

Section V.   OUTCOMES MEASUREMENT
IN SPECIAL SETTINGS

Chapter 19. Outcomes Measurement in the Schools   438
Diane L. Eger

Chapter 20. Outcomes Measurement in Health Care Settings   453
Becky Sutherland Cornett

Chapter 21. Outcomes Measurement in Universities   477
Judith A. Rassi

Chapter 22. Outcomes Measurement in Private Practice   503
Christie-Ann M.Conrad

Section VI.   STATE, NATIONAL, AND
INTERNATIONAL INITIATIVES

Chapter 23. State Initiatives in Outcomes Measurement   514
Melinda K. Harrison

Chapter 24. National Initiatives in Outcomes Measurement   527
Tanya M. Gallagher

Chapter 25. International Initiatives in Outcomes Measurement:
A Perspective from the United Kingdom   558
Sally Byng,
Anna van der Gaag, and
Susie Parr

INDEX   579

To Dr. Audrey L. Holland

Foreword

As I read this text on measuring outcomes in speech-language pathology, three words come to mind: assumption, value, and change.

Twenty years ago, when I began teaching clinical courses in a variety of disorders, I assumed that my students, when they became professionals, would monitor carefully what they did in therapy and convey this information in a clear and sensitive manner to their patients, the patients' families, other professionals, and insurers. We all assumed that the professional speech-language pathologist would be best qualified to determine what to work on, what methods to use, for how long, and to what degree of success. We never assumed that anyone would question our professional judgment. We took comfort in our knowledge, training, and empathetic natures.

Today, I teach the same coursework, but from a different perspective. We have moved from assuming that professional judgment will convince patients and others of the value of our services to approaching each therapy session from an outcomes-based model. Goals must be functional for each patient; methods must be theoretically sound, empirically based, and facilitate learning; and outcomes must be meaningful, measurable, and cost effective. I encourage my students to ask at the end of each session: "How is what I have done today going to make a real difference to the patient and his or her communication partners?"

The demands on today's clinicians are great. They must assess a patient's skills quickly yet comprehensively and amalgamate these findings with the patient's/payer's expectations into a plan of care that can be accomplished in a reasonable amount of time. My future clinicians now understand that it is not enough to document that the patient is communicating better in therapy, but that therapy has helped the patient communicate better in everyday life with a variety of people and for a variety of purposes. They also know that there is limited time in which to achieve goals. I now teach my students not to assume that others will readily accept their care plans, their therapy approaches, or their documentation. Now, our comfort is in the increasing number of studies that demonstrate the benefit of our intervention. We are further bolstered by the growing numbers of tools across disorders, populations, and settings that will help us document our outcomes.

As I read this text, I also think of value. Several years ago, I attended a convention session titled "What Is a Word Worth?" I was intrigued by this topic because I like to frame value in terms such as increased self-esteem and socialization. How could someone put a monetary value on such life-fulfilling goals? Another part of me, the taxpayer and consumer, was also intrigued. Therapy should result in measurable gains, such as improvement in communication skills, changes in communication partners' ability to facilitate effective interaction, and increased opportunities to communicate in activities of choice. Value might further be measured in reduction of burden on family members or by cost-effective treatments.

Finally, as I read this text, I think of change. Most of us like to think that we are current in our therapy approaches and individualize treatment to meet the differing needs of patients. But the change that this text calls for is more fundamental and challenging. Our therapy is now under scrutiny, and its results are being used to make decisions about who will receive therapy, for how long, and at what financial burden. Therapy results are being logged into databases that are statistically analyzed to demonstrate our worth. Unless we understand the analyses and their implications, and unless we initiate what to analyze and how, decisions will be made by others. As Marjorie Kelly, in *Taming the Demons of Changes,* states: "It comes down simply to this: we can't advance as long as we're holding tight to what no longer works. And we have to break the mold before a new form can emerge."

In this text, *Measuring Outcomes in Speech-Language Pathology,* Carol Frattali and her colleagues help us to break the traditional mold of service delivery. Dr. Frattali has conceptualized a book that provides a comprehensive model for understanding outcomes and their measurement. It begins with an historical overview of outcomes, measurement in medicine, rehabilitation, and speech-language pathology. Dr. Frattali realizes that to effect change in our thinking and eventually our practice, we must be familiar with the various conceptual models, outcome measures, and measurement methods currently available. She also realizes that we will be better able to document outcomes if we have valid and reliable tools. The text is a state-of-the-art approach to measuring outcomes that cross the age span, a multitude of settings, and national and international boundaries. Perhaps most importantly, Dr. Frattali and her colleagues have provided information that will help you and me to develop new and better ways to measure outcomes. Dr. Frattali herself challenges us to break our assumptions about the value of what we do with her comment, "In the long term, practitioners who can prove both cost-effectiveness and quality of care will gain a strategic advantage in what has become a competitive game of service delivery."

Rosemary Lubinski, Ed.D.
Professor
State University of New York
at Buffalo

Preface

It was Dr. Robert T. Wertz who introduced me to a useful way of thinking about outcomes. The process requires answers to three fundamental questions:

- What do you mean? (thus, requiring operational definition)
- How do you know? (requiring evidence to support the claim)
- What difference does it make? (placing the claim in a pragmatic context)

Dr. Wertz was passing along the advice of another colleague, the late Dr. Wendell Johnson, to help me in formulating a thought process for coordinating a project to develop technical reports on the efficacy of treatment. It later served as the foundation for organizing the content of this book.

Talking about client outcomes first requires operational definition. As I describe in Chapters 1 and 3, the concept can address specific clinical results, their functional implications, and, by extensions, their effects on the quality of life as judged by clients, families, and their culturally diverse communities. From a student supervisor's point of view, outcomes can address student competencies and supervisor/employee satisfaction. From a payer's point of view, outcomes can address cost effectiveness or client independence that leads to the need for fewer resources.

Once we *know what we mean* and can formulate operational definitions for desired or expected outcomes, the *"how do you know?"* question leads us to search for evidence or collect new data related to the effects of our interventions. This question directs us back to the professional literature in order to uncover what evidence already exists. It also directs us forward to the use of outcomes measures and research methodologies designed to build on the existing level of knowledge about the outcomes of our interventions.

The final question relates to the relevancy of targeted or achieved outcomes. *To whom do they make a difference* and, depending on one's perspective, to what degree of importance? The final of the three questions opens our minds to various and often vastly different points of view about clinical and educational interventions. It discourages us from thinking that we know what is best, and encourages us to integrate the various perspectives of important others into our interventions and expected outcomes. Some of these perspectives are no more apparent than in Kayser's chapter on multicultural populations, which sensitizes the reader to cultural diversity and the range of beliefs about disease, its consequences, its treatment, and its effects.

These three questions and the discussion that ensues as a result of their answers form the essence of this book. Discussing outcomes begins with inquiry. It leads to selection of outcomes measures, the design of research methodologies, and the collection, analysis, and dissemination of data. Finally, the research results spark dialogues of relevance and importance in terms of clinical breakthroughs and meaningful enhancements in patients' lives.

This text was written with two purposes: to create a useful framework within which to discuss outcomes, and to educate the reader about the state of the art of measuring outcomes. The text is organized into six sections. Section I provides an overview of the topic, covering definitions, conceptual frameworks, and current regulatory or accreditation requirements. Section II focuses on outcomes measures designed to measure modality-specific behaviors, functional status, and general well-being or quality of life. In addition, separate chapters are devoted to reviewing measures of patient satisfaction and cost effectiveness. Section III covers the various methods used to measure outcomes. These include efficacy research, outcomes research methods embodied by the concepts of program evaluation and quality improvement processes, and the design of automated outcomes management systems. As these methods require their effective use on a continual basis by both clinicians and clinical researchers, a chapter is devoted to the topic of identifying and removing barriers to successful measurement. Section IV reviews outcomes measurement within the context of defined client populations. These populations include multicultural groups and the clinical populations who present with aphasia, cognitive-communication disorders, dysphagia, motor speech disorders, voice disorders, fluency disorders, and child language and phonological disorders. Each chapter frames outcomes measurement within a conceptual model, summarizes current research findings, reviews pertinent outcomes measures, and identifies efficacy and outcomes research needs. Section V defines outcomes measurement by particular work settings, including schools, health care settings, universities, and private practice. The book closes with Section VI, which describes state, national, and international outcomes measurement initiatives. Of particular note is that outcomes measurement is a universal issue in the field, which has led to large-scale initiatives and ambitious collaborative efforts between states, regions, and countries intended to shape public health care and education policies and influence patterns of practice.

As with any in-depth treatment of a subject or formative stage in the development of a field of study, however, caveats can be made. One is of vital importance here: Even the most sensitive outcome measure or robust body of data may miss what only the trained eye can see. The advice of Dr. Muriel Lezak, whose description of "tests" can also refer to outcomes measures, appropriately provides a prologue to this book:

> Tests are simply a means of enhancing (refining, standardizing) our observations. They can be thought of as extensions of our organs of perception—the seven-league boots of clinical behavioral observation. If we use them properly, as extensions of our observational end-organs, like seven-league boots they enable us to accomplish much more with greater speed. When tests are misused as substitutes of rather than extensions of clinical observations, they can obscure our view of the patient much as seven-league boots would get in the way if worn over the head.

Measurement will never replace our keen observations or our sharpened professional sense of both the needs and gains of those whom we serve. In the end, to lose the art of behavioral observation is to lose the human sense of connectedness with our clients, our students, and ultimately ourselves.

Acknowledgments

I wish to recognize the following individuals without whose assistance the development of this book or the accuracy of its contents would not have been possible. I am grateful to Andrea Seils, Medical Editor of Thieme, whose high level of skill, competency, and professionalism facilitated the process of development and simplified an otherwise formidable task. I extend appreciation also to Robin Cook, Jinnie Kim, and Adam Weiss of Thieme for their expert technical assistance. I thank Drs. Audrey Holland, Lesley Olswang, Martha Taylor Sarno, and Robert T. Wertz for their insightful views, philosophies, and models of measuring client outcomes, which have both influenced and crystallized my thinking on the subject. I am indebted to this book's contributing authors, who have provided the substance that allowed this field of study to take shape. Finally, I thank my dear family, Mike, Greg, Sara, and Ian, for supporting this project with considerable selflessness, patience, and sufficient doses of humor.

Contributors

Brenda L. B. Adamovich, Ph.D.
Vice President
Clinical Services
Wheeling Hospital
Wheeling, West Virginia

David R. Beukelman, Ph.D.
Director of Research and Education
Munroe-Meyer Institute for Genetics
  and Rehabilitation
University of Nebraska Medical Center
Omaha, Nebraska

Gordon W. Blood, Ph.D.
Professor and Chair
Department of Communication
  Disorders
Penn State University
University Park, Pennsylvania

Jean Blosser, Ed.D.
Director
Speech and Hearing Clinic
Department of Communication
  Disorders
The University of Akron
Akron, Ohio

Michelle Bourgeois, Ph.D.
Associate Scientist/Scholar
Department of Communication
  Disorders
Florida State University
Tallahassee, Florida

Sally Byng, Ph.D.
Chair of Communication Disability
Head of Department of Clinical
  Communication Studies
City University
London, United Kingdom

Christie-Ann M. Conrad, M. A.
Director
Crossroads Speech & Hearing Center
McMurray, Pennsylvania

Edward G. Conture, Ph.D.
Professor
Department of Hearing and Speech
  Sciences
Vanderbilt University
Nashville, Tennessee

Becky Sutherland Cornett, Ph.D.
Director
In-patient Rehabilitation Programs and
  Services
The Ohio State University Medical
  Center
Columbus, Ohio

Diane L. Eger, Ph.D.
Director
Speech-Language, Hearing, and Vision
  Programs
Allegheny Intermediate Unit
Pittsburgh, Pennsylvania

Carol M. Frattali, Ph.D.
Research Coordinator
Speech-Language Pathology Section
W. G. Magnuson Clinical Center
National Institutes of Health
Bethesda, Maryland

Tanya M. Gallagher, Ph.D.
Associate Dean
Planning and Resources
Faculty of Medicine
McGill University
Quebec, Canada
Co-Project Officer
ASHA Task Force on Treatment Outcome
and Cost Effectiveness

Judith Gierut, Ph.D.
Associate Professor
Department of Speech and Hearing
Sciences
Indiana University
Bloomington, Indiana

Howard Goldstein, Ph.D.
Professor and Chair
Department of Communication
Disorders
Florida State University
Tallahassee, Florida

Melinda K. Harrison, MS, MBA
Director
Clinical Services
The Watson Clinic
Lakeland, Florida

Patricia Larkins Hicks, Ph.D.
President and Founder
The Outcomes Management Group, Ltd.
Columbus, Ohio

Audrey L. Holland, Ph.D.
Professor
Department of Speech and Hearing
Sciences
Institute for Neurogenic Communication
Disorders
University of Arizona
Tucson, Arizona

Nancy P. Huffman, M. A.
Chairperson
Speech-Language & Audiology Service
Board of Cooperational Education
Services #1
Monroe County, New York

Barbara Jacobson, Ph.D.
Director, Speech Production Laboratory
Division of Speech-Language Sciences
and Disorders
Henry Ford Hospital
Detroit, Michigan

Alex F. Johnson, Ph.D.
Director
Division of Speech-Language Sciences
and Disorders
Henry Ford Hospital
Detroit, Michigan

Hortencia Kayser, Ph.D.
Associate Professor
Special Education and Communication
Disorders
New Mexico State University
Las Cruces, New Mexico

Mary Ann Keatley, Ph.D.
President
Evaluation Systems, International
Boulder, Colorado

Margaret T. Lehman, M. S.
Communication Sciences and Disorders
University of Pittsburgh
Pittsburgh, Pennsylvania

Jeri A. Logemann, Ph.D.
Ralph and Jean Sundin Professor
Department of Communication Sciences
  and Disorders
Northwestern University
Evanston, Illinois

Pamela Mathy, Ph.D.
Munroe-Meyer Institute for Genetics
  and Rehabilitation
University of Nebraska Medical Center
Omaha, Nebraska

Richard M. Merson, Ph.D.
Speech-Language Pathology Department
William Beaumont Hospital
Royal Oak, Michigan

Thomas I. Miller, Ph.D.
Vice President
Evaluation Systems, International
Boulder, Colorado

Lesley B. Olswang, Ph.D.
Professor
Department of Speech and Hearing
  Sciences
University of Washington
Seattle, Washington

Susie Parr, Ph.D.
Research Fellow
Department of Clinical Communication
  Studies
City University
London, United Kingdom

Lorraine Olson Ramig, Ph.D.
Associate Professor
Department of Speech, Language, and
  Hearing Sciences
University of Colorado at Boulder
Boulder, Colorado

Paul R. Rao, Ph.D.
Executive Director, Clinical Services
Director, Quality Improvement
Co-Director, Stroke Recovery Program
National Rehabilitation Hospital
Washington, D. C.

Judith A. Rassi, M. A.
Associate Professor and Director
Department of Hearing and Speech
  Sciences
Vanderbilt University School of Medicine
Nashville, Tennessee

Michael I. Rolnick, Ph.D.
Director
Speech-Language Pathology Department
William Beaumont Hospital
Royal Oak, Michigan

Cynthia K. Thompson, Ph.D.
Associate Professor
Department of Communication Sciences
  and Disorders, and Neurology
Northwestern University
Evanston, Illinois

Connie A. Tompkins, Ph.D.
Professor
Communication Sciences and Disorders
University of Pittsburgh
Pittsburgh, Pennsylvania

Anna van der Gaag
Lecturer in Speech and Language Therapy
Department of Speech and Language
  Therapy
University of Strathclyde
Glasgow, United Kingdom

Katherine Verdolini, Ph.D.
Director
Voice/Speech/Swallowing Division
Joint Center for Otolaryngology
Beth Israel Deaconess Medical Center and
Brigham & Women's Hospital
Boston, Massachusetts

Reg Warren, Ph.D.
Vice President
Outcomes Research
The Polaris Group
Hingham, Massachusetts

Deborah L. Wilkerson, M. A.
Director
Research and Quality Improvement
CARF...The Rehabilitation Accreditation
  Commission
Tucson, Arizona

Kathryn M. Yorkston, Ph.D.
Professor
Head, Division Of Speech Pathology
Department of Rehabilitation Medicine
University of Washington
Seattle, Washington

Measuring Outcomes in Speech-Language Pathology

CHAPTER 1

Outcomes Measurement: Definitions, Dimensions, and Perspectives

CAROL M. FRATTALI

INTRODUCTION

We know surprisingly little about what works in clinical care. Many treatments and technologies in common use have never been evaluated. Many others that have been evaluated remain of uncertain benefit to large patient populations. Why, in this age of technology and information, haven't we learned more about the outcomes of our interventions?

Ellwood (1988) believes that moving even a substantial fraction of the service delivery system in a common direction of data collection is difficult. He describes hard-held practitioner notions of patient care (more care; less paperwork) and the begrudging attitude to adopt outcomes technology only to preempt the threat of losing professional control. Iezzoni (1994) says "the devil is in the details" (p. 3). She suggests that meaningful measurement of patients' outcomes requires vigilant application of two basic methodologies: a measure of the outcome itself (few good outcome measures exist), and a way to adjust for patient's risks for various outcomes (often outside experimental control). Deming (1982) blames managers unwilling to break habits of decision making based on hunches instead of data. He labels this prevailing style of management "tyranny" and calls for a transformation routed toward profound knowledge.

We enter an era rich with pioneering deacons and seminal tomes crossing the disciplines of health care, education, economics, engineering, business, and management in a field increasingly known as outcomes measurement and, if we are to apply outcomes measurement to improving interventions and decision making, outcomes management. Yet, despite advances in computer technology, measures, and methods, knowledge about the effects of clinical interventions has not accrued at the speed the problem demands.

Paul Ellwood (1988) believes it is timing. He quotes Sir Francis Darwin: "In science the credit goes to the [one] who convinces the world, not to the [one] to whom the idea first occurs." He cites ambitious efforts to install integrated management information systems that capture outcomes, help practitioners in making decisions, and feed the results back to decisionmakers. Yet, most efforts have lost momentum, and have been successful only in capturing the imaginations of the media and the health care professions. None have yet to convince the world.

Nevertheless, strands of optimism are laced in current thinking on outcomes measurement. The time is right for widespread application—an opinion based largely on improvements in our ability to manage information with computers and the demonstration (e.g., by Medicare's diagnosis related groups or DRGs) of the effect an expanded data base can have on integrating service and financial information. Ellwood affirms, "We have the opportunity to proceed immediately" (p. 6).

The purposes of this chapter are to give you a sense of history about outcomes measurement; offer definitions and classification schemes that can serve to organize your thoughts; and provide an overview of the various methods in use. The chapter constructs a framework intended to unify the book's content.

HISTORICAL PERSPECTIVE

Popular opinion holds outcomes measurement as a contemporary concept in service delivery. Outcomes measurement, in fact, actually emerged in the mid-nineteenth century. The leading pioneer of the time was Florence Nightingale (in Iezzoni, 1994). Her motivation was the finding that hospital patients died at higher rates than their cohorts treated elsewhere. Even more troublesome were the comparisons of mortality rates across the principal hospitals of England in 1861. The in-hospital mortality rate in London hospitals was close to 91%, compared to a mortality rate of close to 16% in naval and military hospitals. Nightingale explained the discrepancy, in part, by variations in patient risks (such as age and "state of the cases at admissions"). Her more important findings, however, were her observations that facilities with better outcomes also had better sanitation, less crowding of patients in wards, and a location distant from sewage disposal. In response, Nightingale proposed changes in ward configurations, sanitation, and hospital location that led to reductions in hospital mortality rates. This example became the earliest known account of outcomes measurement (collecting, analyzing, and reporting outcomes data) and management (making changes based on data to improve outcomes).

Ernest A. Codman, a prominent Boston surgeon of the late nineteenth century, also holds a space in history as a proponent of monitoring outcomes of care (Berwick, 1989; Iezzoni, 1994). His contribution was his effort to link specific interventions with their effects on patients. Called the "end-results idea," Codman described it as

> . . . merely the common-sense notion that every hospital should follow *every* patient it treats, long enough to determine whether or not the treatment has been successful, and then to inquire "if not, why not" with a view to preventing similar failures in the future [Codman, 1934, p. xii].

Unfortunately, Codman's idea led to his fall from grace among his medical colleagues at The Massachusetts General Hospital, who viewed his practices of tracking patients as extreme. Codman reacted:

So I am called eccentric for saying in public: that Hospitals, if they wish to be sure of improvement,

1. Must find out what their results are.
2. Must analyze their results, to find their strong and weak points.
3. Must compare their results with those of other hospitals . . .

Such opinions will not be eccentric a few years hence [Codman, 1917, p. 137].

Codman eventually left The Massachusetts General Hospital and opened his own hospital in Boston's Beacon Hill, where he completely installed his end-results tracking system. He categorized, as a result of scanning volumes of data for each patient, types of causes of treatment errors or failures, including (Codman, 1917):

- Errors due to lack of technical knowledge or skill
- Errors possibly due to a lack of judgment
- Errors due to lack of care or equipment
- Errors due to incorrect diagnosis
- Cases in which the nature and extent of the disease was the main cause of failure
- Cases who refused to accept treatment

Thus, Codman linked specific outcomes to specific interventions. He later resigned from The Massachusetts General Hospital, protesting its practice of promotion by seniority (a practice considered antithetical to his end-results idea), and was forced, with few referrals, to close his hospital and live a professional life of discontent.

Where Nightingale succeeded, Codman failed. Today, however, both are recognized for their contributions, which form the conceptual foundation of outcomes measurement and management. The lesson learned here is that it is not enough to know simply about end results, but to know *why* these events occurred (Iezzoni, 1994). Thus, the link of patient characteristics and specific interventions with specific outcomes is crucial to knowledge.

Modern-Day Leaders in the Outcomes Movement

Two current-day leaders in outcomes measurement, whose contributions largely founded the field of quality improvement, are Avedis Donabedian (1980) and the late W. Edwards Deming (1982). Donabedian, a physician and professor of public health at the University of Michigan, spread his knowledge across three volumes exploring approaches to quality assessment and monitoring. He is best known for establishing a unifying framework of quality of care, and coining the terms *structure, process,* and *outcome* in his approaches to its assessment. He defines these terms:

Structure: The relatively stable characteristics of the providers of care, of the tools and resources they have at their disposal, and of the physical and organizational settings in which they work. Thus, the concept of structure includes the human, physical, and financial resources needed to provide care. [pp. 81–82]

Process: The set of activities that go on between and within practitioners and patients. These include technical management (e.g., diagnostic and treatment methods), and interpersonal aspects of care (e.g., the psychosocial interactions between practitioner and patient). [pp. 79–80]

Outcome: A change in a patient's current and future health status that can be attributed to antecedent health care. Change includes improvement of social and psychological function in addition to the more usual emphasis on the physical and physiological aspects of performance. By still another extension I shall add patient attitudes (including satisfaction), health-related knowledge acquired by the patient, and health-related behavioral change. All of these can be seen either as components of current health or as contributions to future health. [pp. 82–83]

Donabedian's teachings were introduced during a time of intense debate over which approach to quality assessment—process or outcome—was superior. Like his predecessors, he found, through conceptual and empirical study, that process and outcome are inextricably linked:

> . . . Process and outcome are fundamentally linked in a single, symmetrical structure that makes of one almost a mirror image of the other, no matter how many attributes are used to test the relationship. Thus, the emphasis shifts to a more thorough understanding of the linkages between process and outcome, and away from the rather misguided argument over which of the two is the superior approach to assessment. [p. xi]

Donabedian's (1980) triad of structure-process-outcome mirrors the notion of systems thinking by recognizing the fundamental relationship among all three elements.

During the same time period, a similar movement was underway, but in the manufacturing industry. The attention of large corporations in the United States, such as Ford and General Electric, was being diverted to the work of W. Edwards Deming (1982). Deming was an internationally renowned statistician and consultant, based in Washington, D.C., whose work led Japanese industry into new principles of management and revolutionized the quality of their products and service. He called for nothing short of a transformation of the American style of management, one that neglects to plan for the future and foresee problems through use of a systematic process of data collection and analysis to increase knowledge. Deming states, "Anyone in management requires, for transformation, some rudimentary knowledge about science—in particular, something about the nature of variation and about operational definitions" [p. xi].

His work spilled into the industries of education and health care, although the impatience of managers, oriented toward quick fix and pressured by economic constraints, quelled the movement. A wise Deming predicted:

> Long-term commitment to new learning and new philosophy is required of any management that seeks transformation. The timid and the fainthearted, and people that expect quick results, are doomed to disappointment. [p. x]

Among Deming's principles for transformation is the fifth of his 14 points for management: Improve constantly and forever the system of production and service. Through a use of statistical tools and knowledge of systems and process variation, he proposes cycle of Plan (study a work process to decide what change might improve it), Do (make the change), Study (observe the effects or outcomes), Act (standardize the change if it resulted in improvement; if not, decide what other changes might result in improvement and begin the cycle again) to improve continually the quality of products and services. Deming also emphasizes consumer research as the hallmark of innovation. Thus, quality is aimed at the needs of the consumer, present and future. His vigilant focus on systematic and scientifically based process improvement invariably leads to better outcomes at a lower cost, which he believes should be the aim of any service provider who works for the common good of an industry as a whole.

In the field of medicine, the work of John Wennberg is also noteworthy from an historical perspective. John Wennberg, a professor at Dartmouth Medical School, conducted a landmark study of unacceptable variation in performing hysterectomies in the state of Maine (Wennberg & Gittelsohn, 1973). In one county, 70% of women had had hysterectomies by the age of 70; in a nearby county the figure was only 20%. The measured variation passed all tests of statistical analysis to adjust for possible explanatory factors, including age, diagnosis, socioeconomic status, and severity level. If Wennberg is right, states Berwick and colleagues (1990), "then the health care dollar is not only inflating, it is being spent largely in some colossal game of dice" (p. 8). The study confirmed suspicions of "for-profit" medicine and dissolved consumer trust in the quality of care.

It is perhaps this study that has spurred payers, managed care systems, accreditation bodies, and government agencies to approach any provider with scepticism and scrutinize the care rendered in the service delivery system. Thus, the 1970s marked the end of the practitioner's "our word is our honor," and the beginning of the payer's "prove it."

Advances in Outcomes Measurement

Another study is credited with accelerating the outcomes movement, at least from a position of public protection. This time it was the release of mortality data by the U.S. Department of Health and Human Services' Health Care Financing Administration (HCFA) (Brinkley, 1986). Its only value is found in a lesson learned about the consequences of looking at outcomes alone.

In the mid-1980s, HCFA was compelled to publicly release death rates of Medicare beneficiaries by reporters' demands under the federal Freedom of Information Act. Based on governmental predictions, 142 hospitals had significantly higher death rates, while 127 had significantly lower rates. One facility had a death rate of 86.7% compared to a predicted 22.5%. The hospital administrators, infuriated by the data and media interpretations regarding quality of care that followed, argued rightfully that HCFA failed to standardize adequately for severity of illness. What the public did not know was that many of the hospitals with high mortality rates were tertiary care centers treating more medically complex patients, and the facility with the most aberrant death rate was a hospice caring for terminally ill patients.

The release of HCFA data spurred the development of other systems that incorporate severity adjustments in order to level the playing field and allow fair comparisons of "apples to apples." At the same time, systems were becoming more sophisticated with advances in computer technology. Several severity measurement systems were introduced in the health care field. Examples include APACHE (Acute Physiology, Age, and Chronic Heath Evaluation) (Knaus et al., 1981); CSI (Computerized Severity Index) (Horn et al., 1991); MedisGroups (Brewster et al., 1985; Iezzoni & Moskowitz, 1988);

and DRGs (Diagnosis-related Groups) (Fetter et al., 1980; Vladeck, 1984). While severity is defined differently by each system, all defined "severity" by linking it to a specific outcome or clinical state. For example, APACHE linked severity to in-hospital mortality; CSI to treatment difficulty based on diagnosis and disease-specific signs and symptoms; MedisGroups to clinical instability as indicated by in-hospital death; and DRGs to total hospital charges or length of stay. Severity is rated by factors such as diagnosis, separate ratings of severity for all diagnoses, and categories of major surgery. While medically based in their designs, these outcomes measurement systems influenced activities in other areas of the service delivery system.

Advances in the Field of Rehabilitation

Outcomes measurement in the multidisciplinary field of rehabilitation is particularly interesting to us as rehabilitation providers. Of perhaps greatest significance was the introduction of the Functional Independence Measure (FIM) (State University of New York at Buffalo, 1993) as an outcome instrument designed to quantitatively measure the burden of care and written in a language understandable to the payer. This minimum data set, which measures communication among other rehabilitation variables, rates functional abilities on a 7-point scale of independence. Due to its ease and efficiency of use, as well as its appeal to payers, the FIM has become an industry standard worldwide. Another data base, the Uniform Data System for Medical Rehabilitation (UDS mr), which incorporates the FIM and has catalogued the functional outcomes of hundreds of thousands of patients, has become potentially powerful in its capacity to establish a payment system for rehabilitation. Yet, the data base suffers from its neglect in linking specific processes to specific outcomes. Thus, the claims of treatment effectiveness remain largely unfounded. Nevertheless, outcomes measurement studies using the FIM are proceeding in order to create Function-related Groups (FRGs) to determine resource use and, thus, set reimbursement rates for rehabilitation (Stineman, Escarce, Goin, Hamilton, Granger, & Williams, 1994; Wilkerson, Batavia, & DeJong, 1992).

In the meantime, other rehabilitation outcome measures and automated systems were being designed or refined as outcomes measurement and management became a primary means for survival in a cost-constrained system. These measures or systems include the Level of Rehabilitation Scale III—LORS III (Parkside Associates, 1986), Patient Evaluation and Conference System—PECS (Harvey & Jellinek, 1979, 1981), and Rehabilitation Institute of Chicago Functional Assessment Scale '95—RICFAS (Cichowski, 1995). Some have been designed to overcome some of the weaknesses of the FIM, particularly the problem of low sensitivity in capturing functionally important change. Yet, many continue to lack sufficient reliability and validity that allow sound interpretations of derived data.

Advances in Speech-Language Pathology

Fueled by flaws in current research activities, accreditation agency outcomes initiatives (e.g., the Joint Commission on Accreditation of Healthcare Organizations' [JCAHO's] Agenda for Change and the Rehabilitation Accreditation Commission's [CARF's] outcomes management focus in its standards for medical rehabilitation), managed care and regulatory agency demands for data, and consumer choice, professionals began looking to their membership organizations for needed leadership and direction. In response, the American Speech-Language-Hearing Association (ASHA), in 1993, established the Task Force on Treatment Outcomes and Cost Effectiveness (ASHA, 1995). It was established to generate an outcomes data base to assist in meeting current public demands. Among its many initiatives, the task force packaged cost data for use in negotiating managed care contracts, supported the development and dissemination of 10 technical reports summarizing the efficacy of treatment in key clinical areas, and designed a data collection system to aggregate outcomes data in the areas of cost, consumer satisfaction, and functional status. It continues its work in validating new outcome measures, focusing more recently on pediatric measures and measures that can be used by school systems. Concurrently, ASHA completed a 3-year grant project to develop the *ASHA Functional Assessment of Communication Skills for Adults (ASHA FACS)* (Frattali, Thompson, Holland, Wohl, & Ferketic, 1995), and reorganized its research structure (i.e., elevated the Research Division to a Scientific Affairs and Research Department) for, among other important activities, the pursuit of multisite clinical trials research (see Chapter 24 by Gallagher for further discussion).

Predating ASHA's aggressive outcomes initiative, however, was a landmark conference sponsored by the American Speech-Language-Hearing Foundation, titled *Treatment Efficacy Research in Communication Disorders* (Olswang, Thompson, Warren, & Minghetti, 1990). This conference injected new life into our field in the area of efficacy research, and, by extension, outcomes measurement. Leija McReynolds, assigned to present an historical perspective of treatment research, admitted:

> . . . there is not much history to report. Applied research in the behavioral sciences only began in earnest in the 1960s, and even later than that in speech, language, and hearing. Treatment efficacy research has an even shorter history than applied research in general. . . . So, the history is sparse and short. Very little treatment research has been conducted. [p. 5]

But, McReynolds (1990), in the same stream of thought, continued:

> . . . "There is a new breeze blowing." Certainly it is a gentle breeze, not a strong wind, but it is a kinder wind than it was just a few years ago, and I believe our profession is gradually becoming aware of the need for evaluating our treatment in a controlled manner. [p. 5]

McReynolds (1990) was right. Today, we are hearing about new outcome measures, such as the Voice Handicap Index (Jacobson, Johnson, & Grywalski, 1995), the National Outcomes Measures (NOMS) (ASHA, 1995), and the ASHA FACS (Frattali et al., 1995). New automated outcomes management systems, such as the OUTCOME (Evaluation Systems International, Inc., 1994), Beaumont Outcome Software System (BOSS) (Merson, Rolnick, & Weiner, 1995), and The Functional Outcome and Utilization System (F.O.C.U.S.) (Focus Rehab, Inc., 1995) recently were made commercially available. Refereed journals devoted to scientifically based clinical practice (e.g., *The American Journal of Speech-Language Pathology: A Journal of Clinical Practice*) were created, thus inviting the conduct and publication of efficacy and outcomes research. National and international efforts in outcomes measurement are mounting, as evidenced by the number of scientific meetings and workshops addressing the topic, and the creation of related professional organizations (e.g., The Treatment Efficacy

Research Group in Communication Disorders), and study sections (e.g., Quality Improvement Study Section of ASHA Special Interest Division 11: Administration and Supervision), whose missions include the advancement of clinical research or data-based quality of care.

But a caveat is offered with recent advances in outcomes measurement. The problem easily could shift from one of "too little evidence," to another of "too much weak evidence." We soon could suffer from division of purpose in outcomes measurement in general, and flawed methods of data collection, analysis, and interpretation in specific. These pitfalls are all too possible in the current environment that is operating with differing, and sometimes conflicting, terminology and conceptual frameworks from which to create new knowledge. Further, various measurement methodologies are being applied, some correctly; some incorrectly, with less than vigilant efforts at acknowledging study limitations and making valid interpretations. Consequently, we must devote considerable attention at the outset to how we are defining our terms and applying our methodologies so that the data collected and interpretations made are both useful and meaningful.

TERMINOLOGY

I have chosen the term *outcomes measurement* as the topic of this book, but not without considering the terms *outcomes research, efficacy research,* and *outcomes management.* Often used either loosely or interchangeably, these terms and their offshoots (e.g., *treatment efficacy, treatment effectiveness, treatment efficiency, program evaluation, quality improvement*) cause many professionals to stumble in discussions on the topic. I use the term outcomes measurement as a broad term that encompasses both outcomes research and efficacy research. Outcomes management, however, overlaps the boundaries of measurement because it involves taking next steps of using outcomes data to improve or make decisions about care. Although outcomes management is addressed throughout this book, particularly in the Methods and Special Settings sections, measurement is the central theme.

I also use the term outcomes measurement with no intention of minimizing *process measurement.* Outcomes measurement, as described by its proponents, is meaningful only if linked to facility, client, and clinician characteristics (to allow comparison of "apples to apples"), and the various processes of care (to allow us to make relational statements about the effects of specific interventions).

What Is an Outcome?

Given the above qualifications, an *outcome* is simply a result of an intervention. I intentionally use the plural term, *outcomes,* because it is a multidimensional concept defined only in terms of the agent. Agents can be clinicians, teachers, employers, administrators, payers, and the clients/families themselves—all consumers of care. Thus, outcomes can be

- *clinically derived* (e.g., ability to sustain phonation, accuracy in naming, type and frequency of disfluencies in a speech sample, integrity of the swallowing mechanism);

- *functional* (e.g., ability to communicate basic needs, telephone use);
- *administrative* (e.g., client referral patterns, productivity levels in direct client care, rates of missed sessions);
- *financial* (e.g., cost-effective care, rate of rehospitalizations, average lengths of stay;
- *social* (e.g., employability, ability to learn, community reentry); and
- *client-defined* (e.g., satisfaction with services; quality of life).

Donabedian (1985) offers a definition of *outcome* in the context of health care:

> Outcomes are those changes, either favorable or adverse, in the actual or potential health status of persons, groups, or communities that can be attributed to prior or concurrent care. What is included in the category of "outcomes" depends, therefore, on how narrowly or broadly one defines "health" and the corresponding responsibilities of . . . practitioners or the health care system as a whole. [p. 256]

If we use this example in other contexts, we can easily replace the term *health* with terms such as *learning ability* (from the standpoint of education), *costs* (from the standpoint of the payer), and *quality of life* and *satisfaction* (from the standpoint of clients or their families). We quickly understand that we as clinicians are not striving for one outcome only, but for a range of outcomes, as defined by the interests or needs of any given stakeholder, and at any given point in time during or after the provision of care. While a clinician might show initial interest in short-term outcomes (e.g., articulation accuracy from session to session), a client might be more interested, even at the start, in long-term outcomes (e.g., returning to work as a result of improved communication skills required by the job).

If we extend beyond the clinical model, outcomes measurement also can be applied to other contexts, including the professional preparation level in university programs. Methods can allow, for example, investigation of educational outcomes and related outcomes such as student satisfaction with curricula, employer's appraisal of graduates' on-the-job performance, and clinical competency (see Chapter 21 by Rassi). Management of these outcomes would have strong implications for revising or improving academic programs.

When Do Outcomes Occur?

The temporal order of outcomes gives rise to three terms, coined by Rosen and Proctor (1981): intermediate, instrumental, and ultimate outcomes. *Intermediate outcomes* let us know, from session to session, whether treatment is benefiting the client. These outcomes allow exploration of the treatment process. Thus, they are of prime interest to clinicians who use them as barometers of adjustment in treatment plans. Studies that investigate intermediate outcomes are designed to answer questions such as, What makes a good session? How important is this to the overall goal of treatment (or the ultimate outcome)? Olswang (1990) gives the example of a clinician questioning whether practicing sounds in isolation, syllables, words, and/or phrases is necessary to achieve sound production in conversation.

Instrumental outcomes are outcomes that activate the learning process. These are outcomes that, when reached, trigger the ultimate outcome. Once an instrumental outcome is reached, treatment is no longer necessary, for the individual will continue to improve on his or her own. The focus is on how long to treat—a question of particular interest to payers. Citing phonology treatment again, Olswang (1990) recommends that the clinician question at what level of correct production of the target sound is sufficient to trigger correct production in conversation.

Ultimate outcomes are those that demonstrate the social or ecological validity of our interventions, such as functional communication, employability, ability to learn, social integration, and so on. Research designed to study ultimate outcomes explores questions about the meaningfulness of treatment. What does it mean to attain functional communication, and how much direct treatment is necessary? Ultimate outcomes are of prime interest to payers and regulators as well as clients and their families: How will this treatment make me a more effective communicator? How will it enhance my ability to learn in school? To get a job? (See Chapter 6 by Olswang for further discussion.)

How Are Outcomes Defined?

Once outcomes are identified, they must be defined operationally if they are to be measured. For example, if we are measuring functional communication, what do we mean by functional? Do we mean common everyday skills (e.g., telephone interactions, responding in an emergency) that allow one to convey basic needs or interests? Or do we mean more individually defined or higher level skills (e.g., writing business letters, completing forms, reading and comprehending a book) that allow one to return to work, school, or community activities? What do we mean by communication? Do we mean understanding and speaking only, or do we include nonverbal skills? With a partner? In a group? Do we include speech intelligibility? Do we include reading and writing? Very quickly, the business of outcomes measurement becomes weighted in definition.

Deming (1982) devotes an entire chapter of his book, *Out of the Crisis,* to operational definitions: "An operational definition puts communicable meaning into a concept" (p. 276). Deming continues:

> Adjectives like good, reliable, uniform, round, tired, safe, unsafe . . . have no communicable meaning until they are expressed in operational terms of sampling, test, and criterion. . . . We have seen in many places how important it is that buyer and seller understand each other. They must both use the same kind of centimetre. . . . This requirement has meaning only if instruments are in statistical control. Without operational definitions, a specification is meaningless. [p. 277]

Indeed, if we are to be consistent in our measurement of physical, physiologic, or behavioral changes, we must operationally define "changes" by way of measurement instruments. Further, these instruments must be reliable and valid (i.e., in statistical control) if the data derived are to be meaningful. In addition, current demands add to the requirement of sound psychometric properties. Given current payer demands, our instruments should also be quantitative and comprehensible. That is, they should be interpretable in numeric terms (e.g., by means of scores) to objectively and efficiently document or measure change, and the test results must be interpretable by the lay person (often the person who is making decisions about payment or continuation of services).

Classification Schemes

Useful frameworks in which to define outcomes are found if you consider outcomes along a continuum of the consequences of disease, disorder, injury, or active pathology. Both medical and social models are advanced by the health care community. No one model has yet to be universally accepted; thus, the lack of a uniformly accepted conceptual famework presents one obstacle to development and application of outcome measures, as well as outcomes measurement methods and interpretations. Three frameworks are described.

World Health Organization Classifications

The most well-known conceptual framework, the *International Classification of Impairments, Disabilities, and Handicaps (ICIDH)* comes from the World Health Organization (WHO) (1980). The ICIDH acknowledges a chain of principal events that occur in the development of illnesses:

1. Something abnormal happens (a pathology occurs).
2. Someone becomes aware of such an occurrence (thus, heralding recognition of impairment).
3. The individual's performance or behavior may be altered and common activities may be restricted (giving rise to a disability).
4. The individual is placed at a disadvantage relative to others, thus socializing the experience (creating a handicap).

The pathology, according to the WHO, is an intrinsic situation which becomes exteriorized by an impairment. The impairment becomes objectified (i.e., the process through which a functional limitation expresses itself as a reality in everyday life) by disability and, in turn, socialized by handicap. The WHO defines the consequential phenomena as follows:

Impairment. Any loss or abnormality of psychological, physiological, or anatomical structure or function. It represents deviation from a norm.

Disability. Any restriction or lack of ability (resulting from an impairment) to perform an activity in a manner or within a range considered normal for a human being. A disability is the functional consequence of an impairment manifested in integrated activities represented by tasks and skills.

Handicap. A disadvantage resulting from an impairment or disability that limits or prevents the fulfillment of a role that is normal (depending on age, sex, and social and cultural factors) for that individual. A handicap is the social consequence of an impairment or disability, defined by the attitudes and responses of others. Thus, the state of being handicapped is relative to other people.

As Figure 1–1 illustrates, impairment, disability, and handicap can be linked. Although suggesting a simple linear progression along the full sequence, the situation can become more complex. Handicap may result from impairment without the media-

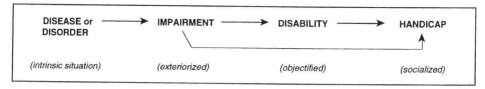

Figure 1–1. The World Health Organization's Consequences of Disease or Disorder

SOURCE: World Health Organization. (1980). *International classification of impairments, disabilities & handicaps.* Geneva: Author. Used by permission.

tion of a disability. For example, an individual who uses an augmentative communication device may not have difficulty with everyday communication (a disability), but may, in fact be socially stigmatized, which leads to social isolation (handicap). Also, one can be impaired without being disabled, and disabled without being handicapped—for example, the individual with a lisp who experiences no problems with communication, or the augmentative communication user whose social and work environments make the necessary accommodations to prevent handicap. If we are to apply the framework to the field of speech-language pathology, we can use the example of the person with cerebral vascular disease who sustains a stroke (disease and disorder). The resultant impairment is aphasia, which leads to a communication disability manifested in the performance of daily life activities such as communicating with family and friends, using the telephone, making grocery lists, and reading the newspaper. The disability leads to social isolation, interruption of community activities (e.g., bridge club, holiday celebrations), and loss of a job as an office assistant.

The WHO framework portrays a problem-solving sequence in the context of clinical intervention. Intervention at the level of one element has the potential to modify or prevent succeeding elements. As Batavia (1992) explains, "with appropriate rehabilitative interventions, an impairment does not necessarily result in a disability. Similarly, with appropriate social and environmental interventions, a disability does not necessarily result in a handicap" (p. 3).

Because each stage along the WHO continuum can be classified as an outcome, three classes of outcome measures are identified. Impairment instruments include our traditional diagnostic and instrumental measures, designed for differential diagnosis and identification of specific phonological, voice, fluency, language, cognitive, and swallowing deficits. Disability measures include the functional status instruments that measure communication in everyday contexts, and also include swallowing measures that assess, for example, independence during meals and adequate nutrition. Handicap measures include health-related quality of life measures or handicap inventories, usually designed as self-administered questionnaires that capture social, environmental, and economic disadvantages from the perspective of the client or family.

The WHO framework, while useful universally, has suffered from its simplicity (e.g., excluding certain scenarios of the consequences of disease) and terminology (e.g., use of the term handicap). It also has been criticized for its alignment with a medical rather than social model, and its internal inconsistencies and lack of clarity of the terms disability and handicap. In recent years the term "handicap" has fallen into disuse in the United States, primarily because individuals with disabilities consider the term to have socially imposed negative connotations. Numerous proposals have suggested revisions to the WHO model and an ICIDH-2 model is currently in Beta testing. (Placek, personal communication 1996). In the meantime, however, other classification schemes, aimed at solving some of the problems of the WHO typology, have been described.

Nagi Classifications

Saad Nagi (1965) constructed a framework of four distinct but interrelated concepts: active pathology, impairment, functional limitation, and disability. His model is a close variant of the Institute of Medicine Model of Disability and Disability Prevention (Pope & Tarlov, 1991) as well as the Disablement Model of the National Institutes of Health, National Center for Medical Rehabilitation Research (NIH, 1993). Nagi's concepts are described as follows:

Active pathology. Interruption or interference with normal processes and efforts of the organism to regain normal state. It refers to cell and tissue changes. Indicators include signs and symptoms and are found in attributes of the individual.

Impairment. Anatomical, physiological, mental, or emotional abnormalities or loss. Indicators, again, include signs and symptoms and are found in attributes of the individual.

Functional limitation. Limitation in performance at the level of the whole organism or person. Indicators include limitations in various activities such as walking, reasoning, and communicating. Indicators are found in attributes of the individual.

Disability. Limitation in performance of socially defined roles and tasks within a sociocultural and physical environment. Indicators include limitations in performance of such roles and tasks as related to family, work, community, school, and recreation. Indicators are found in these relations on the one hand, and in the conditions in the sociocultural and physical environment on the other.

When compared to the ICIDH, many would say that Nagi's "functional limitation" is synonymous with the WHO's "disability"; likewise, Nagi's "disability" is synonymous with the WHO's "handicap." Both frameworks recognize that whether or not a person performs a socially expected activity depends not simply on the characteristics of the person, but also on the larger context of social and physical environments.

According to the Nagi framework, all pathology is associated with impairment, but not all impairments lead to functional limitations. Similarly, all functional limitation and disability are associated with impairment, but not all functional limitations lead to disability. Disability can also exist in the absence of functional limitation (e.g., disfigurement). Figure 1–2 illustrates the conceptual relationship among the categories in Nagi's framework.

Wilson and Cleary's Conceptual Model of Patient Outcomes

Wilson and Cleary (1995) recognize that as therapeutic efforts focus more on improving patient function and well-being, the need to understand these relationships will increase. They also recognize the problem that has hampered progress in this area—the

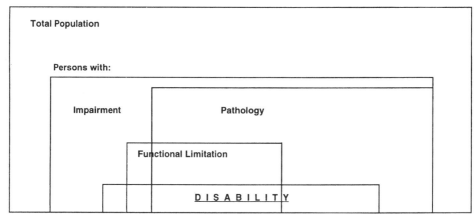

Figure 1–2. Nagi Framework

SOURCE: Institute of Medicine. (1991). *Disability in America.* Washington, DC: National Academy Press. Used by permission.

lack of conceptual models that specify how different types of outcome measures interrelate. They believe that such a conceptualization involves the integration of medical and social paradigms of health: the former held by clinicians and basic science researchers; the latter by social scientists.

In the clinical paradigm, the focus is on etiologic agents, pathological processes, and biological, physiological, and clinical outcomes. The principal goal is to understand causation in order to guide diagnosis and treatment. Controlled experiments are its principal methodology. In contrast, the social science paradigm (i.e., the "quality-of-life model"), focuses on dimensions of functioning and overall well-being. Experimental research designs are rarely possible because the focus is on the way numerous social structures influence individuals.

Wilson and Cleary (1995) conclude that none of the current conceptual models include the full range of variables that are typically included in health-related quality-of-life assessments. Furthermore, they attest that most models do not specify the links between biological and other types of measures, nor have they been tested empirically. Thus, Wilson and Cleary propose a conceptual model, a taxonomy of patient outcomes, that categorizes measures of patient outcome according to the underlying health concepts they represent. They also propose different specific causal relationships between different health concepts, thereby integrating medical and social models of health (Figure 1–3).

According to the model, measures of health can be thought of as existing on a continuum of increasing biological, social, and psychological complexity. At one end of the continuum are biological measures; at the other end are more complex and integrated measures such as functioning and general health perceptions. Dominant causal associations with each level are specified. The five levels in the model are described:

Biological and physiological variables. These include the function of cells, organs, and organ systems. Measures include those of physiological function (e.g., pulmonary function, reflexes), and physical examination findings.

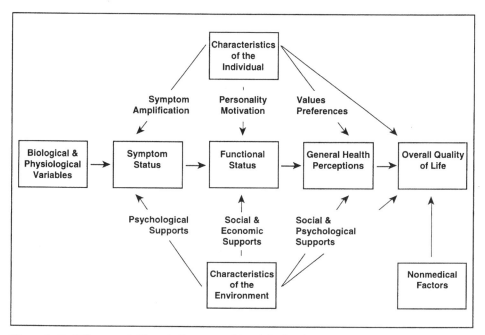

Figure 1–3. Wilson and Cleary's Conceptual Model of Patient Outcomes

SOURCE: Wilson, I. B., & Cleary, P. D. (1995). Linking clinical variables with quality of life: A conceptual model of patient outcomes. *JAMA, 273*(1), 59–65. Used by permission.

Symptom status. Assessment focuses not on specific cells and organs, but on the organism as a whole. These include physical, psychological, or emotional symptoms (e.g., weakness, confusion, speech difficulty, fear, worry). Thus, a symptom is a patient's perception of an abnormal physical, emotional, or cognitive state.

Functional status. Measures of function assess the ability of the individual to perform particular defined tasks. Four domains of function include physical function, social function, role function, and psychological function. Functional status can vary depending on personality and motivation (e.g., a determination to be self-sufficient), as well as social and economic supports (e.g., supportive family, access to care). Thus, two individuals with similar conditions may function very differently.

General health perceptions. These represent an integration of previous health concepts, discussed above, as well as others such as mental health. Thus, they are, by definition, a subjective rating. Variations in health perceptions are associated with individual values and preferences, as well as social and psychological supports.

Overall quality of life. This concept involves subjective measures of a patient's well-being. These general measures often assess how happy and/or satisfied respondents are with their life as a whole. They represent a synthesis of a wide range of experiences and feelings that people have. Overall quality of life, too, is associated with individual values and preferences, and social and psychological supports.

The Wilson and Cleary model (1995) perhaps does the best job of integrating a social model of health with a medical model. As you move from left to right in the model, you move outward from the cell to the individual to the interaction of the individual as a member of society. The concepts at each level are increasingly integrated and increasingly difficult to define and measure. At each level, there are a growing number of inputs that cannot be controlled by clinicians or the health care system as it is traditionally defined.

How Are Outcomes Measured?

Outcomes measurement involves a range of measures (from physical to physiologic to behavioral to self-perceived, and including financial and administrative measures) and methodologies (from experimental, to quasi-experimental, to non-experimental). These latter classifications have attempted to give order to the multiplicity of methods that can be applied, and the conclusions that can be drawn about the outcomes of clinical interventions. An appropriate precursor to describing these classifications is a discussion of the distinction between outcomes research and efficacy research, which has led to differing views about treatment efficacy and treatment effectiveness.

Outcomes Research versus Efficacy Research

The terms *outcomes research* and *efficacy research* are found under the umbrella of outcomes measurement. Typically, research carries a definition of scientific or scholarly investigation that implies explicit protocols and well controlled conditions aimed at proving causation. Not all research, however, is aimed at questions of causation. Thus, important differences have evolved between outcomes research and efficacy research.

Benninger et al. (1997) draw a distinction between efficacy research and outcomes research. Treatment efficacy is the ability of an applied treatment to produce a predicted result. Treatment efficacy is what drives controlled clinical studies. Conceptually, it is distinct from outcomes research that measures the effectiveness of a specific treatment as it is applied to a typical circumstance. Outcomes studies seldom incorporate experimental research designs because their focus is on the influence of the applied treatment over numerous facets of the patient's life that typically cannot be experimentally controlled. Benninger and his colleagues conclude:

> In simple terms, outcomes research attempts to demonstrate treatment effectiveness by relating clinical and more objective measures of treatment results to the subjective experiences and responses of patients who have had those treatments.

Efficacy versus Effectiveness

As noted above, a distinction is made between studies of treatment *efficacy* and *effectiveness*. The U.S. Department of Health and Human Services' Agency for Health Care Policy and Research (AHCPR) (1994), borrowing from the original definitions of the Congressional Office of Technology Assessment (1978), also distinguishes the concepts of efficacy and effectiveness in terms of the different research methodologies applied (Table 1–1). *Treatment efficacy* involves the extent to which an intervention can be

Table 1–1. Outcomes Measurement Classifications

CLASSIFICATION	DESCRIPTION	EXAMPLES
Experimental or Class I	Random assignment to intervention and control groups/phases	Randomized controlled clinical trials
		Time series research (single-subject designs)
Quasi-experimental or Class II	Nonrandom assignment to intervention and control groups/phases	Case-control studies
		Cohort studies
		Program evaluations
		Quality improvement studies
Non-experimental or Class III	No clear comparison groups, or non-randomized historical controls	Case studies or reports
		Registries and data bases
		Group judgments or expert opinion

SOURCES: Adapted from Fineburg, H.V. (1990, May). The quest for causality in health services research. *Research methodology: Strengthening causal interpretations of nonexperimental data.* Rockville, MD: Agency for Health Care Policy and Research, U.S. Department of Health and Human Services; American Academy of Neurology. Therapeutics and Technology Assessment Subcommittee. (1994). Assessment: Melodic intonation therapy. *Neurology,* 44, 566–568.

shown to be beneficial under optimal (or ideal) conditions; *treatment effectiveness* involves the extent to which services are shown to be beneficial under typical (or real-world) conditions. In this sense, treatment effectiveness involves the extent to which optimal benefits are actually achieved.

Palmer (1990) suggests that the distinction between efficacy and effectiveness was made in medical treatment research because of awareness of the loss of control when moving from animal to human experiments. As summarized by AHCPR (1994), efficacy research is reserved exclusively for well-controlled clinical studies; it is only efficacy research that can prove cause-effect. The real-world limitations of "effectiveness" research prevents complete control of conditions and reduces confidence in conclusions about causality. Consequently, studies of effectiveness (i.e., outcomes research) are better suited for making statements about trends, associations, and estimates.

The efficacy-effectiveness distinction is captured in Sackett's dichotomy of randomized controlled clinical trials into *explanatory* and *management trials* (Sackett & Gent, 1979). Explanatory trials measure efficacy by ensuring ideal conditions in subject selection, strict adherence to an experimental protocol, and only counting outcomes that are predicted by theory to relate to the treatment process. In contrast, in management trials that measure effectiveness, all comers are accepted as subjects, treatment is given according to usual practice, and all outcomes occurring after randomization are counted. Lipsey (1990), however, argues that it becomes essential to deal with the reality of conditions that cannot be controlled. Therefore, clinical trials increasingly include quasiexperimental features, are conducted in multiple phases, and are accompanied by side studies (in Palmer, 1990).

So far in the discussion, there is agreement that efficacy research is designed to *prove;* outcomes research can only *identify trends, describe, or make associations or estimates.* But, if we are to extend the difference to the research concepts of efficacy and effectiveness, there is a parting of the ways. Proponents of efficacy research, as conceptualized by Kendall and Norton-Ford (1982), regard efficacy research as research that can prove treatment *effectiveness,* as well as other characteristics of efficacy, such as treatment *efficiency* and treatment *effects.* Thus, the concept of efficacy vs. effectiveness research, in terms of differences in experimental control, becomes illogical. The terms that characterize treatment efficacy are described by Kendall and Norton-Ford as follows:

- Treatment effectiveness: Whether treatment does or does not work
- Treatment efficiency: Whether one treatment works better than another/whether all components are necessary in a treatment
- Treatment effects: Which aspects of treatment differentially influence which behaviors

(See Chapter 6 by Olswang for further discussion.)

Treatment efficacy *is* effectiveness; it, too, is efficiency and effects if we ascribe to the nomenclature of Kendall and Norton-Ford (1982). Treatment effectiveness does not, then, suggest research method (both outcomes research and efficacy research can investigate treatment effectiveness, only at differing degrees of experimental control and levels of confidence in interpretations of causality). It does characterize the aspect of treatment efficacy being investigated (i.e., whether or not the specified treatment works).

The term *treatment efficiency* finds yet a different spin on Kendall and Norton-Ford's (1982) definition, if viewed from the vantage of economics. According to JCAHO (1994), treatment efficiency is the proportion of total cost (money, resources, time) that can be related to actual benefits received. Thus, efficiency refers to cost effectiveness. Studies of this type link costs to clinical outcomes, and are sought by many payers who want to know what kind of value they are getting for the money spent.

Classifications of Outcomes Measurement Methods

Outcomes measurement methodologies usually involve primary analysis of data (i.e., data from those sources that produce original knowledge about an intervention) and can be classified as *experimental, quasi-experimental,* or *nonexperimental.* Fineburg (1990), who views methodologies from the vantage of group designs, offers definitions:

Experimental: Studies that involve random or fully specifiable assignment to intervention and control groups. Randomized controlled clinical trials are included in this category.

Quasi-experimental: Studies that involve non-random (and not fully specified) assignment to intervention and control groups. Examples include program evaluation and quality improvement studies.

Nonexperimental: Studies that involve no clear comparison groups. Case studies and data registries are examples.

Outcomes studies have also been classified, according to the quality of evidence yielded by various measurement methods, as *Class I, Class II*, and *Class III evidence* [Therapeutics and Technology Assessment Subcommittee of the American Academy of Neurology (AAN) (1994)]. Holland and colleagues (1996) summarize these categories in a brief synopsis of the efficacy of the treatment of aphasia as follows:

Class I: Evidence provided by one or more well-designed randomized controlled clinical trials.

Class II: Evidence provided by one or more well-designed randomized clinical studies such as case-control, cohort studies, and so forth.

Class III: Evidence provided by expert opinion, nonrandomized historical controls, or one or more case reports.

Efficacy research, as described above, could be regarded as experimental or Class I; outcomes research as quasi- or nonexperimental, or Class II or Class III. Table 1–1 organizes various research methods used by clinical researchers, clinicians, or managers into these classifications. These design methodologies, however, cannot be so neatly cataloged. While we can differentiate efficacy and outcomes research methods, "they more accurately exist on a continuum where at some point in the middle, they overlap" (Olswang, personal communication; see Chapter 6 by Olswang for further discussion). Even at the "low end" of outcomes research, certain methods (e.g., case studies), if well controlled, can constitute efficacy research. In addition, criticism has been directed toward study implications in terms of the quality of the methods categorized. Holland et al. (1996) identify a weakness of the AAN classifications in that they are based solely on the design of a study and do not guarantee the quality of the study itself. For example, they cite a study by Lincoln (1984), classified as a Class I study, which seriously questions quality of evidence. First, its lack of treatment effects "was likely attributable to the facts that the 'treated' patients received less than 2 hours of treatment per week, given over a very short period of time, and the subjects were heterogeneous and included individuals with dementia and brain tumor" (p. 5). In contrast, a study by Poeck et al. (1989), classified as a Class II study, "incorporated an ingenious method of partialing out the effects of spontaneous recovery in both treated and untreated groups, thereby solving a particularly troublesome issue in relation to the effects of treatment" (p. 5). The same weakness can be extended to experimental, quasiexperimental, and nonexperimental studies because they, too, are classified by study design.

Experimental (or Class I) Methods

Traditional thinking (Fineburg, 1990) in the medical field reserves randomized controlled clinical trials as the only accepted method of experimental research—a position refuted by clinical researchers who employ small-group or single-subject designs. Holland and colleagues (1996) remind us that large studies may not provide us with much information concerning the results of treatment for excluded subjects with comorbidities or unusual forms of disorders. So too, they may not provide information on how the treatment works, the duration or intensity of treatment that might affect the efficacy of treatment, or the specific nature and quality of treatment that may or may not be effective with certain patients. These important efficacy questions may be answered more appropriately and economically by small-group or single-subject experimental studies.

According to Olswang (1990), efficacy research involves the use of *group (large or small)* or *single-subject experimental methods.* Group designs allow for the study of subject populations, thus permitting the generalization of results. They typically involve a treatment group and no-treatment or other-treatment control group. Behaviors between the groups are compared to note any differences. These designs, however, often suffer from problems associated with subject homogeneity, thereby threatening the validity of experimental findings.

Single-subject designs solve the problems associated with subject homogeneity in that a subject serves as his or her own control, or heterogeneity among subjects is systematically investigated. These designs methodologically rely on tight experimental control and replication within and across subjects to allow for enhanced generalizability of results. Thus, this type of efficacy research, unlike between-group designs, can reveal the nature of the interaction between the independent variable (treatment) and subject characteristics. The ways in which a subject, or different subjects, respond to different amounts and types of treatments become a rich source of information about the intervention process.

Quasi-experimental (or Class II) Methods

Most investigators would agree that any inferences made about causal relationships are impaired when the premises of the true experiment are breached (Sechrest & Hannah, 1990). But there are several reasons why experimental data are not always available, and why it may not be possible to produce them. Some experiments may not be ethical (e.g., an experiment that withholds treatment for a control group); some experiments are administratively and logistically impossible; some may be too expensive; some may require too much time to complete; some experiments may fail (e.g., due to loss of subjects); and some experiments may lack the ability to control all variables in order to draw conclusions. A quasiexperiment is one in which the researcher falls short of meeting all the parameters of the experimental research design, but with much of the study methodology in place.

The methodological and ethical dilemmas that underlie randomized clinical trials research have given rise to the slow but steady acceptance of less rigorous or quasiexperimental methods of outcomes measurement, including methods in the realms of program evaluation and quality improvement.

Program Evaluation and Quality Improvement Methods

Program evaluation methods were designed primarily to determine whether a program is meeting its goals. Both clinical and administrative goals are monitored. Program evaluation is defined in The Rehabilitation Accreditation Commission Standards Manual for Medical Rehabilitation (CARF, 1997) as a system that enables the organization to identify the outcomes of its programs, the satisfaction of persons served, and follow-up on outcomes achieved by persons served.

As implied by CARF's definition, program evaluation activities must be outcome-oriented. Patton (1982) describes program evaluation as the systematic collection of information about the characteristics (structure), activities (process), and outcomes of programs and services that help administrators reduce uncertainty in the decisions they make regarding those same programs and services that they administer. Thus, program evaluation is a planned process of gathering and analyzing data to help reduce the risk of decisions (see Chapter 7 by Wilkerson for further discussion).

Quality improvement methods were designed to determine primarily whether actual services comply with pre-established gold standards (e.g., accepted practice parameters). In this sense, the methods constitute comparison testing. However, with recognition that methods also can be designed to acquire new knowledge, quality improvement activities can result in establishing or refining gold standards. Quality assessment and improvement are defined broadly by the JCAHO (1997) in its standards for improving organization performance:

> PI.1 The hospital has a planned, systematic, hospitalwide approach to process design and performance measurement, assessment, and improvement.

> PI.3.1 The hospital collects data on important processes and outcomes related to patient care and organization functions.

> PI.5 The hospital systematically improves its performance (pp 134–136).

The methods typically involve a systematic process, as described above, of Plan-Do-Study-Act. With the introduction of systems thinking in quality improvement activities, all structural inputs and processes (including clinical, organizational, support, and administrative) share equal importance in influencing positive outcomes. As managers acquire advanced computer technologies and statistical knowledge, both program evaluation and quality improvement methods are becoming more sophisticated from theoretical and scientific standpoints (see Chapter 8 by Frattali for further discussion).

Other Methods

Other quasi-experimental methods include case-control studies and cohort studies, often catalogued in the field of epidemiology (i.e., the study of the nature, cause, control, and determinants of the frequency and distribution of disease, disability, and death in human populations) (Timmreck, 1994). Both studies are considered observational studies because no one attempts to intervene or to alter the course of the disease.

Case-control studies are retrospective studies because they are conducted after the onset of an outbreak and "look backward" to the possible causes of the outbreak. Case-control refers to the way in which the study group is put together. These studies begin with assessment of the persons or groups with a disease, condition, or disorder (cases) and identify a separate control group that has not been affected (controls). The possible causes of the disease, condition, or disorder constitute the outcome under study (Riegelman & Hirsch, 1989).

Cohort studies are prospective studies because they are conducted before the onset of an outbreak and "look forward" to assess morbidity and mortality. "Cohort" means a group of persons who share a common characteristic, especially age. Cohort studies begin with a study group that possesses the characteristic(s) under study and a control group that is free of this characteristic. Both groups are followed forward in time to determine whether they will develop a particular condition. The occurrence of the condition is the outcome under study (Riegelman & Hirsch, 1989).

Nonexperimental (or Class III) Methods

Case reports, use of *data bases* or *registries, group judgments,* and *expert opinion* are among the nonexperimental methods. These methods, while subjective and fraught with a lack of experimental controls, are useful in that they can be conducted by clinicians and managers for large groups of clients, and lend support to quasi- and experimental studies of treatment efficacy or outcome. These methods can also help to prompt and shape causal hypotheses.

Synthetic Analysis

In contrast to outcomes measurement methods that involve primary analysis of data, methods that involve synthetic analysis (i.e., studies that refer to available knowledge, which involve synthesis of information in order to gain new insights) should be mentioned. Some of these methods include meta-analysis, cost-benefit or cost-effectiveness analyses, and technology assessment.

Meta-analysis is a method for reviewing and summarizing clusters of prior studies, irrespective of their differences. The results of studies are statistically combined, thus producing a single estimate of an intervention effect from studies that use different scales to measure the effectiveness of an intervention (Eddy, 1990; Smith & Glass, 1977).

Cost-benefit or *cost-effectiveness analyses* are conducted to determine how outcomes compare to their costs. They also are conducted for comparative purposes in determining which provider can achieve the same outcomes at a lower cost. Thus, costs and outcomes are linked in data analysis, often via use of automated management information systems or existing data banks available from large payers, such as Medicare, Medicaid, or Blue Cross/Blue Shield. A cost-benefit analysis determines the economic efficiency of a program expressed as the relationship between dollars spent and dollars saved. A cost-effectiveness analysis explores the effectiveness of a program in achieving targeted intervention outcomes in relation to the program costs (e.g., dollars spent per points on a functional outcome measure) (Rossi & Freeman, 1982).

Technology assessment denotes any process of examining and reporting properties of a technology used in clinical care, such as safety, efficacy, feasibility, and indications for use, cost, and cost-effectiveness, as well as social, economic, and ethical consequences. Assessment ideally includes evaluation of immediate results of the technology as well as its long-term consequences. A comprehensive assessment of a technology may also include an appraisal of problems of personnel training and licensure, new capital expenditures for equipment and buildings, and possible consequences for the health insurance industry and social security system. Currently, the predominant assessment methods are literature reviews and consultation with experts.

Technology assessments historically have been conducted on a reactive, ad hoc basis (e.g., in reaction to inquiries by third-party payers) rather than by systematic review and priority setting. Consequently, rigorous clinical evaluation of technologies (e.g., clinical trials research) largely has been confined to the final regulatory step of premarket approval (Institute of Medicine, 1985).

Multiple-Attacks Approach

Perhaps the most effective approach to outcomes measurement is one of multiple attacks. By this I mean the measurement of outcomes from multiple but independent sources using various methods. Mosteller (1990) believes a multiple attacks approach is more influential in shaping public policy than outcomes data from one study or a collection of studies using the same method. Considering the spectrum of methods, the concept of multiple attacks has appeal for both the researcher and the clinician.

As explained in an earlier publication (Frattali, 1996), we have looked historically to our scientists to conduct the needed experimental research to amass outcomes data and prove that what we do makes a difference. Given the various outcomes measurement methods either advanced or in use today, such a view is myopic. Outcomes research methodologies, because of their less stringent design characteristics, are amenable for use in real-world settings with large patient populations. While causal interpretations must be qualified by study design limitations, findings can lend support to experimental evidence of efficacy. Outcomes research methdologies, in fact, may be a bridge to the longstanding schism between clinicians (who argue that research is seldom clinically relevant) and researchers (who argue that clinicians seldom apply research findings to clinical practice).

How Are Outcomes Managed?

Once we measure outcomes, we must manage them if they are to have any purpose at all. The management of outcomes gives rise to the development of new standards of practice and management tools such as critical paths (i.e., treatment regimes, supported ideally by patient outcomes research, that include only those vital elements that have been proved to affect patient outcomes) to increase both treatment- and cost effectiveness. Thus, we can move from assumption-driven to data-driven clinical methods. Ellwood (1988) concisely defines the field of *outcomes management* in the context of health care:

> Outcomes Management is a technology of patient experience designed to help patients, payers, providers make rational [health care]-related choices based on better insight into the impact of these choices on the patient's life. Outcomes Management consists of:
>
> - Common patient-understood language of health outcomes;
> - A national data base containing clinical, financial and health outcome information and analysis that estimates as best we can the relationship between [health care] interventions and health outcomes, as well as the relationship between health outcomes and money;
> - An opportunity for each decision maker to have access to those analyses that are relevant to the choices they must make. [p. 4]

The best outcomes data can exist without anyone knowing and, thus, without any influence on clinical practice. In order for us to manage outcomes, outcomes data must be translated into practice guidelines and protocols, which in turn should be distributed widely in efforts to change practitioners' ways of doing things and, thus, reach desired outcomes in a more predictable manner.

CONCLUSION

There is no need for euphemism on what is driving the need for outcomes data. We all know it is cost pressures. But it was costly, under a retrospective payment system, to support practitioners who were paid for any service they wished to provide with no accountability for the end result. It is equally worrisome to wonder if practitioners in a prepaid system might withhold needed care because they stand to gain financially from doing so (Berwick, Godfrey, & Roessner, 1990). Outcomes data, then, become the link to knowledge about the appropriateness and quality of care.

Many practitioners believe that in a cost-driven system, money saved, not outcomes gained, is the object. This view is short-sighted. As quality of care suffers, consumers (e.g., clients, families, managed care systems, regulators) will not remain passive, particularly if given a choice of providers. In the long-term, practitioners who can prove both cost effectiveness and quality of care will gain a strategic advantage in what has become a competitive game of service delivery.

We have a task before us—to cumulate outcomes data, not only to prove that what we do works, but to continually upgrade what we do. Thus, we have a second task—to apply new knowledge to new practice patterns. Fineburg (1990) speaks about the connections of causality, convincingness, and change. He explains that one measure of success in research is the extent to which the knowledge produced by researchers leads to action. In the design of studies, analysis of data, and presentation of findings, we should never lose sight of the purposes of the investigation and what audiences we want to convince. For whom is the investigation being conducted? What are their needs, beliefs, interests, and incentives? It is naive not to recognize that surprising or unwelcome results will be met with much more skepticism and scrutiny than will results that confirm preconceptions or satisfy political agendas. But, if we are to do our jobs, we must engage controversial and political topics.

Holland (cited in Goldberg, 1993) believes we must be masters of our fate—for our professional integrity and for the sake of our clients. To do that, "we must take what we know from efficacy studies, see that the results are translated into practice guidelines, and make sure that those guidelines are widely disseminated and followed" (p. 45). Every individual has the right to expect the best of what exists in clinical practice.

Outcomes measurement begins with inquiry. Clinical questions are subjected to systematic study. The findings lead to yet other questions that are explored, answered, and generate more questions. Clinical inquiry and its subsequent study form the foundation of any clinical discipline. We must ask the questions, and seek to answer them intelligently using various methodologies under the rubric of outcomes measurement.

REFERENCES

Agency for Health Care Policy and Research. (1994). *Distinguishing between efficacy and effectiveness.* Rockville, MD: Author.

American Academy of Neurology, Therapeutics and Technology Assessment Subcommittee. (1994). Assessment: Melodic intonation therapy. *Neurology, 44,* 566–568.

American Speech-Language-Hearing Association. (1995). *ASHA Task Force on Treatment Outcomes and Cost Effectiveness: Project overview and status.* Rockville, MD: Author.

Batavia, A.I. (1992). Assessing the function of functional assessment: A consumer perspective. *Disability and Rehabilitation,* 14, 156–160.

Benninger, M.S., Gardner, G.M., Jacobson, B.H., & Grywalski, C. (1997). New dimensions in measuring voice treatment outcomes. In R. T. Sataloff (Ed.), *Professional voice: The science and art of clinical care* (2nd ed, pp. 789–794). San Diego, CA: Singular Publishing Group.

Berwick, D.M. (1989). E.A. Codman and the rhetoric of battle: A commentary. The *Milbank Quarterly, 67*(2), 262–267.

Berwick, D.M., Godfrey, A.B., & Roessner, J. (1990). *Curing health care: A report on the National Demonstration Project on Quality Improvement in Health Care.* San Francisco: Jossey-Bass.

Brewster, A.C., Karlin, B.G., Hyde, L.A., Jacobs, C.M., Bradbury, R.C., & Chae, Y.M. (1985). MEDISGRPS: A clinically based approach to classfying hospital patients at admission. *Inquiry, 22*(4), 377–387.

Brinkley, J. (1986). U.S. releasing lists of hospitals with abnormal mortality rates. *New York Times.* 12 March: 1.

CARF . . . The Rehabilitation Accreditation Commission. (1997). *Standards manual and interpretive guidelines for medical rehabilitation.* Tucson, AZ: Author.

Cichowski, K. (1995). *Rehabilitation Institute of Chicago Functional Assessment Scale—Revised.* Chicago, IL: Rehabilitation Institute of Chicago.

Codman, E.A. (circa 1917). A study in hospital efficiency as demonstrated by the case report of the first five years of a private hospital. Boston: Thomas Todd Company.

Codman, E.A. (1934). The shoulder: Rupture of the supraspinatus tendon and other lesions in or about the subacromial bursa. Boston: Thomas Todd Company.

Deming, W. E. (1982). *Out of the crisis.* Cambridge: Massachusetts Institute of Technology, Center for Advanced Engineering Study.

Donabedian, A. (1980). *Explorations in quality assessment and monitoring. Volume 1: The definition of quality and approaches to its assessment.* Ann Arbor, MI: Health Administration Press.

Donabedian, A. (1985). *The methods and findings of quality assessment and monitoring: An Illustrated analysis. Volume 3.* Ann Arbor, MI: Health Administration Press.

Eddy, D. M. (1990). The role of meta-analysis. In L. Sechrest, E. Perrin, & J. Bunker (Eds.), *Conference proceedings: Strengthening causal interpretation of nonexperimental data* (pp. 173–176). Rockville, MD: U.S. Department of Health and Human Services, Public Health Service, Agency for Health Care Policy and Research.

Ellwood, P. (1988). Shattuck Lecture—Outcome management: A technology of patient experience. *New England Journal of Medicine, 318*(23), 1549–1556.

Evaluation Systems International, Inc. (1994). *OUTCOME TM.* Denver, CO: Author.

Fetter, R.B., Shin, Y., Freeman, J.L., Averill, R.G., & Thompson, J.D. (1980). Case mix definition by diagnosis related groups. *Medical Care, 18* (Suppl. 2), 1–53.

Fineburg, H.V. (1990). The quest for causality in health services research. In L. Sechrest, E. Perrin, & J. Bunker (Eds.), *Conference proceedings: Strengthening causal interpretation of nonexperimental data* (pp. 215–220). Rockville, MD: U.S. Department of Health and Human Services, Public Health Service, Agency for Health Care Policy and Research.

Focus Rehab, Inc. (1995). The Functional Outcome and Utilization System (F.O.C.U.S.). Nashville, TN: Author.

Frattali, C.M. (1996). Childhood language perspectives: Clinical outcome perspectives. In M.D. Smith & J.S. Damico (Eds.), *Childhood language disorders.* (pp. 3–16). New York: Thieme Medical Publishers.

Frattali, C.M., Thompson, C.K., Holland, A.L., Wohl, C.B., & Ferketic, M.M. (1995). *The American Speech-Language-Hearing Association functional assessment of communication skills for adults (ASHA FACS).* Rockville, MD: ASHA.

Goldberg, B. (1993). Translating data into practice. *Asha, 35,* 45–47.

Harvey, R.G., & Jellinek, H.M. (1979). *Patient evaluation and conference system: PECS.* Wheaton, IL: Marianjoy Rehabilitation Center.

Harvey, R.F., Jellinek, H.M. (1981). Functional performance assessment: A program approach. *Archives of Physical Medicine and Rehabilitation, 63,* 43–52.

Holland, A.L., Fromm, D.S., DeRuyter, F., & Stein, M. (1996). Efficacy of treatment for aphasia: A brief synopsis. *Journal of Speech and Hearing Research.* 39 (5), S27-S36.

Horn, S.D., Sharkey, P.D., Buckle, J.M., Backofen, J.E., Averill, R.F., & Horn, R.A. (1991). The relationship between severity of illness and hospital length of stay and mortality. *Medical Care, 29*(4), 305–317.

Iezzoni, L. I. (Ed.) (1994). *Risk adjustment for measuring health care outcomes.* Ann Arbor, MI: Health Administration Press.

Iezzoni, L.I., & Moskowitz, M.A. (1988). A clinical assessment of MedisGroups. *Journal of the American Medical Association, 260*(21), 3159–3163.

Institute of Medicine, Committee for Evaluation of Medical Technologies. (1985). *Assessing medical technologies.* Washington, DC: National Academy Press.

Jacobson, B.H, Johnson, A., & Grywalski, C. (1995). *The Voice Handicap Index.* Detroit, MI: Henry Ford Hospital, Division of Speech-Language Sciences & Disorders, Department of Neurology.

Joint Commission on Accreditation of Healthcare Organizations. (1997). *Hospital accreditation standards.* Oakbrook Terrace, IL: Author.

Kendall, P., & Norton-Ford, J. (1982). Therapy outcome research methods. In P. Kendall & J. Butcher (Eds.), *Handbook of research methods in clinical psychology* (pp. 429–460). New York: John Wiley and Sons.

Knaus, W.A., Zimmerman, J.E., Wagner, D.P., Draper, E.A., & Lawrence, D.E. (1981). APACHE— Acute physiology and chronic health evaluation: A physiologically based classification system. *Critical Care Medicine, 9*(8), 591–597.

Lincoln, N., McGuirk, E., Mulley, G., Lendrem, W., Jones, A., & Mitchell, J. (1984). Effectiveness of speech therapy for aphasic stroke patients: A randomised controlled trial. *Lancet, 1,* 1197–1200.

Lipsey, M. W. (1990). Theory as method: Small theories of treatments. In L. Sechrest, E. Perrin, & J. Bunker (Eds.), *Conference proceedings: Strengthening causal interpretation of nonexperimental data* (pp. 33–52). Rockville, MD: U.S. Department of Health and Human Services, Public Health Service, Agency for Health Care Policy and Research.

McReynolds, L. (1990). Historical perspective of treatment efficacy research. In L.B. Olswang, C.K. Thompson, S.F. Warren, & N.J. Minghetti (Eds), *Treatment efficacy research in communication disorders* (pp. 5–14). Rockville, MD: American Speech-Language-Hearing Foundation.

Merson, R.M., Rolnick, M.I., & Weiner, R. (1995). *The Beaumont Outcome Software System (BOSS).* West Bloomfield, MI: Parrot Software.

Mosteller, F. (1990). Improving research methodology: An overview. In L. Sechrest, E. Perrin, & J. Bunker (Eds.), *Conference proceedings: Strengthening causal interpretation of nonexperimental data* (pp. 221–230). Rockville, MD: U.S. Department of Health and Human Services, Public Health Service, Agency for Health Care Policy and Research.

Nagi, S.Z. (1965). Some conceptual issues in disability and rehabilitation. In M.B. Sussman (Ed.), *Sociology and rehabilitation* (pp. 100–113). Washington, DC: American Sociological Association.

National Institutes of Health (1993 March). Research plan for the National Center for Medical Rehabilitation Research. [NIH Pub. No. 93-3509]. Bethesda, MD: U.S. Department of Health and Human Services.

Office of Technology Assessment. (1978). *Assessing the efficacy and safety of medical technologies.* (OTA Publication No. OTA-H-75). Washington, DC: Author.

Olswang, L. (1990). Treatment efficacy: The breadth of research. In L.B. Olswang, C.K. Thompson, S.F. Warren, & N.J. Minghetti (Eds.), *Treatment efficacy research in communication disorders* (pp. 99–103). Rockville, MD: American Speech-Language-Hearing Foundation.

Olswang, L.B., Thompson, C.K., Warren, S.F., & Minghetti, N.J. (Eds.). (1990). *Treatment efficacy research in communication disorders.* Rockville, MD: American Speech-Language-Hearing Foundation.

Palmer, R.H. (1990). Small theories of programs. In L. Sechrest, E. Perrin, & J. Bunker (Eds.), *Conference proceedings: Strengthening causal interpretation of nonexperimental data* (pp. 57–60). Rockville, MD: U.S. Department of Helath and Human Services, Public Health Service, Agency for Health Care Policy and Research.

Parkside Associates, Inc. (1986). *Level of Rehabilitation Scale III.* Park Ridge, IL: Author. (Now available from Formations in Health Care, Chicago.)

Patton, M.Q. (1982). *Practical evaluation.* Beverly Hills, CA: SAGE Publications.

Poeck, K., Huber, W., Willmes, K. (1989). Outcome of intensive language treatment in aphasia. *Journal of Speech and Hearing Disorders, 54,* 471–479.

Pope, A.M., & Tarlov, A.L. (Eds.). (1991). *Disability in America: Toward a national agenda for prevention.* Washington, DC: National Academy Press.

Riegelman, R.K., & Hirsch, R.P. (1989). *Studying a study and testing a test.* Boston: Little, Brown and Company.

Rosen, A., & Proctor, E. (1981). Distinctions between treatment outcome and their implications for treatment evaluation. *Journal of Consulting and Clinical Psychology, 49,* 418–425.

Rossi, P.H., & Freeman, H.E. (1982). *Evaluation: A systematic approach* (2nd ed.). Beverly Hills: Sage Publications.

Sackett, D.L., & Gent, M. (1979). Controversy in counting and attributing events in clinical trials. *New England Journal of Medicine, 301,* 1410–1412.

Sechrest, L., & Hannah, M. (1990). The critical importance of nonexperimental data. In L. Sechrest, E. Perrin, & J. Bunker (Eds.), *Conference proceedings: Strengthening causal interpretation of nonexperimental data* (pp. 1–8). Rockville, MD: U.S. Department of Health and Human Services, Public Health Service, Agency for Health Care Policy and Research.

Sechrest, L., Perrin, E., & Bunker, J. (Eds.). (1990). *Conference proceedings: Strengthening causal interpretation of nonexperimental data.* Rockville, MD: U.S. Department of Health and Human Services, Public Health Service, Agency for Health Care Policy and Research.

Smith, L.M., & Glass, G. (1977). Meta-analysis of psychotherapy outcome studies. *American Psychologist, 32,* 752–760.

State University of New York at Buffalo, Research Foundation. (1993). *Guide for use of the Uniform Data Set for Medical Rehabilitation: Functional Independence Measure.* Buffalo: Author.

Stineman, M.G., Escarce, J.J., Goin, J.E., Hamilton, B.B., Granger, C.V., & Williams, S.V. (1994). A case-mix classification system for medical rehabilitation. *Medical Care, 32*(4), 366–379.

Timmreck, T.C. (1994). *An introduction to epidemiology.* Boston: Jones and Bartlett Publishers.

Vladeck, B.C. (1984). Medicare hospital payment by diagnosis-related groups. *Annals of Internal Medicine, 100*(4), 576–591.

Wennberg, J., & Gittelsohn, A. (1973). Small area variations in health care delivery. *Science, 182*(117), 1102–1108.

Wilkerson, D.L., Batavia, A.I., & DeJong, G. (1992). Use of functional status measures for payment of medical rehabilitation services. *Archives of Physical Medicine and Rehabilitation, 73,* 111–120.

Wilson, I.B., & Cleary, P.D. (1995). Linking clinical variables with health-related quality of life: A conceptual model of patient outcomes. *Journal of the American Medical Association, 273*(1), 59–65.

World Health Organization. (1980). *International classification of impairments, disabilities, and handicaps.* Geneva: Author.

CHAPTER 2

Outcomes Measurement Requirements

PATRICIA LARKINS HICKS

INTRODUCTION

The U.S. health care and education systems are in the midst of changes that are rapid, dramatic, and unprecedented. As a result of this fast-paced, market-driven transformation, practitioners are being challenged to deliver quality care for a reasonable price. In health care, patients are being given a key role in provider selection. If dissatisfied, they are expected to vote by changing providers. Payers are moving to center stage demanding quality care at the lowest cost and convenient, "one-stop shopping." They expect coordinated services, facilities, systems, and providers that are willing to be accountable, and demonstrate quality and value-added services. Services must be justified to patients, providers, and payers by demonstrating that they improve patient outcomes. In education, students are being expected to demonstrate their mastery of concepts and skills that will facilitate their doing business or working in the "real world." For example, students must pass proficiency tests in order to receive their high school diploma. This focus on learning outcomes is transforming teaching and learning. It is requiring a shift in classroom practices and coordinating support among members of the learning team including students, parents, teachers, school administrators, board members, and policymakers.

Accrediting bodies, payers, and government agencies alike are requiring, in one form or another, outcomes measurement. Demands for outcomes data are most prevalent currently in the health care system. These requirements will increase as fee-for-service health insurance plans are replaced by capitated systems, not-for-profit managed care organizations decrease and for-profit managed care organizations increase, stand-alone hospital hubs are replaced with integrated health care systems and networks, and Medicaid/Medicare beneficiaries increase their enrollment in managed care plans. Gone are the days of subjective information and a focus on individually defined procedures. Here to stay is the demand for objective data that can be used to create benchmarks and manage resources for populations and communities.

Speech-language pathology services can improve the quality of life of many individuals and often lower other health care or special education costs. Speech-language pathologists (SLPs) then must ensure that persons in need of rehabilitation services will have access to appropriate services. In addition, it will become equally important to position the profession to capture the many new opportunities that will arise as a result of this service delivery transformation.

In order to accomplish the above-stated goals, SLPs will need outcomes data that are required by various entities. The purposes of this chapter are to acquaint you with some key agencies that are requiring outcomes measurement, review their requirements, and provide suggestions that will assist you in preparing to meet the requirements. The information presented will facilitate your becoming a more informed professional equipped to participate effectively in the current service delivery environment.

REQUIREMENTS OF ACCREDITING AGENCIES

Today's marketplace is competitive. Why should a network want you to be among its providers? Why should consumers choose you as their preferred provider of speech-language pathology services? Why should a purchaser of speech-language pathology services select you as a vendor?

One credential that signifies good practice procedures and outcomes is *accreditation.* Payers, consumers, and government regulators perceive organizations that are accredited as leaders in quality. This certificate also enhances your marketing capabilities. It communicates to others that you were able to undergo a rigorous review process and pass the scrutiny of reviewers (surveyors) outside of your immediate organization.

The following accrediting agencies (see Appendix 2-A for addresses) have outcomes measurement requirements that you need to be aware of:

- The Rehabilitation Accreditation Commission, formerly the Commission on Accreditation of Rehabilitation Facilities (CARF)
- American Speech-Language-Hearing Association's Professional Services Board (PSB)
- Joint Commission on Accreditation of Healthcare Organizations (JCAHO)

A description of each agency and its requirements* follows. For each requirement, questions are provided to give you an opportunity to assess your organization's accreditation readiness. Recommendations are provided that will assist you in preparing for accreditation.

The Rehabilitation Accreditation Commission (CARF)

Description of the Agency: Key Facts

CARF, a national not-for-profit organization, was founded in 1966 to serve as the preeminent standards-setting accrediting body, promoting the delivery of quality services to people with disabilities and others in need of rehabilitation.

---

*At the time of this writing, 1996 requirements were in place. The requirements as described in this chapter will likely change in future years. Therefore, refer to the most current standards manuals for up-to-date information.

The standards are "national consensus standards" defined with the active support and involvement of providers, consumers, and purchasers of services rather than being derived from a research base. Usually about 10,000 people have the opportunity to review and comment on the proposed standards.

Because CARF provides an opportunity for input into its standards development process, SLPs should make sure that their feedback is included. Participation will become increasingly important as changes occur in the health care marketplace.

Once standards are published in the new *Standards Manual and Interpretive Guidelines for Medical Rehabilitation,* they become effective after a 6-month period has elapsed to provide organizations with time to incorporate the changes into their operations.

Description of Outcomes Measurement Requirements

The following requirements are found in the Standards Manual and Interpretive Guidelines for Medical Rehabilitation (CARF, 1996).

Accreditation Principle #4

Based on the informed choices of the persons served, the organization, using a team approach, provides coordinated, individualized, goal-oriented services leading to desired outcomes (CARF, p. 5).

CARF expects your organization to have defined outcomes for the services provided. Answer the following questions to determine if your organization can meet this requirement:

- Does your organization provide its patients with information that allows them to make appropriate choices? Yes [ ] No [ ]
- Does your organization use a team approach to care? Yes [ ] No [ ]
- Does your organization have a process for ensuring its services are coordinated? Yes [ ] No [ ]
- For each patient served, were the goals for the services provided? Yes [ ] No [ ]
- For each patient's goals, were expected results defined? Yes [ ] No [ ]

If you answered "Yes" to *all* the questions, then your organization meets this overall requirement. If you answered "No" to *any* of the questions, then these are areas that your organization must address.

Accreditation Criteria #3: The Organization Meets the Policy on Outcomes

The organization should demonstrate that systems are in place to measure outcomes including effectiveness, efficiency, satisfaction of persons served, and status of the persons served after discharge (follow-up). These outcome measures should be in place for all programs for which the organization is seeking accreditation. The organizations should demonstrate the utilization of outcome information throughout its planning activities. This information should be provided to the persons served, personnel, payers, and if requested.

To conform to this policy, at a minimum, the following should be demonstrated:

- there should be established measures for effectiveness, efficiency, consumer satisfaction, and follow-up. If one of these measures is missing from the system or if there is not a system for each program submitted for accreditation, the organization should be placed on 60-day hold.

- for each program submitted for accreditation, data should be collected to gauge how the program is meeting the established measures for effectiveness, efficiency, consumer satisfaction, and follow-up. If data are not being collected for any one of these measures or programs, the organization should be placed on a 60-day hold.

- there should be a written management report for each program submitted for accreditation. This report should describe the extent to which the program is meeting or not meeting the established measures for effectiveness, efficiency, consumer satisfaction, and follow-up. The report should be available at the time of the site survey. If this report is not available, the organization must submit a copy of it to CARF within 6 months following notification of the accreditation outcome. Failure to submit the report could result in loss of accreditation.

- the organization should demonstrate that it utilizes the results of the system at the time of the site survey. If utilization cannot be demonstrated, the organization must submit written evidence of how it has used the information to CARF within 6 months following notification of the accreditation outcome. Failure to submit this evidence could result in the loss of accreditation (CARF, p. 8).

CARF expects that your organization will be measuring to: determine what works; ensure results are achieved in the shortest period of time; and determine if your consumers are satisfied. Additionally, CARF expects that your organization will have documented its results and more importantly are using them to improve the quality of its services. Answer the following questions to determine if your organization can meet these requirements:

- Does your organization have effectiveness measures? Yes [ ] No [ ]
- Does your organization have efficiency measures? Yes [ ] No [ ]
- Does your organization have consumer satisfaction measures? Yes [ ] No [ ]
- Does your organization have outcome follow-up measures? Yes [ ] No [ ]
- Does your organization have regularly scheduled planning activities?
  Yes [ ] No [ ]
- When your organization meets to plan, are the outcomes data used?
  Yes [ ] No [ ]
- Does your organization communicate its outcomes data with its patients?
  Yes [ ] No [ ]
- Does your organization communicate its outcomes data with all staff?
  Yes [ ] No [ ]
- Does your organization communicate its outcomes data with payers?
  Yes [ ] No [ ]

- Does your organization have a written report that summarizes its performance against results? Yes [ ] No [ ]

Promoting Outcomes Measurement and Management Principle

Outcomes measurement and management and the utilization of outcomes information in planning should reflect the organization's ability to achieve outcomes that meet the identified needs of past, current, and prospective consumers. This process is dynamic and should demonstrate the value of rehabilitation.

Information from outcomes measurement should be managed and utilized in planning, modifying, adding, or deleting programs and services. Results of outcomes measurement should be communicated internally throughout the organization and externally to those concerned in the communities served (CARF, p. 61–3c).

CARF expects that your organization will use its data to ensure that it meets consumer needs and that it will make programmatic changes when necessary. Answer the following questions to determine if your organization can meet these requirements:

- Does your organization identify the needs of past consumers? Yes [ ] No [ ]
- Does your organization identify the needs of current consumers? Yes [ ] No [ ]
- Does your organization identify the needs of prospective consumers? Yes [ ] No [ ]
- When your organization plans, are outcomes data used to ensure consumers' needs are met? Yes [ ] No [ ]
- Does your organization make changes in its program based upon outcomes data and consumer needs? Yes [ ] No [ ]
- Does your organization share its results with appropriate persons within the community? Yes [ ] No [ ]

Program Evaluation Principle

The program evaluation system should enable the organization to identify the outcomes of its programs, the satisfaction of the persons served, and follow-up on outcomes achieved by the persons served.

There should be a written description of the program evaluation system. It should include:

- admission criteria
- a listing of services provided
- measurable objectives
- a specification of the time for which each measure is applied
- a priority ranking and weighting of objectives
- measures of effectiveness and efficiency
- measures of satisfaction of the persons served with the program follow-up information

The follow-up information gathered by the organization concerning the status of the persons served should be integrated into the program evaluation system. The focus should be on the aggregate outcomes of the persons served in a specific program. This information will assist the organization and the program to determine their success in achieving and maintaining appropriate and desirable outcomes (CARF, p. 61–3a).

The system should track and maintain at a minimum:

- characteristics of persons served
- lengths of stay
- measures of effectiveness (eg., outcomes achieved by persons served)
- measures of efficiency (eg., time, cost, resource utilization)
- measures of satisfaction of the persons served

There should be a follow-up system that collects the same data at admission, discharge, and a date(s) after discharge, determined by the program (CARF p.62–3b).

CARF expects your organization to have a program evaluation system. This system should track information about patients' aggregate outcomes at admission, discharge, and follow-up. Answer the following questions to determine if your organization can meet these requirements:

- Does your organization have a written description of its program evaluation system? Yes [ ] No [ ]
- Does your organization have written admission criteria? Yes [ ] No [ ]
- Has your organization identified in writing the services it provides? Yes [ ] No [ ]
- Does your organization have measurable objectives? Yes [ ] No [ ]
- Are your organization's objectives prioritized? Yes [ ] No [ ]
- Does your organization have a specified time for which each measure is applied? Yes [ ] No [ ]
- Does your organization track its patients' demographics? Yes [ ] No [ ]
- Does your organization track its patients' lengths of stay? Yes [ ] No [ ]
- Does your organization track the results of its effectiveness measures? Yes [ ] No [ ]
- Does your organization track the results of its efficiency measures? Yes [ ] No [ ]
- Does your organization track the results of its consumer satisfaction measures? Yes [ ] No [ ]
- Does your organization track the results of its follow-up measures? Yes [ ] No [ ]
- Are there written data collection protocols? Yes [ ] No [ ]
- Are there written outcomes reports requirements? Yes [ ] No [ ]

Assessing Quality of Services Provided to the Persons Served

The reviews should determine whether:

- services provided relate to goals
- services were provided for an appropriate duration and intensity

- services produced the desired results in terms of the stated goals of the individual plans of the persons served
- there were unexpected results/complications

Each review should involve a representative sampling which includes current records and records of persons discharged within the last quarter. The system should provide for reviews to be performed at least semiannually (CARF, p.63–3c).

CARF expects your organization to conduct periodic reviews to determine the quality of services provided. Answer the following questions to determine if your organization can meet these requirements:

- Does your organization have established timelines for program reviews? Yes [ ] No [ ]
- Does your organization review its program(s) at least twice a year? Yes [ ] No [ ]
- Does your organization use a representative sample for each review? Does this sample include both current patients and patients discharged within the last quarter? Yes [ ] No [ ]
- When your organization reviews its program(s), does it determine if services provided related to the goals? Yes [ ] No [ ]
- When your organization reviews its program(s), does it determine if services were provided for an appropriate duration and intensity? Yes [ ] No [ ]
- When your organization reviews its program(s), does it determine if the results achieved were consistent with patients' goals? Yes [ ] No [ ]
- When your organization reviews its program(s), does it determine that unexpected results were obtained? Yes [ ] No [ ]
- When your organization reviews its program(s), does it determine that complications occurred? Yes [ ] No [ ]

Analysis and Utilization of Information

The organization should be involved in a continuous analysis and utilization of information gathered from various sources. This process should include results from the organization's program evaluation system, planning process, the delivery of services, and the review of the organization's fiscal management.

There should be documentation that demonstrates:

- analysis of internal and external information reports
- actions taken based on this analysis
- ongoing utilization of information to create new programs as needed to improve, modify, and/or delete existing programs
- continual review of all information gathered by the program

The analysis of the information gathered from the systems and reports should enable the organization to:

- determine when performance is less than acceptable

- identify the reasons why the performance fell below the acceptable level
- take action to improve program performance to an acceptable level
- follow up on and monitor corrective actions performed at specific times, with the results documented (CARF, p.64–3c).

CARF expects your organization to use its outcomes data as a means of assessing and improving performance. Answer the following questions to determine if your organization can meet these requirements:

- After your organization collects its outcomes data, does it analyze it to determine what needs improvement? Yes [ ] No [ ]
- After your organization collects its outcomes data, does it analyze it to determine what new programs can be developed? Yes [ ] No [ ]
- After your organization collects its outcomes data, does it analyze it to determine what needs to be deleted? Yes [ ] No [ ]
- After your organization collects its outcomes data, does it determine when performance was unacceptable? Yes [ ] No [ ]
- After your organization collects its outcomes data, does it use the data to establish corrective action? Yes [ ] No [ ]
- After your organization collects its outcomes data, does it use the data to establish timelines to follow up until problems have been resolved? Yes [ ] No [ ]

CARF has program standards that are specific for Medical Rehabilitation Programs. These programs are: comprehensive inpatient, spinal cord rehabilitation, comprehensive pain management, brain injury, outpatient medical rehabilitation, and home- and community-based rehabilitation.

If your organization has one of these programs, then, in addition to the previous requirements, it should demonstrate that:

the persons served are making reasonable improvement toward accomplishment of functional goals. The organization should adopt measurable criteria for initiation and termination of specific rehabilitation treatments.

the program evaluation system should address at minimum: functional outcomes, medical outcomes, disposition at discharge, and status post-discharge functional abilities (CARF, p. 70–4a).

CARF expects Medical Rehabilitation Programs to establish functional goals for their patients. Additionally, CARF expects these programs to assess the functional status of their patients at admission, discharge, and follow-up. Answer the following questions to determine if your organization can meet these requirements:

- Does your organization identify functional goals for its patients? Yes [ ] No [ ]
- Does your organization use functional status measures with its patients at admission, discharge, and follow-up? Yes [ ] No [ ]
- For each treatment provided, does your organization have criteria established to indicate when to initiate/terminate the treatment? Yes [ ] No [ ]

Promoting Program Quality

Assessment—Medical Rehabilitation Programs are expected to include the desired outcomes and expectations of the persons served and the outcomes anticipated by the persons conducting the assessment. They are expected to provide for the reporting of the assessment outcomes to appropriate personnel and to the persons served (CARF, p. 49–2d).

Individual Plan—it should include an overall plan that addresses the desired outcomes and expectations of the persons served based on his or her strengths, abilities, needs, and preferences as well as the outcomes expected by the team (CARF, p. 50–2d).

Referral—this should include tracking information about the reason for referral and report of outcome (CARF, p. 52–2d).

Discharge Planning and Implementation—this should include establishing desired outcomes and expectations, identifying services provided, desired outcomes and expectations achieved or not achieved, reason for discharge, and referrals and recommendations to assist the persons to maintain and/or improve functioning (CARF, p. 53–2e).

Follow-Up—these reports should be prepared, which specifically relate each person's current status to his or her discharge status (CARF, p. 54–2e).

CARF expects medical rehabilitation programs to establish desired outcomes and expectations upon assessment, during discharge planning and implementation and when developing individual plans. CARF further expects these programs to determine if functional status has been maintained and/or improved after the patient has been discharged. Answer the following questions to determine if your organization meets these requirements:

- During assessments, does your organization document the patient's desired outcomes and expectations? Yes [ ] No [ ]
- During assessments, does your organization document the person conducting the assessment and anticipated outcomes? Yes [ ] No [ ]
- Are assessment outcomes reported to patients? Yes [ ] No [ ]
- Are assessment outcomes reported to appropriate staff? Yes [ ] No [ ]
- When individual plans of care are developed, do they include the desired outcomes and expectations of patients based upon their ability, needs, and preferences? Yes [ ] No [ ]
- When individual plans of care are developed, do they include the team's expected outcomes? Yes [ ] No [ ]
- Does your organization track reasons for referral? Yes [ ] No [ ]
- Does your organization track when outcomes are reported to referral sources? Yes [ ] No [ ]
- During discharge planning, does your organization establish desired outcomes? Yes [ ] No [ ]

- During discharge planning, does your organization identify services needed? Yes [ ] No [ ]

- During discharge implementation, does your organization document what has been achieved/not achieved? Yes [ ] No [ ]

- Does your organization prepare follow-up reports that relate current status to discharge status? Yes [ ] No [ ]

Wilkerson (1996) reports that as part of a strategic outcomes initiative, CARF is examining the integrity of data, validity, and reliability of tools used by rehabilitation providers. Specific requirements for outcome measures will be developed in the near future for inclusion in revised medical rehabilitation accreditation standards.

In the future, CARF also plans to address issues such as a common set of measures or performance indicators for rehabilitation services, the use of scorable standards for quantifying survey results, and education and technical assistance activities.

American Speech-Language-Hearing Association's Professional Services Board (PSB)

Description of the Agency: Key Facts

The Professional Services Board (PSB) of ASHA was established in 1959 to assure the best possible service to the public, encourage effective clinical management and high quality services, and provide a nationally recognized accreditation mechanism for professional clinical service programs in audiology and speech-language pathology (ASHA, 1996).

The PSB standards represent the input of numerous professionals in the fields of speech-language pathology and audiology, as well as the current trends in service delivery. They are established by the Council on Professional Standards in Audiology and Speech-Language Pathology. Generally, at the annual ASHA convention, the Council on Professional Standards provides an update to the membership, answers questions, and solicits input regarding standards issues.

PSB standards are the model for the delivery of quality services in audiology and speech-language pathology. PSB accreditation is ASHA's official recognition and declaration to others that a program meets professional standards of quality. Currently, state funding agencies use PSB accreditation for selection of audiology and speech-language pathology service providers.

Description of Outcomes Measurement Requirements

The following requirements are found in ASHA (1996):

Standard 3.0 Quality Improvement and Program Evaluation

> The quality of services provided is evaluated and documented on a systematic and continuing basis.

    3.1 There are written policies and procedures for evaluating the effectiveness and efficiency of client care and other key areas of program operation.

    3.2 Evaluation results are used to improve quality of care and program operation.

    3.3 The evaluation process is reviewed and updated on a regular and systematic basis. (p. 106)

Implementation

a. The program has a written plan for continuously improving quality that includes at least:

- the areas and indicators to be addressed or monitored.
- the process for ongoing assessment, including schedules of monitoring, potential methods for data collection and analysis, and the reporting of results.
- the ways in which results will be used to achieve improvements in areas of concern.

b. The plan for ongoing quality improvement periodically addresses all standards, with particular attention to services that are of high volume or that carry added risk, and emphasizing:

- client evaluation or treatment outcomes; these may include, but are not limited to, identification of disorder, acceptance of recommendations, functional change in status, client/family satisfaction, and others appropriate to the population. (p. 109)

The ASHA PSB expects your organization to have effectiveness and efficiency measures and written policies and procedures. It also expects your organization to use its outcomes data to improve the quality of care provided. Answer the following questions to determine if your organization meets these requirements:

- Does your organization have written policies and procedures for evaluating the effectiveness and efficiency of client care and other key areas of program operation? Yes [ ] No [ ]
- Has your organization identified potential methods for data collection and analysis? Yes [ ] No [ ]
- Does your organization have defined outcomes reporting requirements? Yes [ ] No [ ]
- Does your organization use its outcomes data to make improvements? Yes [ ] No [ ]
- Does your organization have measures to determine clinical outcomes? Yes [ ] No [ ]
- Does your organization have measures to determine functional outcomes? Yes [ ] No [ ]
- Does your organization have measures to determine social outcomes? Yes [ ] No [ ]
- Does your organization have measures that are client-defined? That is, did your clients assist you in defining your desired outcomes? Yes [ ] No [ ]

Since August 1996, any program seeking accreditation as a Medical Rehabilitation

Program may be surveyed simultaneously and receive accreditation by CARF and ASHA's PSB as part of a joint survey process (CARF, 1996).

The CARF administrative surveyor will be a speech-language pathologist or audiologist who is trained as both a CARF and PSB surveyor. The survey report, using the CARF format, will be reviewed by ASHA/PSB staff, CARF staff, the CARF Board of Trustees and the Professional Services Board of ASHA. There will be one accreditation outcome, and the CARF accreditation cycle will be followed. The surveys will be conducted using CARF procedures with additions for the standards that are specific to PSB.

This joint venture provides a unique opportunity for SLPs in that one survey can result in accreditation by two agencies.

Joint Commission on Accreditation
of Healthcare Organizations (JCAHO)

Description of the Agency: Key Facts

The Joint Commission has standards for, and conducts surveys of:

- hospitals;
- nonhospital-based psychiatric and substance abuse organizations, including mental health centers, freestanding chemical dependency providers, and organizations that serve persons with mental retardation or other developmental disabilities;
- long-term care organizations;
- home care organizations;
- ambulatory care organizations;
- pathology and clinical laboratory services; and
- health care networks

The Joint Commission tailors its survey to reflect the services offered by the organization. The standards for each accreditation program are published in accreditation manuals.

In 1995, JCAHO unveiled its performance-based, functionally organized standards. These standards constitute a stable standards framework that describes the eventual basic foundation for providing quality care and continuously improving that care over time (JCAHO, 1996). The patient is at the center of activities from admission through discharge. Consequently, the standards are organized around specific functions, under one of three headings: Care of the Patient, Organizational Functions, and Essential Structural Components.

Description of Outcomes Measurement Requirements

The following standards that relate to outcomes measurement are found in the section titled Care of the Patient (JCAHO, 1996).

Assessment of patient function (PE). The goal of the patient assessment function is to determine what kind of care is required to meet a patient's initial needs as well as his or her needs as they change in response to care.

> PE.1.3 Functional status is assessed when warranted by the patient's needs or condition.

> PE.1.3.1 All patients referred to rehabilitation services receive a functional assessment. (p. PE7)

JCAHO expects your organization to determine during assessment the functional status of its patients. Answer the following questions to determine if your organization meets these requirements:

- Does your organization assess the functional status of its patients? Yes [   ] No [   ]
- Do all patients receive a functional assessment? Yes [   ] No [   ]

Care of patients (TX). The goal of the care function is to provide individualized care in settings responsive to specific patient needs.

> TX.6.3 Rehabilitation restores, improves, or maintains the patient's optimal level of functioning, self-care, self-responsibility, independence, and quality of life.

JCAHO expects your organization to determine the impact of its services; that is, patients' functioning at optimal and more independent levels. (p.TX4.4)

Answer the following questions to determine if your organization meets this requirement:

- Does your organization use measures to assess clinical outcomes? Yes [   ] No [   ]
- Does your organization use measures to assess functional outcomes? Yes [   ] No [   ]
- Does your organization use measures to assess social outcomes? Yes [   ] No [   ]

Rehabilitation hospitals seeking accreditation from JCAHO must be actively participating in at least one form of external performance data comparison. Scalenghe (1996) reports that this means "getting some experience in collecting data, sending it to an outside organization, comparing it, and making judgments about it" (p. 3611). This is one component of JCAHO's multiyear project to incorporate performance measures requirements into its accreditation process.

Scalenghe (1996) indicates that the requirement can be met by participating in a provider chain or network that shares information. An informal effort of collecting data on lengths of stay and comparing these findings to those of other community providers will also work.

JCAHO has launched a new initiative called ORYX which will require accredited hospitals and long-term care organizations to collect outcomes data and submit the data on a continuing basis to JCAHO.

By December 31, 1997, accredited organizations must select a system and measures. JCAHO has contracted with 60 performance measurement systems to date. A profile of each will be included in its new accreditation manual.

Each accredited facility will begin collecting data and submitting to the system no later than the first quarter of 1999. For additional information about the ORYX initiative refer to Internet at www.jcaho.org.

JCAHO is reviewing its performance measures in an attempt to expand the types of healthcare providers to which it offers accreditation. In order to accomplish this, JCAHO is exploring ways to make its survey process flexible, based upon how providers are organized.

With the passage of federal legislation expanding the use of "deemed" status for Medicare providers, JCAHO's expansion efforts will have increased importance. That is, rehabilitation providers may be able to use their JCAHO accreditation when seeking Medicare certification if JCAHO receives the necessary approval from the U.S. Department of Health and Human Services.

Providers must be mindful that the JCAHO is embarking upon a process of change over time. Consequently, new requirements may emerge and providers will need to be flexible.

General Recommendations

In order to meet the requirements of accrediting agencies, it will become increasingly important to institute outcomes measurement activities. You might suggest that your organization or your state speech-language-hearing association appoint an accreditation team or committee.

Some of the responsibilities of an accreditation team or committee may be to:

- review standards of accrediting agencies on an ongoing basis to remain current;
- conduct self assessments to determine the organization's accreditation readiness;
- develop corrective plans for areas needing improvement and follow-up until areas have improved;
- scan the marketplace for information on outcomes measurement tools including software;
- provide input to accrediting agencies' requests regarding standards development and outcomes measurement;
- identify new accreditation organizations and their requirements.

One new accreditation organization targeted to launch its accreditation program in the near future is the Council on Healthcare Provider Accreditation (CHPA). This Wayland, Massachusetts-based organization plans to develop accreditation standards that are customized for rehabilitation, assistive technology, and home medical equipment suppliers. The survey process will include customer survey programs, mandatory self-assessment, educational programs, mock surveys, consultation services, and special programs for organizations with multiple sites.

New players are certain to enter the marketplace. Current players will be continually changing in order to remain competitive. Providers will need to monitor the marketplace regularly for both new players and new requirements.

PAYER REQUIREMENTS

There are several factors affecting the reimbursement of speech-language pathology services. From a health care perspective, they include:

- the shifting from a fee-for-service to a capitated payment structure;
- change in economic incentives (i.e., a "do more" versus "do less" mindset);
- transformation from a largely nonprofit industry to a domination by for-profit systems of care;
- new organizational forms replacing the more traditional group and staff model health maintenance organizations;
- shifting from solo practices to large networks of care; and
- increase in Medicaid recipients and Medicare beneficiaries enrolled in managed care plans.

As a result of these shifts, SLPs are finding that their profit margins are shrinking while they are being demanded to do more. To ensure adequate payment, they are finding that payers are beginning to ask for outcomes data.

This section focuses on the Medicare and Medicaid programs, and managed care organizations. An overview of each payer is provided along with a discussion about its outcomes measurement requirements. Suggestions for meeting these requirements are provided.

The Medicare Program

Description of the Program: Key Facts

In 1965, Congress enacted two new programs of medical care as part of the Social Security Amendments. The first of these programs that provides basic protection against the costs of inpatient hospital and other institution-provided inpatient or home health care is "Part A Medicare." Officially, this program is called "Hospital Insurance Benefits for the Aged and Disabled."

The second of these programs covers the costs of physicians' services and a number of other items and services not covered under the basic program. It is called "Part B Medicare." Officially, this program is called "Supplementary Medical Insurance Benefits for the Aged and Disabled."

Both programs are known officially as "Health Insurance for the Aged and Disabled," the name of Title XVIII of the Social Security Act. The Medicare Program is administered by the HCFA of the U.S. Department of Health and Human Services and through its regional offices. Private health insurance organizations (i.e., fiscal intermediaries or carriers) contract with HCFA to process claims and to make Medicare decisions regarding covered services and reimbursement.

Outcomes Measurement Requirements

The following guidelines instruct Medicare providers in billing for outpatient speech-language pathology services (Medicare Intermediary Manual Part 3, Claims Process Section 3905, Medical Review Part B, Intermediary Outpatient Speech-Language Pathology Bills, June, 1991). These same guidelines are used by intermediaries to conduct focused medical review claims.

While the guidelines are for outpatient Part B claims, the same general principles apply to Part A claims and to any Medicare provider setting. The guidelines were developed by HCFA with input from ASHA.

3705.2 Assessment. Submit an initial assessment when it is reasonable and necessary for the SLP to determine if there is an expectation that either restorative services or establishment of a maintenance program will be appropriate. . . .

The assessment establishes the baseline data necessary for assessing expected rehabilitation potential, setting realistic goals, and measuring communication status at periodic intervals.

The initial assessment is a collection of data concerning the patient's functional limitations and identification of problems to be addressed in the treatment plan. The SLP must identify factors that may be contributing to or causing functional losses or limitations found. It is important that the patient's prior level of function is included (Hicks & Hartman, 1995).

3905.3 Plan of treatment. The plan of treatment must contain . . . functional goals and estimated rehabilitation potential.

A. *Functional Goals* must be written by the SLP to reflect the level of communicative independence the patient is *expected* to achieve outside of the therapeutic environment. The functional goals must reflect the final level the patient is expected to achieve, be realistic, and have a positive effect on the quality of the patient's everyday functions. . . .

Examples of functional communication goals in achieving optimum communication independence are the ability to:

- communicate basic physical needs and emotional status.
- communicate personal self-care needs.
- engage in social communicative interactions with immediate family or friends.
- carry out communicative interactions in the community.

Medicare requires SLPs to develop functional goals for their patients. Specifically, SLPs must justify that these goals can be realized and will have an impact on the patients' ability to function in daily activities.

3905.4 Progress reports. Document and report:

- the initial functional communication status of the patient at [your] provider setting;
- the present functional status of the patient for [the] reporting period;
- the patient's expected rehabilitation potential; and
- changes in the plan of treatment.

Where a valid expectation of improvement exists at the time services are initiated, or thereafter, the services are covered even though the expectation may not be realized. However, in such instances, they are covered only until no further significant practical improvement can be expected. Your progress reports must document a continued expectation that the patient's condition will continue to improve significantly in a reasonable and generally predictable period of time.

The SLP may choose how to demonstrate progress. However, the method chosen and the measures used generally remain the same for the duration of treatment.

Medicare reviewers focus primarily on progress reports when reviewing claims. Outcomes data, therefore, are necessary to justify that the services provided were reasonable and necessary.

The Medicare Outpatient Rehabilitation Services Form 700 (Plan of Care and Assessment; see Appendix 2–B) requires an initial assessment that includes: patient's prior functional level, functional losses that justify therapy now, and all pertinent functional deficits and clinical findings identified on the initial assessment.

The 700 Form also requires the you document the patient's functional level at the end of the billing period. According to Hicks and Hartman (1995), functional level should also include:

- End-of-month functional levels and progress in objective terminology.
- Include test results and measurements as appropriate.
- A comparison of results to those shown on the initial assessment.
- An indication of whether or not the goals have been met.

Medicare Outpatient Rehabilitation Services Form 701 (Updated Plan of Care and Patient Progress; see Appendix 2–C) requires an update of functional goals and a statement of functional level at the end of the billing period as compared to the previous month or initial assessment. Indicate the date when function can be consistently performed, when meaningful functional improvement is made, or when significant regression in function occurs.

According to Hicks and Hartman (1995), information in this section should also include:

- documented functional levels and progress in objective terminology.
- comparison of objective measures to those on the initial assessment.
- documented goals met and not met.
- justification of lack of progress by documenting medical complications that interfered with the patient meeting goals.
- documented changes in plan of treatment.

Not all fiscal intermediaries currently require the 700 and 701 forms, but they and other payers may do so in the future. HCFA is presently piloting the electronic transfer of these forms.

In summary, HCFA is increasing its scrutiny of speech-language pathology services. Proper documentation is critical to pass these focused reviews. Outcomes data must be included in the documentation to justify payment for services.

Medicaid Program

Description of Program: Key Facts

Medicaid is the largest program providing medical and health-related services to America's poorest people. This program became law in 1965 as a jointly funded cooperative venture between Federal and State governments to assist states in the provision of adequate medical care to eligible needy persons. Within broad national guidelines which the Federal government provides, each of the states:

- establishes its own eligibility standards;
- determines the type, amount, duration, and scope of services;
- sets the rate of payment of services; and
- administers its own program.

Increasingly, Medicaid has become a payer for speech-language services provided to children enrolled in public schools. The most significant trend in service delivery is the rapid growth in managed care enrollment within Medicaid. In 1994, almost a quarter of all Medicaid recipients were enrolled in managed care plans. One vehicle for the expansion of managed care is the 1115 waiver process, which allows states increased flexibility to research health care delivery alternatives while controlling program costs. Another vehicles is the section 1115(b) waiver authority, which permits states to implement managed care delivery systems within prescribed parameters.

Outcomes Measurement Requirements

Currently, reimbursement for speech-language services by the Medicaid program is not contingent upon outcomes data. However, as managed care plans continue to increase their Medicaid enrollments, outcomes data for speech-language services will become necessary.

For example, Arizona implemented its managed competition model for Medicaid recipients in 1982. It is the only state to run its Medicaid program entirely on the basis of managed care plans.

Under the terms of the plan, each patient is enrolled in a health plan that contracts with the state to deliver care to patients. A fixed capitation payment is provided regardless of the number or type of services provided. Providers are expected to control utilization and costs.

Another example, the Oregon Medicaid plan (1993) ranks health services based on factors that include medical effectiveness of a particular treatment and the cost and social value of the treatment. Individuals below the poverty line are covered by Medicaid and guaranteed a basic benefits package based on the prioritized list of health services.

Because the Medicaid program varies considerably from state to state, as well as within each state, you will need to contact your state agency to determine its specific outcomes measurement requirements.

Managed Care Organizations (MCOs)

Description of These Organizations:
Key Facts You Need To Know

Within 10 years, enrollment in managed care organizations has doubled. As of 1994, there were 572 health maintenance organizations (HMOs) representing 51 million persons, or approximately 21% of the population. Part of this growth can be attributed to the failed efforts to enact universal coverage (Davis & Schoen, 1996).

In managed care plans, the provider agrees to provide a defined set of services to a defined patient population. While different payment arrangements exist currently, the payer will increasingly agree to pay a predetermined payment per member per month (i.e., a capitated payment). The provider agrees to be accountable for a defined level of quality of care. The financial risk, then, shifts to the provider.

Managed care entities purport to improve efficiency and effectiveness of care, reduce costs, and maintain quality. Additionally, managed care expects to improve outcomes of care and reduce unnecessary use of expensive resources and duplication of services.

Outcomes Measurement Requirements

Outcomes research, finding out what works and what doesn't, is being conducted to varying degrees by HMOs nationwide. Foster and Higgins (1994) reported that 87% of HMOs conduct outcomes studies to identify problems pertaining to quality. Approximately 86% shared their outcomes data with providers. About 61% used their data to develop practice guidelines.

It is essential that SLPs contracting with managed care organizations collect outcomes data. These data are essential because the financial risk under the managed care contract can likely shift to the SLP. Specifically, SLPs will need to use both efficiency and effectiveness measures. Also, they will need measures that will provide clinical, functional, administrative, financial, and social outcomes data.

Because the patient has significant influence over the purchaser, it will be necessary for SLPs to collect patient satisfaction data. DeJong (1996) suggests that therapists' perceptions of what the patient needs or wants may not necessarily be consistent with what the patient expects.

Because managed care organizations are transforming the delivery of health care and more risks to the provider of care are involved, the importance of outcomes measurement cannot be overemphasized.

General Recommendations

In order to meet payer demands, it is important that your organization utilizes an information system that integrates financial, clinical, and human resource information. You must understand what it costs and how much staff power it took to obtain your results. Using an information system that is integrated will facilitate easy access to the information you need.

It is essential that you take the time to engage in educational experiences that will facilitate the development of your computer skills. You will need to have the ability to enter and access data quickly. Efficiency of data use will allow you to be responsive to both payers and consumers of your services.

Entities requesting your outcomes data will be increasingly concerned about its integrity. You will need to ensure that your data are reliable and accurate. One means by which you can accomplish this is to collect your data at the point of service (i.e., while you are providing a service, enter data into your information system). Hand-held, pen-based computers and bar coding are examples of technology that facilitate point of service data entry. You should investigate these technologies and stay abreast of emerging technologies.

Because managed care organizations are evaluating the effectiveness of health care providers, it is important that you begin to make performance comparisons within your organization and between similar organizations. This comparative data will allow you to identify gaps in performance. You can then target your focus on these gaps for improving performance. Additionally, in order to be competitive in the marketplace, you will need to know how your performance compares to your competition. A basic premise of competition is that providers of the highest quality and lowest cost services will gain the largest market share.

Increasingly, you will need to improve your performance (i.e., provide services that will result in the best outcome at the lowest cost) if you are to remain an active player with managed care organizations.

LEGISLATIVE AND REGULATORY REQUIREMENTS

An example of legislation and regulations that require outcomes measurement are: the Omnibus Budget Reconciliation Act of 1987 (OBRA), Public Law 100-203, and the Social Security Act, Part 484. An overview of these follows.

Omnibus Budget Reconciliation Act of 1987 (OBRA). This act represents major revisions to Medicare regulations. Section 9305 requires development of the Uniform Needs Assessment to evaluate the individual's functional capacity and health care needs to assist with functional incapacities. Specifically:

> OBRA requires residents in long-term care facilities to receive a comprehensive assessment initially and periodically, and after a significant change occurs in a resident's physical or mental status.

> OBRA provides a legal basis for providers and clinicians to attain and maintain the highest possible mental and physical functioning status of resident in nursing facilities.

> OBRA requires residents to receive care in a manner and environment that maintains or enhances high quality of life (Hicks & Hartman, 1995).

As a result of this legislation, SLPs providing services in long-term care facilities are finding that they must conduct functional assessments. Their outcome measures have focused on clinical and functional outcomes. Increasingly, they are also collecting client-centered outcomes data.

Social Security Act, Part 484, Subpart B: 483.20 Resident Assessment. This long-term care regulation requires the facility to conduct initially and periodically a comprehensive, accurate, standardized, reproducible assessment of each resident's functional capacity (pp. 8551–8624).

With the advent of the Resident Assessment Instrument and its Minimum Data Set (MDS) of core elements, nursing facilities may be able to monitor outcomes in a multidimensional way (American Health Care Association, 1990).

The Resident Assessment Instrument (RAI) is to provide "comprehensive, accurate, standardized, reproducible assessment of each resident's functional capacity." Additionally, a uniform minimum data set, MDS, forms the core of the required resident assessment instrument. The assessment is to be conducted or coordinated by a registered nurse with participation of appropriate health professionals, including SLPs. These assessments are conducted upon admission, after any significant change in mental and physical condition, and at least every year with a partial reassessment every quarter. Assessments are conducted on all residents, regardless of payer (Omnibus Budget and Reconciliation Act, 1987).

Communication represents one of the areas assessed by the MDS. This assessment includes the following domains: hearing, communication devices/techniques, modes of expression, making self understood, ability to understand others, and change in communication and hearing.

It is expected that as service delivery continues to change, new legislation and regulations will be introduced that will require outcomes measurement. In order to monitor proposed legislation, the Thomas Web site provides easy access to this information. You can obtain the full text or summaries by accessing the Web Page: http://thomas.loc.gov/.

Increasingly, states are becoming more active in sponsoring health care and education legislation. You will need to monitor regularly proposed legislation within your state.

CONCLUSION

Accrediting agencies, payers, and government entities are demanding that we justify the need for our services. Therefore, we can no longer wait to begin outcomes measurement and management activities.

We must also stay informed on a continual basis. Changes are rapid and significant. If we do not monitor the activities of accrediting bodies, payers, and government agencies, we may find that our profession is no longer a viable player in the current service delivery environment.

We must also become computer literate. Utilizing computer services such as the Internet is essential. It will allow us to more easily access the vital information we need to function effectively in today's fast-paced world. Hence, we must venture out on the World Wide Web.

In addition, we must begin to utilize integrated data systems that link clinical, cost, utilization, and patient satisfaction data, which will assist us in demonstrating the value of our services. Doing so will allow us to more effectively position our profession in the current environment, ensure that we get adequately reimbursed, ensure that persons who can benefit from our services have appropriate access to them, and ensure that we continuously improve the quality of our services.

Those providers who can meet the requirements detailed above in a timely manner will be best equipped to stay afloat in a dynamic service delivery system that depends on data for decision making.

REFERENCES

American Health Care Association (1990). *Resident assessment instrument (RAI) training manual and resource guide.* Washington, DC: Author.

American Speech-Language-Hearing Association (1996). *Desk reference* (vol. 1). Rockville, MD: Author.

Arizona Health Care Cost Containment System Overview (1993). The Arizona cost containment system: Arizona's health care program for the indigent. Phoenix, AZ: Author.

CARF. . . The Rehabilitation Accreditation Commission (formerly the Commission on Accreditation of Rehabilitation Facilities). (1996). Standards manual and interpretive guidelines for medical rehabilitation. Tucson, AZ: Author.

Davis, K., & Schoen, C. (1996). Health services research and the changing health care system. Commonwealth Fund Publication, New York, NY.

DeJong, G. (1996). Improved outcomes measures, patient-centered focus needed in geriatric rehab, conference finds. *Eli Rehab Report.* Vol. III, No. 6, 3608–3610.

Foster Higgins (1994). *Survey on outcomes management.* Princeton, NJ: Author.

Hicks, P., & Hartman, N. (1995). Medicare documentation manual. Outcomes Management Group. Columbus, OH.

Joint Commission on Accreditation of Healthcare Organizations. (1996). Comprehensive Accreditation Manual for Hospitals. Oakbrook, IL: Author.

Omnibus Budget and Reconciliation Act of 1987. Pub L. 100–203.

Oregon Department of Human Resources, Office of Medical Assistance Program (1993). The Oregon health plan. Salem, OR: Author.

Scalenghe, R. (1996). Joint Commission ramping up performance measure requirements for accreditation. *Eli Rehab Report.* Vol. III, No. 6, 3611–3612.

State University of New York at Buffalo, School of Medicine and Biomedical Sciences, Center for Functional Assessment Research (1993). *Uniform Data System for Medical Rehabilitation. Guide for the uniform data set for medical rehabilitation (Adult FIM),* Version 4.0. New York: State University of New York.

Wilkerson, D. (1996). CARF responding to rehab provider questions about outcomes measures. *Eli Rehab Report.* Vol. III, No. 8, 3654–3655.

Accrediting Organizations

American Speech-Language-Hearing Association (ASHA)
Professional Services Board (PSB) Accreditation
10801 Rockville Pike
Rockville, MD 20852
(301) 897-5700

CARF. . . The Rehabilitation Accreditation Commission, formerly
Commission on Accreditation of Rehabilitation Facilities
4891 East Grant Road
Tucson, AZ 85712
(520) 325-1044

Council on Healthcare Provider Accreditation (CHPA)
21 Cochituate Rd.
Wayland, MA 01778

Joint Commission on Accreditation of Healthcare Organizations (JCAHO)
One Renaissance Boulevard
Oakbrook Terrace, IL 60181
(708) 916-5909

HCFA 700 Form

DEPARTMENT OF HEALTH AND HUMAN SERVICES
HEALTH CARE FINANCING ADMINISTRATION

FORM APPROVED
OMB NO. 0938-0227

PLAN OF TREATMENT FOR OUTPATIENT REHABILITATION *(COMPLETE FOR INITIAL CLAIMS ONLY)*

1. PATIENT'S LAST NAME	FIRST NAME	M.I.	2. PROVIDER NO.	3. HICN

4. PROVIDER NAME	5. MEDICAL RECORD NO. *(Optional)*	6. ONSET DATE	7. SOC. DATE

8. TYPE: ☐ PT ☐ OT ☐ SLP ☐ CR ☐ RT ☐ PS ☐ SN ☐ SW

9. PRIMARY DIAGNOSIS *(Pertinent Medical D.X.)*	10. TREATMENT DIAGNOSIS	11. VISITS FROM SOC.

12. PLAN OF TREATMENT FUNCTIONAL GOALS

GOALS *(Short Term)*

OUTCOME *(Long Term)*

PLAN

13. SIGNATURE *(professional establishing POC including prof. designation)*

14. FREQ/DURATION *(e.g., 3/Wk x 4 Wk.)*

I CERTIFY THE NEED FOR THESE SERVICES FURNISHED UNDER THIS PLAN OF TREATMENT AND WHILE UNDER MY CARE   ☐ N/A

15. PHYSICIAN SIGNATURE

16. DATE

17. CERTIFICATION   ☐ N/A
FROM   THROUGH

18. ON FILE *(Print/type physician's name)*
☐

20. INITIAL ASSESSMENT *(History, medical complications, level of function at start of care. Reason for referral)*

19. PRIOR HOSPITIALIZATION   ☐ N/A
FROM   TO

21. FUNCTIONAL LEVEL *(End of billing period)* PROGRESS REPORT   ☐ CONTINUE SERVICES *OR* ☐ DC SERVICES

22. SERVICE DATES
FROM   THROUGH

FORM HCFA-700 (11-91)

*U.S. Government Printing Office: 1993 — 771-861

INSTRUCTIONS FOR COMPLETION OF FORM HCFA-700
(Enter dates as 6 digits month, day, year)

1. **Patient's Name** - Enter the patient's last name, first name and middle initial as shown on the health insurance Medicare card.

2. **Provider Number** - Enter the number issued by Medicare to the billing provider *(i.e., 00-7000)*.

3. **HICN** - Enter the patient's health insurance number as shown on the health insurance Medicare card, certification award, utilization notice, temporary eligibility notice, or as reported by SSO.

4. **Provider Name** - Enter the name of the Medicare billing provider.

5. **Medical Record No.** - *(optional)* Enter the patient's medical/clinical record number used by the billing provider.

6. **Onset Date** - Enter the date of onset for the patient's primary medical diagnosis, if it is a new diagnosis, or the date of the most recent exacerbation of a previous diagnosis. If the exact date is not known enter 01 for the day *(i.e., 120191)*. The date matches occurrence code 11 on the UB-82.

7. **SOC** *(start of care)* **Date** - Enter the date services began at the billing provider (the date of the first Medicare billable visit which **remains the same on subsequent claims** until discharge or denial corresponds to occurence code 35 for PT, 44 for OT, 45 for SLP and 46 for CR on the UB-82).

8. **Type** - Check the type therapy billed i.e., physical therapy (PT), occupational therapy (OT), speech-language pathology (SLP), cardiac rehabilitation (CR), respiratory therapy (RT), psychological services (PS), skilled nursing services (SN), or social services (SW).

9. **Primary Diagnosis** - Enter the pertinent written medical diagnosis resulting in the therapy disorder and relating to 50% or more of effort in the plan of treatment.

10. **Treatment Diagnosis** - Enter the written treatment diagnosis for which services are rendered. For example, for PT the primary medical diagnosis might be Degeneration of Cervical Intervertebral Disc while the PT treatment DX might be Frozen R Shoulder or, for SLP, while CVA might be the primary medical DX, the treatment DX might be Aphasia. If the same as the primary DX enter SAME.

11. **Visits From Start of Care** - Enter the **cumulative total** visits *(sessions)* completed since services were started at the billing provider for the diagnosis treated, through the last visit on this bill. *(Corresponds to UB-82 value code 50 for PT, 51 for OT, 52 for SLP, or 53 for cardiac rehab on the UB-82)*.

12. **Plan of Treatment/Functional Goals** - Enter brief current plan of treatment goals for the patient for this billing period. Enter the major short-term goals to reach overall long-term outcome. Enter the major plan of treatment to reach stated goals and outcome. Estimate time-frames to reach goals, when possible.

13. **Signature** - Enter the signature *(or name)* and the professional designation of the professional establishing the plan of treatment.

14. **Frequency/Duration** - Enter the current frequency and duration of your treatment, e.g., 3 times per week for 4 weeks is entered 3/Wk x 4Wk.

15. **Physician's Signature** - If the form HCFA-700 is used for certification, the physician enters his/her signature. **If certification is required and the form is not being used for certification, check on ON FILE box in item 18.** If the certification is not required for the type service rendered, check the N/A box.

16. **Date** - Enter the date of the physician's signature only if the form is used for certification.

17. **Certification** - Enter the inclusive dates of the certification, **even if the ON FILE box is checked in item 18.** Check the N/A box if certification is not required.

18. **ON FILE** (Means certification signature and date) - Enter the **typed/printed name of the physician** who certified the plan of treatment that is on file at the billing provider. If certification is not required for the type of service checked in item 8, type/print the name of the physician who referred or ordered the service, **but do not check the ON FILE box.**

19. **Prior Hospitalization** - Enter the inclusive dates of recent hospitalization *(1st to DC day)* **pertinent** to the patient's current plan of treatment. Enter N/A if the hospital stay does not relate to the rehabilitation being rendered.

20. **Initial Assessment** - Enter **only current relevant history** from records or patient interview. Enter the major functional limitations stated, if possible, in objective measurable terms. Include only relevant surgical procedures, prior hospitalization and/or therapy for the same condition. Include only pertinent baseline tests and measurements from which to judge future progress or lack of progress.

21. **Functional Level** (end of billing period) - Enter the pertinent progress made and functional levels obtained at the end of the billing period compared to levels shown on initial assessment. Use objective terminology. Date progress when function can be consistently performed. When only a few visits have been made, enter a note indicating the training/treatment rendered and the patient's response if there is no change in function.

22. **Service Dates** - Enter the from and through dates which represent this billing period *(should be monthly)*. Match the From and Through dates in field 22 on the UB-82. DO NOT use 00 in the date. Example: 01 08 91 for January 8, 1991.

Public reporting burden for this collection of information is estimated to average 15 minutes per response, including time for reviewing instructions, searching existing data sources, gathering and maintaining data needed, and completing and reviewing the collection of information. Send comments regarding this burden estimate or any other aspect of this collection of information, including suggestions for reducing the burden, to HCFA, Office of Financial Management, P.O. Box 26684, Baltimore, MD 21207; and to the Office of Management and Budget, Paperwork Reduction Project (0938-0227), Washington, D.C. 20503.

HCFA 701 Form

DEPARTMENT OF HEALTH AND HUMAN SERVICES
HEALTH CARE FINANCING ADMINISTRATION

FORM APPROVED
OMB NO. 0938-0227

UPDATED PLAN OF PROGRESS FOR OUTPATIENT REHABILITATION
(Complete for Interim to Discharge Claims. Photocopy of HCFA-700 or 701 is required)

1. PATIENT'S LAST NAME	FIRST NAME	M.I.	2. PROVIDER NO.	3. HICN

4. PROVIDER NAME	5. MEDICAL RECORD NO. *(Optional)*	6. ONSET DATE	7. SOC. DATE

8. TYPE:
☐ PT ☐ OT ☐ SLP ☐ CR
☐ RT ☐ PS ☐ SN ☐ SW

9. PRIMARY DIAGNOSIS *(Pertinent Medical D.X.)*

10. TREATMENT DIAGNOSIS

11. VISITS FROM SOC.

12. FREQ/DURATION *(e.g., 3/Wk x 4 Wk.)*

13. CURRENT PLAN UPDATE, FUNCTIONAL GOALS *(Specify changes to goals and plan)*

GOALS *(Short Term)*

PLAN

OUTCOME *(Long Term)*

I HAVE REVIEWED THIS PLAN OF TREATMENT AND RECERTIFY A CONTINUING NEED FOR SERVICES. ☐ N/A ☐ DC

14. RECERTIFICATION
FROM   THROUGH   ☐ N/A

15. PHYSICIAN'S SIGNATURE

16. DATE

17. ON FILE *(Print/type physician's name)*
☐

18. REASON(S) FOR CONTINUING TREATMENT THIS BILLING PERIOD *(Clarify goals and necessity for continued skilled care)*

19. SIGNATURE *(or name of professional, including prof. designation)*

20. DATE

21.
☐ CONTINUE SERVICES *OR* ☐ DC SERVICES

22. FUNCTIONAL LEVEL *(at end of billing period - Relate your documentation to functional outcomes and list problems still present)*

23. SERVICE DATES
FROM   THROUGH

FORM HCFA-701 (11-91)

☆ U.S. GOVERNMENT PRINTING OFFICE: 1993 771-862

INSTRUCTIONS FOR COMPLETION OF FORM HCFA-701
(Enter dates as 6 digits month, day, year)

1. **Patient's Name** - Enter the patient's last name, first name and middle initial as shown on the health insurance Medicare card.

2. **Provider Number** - Enter the number issued by Medicare to the billing provider *(i.e., 00-7000)*.

3. **HICN** - Enter the patient's health insurance number as shown on the health insurance Medicare card, certification award, utilization notice, temporary eligibility notice, or as reported by SSO.

4. **Provider Name** - Enter the name of the Medicare billing provider.

5. **Medical Record No.** - *(optional)* Enter the patient's medical/clinical record number used by the billing provider. *(This is an item which you may enter for your own records)*

6. **Onset Date** - Enter the date of onset for the patient's primary medical diagnosis, if it is a new diagnosis, or the date of the most recent exacerbation of a previous diagnosis. If the exact date is not known enter 01 for the day *(i.e., 120191)*. The date matches occurrence code 11 on the UB-82.

7. **SOC** *(start of care)* **Date** - Enter the date services began at the billing provider *(the date of the first Medicare billable visit which **remains the same on subsequent claims** until discharge or denial corresponds to occurrence code 35 for PT, 44 for OT, 45 for SLP and 46 for CR on the UB-82)*.

8. **Type** - Check the type therapy billed i.e., physical therapy (PT), occupational therapy (OT), speech-language pathology (SLP), cardiac rehabilitation (CR), respiratory therapy (RT), psychological services (PS), skilled nursing services (SN), or social services (SW).

9. **Primary Diagnosis** - Enter the pertinent written medical diagnosis resulting in the therapy disorder and relating to 50% or more of effort in the plan of treatment.

10. **Treatment Diagnosis** - Enter the written treatment diagnosis for which services are rendered. For example, for PT the primary medical diagnosis might be Degeneration of Cervical Intervertebral Disc while the PT treatment DX might be Frozen R Shoulder or, for SLP, while CVA might be the primary medical DX, the treatment DX might be Aphasia. If the same as the primary DX enter SAME.

11. **Visits From Start of Care** - Enter the **cumulative total** visits *(sessions)* completed since services were started at the billing provider for the diagnosis treated, through the last visit on this bill. *(Corresponds to UB-82, value code 50 for PT, 51 for OT, 52 for SLP, or 53 for cardiac rehab)*.

12. **Current Frequency/Duration** - Enter the current frequency and duration on treatment, e.g., 3 times per week for 4 weeks is entered 3/Wk x 4Wk.

13. **Current Plan Update, Functional Goals** - Enter the current plan of treatment goals for the patient for this billing period. *(If the same as shown on the HCFA-700 or previous 701 enter "same")*. Enter the short-term goals to reach overall long-term outcome. Justify intensity if appropriate. Estimate time-frames to meet goals, when possible.

14. **Recertification** - Enter the inclusive dates when recertification is required, **even if the ON FILE box is checked in item 17.** Check the N/A box if recertification is not required for the type of service rendered.

15. **Physician's Signature** - If the form HCFA-701 is used for recertification, the physician enters his/her signature. If recertification is not required for the type of service rendered, check N/A box. **If the form HCFA-701 is not being used for recertification, check the ON FILE box - item 17.** If discharge is ordered, check DC box.

16. **Date** - Enter the date of the physician's signature only if the form is used for recertification.

17. **On File** *(means certification signature and date)* - Enter the **typed/printed name of the physician** who recertified the plan of treatment that is on file at the billing provider. If recertification is not required for the type of services checked in item 8, type/print the name of the physician who referred or ordered the service, **but do not check the ON FILE box.**

18. **Reason(s) For Continuing Treatment This Billing Period** - Enter the **major reason(s)** why the patient needs to continue skilled rehabilitation **for this billing period** *(e.g., briefly state the patient's need for specific functional improvement, skilled training, reduction in complication or improvement in safety and how long you believe this will take, if possible, or state your reasons for recommending discontinuance)*. Complete by the rehab specialist prior to physician' recertification.

19. **Signature** - Enter the signature *(or name)* and the professional designation of the individual justifying or recommending need for care *(or discontinuance)* for this billing period.

20. **Date** - Enter the date of the rehabilitation professional's signature.

21. Check the box if services are continuing or discontinuing at end of this billing period.

22. **Functional Level** *(end of billing period)* - Enter the pertinent progress made through the end of this billing period. Use objective terminology. Compare progress made to that shown on the previous HCFA-701, item 22, or the HCFA-700, items 20 and 21. Date progress when function can be consistently performed or when meaningful functional improvement is made or when signification regression in function occurs. Your intermediary reviews this progress compared to that on the prior HCFA-701 or 700 to determine coverage for this billing period. Send a photocopy of the form covering the previous billing period.

23. **Service Dates** - Enter the from and through dates which represent this billing period *(should be monthly)*. Match the From and Through dates in field 22 on the UB-82. DO NOT use 00 in the date. Example: 01 08 91 for January 8, 1991.

Public reporting burden for this collection of information is estimated to average 15 minutes per response, including time for reviewing instructions, searching existing data sources, gathering and maintaining data needed, and completing and reviewing the collection of information. Send comments regarding this burden estimate or any other aspect of this collection of information, including suggestions for reducing the burden, to HCFA, Office of Financial Management, P.O. Box 26684, Baltimore, MD 21207; and to the Office of Management and Budget, Paperwork Reduction Project (0938-0227), Washington, D.C. 20503.

CHAPTER 3

Measuring Modality-Specific Behaviors, Functional Abilities, and Quality of Life

CAROL M. FRATTALI

INTRODUCTION

A clinician, when applying a clinical intervention, expects an effect. The effect is either discovery, in the case of assessment; or improvement, in the case of treatment. Discovery involves differential diagnosis and identification of specific strengths and weaknesses; improvement involves positive change in modality-bound behaviors and, by extension, functional ability and quality of life. The focus of this chapter is on measures of improvement (or change, if you consider both positive and adverse outcomes), designed to capture the effects of our clinical interventions.

Clinical intervention begins with expectations or desired outcomes. Cure, of course, is the ideal. But, in many cases, expectations must be tempered to ones of symptom reduction, optimization of function, and attainment of quality of life, even though problems may persist. Our expectations for improvements, thus, are rooted in diagnosis and prognosis. Consequently, clinicians must also be judges. Given a clinical picture, what expectations are the most realistic for the client? And, along a clinical timeline, when should our attempts at cure shift to care that enhances the ability to live with residual deficits?

Using the World Health Organization (WHO) International Classification of Impairments, Disabilities, and Handicaps (WHO, 1980), I frame the discussion that follows into three classes of desired outcomes for our clients: *modality-specific behaviors, functional abilities,* and *quality of life.* Each class is defined along a continuum of outcomes, and their interrelationships discussed before various measures within each class are characterized. Measurement selection considerations are detailed in order to maximize the ability to capture targeted outcomes in a reliable, valid, and practical way.

DESIRED OUTCOMES: A CURE-CARE CONUNDRUM?

Wertz (1984) defines treatment as that which improves whatever is being treated. But given the range of circumstances of those whom we treat, we may or may not improve what we set out to improve. Treatment still does not come with a guarantee. Perhaps the key to improvement is found in how we define "improvement." If we set out to *cure* clients, we often will fail. But, depending on the client's circumstances, if we set out to *optimize performance of daily life activities,* or *enhance quality of life,* we may be on to something that is more meaningful to clients, more reimbursable to payers, and more feasible to clinicians. We would be naive to think that we could, in all cases, cure communication disorders and related disorders of swallowing and cognition. But even more egregious are blinded attempts to try and a refusal to continually ask the question, "Are our treatments making a difference?" Thus, the need to know becomes the basis of ethical practice.

Wertz (1984) emphasizes the need to determine whether our treatment is treatment; "that we have something to do for [communication and related] disorders . . . and that that something works" (p. 65). Wertz continues,

> Some—usually speech and language clinicians—tell me what we do is efficacious. Others—usually physicians and biostatisticians—tell me there is no unassailable evidence that treatment works. I can agree with both. . . . Those I cannot agree with are the ones who suggest we should stop asking the question. The test of repair is whether the broken gets fixed. We ask this of our mechanics, and our patients ask it of us. And, we have some answers for the treatment of aphasia. But, we have little data to back the need for our deeds with other . . . disorders. [p. 65]

Treatment is still treatment even if it does not cure. Once we move beyond the notion of cure, new avenues of care open. I learned this early on from a client—a man with severe verbal apraxia of 2 years duration. During three-times-a-week therapy on a clinical path aimed at cure, I subjected him to persistent demands to "tell me." "Tell me today's date." "Tell me what you did over the weekend." The verbal struggles were all too predictable and painful. Until one day—instead of verbalizing the date, he smiled, reached into his pocket, retrieved a wallet, pulled out a calendar, pointed to the date and said, "Why not?" He then drew a picture of a pond with a man sitting next to a small boy, both holding fishing poles. Without spoken words, the client communicated that he went fishing with his grandson over the weekend. What he was demonstrating to me was his ability to compensate for his residual deficits.

I agree with Wertz (1984). There is a part of clinical management that we have largely ignored. Speaking about treatment for aphasia, Wertz says,

> We tend to treat the language deficit, and when improvement in language slows or stops, we consider terminating treatment or moving the patient to a maintenance group. Perhaps we owe our patients more than just an attempt to improve their lan-

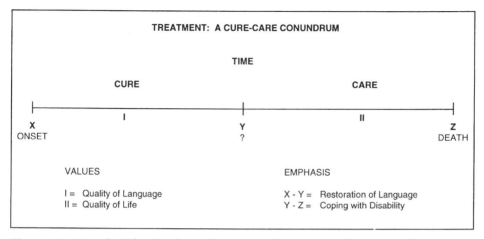

Figure 3–1. How the Value Emphasized in Aphasia Therapy May Change over Time

SOURCE: Wertz, R. T. (1984). Language disorders in adults: State of the clinical art. In A. L. Holland (Ed.), *Language disorders in adults* (pp. 1–78). San Diego, CA: College-Hill. Used by permission.

guage skills. Perhaps we need to assist them in coping with the language deficit that remains after direct language therapy has done what it can. [p. 60]

Wertz's (1984) Cure-Care Conundrum, illustrated as Figure 3–1, implies that two values may be emphasized in client management. At one point, usually early post-onset, we value the quality of language, and seek its restoration. But at another point along the time continuum, our value may change because improvement in the client's language slows or stops. We change our value to the quality of the client's life and emphasize coping with the language deficit that remains. We seek ways for clients to live the best they can with their residual deficits. Wertz believes we do a lot of the former (attempts to restore specific skills); he is not certain we do much of the latter (assist in coping with disability).

Little has changed in the years since Wertz (1984) wrote these words. But clinicians today are becoming more receptive to treatment that emphasizes care, not cure. Our discussion, then, proceeds to the outcomes of specific improvements in modality-bound behaviors (e.g., speech, language, voice, fluency, cognition, or swallowing), as well as outcomes of functional abilities and quality of life in the presence of residual deficits.

INTERRELATIONSHIPS AMONG MODALITY-SPECIFIC BEHAVIORS, FUNCTIONAL STATUS, AND QUALITY OF LIFE

Desired client outcomes and their measurement are easily understood if we consider the consequences of disease, disorder, or injury. To illustrate, I use the WHO's conceptual framework (1980). This framework suggests that measurement of outcomes can occur along a continuum of:

- Impairments: Abnormalities of structure of function at the organ level
- Disabilities: Functional consequences of impairment affecting performance of daily tasks
- Handicaps: Social, economic, or environmental disadvantages resulting from an impairment or disability

The WHO framework (1980) would, for example, represent the consequences of stroke on a continuum of aphasia and dysphagia (impairments), functional communication and eating difficulties manifested in daily life activities (disabilities), and joblessness, feelings of low self-worth, and social isolation (handicaps). Another example is found in the consequences of mental retardation on a continuum of delayed speech and language (impairments), functional communication problems (disability), and inability to learn or develop friendships (handicaps). When the framework is applied to measurement, impairment-level testing would include assessment of auditory comprehension, reading comprehension, verbal expression, speech intelligibility, fluency, voice production, and so forth. Impairment in these areas may lead to, but are not the same as, communication disabilities.

Communication disabilities arising from impairments in auditory or reading comprehension would, for example, include difficulty understanding a telephone message, difficulty engaging in one-on-one or group conversations, and difficulty following a medical prescription or a homework assignment. Thus, measurement shifts to evaluating the *functional* consequences of the impairment, manifested in the performance of daily life activities. In turn, disabilities resulting from impairments can cause handicaps, including, for example, the inability to hold a job that requires understanding conversations or written reports, and the psychosocial limitations associated with feelings of low self-worth. Measurement, then, shifts to evaluating the parameters of handicap and aspects of quality of life, usually from the perspective of the client or his or her family.

Once we conceptualize client outcomes using the WHO typology (1980), we can conclude that:

- Traditional clinical tests and procedures are used for evaluating specific speech, language, voice, fluency, cognitive, or swallowing disorders, focusing on the level of impairment. Thus, they are capable of capturing *modality-specific behaviors.*
- Functional assessment measures are designed to evaluate communication disabilities, exhibited in the performance of everyday activities. They can determine *functional abilities.*
- Measures of handicap include handicap inventories, quality-of-life scales, and well-being measures. These measures, usually designed as self-administered questionnaires or interviews, are used to assess social, economic, and environmental disadvantages, and, thus, the client's or family's perceptions about *quality of life.*

Table 3–1 illustrates this conceptualization and identifies the three classes of outcome measures identified above. Considered together, measures of impairment, disability, and handicap yield a total picture of the client. One class of measurement, therefore, can never replace another. Each class measures a different but related consequential phenomenon.

It seems reasonable, then, that based on the consequences of disease, disorder, or

Table 3–1   World Health Organization Classifications

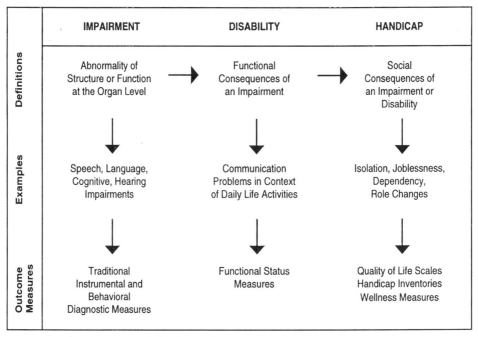

SOURCE: WHO (1980). *International classification of impairments, disabilities & handicaps.* Geneva: Author. Published in Frattali et al. (1995). ASHA Functional Assessment of Communication Skills for Adults. Rockville, MD: American Speech-Language-Hearing Association. Reprinted with permission.

injury, we can draw a straight line across the outcomes of modality-specific behaviors, functional status, and quality of life. One seems to lead to the next. And, the greater the severity of one, the greater the severity of the next. This is not necessarily true. A deficit in one area does not assume a deficit, either in occurrence or degree, in another area. A one-to-one relationship often does not exist. In fact, inverse relationships have been described.

Several writers have documented that an assessment of impairment does not coincide with an assessment of disability or handicap (Sarno, 1965, 1969; Aten, 1986; Murray et al., 1984). Sarno believes the ability to communicate, despite the presence of impairment, is bound by many contributory factors. She uses an example of the highly educated individual with a record of achievement whose communication needs differ from the individual with limited education and vocational goals. These two individuals, if similar speech impairments were acquired, would likely exhibit differing degrees of disability and/or handicap, particularly on the job. Another example is found for two individuals with severe verbal expressive impairment. One may experience only mild disability or no disability at all with adept use of an augmentative and alternative communication (AAC) system. The other may be severely disabled without access to an AAC system, or the inability to use the system effectively. According to Sarno (1965):

> . . . the impact of a verbal impairment on interpersonal interactions, on the use of verbal activities for leisure (e.g., watching TV), on the ability to resume employment, on the overall effect on the quality of life, and on the patient's ability to compensate and/or circumvent the deficits, all play a part in the patient's effectiveness as a communicator.

[p. 77]

From the vantage of aphasia, Aten (1986) states,

> Speaking fluently is not necessarily communicative, as patients with Wernicke's aphasia so vividly demonstrate. Conversely, the essentially mute patient, labeled mixed or Broca's type, may communicate a great deal in his or her animated, head nodding, nonlinguistic way. [p. 266]

In a study to investigate the relationship between language and functional communication skills, Murray and colleagues (1984) tested the hypothesis that clients with Alzheimer's disease appear to have more communicative competence than they actually do, given their ability to talk fluently until the later stages of the disease; and that clients with aphasia appear to have less communicative competence than they actually do, given their impaired language abilities. They administered the *Communicative Abilities in Daily Living* (*CADL;* Holland, 1980) to assess functional communication skills, and the *Porch Index of Communicative Ability* (*PICA;* Porch, 1971) to assess language and communication skills of 10 subjects with aphasia and 10 subjects with dementia. Findings showed that the dementia group scored significantly better than did the aphasia group on the PICA, and the aphasia group scored significantly better than did the dementia group on the CADL, thus confirming the hypothesized inverse relationship between communication and language skills.

Similar to disability, but to an even greater degree, handicap is highly individualized. It brings into play many factors, including societal attitudes, environmental barriers, the client's psychosocial traits, family and community supports, premorbid lifestyle, education, age, gender, vocation, avocations, and cultural and ethnic backgrounds. Quality of life, therefore, is filtered largely by human judgment and dependent on perceptions, attitudes, and social mores. Consequently, a handicap cannot be presumed in the presence of an impairment or disability.

Interrelationships among the concepts of impairment, disability, and handicap have been discussed at length by the WHO (1980). Similar interrelationships and their complexities are identified by Nagi (1965) and Wilson and Cleary (1995), using their respective conceptual frameworks of outcomes (see Chapter 1 for descriptions of these frameworks). All discount the theory of a simple linear progression, and agree that situations can be more complex. For example, a handicap may result from impairment without the mediation of disability. Consider the laryngectomized individual who uses esophageal speech. This person may be able to communicate well in everyday life activities, but may be socially stigmatized by the esophageal sound of the voice. This same person may have an impairment that leads to neither disability nor handicap as a result of a supportive and educated social and occupational network.

A corollary to these consequential patterns is the striking disparities in the degree to which the various elements of the sequence can depart from their norms. As described above, we cannot assume a one-to-one relationship between any two elements.

Further complexity is introduced by other situations. Certain impairments can conceal other abilities. For example, an impairment of language can conceal intelligence, thus creating a disability or handicap. There can also be a degree of influence in a reverse direction. Consider the individual with cognitive impairments resulting from dementia who, as a result of the handicapping condition of social isolation, becomes even more confused and disoriented, thus exacerbating the impairments.

The value of presenting the elements in a linear progression, however, is found in its portrayal of a problem-solving sequence. In other words, intervention at the level of one element has the potential to lessen the severity or prevent the occurrence of succeeding elements. Batavia (1992) tells us that with appropriate rehabilitative interventions, an impairment does not necessarily result in a disability. Similarly, with appropriate social and environmental interventions, a disability does not necessarily result in a handicap. Thus, the focus of rehabilitation and social/environmental interventions is on prevention.

Once we understand these interrelationships, we can select appropriate measures to assess modality-specific behaviors, functional status, or quality of life. We do, however, need to learn much more about how different types of outcome measures interrelate by virtue of their conceptual designs, psychometric properties, and results yielded. For example, we do not yet know how the numbers produced by one instrument (even within the same class of measurement) compare to those of other instruments. Although three classes of measures are identified, many do not fit neatly into categories. Some measures of disability may, in fact, measure impairment. Other measures of disability may be considered measures of handicap. Some measures of handicap are functional status questionnaires. And so the story goes. The rule here is to know precisely what your measures measure, and to what degrees of sensitivity and confidence they capture change.

MEASURING MODALITY-SPECIFIC BEHAVIORS

Outcomes measurement usually begins with identification of specific impairments. Impairment, according to the WHO (1980), represents exteriorization of a pathological state. If the pathological state is cerebral vascular disease resulting in stroke, impairments could include aphasia and dysphagia. If the state is dementia or traumatic brain injury, the impairment could be cognitive disturbances. If it is laryngeal cancer necessitating laryngectomy, aphonia would result. If it is mental retardation, delayed speech and language could be impaired. One can generate many examples.

Inherent in the measurement of impairment is differential diagnosis and identification of specific strengths and weaknesses. We, as clinicians, are skilled at this. The vast majority of our assessment instruments and procedures measures at the level of impairment. Included in this category are our traditional instrumental and behavioral diagnostic tests and procedures that assess distinct anatomical structures, physiological functions, and behavioral processes of speech, language, voice, fluency, cognition, and swallowing.

Available tests and procedures abound. In recent years, technological advances have added to our assessment batteries, including vocal tract visualization and imaging (e.g., flexible fiberoptic nasendoscopy, stroboscopy), instrumental diagnostic procedures for swallowing (e.g., fiberoptic endoscopic examination of swallowing [FEES], electromyography, ultrasonography), and evaluation for tracheoesophageal fistulization/puncture.

Purposes

The purposes of clinical tests of impairments are to determine differential diagnosis, prognosis, and focus for treatment, if treatment is warranted. These tests also can provide information about the client's capability, but not ability, to communicate. Individuals may be capable of communication but, in fact, may not communicate. This distinction is important when we discuss the purposes of functional measures. Traditional clinical tests, according to Sarno (1965), are designed to discover whatever residuals a client may have in each modality. Thus, she believes they are more often a measure of potential than actual use.

Differentiating Features

Impairment-level tests are modality bound. That is, they are designed exclusively to assess separate behavioral processes (e.g., speech, language, voice) that, considered together, constitute the realm of human communication and related areas such as swallowing. A range of behaviors within each modality (e.g., aspects of auditory comprehension and verbal expression for the modality of language) usually is measured by each instrument. Tests of acquired language dysfunction in adults, for example, could measure naming, word fluency, repetition, grammar, content, proverb interpretation, spontaneous speech, auditory comprehension, auditory retention, and so forth. Examples include the *Boston Diagnostic Aphasia Examination* (Goodglass & Kaplan, 1972), *The Minnesota Test for Differential Diagnosis of Aphasia* (Schuell, 1965), the *Porch Index of Communicative Ability* (Porch, 1973), and the *Western Aphasia Battery* (Kertesz, 1982). Tests of written language could include copying, writing words from dictation, writing sentences, spelling, syntax, and legibility. Tests of speech could assess intelligibility, rate, prosody, and fluency.

Separate behaviors within a particular modality can also be assessed by a single test. Examples are found in the area of childhood language assessment, with tests designed to assess specific behaviors involving syntax, semantics, morphology, phonology, and pragmatics. They include the *Peabody Picture Vocabulary Test* (Dunn & Dunn, 1981), *Expressive One-Word Picture Vocabulary Test—Revised* (Gardner, 1990), Mean Length of Utterance, *Developmental Sentence Scoring* (Lee, 1974), and the *Northwestern Syntax Screening Test* (Lee, 1971).

Many tests of impairment are standardized and require administration by skilled speech-language pathologists. Because of their objectivity and psychometric properties, they also are used typically for purposes of controlled clinical studies. Thus, we currently know more about the effects of our interventions on impairment-level phenomena than we do about their effects on functional abilities or quality of life.

The intention here is not to detail the characteristics of impairment measures. We are sufficiently familiar with them. Rather, the emphasis is to detail less well known and formative measures, those of disability and handicap, and their differential features.

MEASURING FUNCTIONAL ABILITIES

If we move along the WHO continuum, we know that a disability can result from an impairment. A disability describes the functional consequences of an impairment, exhibited in the performance of daily life activities. Thus, specific impairments of speech, language, voice, fluency, and cognition can lead to communication disabilities. Similarly, impairments in swallowing can lead to a disability that can interfere with adequate intake and nutrition.

Purposes

Functional measures assess a person's communication abilities in the presence of specific impairments. The ability to receive and convey messages in an individual's natural environments, *regardless of the mode of communication,* is the focus. Functional abilities are determined in the context of daily life activities. These activities include, for example, using the telephone; listening to television/radio; following homework assignments, prescriptions, and recipes; engaging in one-on-one or group conversations; understanding environmental signs; telling time.

Functional measures typically assess performance, not potential. That is, they are designed to capture the client's actual communication rather than the capability to communicate in targeted situations. Thus, most functional communication measures are based on direct observations.

For children, functional communication assessment measures two components: the child's current state of communication development (e.g., comprehension, extant skills), and the child's state of functional communication in various environments and contexts (e.g., at home, at school, with partners, communication opportunities) (Romski & Sevcik, 1996). Damico, Smith, and Augustine (1996) believe that functional assessment of children should be based on authentic observation with one question in mind: "How successful is this [child] as a communicator in the contexts and modalities of interest?" This question is based on how well the child functions on three criteria: the *effectiveness* of meaning transmission, the *fluency* of meaning transmission, and the *appropriateness* of meaning transmission. Thus, the approach transcends the need to divide language proficiency into a variety of skills, modules, or components at the time of assessment.

Clinicians use functional measures primarily for treatment planning aimed at communication in the client's natural environments, to facilitate interdisciplinary team communication, and to document functional gains. This class of measurement, however, has other purposes. Payers and regulators use functional measurement data to determine levels of independence (and thus, to make fiscal decisions about care). They, indeed, are popular among these groups because they are easy to interpret and quantitative. I am reminded of the words of a payer who addressed an audience of rehabilitation providers:

> I'm paying you to maximize the patient's independence. I want a quantitative measure of a qualitative product [i.e., rehabilitation]. I want to know how many points on a functional scale I can get for the money. If another provider can give me more points on the scale after the same treatment time, I'll buy from them. I'm a buyer. I want to get more for my money. [Adamzyk, 1991]

Thus, data yielded from functional measures are being used to select providers, set payment rates, determine eligibility for service, determine treatment cut-offs, and judge the quality of care.

What Is Functional?

Elman and Bernstein-Ellis (1995) pose the question, "What is functional?" They believe it has become virtually impossible to write a treatment plan or submit a health insurance claim without using the word *functional*. A speech-language pathologist must identify functional goals, use functional tasks, and show functional gains, or reimbursement for treatment may be denied. Their fear, however, is that the definition of *functional* has become synonymous with *basic skills*. Thus, the limited definition can, in turn, impose limits on treatment.

Functional *is* basic, some would argue. Yet, others would argue, what is functional for one may not be functional for another. The ability to communicate basic needs and engage in social communication will not, for example, be enough for the radio announcer whose everyday life activities require quick synthesis of information and the ability to transmit information with verbal precision. Thus, *functional* is individually defined, depending on life situations and roles. Nevertheless, functional measures limited to basic skills were not designed so without justification. Often, the intention is that these measures be used with the majority of individuals, regardless of age (within specified age ranges), gender, race/ethnicity, socioeconomic status, and educational/vocational status. The more individualized the test items to cover a wider range of possible skills, the greater the risk of measurement bias, and the more the validity of the measure and scores yielded are threatened. Regardless of differing opinions, any functional measure, whether basic or more comprehensive, should state explicitly what it is intended to measure, and what it does not measure (i.e., its limitations) to prevent either generalizations or undue criticism.

The issues surrounding school or work performance or social reintegration may, indeed, escape detection on a functional measure. Functional ability is not absolute, but relative to the client's expectations, priorities, goals, social supports, and other factors. These considerations lend credence to the notion of assessment with a set of measures capable of capturing a continuum of effects stemming from a clinical condition. For example, the results of a quality-of-life assessment can potentially justify continuation of treatment or social/environmental adaptations to improve learning, employability, and psychosocial well-being—justifications that may not easily be supported with data from measures of impairment or disability alone.

Differentiating Features

Unlike impairment-level measures, functional communication measures typically are not designed to assess separate modality-bound behaviors. Rather, their designs coincide with the concept of communication as an integration of specific behaviors that allow the ability to perform everyday life activities. For example, the ability to communicate socially, communicate basic needs, and use the telephone each require a range of specific skills (e.g., auditory comprehension, verbal and gestural expression, speech intelligibility) that, working together, allow the ability to perform the activity.

A good example that draws the distinction between measures of impairment and measures of disability is found in the development of *The Communicative Effectiveness Index* (Lomas et al., 1989). At the outset, the developers asked several relevant questions: "Are patients' values reflected in the instrument?", and "Is performance in daily living assessed?". In order to ensure that communication situations were representative of patients' values and daily living activities, situations were elicited from the patients themselves. Using a nominal group process, a group of adults with aphasia and their family members were asked for their responses to the question, "In which situations does a stroke survivor have to be able to get his meaning across and to understand what someone else means?" Four categories were generated:

- *Basic need* (e.g., communication required for toileting, eating, grooming, positioning)
- *Life skill* (e.g., telephone use, understanding traffic signals, communication required for shopping)
- *Social need* (e.g., dinner table conversation, writing a letter to a friend)
- *Health threat* (e.g., calling for help, conveying information about one's medical condition)

These assessment domains are necessarily different from the common domains of auditory comprehension, verbal expression, speech intelligibility, and the like, which characterize impairment measures. Functional measures assess a different but related set of behaviors. A review of available measures, however, break the rule of differentiating features when some impairment and disability measures are compared. This is particularly true when measures designed for multildisciplinary rehabilitation or comprehensive health care are considered. Table 3–2 provides examples of these measures and their characteristics.

General Rehabilitation and Global Measures

Numerous functional outcome measures are available, and the numbers are growing, in the multidisciplinary field of rehabilitation. Because the overall goal of rehabilitation is to optimize function, measurement of functional abilities predominates assessment methods.

A sample of widely used measures are reviewed here. Functional communication measures are embedded as sections of these instruments, designed to assess a range of rehabilitative functions (e.g., mobility, activities of daily living). Instruments of this nature include, for example, the *Patient Evaluation and Conference System* (*PECS;* Harvey & Jellinek, 1979, 1981), the *Level of Rehabilitation Scale—III* (*LORS;* Parkside Associates, 1986; Formations in Health Care, 1995), the *Rehabilitation Institute of Chicago Functional Assessment Scale* (*RICFAS;* Cichowski, 1995), the *Neurological Outcome Scale, an Evaluation System for Outpatient Rehabilitation Programs* (Santopoalo & Carey, 1991), and the *Functional Independence Measure* (*FIM;* State University of New York at Buffalo, 1993).

Measures of communication also are embedded as sections of global instruments, such as the *Assessment of Needs for Continuing Care* (Health Care Financing Administration, 1989) and the *Minimum Data Set for Nursing Facility Resident Assessment and Care Screening* (Hawes et al., 1995).

These measures, all of which use rating scales (ranging from 4 to 7 points) along a continuum of independence, were developed to yield a relatively quick estimate of functional communication. The extent to which communication functions are considered,

Table 3–2. Characteristics of Selected Functional Status Measures

Instrument (Reference)	Instrument Type	Assessment Domains	Aspects of Communication and Related Areas Addressed	Assessment Method	Reliability/Validity
Patient Evaluation and Conference System (PECS) (Harvey & Jellinek, 1979, 1981)	General Rehabilitation for Adults	Functions related to rehabilitation medicine, rehabilitation nursing, physical mobility, ADL, communication, medications, nutrition, assistive devices, psychology, neuropsychology, social issues, vocational educational activity, therapeutic recreation, pain, pulmonary rehabilitation, pastoral care	Hearing, comprehension of spoken language, production of verbal language, comprehension of written language, production of written language, production of speech, swallowing, knowledge of assistive devices, skill in speaking with assistive communication devices, utilization of assistive communication devices, impairment in thought processing, comprehension and use of gestures	7-point ordinal scale from dependent to independent function combined into 6 interval Life Scales	Studies are ongoing. Preliminary studies found range of interrater reliability from .68 to .80. Content and construct validity are reported.
Level of Rehabilitation Scale—III (LORS III) (Parkside Associates, 1986; Formations in Health Care, 1995)	General Rehabilitation for Adults	ADL, mobility, communication, cognitive ability	Auditory comprehension, oral expression, reading comprehension, written expression, alternate communication	5-point interval scale	Interrater reliability of item ratings ranges from .53 to .70 at admission and from .64 to .76 at discharge. Face validity based on agreement by experts in the field of rehabilitation is reported.

Measure	Population	Content/Services	Domains	Scale	Reliability/Validity
Rehabilitation Institute of Chicago Functional Assessment Scale '95 (RIC-FAS) (Cichowski, 1995)	General Rehabilitation for Adults	Functions related to the following services: physical medicine, nursing, physical therapy, occupational therapy, communication disorders, psychology, social work, vocational rehabilitation, therapeutic recreation	Hearing, auditory comprehension, oral expression, reading comprehension, written expression, speech production, chewing/swallowing, alternative/augmentative communication, money management	7-point ordinal scale ranging from normal to severe	Interrater reliability for RIC-FAS ranges from .66 to 1 across item scores, with 75 to 100% agreement on most items. Interrater reliability for communication items ranges from .90 to 1 ($<.0001$); 100% on all except written and pragmatic (97% agreement) and speech production (93% agreement).
Neurological Outcome Scale, an Evaluation System for Outpatient Rehabilitation Programs (Santopoalo & Carey, 1991)	General Rehabilitation for Adults	Physical restoration, cognitive retraining, communication skills development, community reentry, social involvement	Expressive skills (written, verbal), comprehension (auditory, reading)	5-point ordinal scale from 0 to 100% function	Based on pilot data from 36 clients, interitem reliability of the scale item ratings range from .81 to .93 (admission) and .47 (for communication skills) to .94 (discharge). Face validity is being tested.
Functional Independence Measure (FIM), Version 4.0 (State University of New York at Buffalo, 1993)	General Rehabilitation for Adults	Self-care, sphincter control, transfers, locomotion, communication, social cognition	Comprehension (auditory), expression (vocal), comprehension (visual), expression (nonvocal), eating, problem solving, memory, social interaction	7-point ordinal scale from complete independence to total assistance	Intraclass correlation coefficients (ICC) range from .89 to .96 for FIM domain scores. FIM item Kappa range: .53 (memory) to .66 (stair climbing). Interrater reliability ranges from .97 to .98 for FIM domain scores; FIM item Kappa range: .69 (memory) to .84 (bladder management). Reported face-, con-

(continued)

Table 3–2. Characteristics of Selected Functional Status Measures (*continued*)

Instrument (Reference)	Instrument Type	Assessment Domains	Aspects of Communication and Related Areas Addressed	Assessment Method	Reliability/Validity
					struct-, and criterion-related (predictive and concurrent validity) for minutes of help per day for stroke, multiple sclerosis, and traumatic brain injury).
WeeFIM (State University of New York at Buffalo, 1991)	General Rehabilitation for Children (6 mos. to 7 years and older)	Self-care, transfers, locomotion, sphincter control, communication, and social cognition	Comprehension (auditory or visual), expression (verbal, nonverbal)	7-point scale from complete independence to total assistance	Reliability and validity studies underway. Statistical comparisons will examine the relationship of ratings on the WeeFIM with scores on the *Battelle Developmental Screening Inventory Test* and the *Vineland Adaptive Behavior Scales*.
Pediatric Evaluation of Disability Inventory (Haley et al., 1992)	General Rehabilitation for Children (6 mos. to 7.5 years)	Self-care, mobility, social function	Comprehension of word meanings, comprehension of sentence complexity; functional use of expressive communication, complexity of expressive communication, problem-resolution, social interactive play,	Part 1: Functional skills (0 = unable; 1 = capable of performing item in most situations) Part 2: Caregiver assistance (5-point scale of independence)	Content validity reported by rehab. professionals; standardized on a normative sample (N = 412); PEDI highly correlated with *WeeFIM* and *Battelle*; PEDI selectively responsive to change in certain clinical sam-

			peer interactions, self-information, time orientation, community function	Part 3: Modifications (N = no modifications; C = child-oriented modifications; R = rehabilitation equipment; E = extensive modifications	ples; reliability data currently unavailable.
Assessment of Needs for Continuing Care (ANCC) (Health Care Financing Administration, 1989)	Global for Adults	Health status, functional status (ADLs, IADLs), communication, environmental factors in post-discharge care, nursing and other care requirements, family and community support, patient/family goals and preferences, options for continuing care	Comprehension, expression, usual mode(s) of communication	4-point ordinal scale from independent to dependent function	Information is currently unavailable.
Minimum Data Set for Nursing Home Resident Assessment and Care Screening (MDS) (Hawes et al., 1995)	Global for Adults	Cognitive patterns, communication/hearing patterns, vision patterns, physical functioning and structural problems (including ADLs), continence, psychosocial well-being, mood and behavior patterns, activity pursuit patterns, disease diagnoses, health conditions, oral/nutritional status, oral/dental status, skin condition, medication use, special treatment and procedures	Hearing, communication devices/techniques, modes of expression, making self understood, ability to understand others, change in communication/hearing	4-point ordinal scale	Based on published field test results, select inter-rater reliability values for key functional indicators are: making self understood, .92; hearing, .78; locomotion, .92; eating, .94; bladder continence, .93; cognitive skills, .93; vision, .85; wandering, .83; weight loss, .85; pressure ulcers, .92.

however, varies considerably across measures. For example, the PECS addresses 12 areas of communication and related abilities, while the FIM, designed as a minimum data set, addresses five areas. More noticeable are how the communication domains are assessed and how they depart from the concept of disability measurement. That is, the measures listed in Table 3–2 do not distinguish clearly between impairment and disability phenomena. They treat, for example, auditory comprehension as a function of communication, rather than a skill underlying communication functions (e.g., understanding face-to-face and telephone conversations, understanding television and radio). Similarly, other skills that underlie functional communication also are treated as functions, such as speech production, impairment in thought processing, and so forth.

Currently, one can find glaring deficiencies in the development of functional outcome measures for pediatric populations. Prevention and treatment programs have been successful in reducing the consequences of most of the formidable infectious diseases, in dramatically reducing the neonatal mortality rate, and in prolonging the survival period for children with many congenital and acquired diseases (Pantell & Lewis, 1987). Unfortunately, measurement development has not kept pace with medical advances. The ability to capture outcomes over time is particularly difficult as we expect children to grow and develop but not in a predictably linear fashion.

The few pediatric measures in the multidisciplinary field of rehabilitation include the *WeeFIM* (State University of New York at Buffalo, 1991), and *The Pediatric Evaluation of Disability Inventory* (*PEDI;* Haley, Coster, Ludlow, Halatiwanter, & Andrellos, 1992). The *WeeFIM,* like the *FIM* from which it was derived, is a minimum data set. Therefore, many clinicians believe it cannot capture all functionally important change. In the area of communication, it measures comprehension (auditory and visual) and expression (verbal and nonverbal) on a 7-point scale of independence. Another measure, the *PEDI,* was designed as a more comprehensive measure of disability. It also contains a section addressing communication, but to a greater level of depth when compared to the *WeeFIM.* The *PEDI,* however, is considered to be overly complex to administer and score. Finally, these pediatric measures (like the adult measures described above) address communication as a set of behavioral processes, rather than as a more integrative construct that addresses communication in various contexts. Thus, they may be better measures of impairment than disability.

Holland (1995) uses a simple rule, related to setting treatment goals, to clarify the difference between impairment and disability phenomena. She tells us to add, to our usual clinical goals (e.g., improve auditory comprehension, speech intelligibility, word retrieval), three words: *In order to . . .* , which brings us to a functional goal. Thus, we improve auditory comprehension *in order to* engage in telephone conversations or understand what is heard on television. The bridge is helpful in understanding the meaning of functional communication and in developing conceptual frameworks for its measurement.

Functional Communication Measures

Several measures have been developed exclusively for assessing functional communication. As Table 3–3 describes, these include the *Functional Communication Profile* (*FCP;*

Sarno, 1965), the *Communicative Abilities in Daily Living* (*CADL;* Holland, 1980; Holland, Frattali, & Fromm, in progress), the *Communicative Effectiveness Index* (*CETI;* Lomas, Pickard, Bester, Elbard, Finlayson, & Zoghaib, 1989), the revised *Edinburgh Functional Communication Profile* (Wirz, Skinner, & Dean, 1990), the *Amsterdam-Nijmegen Everyday Language Test* (Blomert, Kean, Koster, & Schokker, 1994), and the American Speech-Language-Hearing Association *Functional Assessment of Communication Skills for Adults* (*ASHA FACS;* Frattali, Thompson, Holland, Wohl, & Ferketic, 1995).

While the above measures were designed primarily for use with adults with aphasia secondary to stroke, and/or with cognitive-communication disorders secondary to traumatic brain injury, other measures were designed primarily for use with other communicatively disordered populations. For example, the *Performance Status for Head and Neck Cancer Patients* (List et al., 1990) was developed for use with adults with head and neck cancer; the *Functional Linguistic Communication Inventory* (Bayles & Tomoeda, 1994) was developed for use with adults with moderate and severe dementia.

Sarno (1965, 1969) is credited with introducing the concept of functional assessment in the field, and developing sets of integrated communication behaviors organized by modality (i.e., movement, speaking, understanding, reading) for measuring the functional communication of individuals with aphasia. The 45 items that constitute the measure are rated on a 9-point scale (from poor to normal) based on informal interactions with the client. "Normal" is equated with a client's premorbid communication status, rather than an absolute standard. The tool is used primarily with adults, but use with children also has been described. In these cases, "normal" is equated with the child's estimated premorbid language level. The measure offers, at a glance, a view of change over time in functional communication. It has high interrater and test-rest reliability and correlates highly with the *CADL* (Holland, 1980).

Holland (1980) built on the work of Sarno (1965) with development of the CADL. The *CADL* is a standardized test of 68 items designed to elicit aspects of language content/form, cognition, and use. Designed as a highly controlled interview, it was first validated for use with adults with aphasia, and later with adults with mental retardation, Alzheimer's disease, and experienced hearing aid users. Holland introduced a true integrative model of assessment. Scoring represents how successfully an individual communicates a message, rather than how the communication was accomplished. Psychometric properties of the *CADL* are well documented. High interrater reliability and test-retest reliability are reported and the instrument correlates with other tests for aphasia. Perhaps the biggest criticism of the *CADL* has been its role-playing feature, which is considered artificial and distorts the client's actual abilities to communicate functionally. Thus, the *CADL* is being revised and will eliminate role-playing, as well as items considered less central to functional communication.

The *CETI* (Lomas et al., 1989) measures 16 items across four domains on a continuum from "not at all able" to "as able as before the stroke." Similar to the *FCP* (Sarno, 1965), ratings are based on a premorbid standard of functional communication. A unique feature of this measure is its administration requirements; significant others (i.e., spouse, relative, neighbor, or friend) of adults with communication disorders administer it. Interrater and test-retest reliability of the *CETI* are high, and the measure correlates well with global ratings of communication made by spouses and with the *Western Aphasia Battery* (Kertesz, 1982).

Table 3-3. Characteristics of Selected Functional Communication Measures

Instrument (Reference)	Communication Components	Assessment Method	Applicable Populations	Reliability/ Validity
Functional Communication Profile (FCP) (Sarno, 1965)	45 communication behaviors in: movement (e.g., gestures), speaking, understanding, reading, miscellaneous (e.g., writing, calculation)	9-point scale	Adults with aphasia	Concurrent and predictive validity (correlates with measures of auditory memory span and CADL); high interexaminer reliability; test-retest reliability described as significant
Communicative Abilities in Daily Living (CADL) (Holland, 1980)	68 items incorporating everyday language activities in: content/form (production, comprehension), cognition, use (role-playing, speech acts)	3-point scoring system (0 = wrong, 1 = adequate, 2 = correct)	Adults with aphasia, mental retardation or Alzheimer's disease; experienced hearing aid users	Concurrent validity (correlates with Boston Diagnostic Aphasia Examination [Goodglass & Kaplan, 1972], Porch Index of Communicative Ability [Porch, 1971, 1981], FCP, and direct observations of communication behavior); high inter-examiner and test-retest reliability
Communicative Effectiveness Index (CETI) (Lomas et al., 1989)	16 communication items categorized by social need, life skill, basic need, health threat	10-cm visual analogue scale from "not at all able" to "as able as before the stroke"	Adults with aphasia secondary to stroke	Based on evaluation of 22 patients with aphasia (11 recovering, 11 stable); has good test-retest and interrater reliability; face and construct validity (correlates with global ratings of language & communication by spouses)
Revised Edinburgh Functional Communication Profile (EFCP) (Wirz, Skinner, & Dean, 1990)	Communication functions and modalities used: greetings, acknowledging, responding, requesting, initiating	5-point effectiveness scale, and modality used is noted	Adults with aphasia, developmental disorders, mental retardation, cerebral palsy who use AAC systems	Concurrent validity; content validity evaluated by scoring 16-minute language samples and comparing with 10 exchanges;

(continued)

Test				
				interrater reliability based on 14 patients
A Performance Status Scale for Head and Neck Cancer Patients (List, Ritter-Sterr, Lansky, 1990)	Eating in public, understandability of speech, normalcy of diet	Total of 3 ratings (one on each subscale). In each subscale, items are arranged hierarchically to describe a continuum, with total incapacitation at one end to full, normal functioning at the other end	Adults with head and neck cancer	Based on 181 patients, interrater reliability between research team members was .88 for normalcy of diet; .64 for understandability of speech; and .78 for eating in public. Interrater reliability for untrained professionals was .84 (normalcy of diet), .43 (understandability of speech), and .81 (eating in public); moderate correlations were found when compared with Karnofsky Performance Status Rating Scale [Karnofsky & Burchenal, 1949].
Amsterdam Nijmegan Everyday Language Test (ANELT) (Blomert et al., 1994)	Two parallel versions, each consisting of 10 items constructed as scenarios of familiar daily life activities	Two 5-point scales: A-scale (understandability of the message) and B-scale (intelligibility of the utterance). Points on rating scale: not at all, a little, medium, reasonable, and good	Adults with aphasia	Psychometric analysis showed perfect parallelism for both test versions. Based on 60 adult subjects with no history of neurological impairment and 60 subjects with aphasia, interrater reliability ranged from .70 to .92. Concurrent validity (correlates with Aachen Aphasia Test-Communicative Behavior Scale) is reported.
Communication Profile: A Functional Skills Survey (Payne, 1994)	26 daily communication skills involving speaking, reading comprehension, verbal com-	5-point scale (face-to-face interview) that allows clients or family members to rate the importance of communication	Adults with language impairments from diffuse neurological disorders, hearing impair-	On the basis of 65 subjects, internal consistency of items was .95. Internal consistency of

Table 3–3. Characteristics of Selected Functional Communication Measures *(continued)*

Instrument (Reference)	Communication Components	Assessment Method	Applicable Populations	Reliability/Validity
	prehension, writing, and math comprehension	skills from "very important" to "not important at all"	ments, mental retardation, stroke, and traumatic brain injury	subscales was reportedly high. Test-retest reliability was .92. Validity between total score and client self-assessment of severity was .63.
Functional Linguistic Communication Inventory (Bayles & Tomoeda, 1994)	Assessment areas include greeting/naming, answering questions, writing, comprehension of signs/pictures, following commands, conversation, reminiscing, gesture, pantomime, and word reading/comprehension	32 items that require the examiner to judge whether a correct response was provided. The number of correct responses are totaled, and subtest scores can be compared to performance on standardization study subjects by severity level.	Adults with moderate and severe dementia	Test-retest reliability for 20 patients with dementia, using the coefficient of determination and the probability of concordance, were high and significant for all subtests except gesture. Criterion validity using the Arizona Battery for Communication Disorders of Dementia (Bayles & Tomoeda, 1993) was strong, r = .78 (p < .002).
ASHA Functional Assessment of Communication Skills for Adults (Frattali et al., 1995)	43 items within 4 assessment domains: social communication; communication of basic needs; reading, writing, and number concepts; daily planning	7-point scale of independence; 5-point scale of qualitative dimensions of communication (i.e., adequacy, appropriateness, promptness, and communication sharing)	Adults with aphasia secondary to left-hemisphere stroke; adults with cognitive-communication disorders secondary to traumatic brain injury	Interrater reliability ranged from .72 to .95. Intrarater reliability ranged from .94-.99. Moderate correlations with Western Aphasia Battery (Kertesz, 1982) and Scales of Cognitive Ability for Traumatic Brain Injury (Adamovich & Henderson 1992). High internal consistency, measurement sensitivity, and social validity reported.

The revised *Edinburgh Functional Communication Profile* (Wirz et al., 1990) quantifies communication functions at the level of conversational interaction. It has been used with adults with aphasia, cerebral palsy, traumatic brain injury, and severe mental disability; and children with developmental language disorders. First, an interaction analysis is completed; then, communication performance analysis is completed using conversational samples. The conversational samples, however, take place with clinical examiners in a clinical setting, and may not be representative of the client's functional communication skills. In contrast, *the Amsterdam-Nijmegen Everyday Language Test* (Blomert et al., 1994) consists of items (arranged in two parallel versions) constructed as scenarios of familiar life activities (e.g., You have an appointment with the doctor. Something else has come up. You call up and what do you say?). The measure was designed for use with adults with aphasia. It incorporates two 5-point scales: an A-scale that rates the understandability of the message, and a B-scale that rates the intelligibility of the utterance. Points on the rating scale range from "not at all" to "good." The measure is primarily limited to verbal modes of communication, and relies on the ability to comprehend the scenarios presented.

Finally, the *ASHA FACS* (Frattali et al., 1995) was designed as a quick and easily administered measure, based on direct observations either by speech-language pathologists or significant others, which allows the rating (on a 7-point scale of independence) of four assessment domains: social communication; communication of basic needs; reading, writing, and number concepts; and daily planning. Each domain is rated globally on the basis of a Scale of Qualitative Dimensions (i.e., adequacy, appropriateness, promptness, and communication sharing). The measure yields domain and dimension mean scores, overall scores, and profiles of both Communication Independence and Qualitative Dimensions. The measure was found to have strong validity and high reliability with the two client populations for which it was initially field-tested: adults who have sustained left-hemisphere stroke with aphasia, and adults with traumatic brain injury with cognitive-communication disorders. Both paper-and-pencil and computerized versions were developed.

Absent, again, are functional communication measures for children. While a few measures mentioned above can be used with children, they were primarily developed for use with adults. Research activities in the field, however, show promise for the development of pediatric measures in the near future.

While these measures assess functional communication and related functional abilities, they usually do so from the perspective of the clinician and not the client. In addition, they do not extend to the measurement of broader and more individually defined phenomena related to the quality of life. That level of assessment is reserved for the so-called quality-of-life or wellness measures.

MEASURING QUALITY OF LIFE

Perhaps the most important development made during the last 10 years is the growing consensus that the client's point of view is central to measuring clinical outcomes. Few would argue that the long-term goal of clinical intervention is quality of life. And, the client is the best judge. Consequently, measuring quality of life is largely subjective; it is based on personal values, beliefs, and preferences. Environmental factors, such as societal attitudes and social/psychological supports, also directly influence perceptions about the quality of life.

When we think about quality of life, the dimensions of emotional well-being, behavioral competence, sleep and rest, energy and vitality, and general life satisfaction come to mind. The WHO (1980) defines interferences with quality of life (i.e., handicaps) as the social, environmental, or economic disadvantages, resulting from an impairment or disability, that limit or prevent the fulfillment of a role that is normal (depending on age, sex, and social and cultural factors). Birren and Dieckmann (1991) offer a global definition of *overall* quality of life:

> The concept of quality of life is complex, and it embraces many characteristics of the social and physical environments as well as the health and internal states of individuals. There are two approaches to the measurement of quality of life: One is based upon the subjective or internal self perceptions of the quality of life; the other approach is objective and based upon external judgments of the quality of life [in Jette, 1993, p. 530].

Thus, Lawton (1983) believes quality-of-life measures should include evaluation of both interpersonal and social-normative criteria including (1) psychological well-being, (2) perceived quality of life, (3) behavioral competence in multiple areas (i.e., health, functional health, cognition, time use, and social behavior), and the objective environment itself. The usefulness of this broad definition of measurement, however, has been questioned. The concept invites inclusion of "anything that suits anyone's fancy" (Jette, 1993). A narrower concept, called *health-related* quality of life, requires one to explicitly select and measure only those dimensions of quality of life that are relevant to the clinical interventions applied.

Gotay, Korn, McCabe, and colleagues (1992) recently proposed that quality of life be defined as a state of well-being which is a composite of two components: (1) the ability to perform everyday activities that reflect physical, psychological, and social well-being; and (2) patient satisfaction with levels of functioning and the control of disease and/or treatment-related symptoms.

Thus, we move from measurement of overall quality of life to health-related quality of life (HQL). HQL typically refers to the individuals's ability to function in a variety of roles and to derive satisfaction from them. These measures, however, still assess multiple dimensions of life (the objective component) and attach values to each dimension (the subjective component). The ideal quality-of-life measure, according to Hayes and Shapiro (1992), is one that taps both multiple dimensions of HQL (e.g., physical functioning, emotional well-being, and social interaction) adequately, and allows for integration of these dimensions into an aggregate score. Unfortunately, instruments that do one of these things well tend to be inadequate at the other.

Purposes

Jette (1993) describes the purposes of HQL measures. These measures are used in clinical practice to determine compensation, predict prognosis, plan placement, estimate care requirements, choose different types of specific care, and indicate changes in client status in response to delivered care. Gotay and Moore (1992) believe quality-of-life assessment has the potential to provide vital treatment-related information. For example, quality-of-life ratings may provide a basis for distinguishing between head and neck cancer treatments with equivalent survival rates but different impacts on quality of life. Thus, these measures can aid in clinical decision making.

Differentiating Features

Major measurement dimensions of health-related quality of life, identified in the professional literature, include (1) signs and symptoms of disease, (2) performance of basic activities of daily living, (3) performance of social roles, (4) emotional state, (5) intellectual functioning, and (6) general satisfaction and perceived well-being (Bergner, 1989; Ware, 1984; Levine & Croog, 1984). The concept subsumes the narrower concepts of functional limitations (per Nagi's definition) and disability (per the WHO definition). It usually does not, however, include specific assessment of pathology or impairment (i.e., dimensions at the organ/body system level). In addition, HQL dimensions are broader than disability concepts. Emotional well-being, overall life satisfaction, energy, and vitality are all legitimate components—dimensions that are not traditionally included in definitions of functional status or disability (see Figure 3–2).

The differentiating feature of quality-of-life measures is that their dimensions are on the personal/social level; values are assigned to each quality of life dimension by clients themselves, thus reflecting their personal values and beliefs. These measures, thus, often take the form of self-administered questionnaires, interviewer-administered questionnaires, and open-ended interviewers.

It is interesting to note what clients consider handicapping consequences of impairments and/or disabilities. For example, the handicapping consequences of aphasia, as identified by individuals with aphasia and their significant others, offer some insight into client views as they pertain to quality of life (Le Dorze & Brassard, 1995).

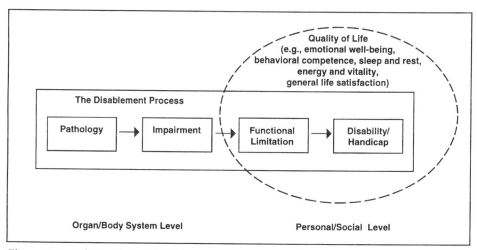

Figure 3–2. Relationship of Disablement Process to Quality of Life

SOURCE: Jette, A. M. (1993). Using health-related quality of life measures in physical therapy outcomes research. *Physical Therapy, 73*(8), 528–537. Used by permission.

Responses of 18 subjects were catalogued with reference to the WHO model (1980) in terms of disabilities and handicaps. Reported handicaps included changes in situations of communication (e.g., frustration when others speak on their behalf, irritation when not finding the right word), changes in interpersonal relationships (e.g., loss of authority over children, loss of friends), loss of autonomy (e.g., loss of employment, feelings of powerlessness), restricted activities (e.g., loss of career objectives, reduced recreational activities), and stigmatization (e.g,. aphasia perceived as mental illness, drunkenness; embarrassment about speaking).

Gotay and Moore (1992), in reviewing head and neck cancer research publications, identified these dimensions of quality of life (with categories from Cella & Tulsky, 1990, and numbers indicating proportions of studies assessing a given dimension): Emotional well-being (4/18; depression, self-concept, general), spirituality (1/18), sexuality/intimacy (5/18), social functioning (7/18; social support, activities/hobbies), occupational functioning (8/18), speech/communication (9/18), eating/swallowing (8/18), functional ability (5/18; performance status, independence in daily activities, strength), physical status (10/18; pain, need for subsequent surgery, survival), treatment satisfaction (1/18), and global ratings (5/18; treatment cost/benefits, self-rated health, quality of life/life satisfaction). It is interesting to note that speech/communication and eating/swallowing were among the most frequently rated dimensions of quality of life for persons with head and neck cancer.

The measures identified in Table 3–4 are primarily general rather than condition-specific measures. In addition, these measures generally were developed to measure outcomes of primary medical care (although they are being used increasingly to measure the outcomes of medical rehabilitation). Two exceptions included in the table are the *Hearing Handicap Inventory for the Elderly* (Ventry & Weinstein, 1982) and the *Voice Handicap Index* (Jacobson, Johnson, Silbergleit, & Benninger, in progress), which measure quality of life in the context of specific conditions of hearing and voice, respectively. A few of the widely known measures are discussed here.

The *Medical Outcomes Study* (*MOS;* Ware & Sherbourne, 1992) was a 4-year observational study designed to examine the influence of specific characteristics of providers, patients, and health systems on outcomes of care. The *SF-36* items were selected to maximize their associations with the long-form MOS scales from which they came. It is perhaps the most widely used general HQL instrument in use today.

The *Quality of Well-Being Scale* (Fanshel & Bush, 1970) summarizes health status in terms of quality-adjusted life years. It quantifies HQL in a single number, ranging from death to complete well-being, on the basis of symptom/problem complexes and ordinal-level classification of functioning. Preference weights are applied to the respondent's scores to obtain the respondent's point-in-time well-being score. These preference weights were obtained in human value studies designed to locate the observable states on a preference continuum ranging from 0 to 1.

The *COOP Charts* (Nelson et al., 1987) (derived from the Dartmouth Primary Care Cooperative Information Project) are similar to Snellen Charts. They are used as quick screens. Each chart comprises a title (e.g., physical, mental, social), a question referring to the status of the patient over the past 4 weeks, and five response choices. Each response is illustrated by a drawing that depicts a level of functioning along a 5-point ordinal scale. The Charts were designed to fit into the standard data collection routine of busy ambulatory practices and can be clinician administered or patient

Table 3–4. Characteristics of Selected Quality of Life Measures

Measure (Reference)	Assessment Domains	Assessment Method	Length	Time Requirements	Reliability/validity
Medical Outcome Study (MOS) Health Status Questionnaire (SF-36) (Ware & Sherbourne, 1992)	Physical; role limitations due to physical and emotional problems; social functioning; general mental health; pain; energy/fatigue; general health perceptions	Self-report	36 items	10 minutes	Reliability estimates for all SF-36 scales were .78 or higher. Multitrait scaling analyses support item convergence for hypothesized scales and item discrimination across scales.
COOP Charts (Nelson, Wasson, Kirk, et al. 1987)	Physical; Mental; role; social; pain; overall health change; social resources; life quality	Self-report or clinical rating	9 items	<10 minutes	Charts correlate with validity indicator variables, indicating convergent and discriminant validity. Reliability data unavailable.
Duke-UNC Health Profile (Parkerson, Gehlbach, Wagner, et al., 1981)	Symptom status; physical function; emotional function; social function	Self-report	64 items	15–20 minutes	Based on 395 ambulatory patients in a family medicine center, temporal stability ranged from .52 to .82. Cronbach's alpha for internal consistency was .85 for emotional function. Convergent and discriminant validity supported by strong associations with the Sickness Impact Profile, and other measures.
Sickness Impact Profile (SIP) (Bergner, Bobbitt, Carter, & Gilson, 1981)	Physical: ambulation, mobility, body care; psychosocial: social interac-	Self-report	136 items	30 minutes	Based on large field trial on a random sample of prepaid group practice

(continued)

Table 3–4. Characteristics of Selected Quality of Life Measures (*continued*)

Measure (Reference)	Assessment Domains	Assessment Method	Length	Time Requirements	Reliability/validity
	tion, communication, alertness, emotional behavior; other: sleep/rest, eating, work, home management, recreational pastimes				enrollees and smaller trials on samples of patients with hyperthyroidism, rheumatoid arthritis, and hip replacements, test-retest reliability (r = .92) and internal consistency (r = .94). Clinical validity (with clinical measures of disease) was moderate to high.
McMaster Health Index Questionnaire (MHIQ) (Chambers, MacDonald, Tugwell, et al., 1982)	Physical: mobility, self-care, communication, global physical function; Social: general well-being, work/social role, performance, social support and participation, global self-function; Emotional: self-esteem, personal relationships, critical life events, global emotional function	Self-report	59 items	20 minutes	Retest reliability coefficients of .53, .70, and .48 for physical, emotional, and social function scores, respectively, were observed in physiotherapy patients. In psychiatry patients, coefficients were .95, .77, and .66, respectively. Scores correlate with global assessment made by health professionals. Physical function scores were responsive to change.
Nottingham Health Profile (NHP) (McEwen, 1988)	Six domains of experience: pain, physical mobility, sleep, emotional reactions, energy, social isolation	Self-report	45 items	10 minutes	High face, content, and criterion validity. NHP scores effectively differentiated between well and ill groups. Intrarater reliability ranged from .44–.89 in groups with chronic illlness. Norms

Instrument	Domains	Format	Items	Time	Reliability/Validity
Quality of Well-being Scale (QWB) (Fanshel & Bush, 1970)	Functional performance: self-care, mobility, institutionalization, social activities; symptoms and problems	Self-report	50 items	12 minutes	for general population and employed population established. Sensitivity to changes over time in patients with AIDS demonstrated in a 52-week multicenter trial.
Functional Status Questionnaire (FSQ) (Jette, Davies, Cleary, et al., 1986)	Physical: basic and intermediate activities of daily living; emotional function: anxiety and depression, quality of social interaction; social performance: occupational function, social activities; other: sexual, global disability, global health satisfaction, social contacts	Self-report	34 items	10 minutes	Intra-rater reliability for the 6 scale scores ranged from .64 to .82. Scale scores correlated with scores on 7 health measures. Inverse relationship found between age and performance on intermediate activities of daily living, and age and social activity. Satisfaction with health is positively correlated with each scale score.
Hearing Handicap Inventory for the Elderly (Ventry & Weinstein, 1982)	Perceived problems caused by hearing loss (i.e., emotional consequences and social and situational effects)	Self-report	25 items	10 minutes	Reported reliability (by assessing internal consistency) as well as construct and content validity
Voice Handicap Index (Jacobson, Johnson, Silbergleit, & Benninger, in progress)	Physical symptamotology, functional factors, emotional factors	Self-report	30 items	15 minutes	Based on 65 subjects, internal consistency of items was .95. Internal consistency of subscales was high. Test-retest reliability was .92. Validity between total score and patient self-assessment of severity was .63.

self-administered. They are used internationally through the endorsement of the World Organization of National Colleges, Academies, and Academic Associations of General Practice/Family Physicians (Hays & Shapiro, 1992).

The *Sickness Impact Profile* (*SIP*; Bergner et al., 1981) was the product of a 6-year research project undertaken to develop a behaviorally based measure of health status. It is widely used and reportedly sensitive enough to detect changes or differences in health status that occur over time or between groups. It was designed to be broadly applicable across types and severities of illness and across demographic and cultural subgroups. The *SIP* contains 136 statements about health-related function in 12 areas of activity. Communication and eating are among the assessment domains. Among the items in the communication section are, "I do not speak clearly when I am under stress," and "I am having trouble writing or typing." The eating section includes these selected items: "I am eating no food at all, nutrition is taken through tubes or intra-venous fluids," and I am eating special or different food." The *SIP* can either be administered by an interviewer or self-administered. Its reliability and validity are well documented.

Two quality-of-life measures developed in the discipline of human communication sciences and disorders are the *Hearing Handicap Inventory for the Elderly* (*HHIE*; Ventry & Weinstein, 1982) and the *Voice Handicap Index* (*VHI*; Jacobson, Johnson, Silbergleit, & Benninger, in progress). The *HHIE* assesses the situational effects and the emotional and social adjustment of elderly people to hearing impairment. Two subscales make up the measure: emotional consequences (13 items) and social and situational effects (12 items). The items are rated on a 3-point scale of yes, sometimes, and no. The *Voice Handicap Index* (Jacobson et al., in progress) measures physical symptoms, functional factors, and emotional factors. The *VHI* uses a 5-point interval-level scale from always to never.

MEASUREMENT SELECTION CONSIDERATIONS

There are many outcome measures from which to choose. Which are best? Some clinicians, working under real-world time demands, would say that quickly administered measures are the best. Other results-oriented clinicians would insist that sensitive measures capable of capturing all important change, no matter how small, are preferred. Payers would say that quantitative measures of independence written in comprehensible terms are the best. Researchers would select measures with documented high reliability and validity. In fact, all opinions are valid.

The first consideration in selecting a measure is the relationship between what you want to know and what information can be captured by a particular measure. Beyond a measure's intended purposes, all measures should possess certain basic characteristics. They should be:

- *Valid*: Measure what they claim to measure. A measure can be reliable, but not valid. For example, the rehabilitation-oriented measures of disability may be administered reliably, but in that functional communication is an integrated construct that should not be measured by specific modalities (e.g., speech intelligibility, auditory comprehension), their validity is questioned.

- *Reliable:* Consistent in their results across time and assessors. We can never completely eliminate error from a measure (e.g., due to client's anxiety level, quality and quantity of observations, time of day and fatigue factors), but to the extent that error is slight, scores derived from that measure are reliable.

- *Sensitive:* Able to detect meaningful change. Instruments must be sufficiently sensitive for their intended purposes. Thus, if it is a screening measure, it should be sensitive enough to identify problems versus no problems. If it is a minimum data set, one should not expect a high degree of sensitivity. Therefore, one should not use tools beyond the limits of their intended purposes. If a measure is sensitive, it must be able to detect change if change occurs.

- *Practical:* Honor the time demands and capabilities of examiners. The feasibility of an instrument typically is determined by the mode of administration required, the time it takes to administer, requirements in use of stimulus materials and other equipment, need for special training of examiners, burden on the respondent, and complexity of scoring.

- *Comprehensible:* Understandable to end users of the information. Often, one makes treatment decisions on the basis of test results. These decisions can include eligibility for services, payment for services, continuation of services, and judgments about the quality of services. Often, decision makers are not clinicians. The information yielded from tests, therefore, should be understandable to the layperson.

Patrick and Erickson (1988) detail practical considerations when selecting quality-of-life measures, which can be applied to selection of any measure. These include acceptability, method of administration, length and cost of administration, method of analysis, and presentation of data. These considerations are detailed as Table 3–5. Bergner, Kaplan, and Ware (1987) agree. To them, the most reliable and valid outcome measure has only limited value to the field if its use is impractical in most outcome studies. They consider also the real dollar and time costs involved in gathering outcomes data and the acceptance of the measure to those involved, including respondents and the audience to be addressed when results are published.

The above considerations should be factored into your evaluation of "best measures." Otherwise, measurement quickly becomes complicated by conceptual, methodological, psychometric, and practical problems, rendering the effort little more than a waste of time and resources.

CONCLUSION

Outcomes measurement can occur along a continuum of the possible consequences of disease, disorder or injury. While our traditional assessment methods have been confined to measurement of modality-specific behaviors (and, thus, impairment), a broader understanding of the consequences of impairment on daily living and quality of life has allowed measurement in the areas of disability and handicap.

Major strides have been made in the past decade in both the development and use of functional status and quality-of-life measures. The coming decade will likely bear

Table 3–5. Practical Considerations When Selecting Quality-of Life-Measures

STANDARDIZED OR NONSTANDARDIZED ASSESSMENT STRATEGY
 o Identification and explanation of real differences among selected clinical populations
 o Resource requirements—time and effort

ACCEPTABILITY
 o Previous experiences in clinical applications
 o Respondent burden
 o Interviewer burden

METHOD OF ADMINISTRATION
 o Direct observation
 o Face-to-face interview
 o Telephone interview
 o Self-administered questionnaire
 o Proxy respondents

LENGTH AND COST OF ADMINISTRATION
 o Other components of interview schedule or questionnaire
 o Completion rates and quality of data

METHOD OF ANALYSIS AND COMPLEXITY OF SCORING
 o Availability of computer scoring
 o Aggregation or disaggregation into component parts

PRESENTATION OF DATA AND USEFULNESS TO DECISION MAKERS
 o Degree of certainty on value
 o Numbers, graphs, and interpretation of data

SOURCE: Patrick, D.L., & Erickson, P. (1988). In S.R. Walker & R.M. Rosser (Eds.), *Quality of life: Assessment and application.* Lancaster, England: MTP Press Limited. Reprinted with permission.

witness to their use in outcomes measurement activities. But these advances should not overshadow the work that must still be done to ensure measurement reliability, validity, sensitivity, and practicality. In addition, we must learn about how these measures interrelate.

Clinicians often search for the perfect measure of functional status, or the perfect measure of quality of life. But, like measures of impairment, a best single or universally accepted instrument does not exist. Measurement of functional status and quality of life often involve complex clinical, behavioral, and culturally bound factors considered within specific contexts. Each instrument, then, will be relevant only to certain groups of clients or to specific research or clinical activities.

In the push towards universality, Carey (1990) warns:

It would, of course, be ideal to have a single instrument that would serve as the perfect clinical assessment tool, the perfect program evaluation tool, and the perfect management information system. It would also be ideal if someone could invent a vehicle that would have the luxury of a big car, the fuel efficiency of a small car, and the flexibility of a truck designed for hauling farm machinery. It is unlikely that such a vehicle will appear in the near future. [p. 234]

Kane (1987) equates the "perfect measure" to the clinical equivalent of the Swiss army knife—something small and easily used with enough blades and attachments to fit any number of circumstances that might arise. He states, "Many of us have been given one of these multipurpose tools that drives nails and tightens screws as well as clips toenails, but it is usually not terribly good for any single one of these tasks" (p. 95S). Consequently, we need to ask, "For whom and in what circumstances is the tool to be used?" The best measure depends on your objectives.

Apart from the difficulties in determining best measures, we have, in fact, reached a turning point in our assessment of clients. We are looking beyond the measurement of impairment. We are reframing client outcomes and their relative importance to the client and other stakeholders in clinical care. The deliberate assessment of functional status and quality of life begins the transformation. Its effective use towards the end of knowledge about meaningful outcomes will complete it.

REFERENCES

Adamovich, B., & Henderson, J. (1992). *Scales of cognitive ability for traumatic brain injury.* Chicago, IL: Riverside.

Adamzyk, J. (1991). Relevance of CIQI measures of quality and outcome to the payer/insurer—How to "buy smart." Presentation at Rehabilitation Medicine: Continuous Interdisciplinary Quality Improvement (CIQI). Conference sponsored by the Buffalo General Hospital and State University of New York at Buffalo, Buffalo, NY.

Aten, J. (1986). Functional communication treatment. In R. Chapey (Ed.), *Language intervention strategies in adult aphasia, 2nd ed.* Baltimore: Williams & Wilkins.

Batavia, A.I. (1992). Assessing the function of functional assessment: A consumer perspective. *Disability and Rehabilitation, 14,* 156–160.

Bayles, K. & Tomoeda, C. (1994) *Functional Linguistic Communication Inventory.* Phoenix, AZ: Canyonlands Publishing, Inc.

Bergner, M.B. (1989). Quality of life, health status, and clinical research. *Medical Care, 27* (Suppl), S148–S156.

Bergner, M.B., Bobbitt, R.A., Carter, W.B., & Gilson, B.S. (1981). The Sickness Impact Profile: Development and final revision of a health status measure. *Medical Care, 19,* 787–805.

Bergner, M.B., Kaplan, R.M., & Ware, J.E. (1987). Evaluation health measures: Commentary: Measuring overall health: An evaluation of three important approaches. *Journal of Chronic Diseases, 40* (Suppl. 1), 23S–26S.

Birren, J., & Dieckmann, L. (1991). Concepts and content of quality of life in the later years: An overview. In J. Birren et al. (Eds.), *Quality of life in the frail elderly* (pp. 344–360). New York: Academic Press, Inc.

Blomert, L., Kean, M.L., Koster, C., & Schokker, J. (1994). Amsterdam-Nijmegen Everyday Language Test: Construction, reliability, and validity. *Aphasiology, 8*(4), 381–407.

Carey, R. (1990). Advances in rehabilitation program evaluation. In M.R. Eisenberg & R.C. Grzesiak (Eds.), *Advances in clinical rehabilitation, Volume 3* (pp. 217–250). New York: Springer, 1990.

Cella, D.F., & Tulsky, D.S. (1990). Measuring quality of life today: Methodological aspects. *Oncology, 4,* 29–38.

Chambers, L.W., MacDonald, L.A., Tugwell, P., et al. (1982). The McMaster health index questionnaire as a measure of quality of life for patients with rheumatoid disease. *Journal of Rheumatology, 9,* 780–784.

Cichowski. (1995). *Rehabilitation Institute of Chicago Functional Assessment Scale—Revised.* Chicago: Rehabilitation Institute of Chicago.

Damico, J.S., Smith, M., & Augustine, L.E. (1996). Multicultural populations and language disorders. In M. Smith & J.S. Damico (Eds.), *Childhood language disorders* (pp. 272–299). New York: Thieme Medical Publishers, Inc.

Dunn, L.M., & Dunn, L.M. (1981). *Peabody Picture Vocabulary Test—Revised.* Circle Pines, MN: American Guidance Service.

Elman, R.J., & Bernstein-Ellis, E. (1995). What is functional? *American Journal of Speech-Language Pathology, 4*(4), 115–117.

Fanshel, S., & Bush, J.W. (1970). A health-status index and its application to health-services outcomes. *Operations Research, 18,* 1021–1066.

Formations in Health Care. (1995). *Level of Rehabilitation Scale—III.* Chicago, IL: Author.

Frattali, C.M., Thompson, C.K., Holland, A.L., Wohl, C.B., & Ferketic, M.M. (1995). *Functional Assessment of Communication Skills for Adults.* Rockville, MD: ASHA.

Gardner, M.F. (1990). *Expressive One-word Picture Vocabulary Test—Revised.* Novato, CA: Academic Therapy Publications.

Goodglass & Kaplan. (1972). *Assessment of aphasia and related disorders, 2nd ed.* Philadelphia: Lea & Febiger.

Gotay, C.C., Korn, E.L., McCabe, M.S., et al. (In press). Quality of life in cancer treatment protocols: Research issues in protocol development. *Journal of the National Cancer Institute.*

Gotay, C.C., & Moore, T.D. (1992). Assessing quality of life in head and neck cancer. *Quality of Life Research, 1,* 5–17.

Haley, S.M., Coster, W.J., Ludlow, L.H., Haltiwanger, J.T., & Andrellos, P.J. (1992). *Pediatric Evaluation of Disability Inventory, Version 1.0.* Boston, MA: New England Medical Center Hospitals, Inc.

Harvey, R.F., & Jellinek, H.M. (1979). *Patient evaluation and conference system: PECS.* Wheaton, IL: Marianjoy Rehabilitation Center.

Harvey, R.F., & Jellinek, H.M. (1981). Functional performance assessment: A program approach. *Archives of Physical Medicine and Rehabilitation, 63,* 43–52.

Hawes, C., Morris, J.N., Phillips, C.D., Mor, V., Fries, B.E., & Nonemaker, S. (1995). Reliability estimates for the Minimum Data Set for Nursing Facility Resident Assessment and Care Screening (MDS). *Gerontologist, 35*(2), 172–178.

Hayes, R.D., & Shapiro, M.F. (1992). An overview of generic health-related quality of life measures for HIV research. *Quality of Life Research, 1,* 91–97.

Health Care Financing Administration. (1989). *Assessment of Needs for Continuing Care.* (Form HCFA-32; 10–89). Baltimore, MD: Author.

Holland, A.L. (1980). *Communicative Abilities in Daily Living.* Baltimore, MD: University Park Press.

Holland, A.L. (1995). Presentation during ASHA teleconference: Developing a functional communication measure. Rockville, MD: ASHA.

Holland, A.L., Frattali, C.M., & Fromm, D. (In progress). *Communicative Abilities in Daily Living—Revised.* Austin, TX: ProEd.

Jacobson, B., Johnson, A., Silbergleit, A., & Benninger, M. (In progress). *Voice Handicap Index.* Detroit, MI: Henry Ford Hospital.

Jette, A.M. (1993). Using health-related quality of life measures in physical therapy outcomes research. *Physical Therapy, 73*(8), 528–537.

Jette, A.M., Davies, A.R., Cleary, P.D., et al. (1986). The Functional Status Questionnaire: Reliability and validity when used in primary care. *Journal of General Internal Medicine, 1*(3), 143–149.

Kane, R.L. (1987). Commentary: Functional assessment questionnaire for geriatric patients—or the clinical swiss army knife. *Journal of Chronic Diseases, 40* (Suppl 1), 95S–98S.

Kertesz, A. (1982). *Western Aphasia Battery.* New York: Grune & Stratton.

Lawton, M.P. (1983). Environment and other determinants of well-being in older people. *Gerontologist, 23,* 349–357.

Le Dorze, G., & Brassard, C. (1995). A description of the consequences of aphasia on aphasic persons and their relatives and friends, based on the WHO model of chronic diseases. *Aphasiology, 9*(3), 239–255.

Lee, L.L. (1971). *Northwestern Syntax Screening Test.* Evanston, IL: Northwestern University Press.

Lee, L.L. (1974). *Developmental Sentence Scoring.* Evanston, IL: Northwestern University Press.

Levine, S., & Croog, S.H. (1984). What constitutes quality of life? A conceptualization of the dimensions of life quality in healthy populations and patients with cardiovascular disease. In N.K. Wenger, M.E. Mattson, C.D. Furberg, & J. Elinson (Eds.), *Assessment of quality of life in clinical trials of cardiovascular therapies* (pp. 25–45). New York: LeJacq Publishing Co.

List, M.A., Ritter-Sterr C., & Lansky, S.B. (1990) A Performance status scale for head and neck Cancer Patients. *Cancer,* 66, 564–569.

Lomas, J., Pickard, L., Bester, S., Elbard, H., Finlayson, A., & Zoghaib, C. (1989). The Communicative Effectiveness Index: Development and psychometric evaluation of a functional communication measure for adults. *Journal of Speech and Hearing Disorders, 54,* 113–124.

McEwen, J. (1988). The Nottingham Health Profile. In S. Walker, & R. Rosser (Eds.), *Quality of life: Assessment and application* (p. 95). Lancaster, England: MTP Press.

Murray, J., Marquardt, T.P., Richardson, A., & Nalty, D. (1984). Differential diagnosis of aphasia and dementia from aphasia test battery scores. *Journal of Neurological Communication Disorders, 1,* 33–39.

Nagi, S.Z. (1965). Some conceptual issues in disability and rehabilitation. In M.B. Sussman (Ed.), *Sociology and rehabilitation* (pp. 100–113). Washington, DC: American Sociological Association.

Nelson, E., Wasson, J., & Kirk, J., et al. (1987). Assessment of function in routine clinical practice: Description of the COOP Chart Method and preliminary findings. *Journal of Chronic Disability, 40* (Suppl) 1, 55S–69S.

Pantell, R.H., & Lewis, C.C. (1987). Measuring the impact of medical care on children. *Journal of Chronic Diseases, 40* (Suppl. 1), 99S–108S.

Parkerson, G.R., Gehlbach, S.H., Wagner, E.H., et al. (1981). The Duke-UNC Health Profile: An adult health status measure. *Medical Care, 19,* 787–805.

Parkside Associates. (1986). *Level of Rehabilitation Scale—III.* Park Ridge, IL: Author. (Now available from Formations in Health Care, Chicago.)

Patrick, D.L., & Erickson, P. (1988). Assessing health-related quality of life for clinical decision making. In S.R. Walker & R.M. Rosser (Eds.), *Quality of life: Assessment and application* (pp. 9–50). Lancaster, England: MTP Press Limited.

Payne, J. (1994). *Communication Profile: A Functional Skills Survey.* San Antonio, TX: Communication Skill Builders.

Porch, B. E. (1971). *Porch Index of Communicative Ability.* Palo Alto, CA: Consulting Psychologists Press.

Romski, M.A., & Sevcik, R.A. (1996). Communication development of children with severe disabilities. In M.D. Smith & J.S. Damico (Eds.), *Childhood language disorders* (pp. 218–234). New York: Thieme Medical Publishers, Inc.

Santopoalo, R.D., & Carey. D. (1991). *Neurological Outcome Scale: An Evaluation System for Outpatient Rehabilitation Programs.* Park Ridge, IL: Parkside Associates. (Now available from Formations in Health Care, Chicago.)

Sarno, M.T. (1965). A measurement of functional communication in aphasia. *Archives of Physical Medicine and Rehabilitation, 46,* 101–107.

Sarno, M.T. (1969). *Functional communication profile.* New York: Institute of Rehabilitation Medicine, New York University Medical Center.

Schuell, H. (1965). *The Minnesota Test for Differential Diagnosis of Aphasia.* Minneapolis, MN: University of Minnesota Press.

State University of New York at Buffalo, Research Foundation. (1991). *Functional Independence Measure for Children (WeeFIM)*, Version 1.5. Buffalo, NY: Author.

State University of New York at Buffalo, Research Foundation. (1993). *Guide for use of the Uniform Data Set for Medical Rehabilitation: Functional Independence Measure.* Buffalo, NY: Author.

Ventry, I., & Weinstein, B.E. (1982). The Hearing Handicap Inventory for the Elderly: A new tool. *Ear and Hearing, 3,* 128–134.

Ware, J. (1984). Methodological considerations in the selection of health status assessment procedures. In N.K. Wegner, M.E. Mattson, C.D. Furberg, & J. Elinson (Eds.), *Assessment of quality of life in clinical trials of cardiovascular therapies* (pp. 87–111). New York: LeJacq Publishing Co.

Ware, J., & Sherbourne, C. (1992). The MOS 36-item Short Form Health Survey (SF-36). *Medical Care, 30,* 473–483.

Wertz, R.T. (1984). Language disorders in adults: State of the clinical art. In A.L. Holland (Ed.), *Language disorders in adults* (pp. 1–78). San Diego, CA: College-Hill.

Wilson, I.B., & Cleary, P.D. (1995). Linking clinical variables with health-related quality of life: A conceptual model of patient outcomes. *Journal of the American Medical Association, 273*(1), 59–65.

Wirz, S., Skinner, C., & Dean, E. (1990). *Revised Edinburgh Functional Communication Profile.* Tucson, AZ: Communication Skill Builders.

World Health Organization. (1980). *International classification of impairments, disabilities, and handicaps: A manual for classification relating to the consequences of disease.* Geneva, Switzerland: Author.

CHAPTER 4

Measuring Consumer Satisfaction

PAUL R. RAO, JEAN BLOSSER, AND NANCY P. HUFFMAN

INTRODUCTION

How do you satisfy the consumer? Who really is the consumer? Since the consumer revolution of the 1970s, consumers have been exerting more and more political pressure and telling hospitals, schools, universities, and other service entities what it is *they* expect. Today's service delivery market has placed an unprecedented emphasis on meeting the consumer's demands and, consequently, providers are increasingly being held accountable for meeting or even exceeding a variety of consumer expectations. In health care, consumers include the recipients of the service (or *patient,* the Latin derivative for receiver), the visitors (family and friends), regulators, payers, the various providers, and the internal customers or partners (e.g., medical records staff or physicians). In schools and universities, consumers consist of the students, parents, other payers, regulators, administrators, and faculty. At a basic level, a *consumer* is defined as a person who receives the results of our work. Speech-language pathologists, therefore, are primarily concerned with their clients, but secondarily concerned with employers, payers, and other key stakeholders in the services provided.

This chapter is intended to assist the reader in understanding the various perspectives of consumers and in how to collect and use consumer data to improve services and ultimately improve outcomes. At the outset of this text, Frattali (Chapter 1) emphasizes that we as clinicians, teachers, administrators, or other service providers are not seeking only one outcome, but rather a range of outcomes defined by the interests or needs of any given stakeholder, and at any given point in time during or after the provision of care. Based on the interests, needs, and expectations of the various customers, we can attempt to measure client-defined satisfaction with services. Deming (1982) emphasized consumer research as the hallmark of innovation—meeting the needs of consumers in the present and future. Gathering and analyzing consumer data

89

in a systematic fashion is perhaps the first step in conducting research on quality of care. This consumer-oriented approach applies to every service setting and to the entire range of persons served by our profession.

CONSUMER SATISFACTION AND ITS IMPLICATIONS

The term *consumer satisfaction,* while part of America's service delivery vernacular for decades, is taking on new and broader significance in the 1990s. The current focus is on quality of service from the consumer's point of view. Therefore, providers are asking whether the creation of a core survey instrument could help today's more educated, sophisticated, and demanding consumers compare and make informed choices about their care. Health care consumers are free to choose from a menu of health plans, hospitals, doctors, and therapists. Education consumers are able to choose schools that meet their standards and vote against, lobby, and persuade those that do not. Leebov and Scott (1994) identify desired features of a consumer-directed health care organization—features that can apply to any organization:

- How well organizations manage to instill a commitment to customer service in every employee;
- How well executives and managers at all levels enlist every manager, physician, and employee in patient retention strategies that have personal meaning for everyone involved;
- How well the organization listens to its customers and makes continuous improvements with the goal of ever-improving levels of customer satisfaction;
- How well customer service commitment can be translated into actions, processes, and performance tracking that everyone understands, shares responsibility for, and embraces wholeheartedly;
- How seriously the organization's leadership is invested in developing employees who excel in fulfilling customer needs and meeting complex challenges of today's changing health care environment. [p. 5]

Consumer Reports surveys and analyzes virtually every consumer good and service that are available in the United States and has for the last several decades been the final arbiter for many consumers on what product, brand, or model to buy. Similarly, the American Association of Retired Persons has embarked on evaluating managed care companies with the expectation that the "top three" that meet this association's criteria of affordability, quality, and service orientation will be endorsed and perhaps supported by the millions of members. Health care organizations, schools, and universities are shifting their attention away from outdoing their competitors toward satisfying their customers. The Forum Corporation (1992) provides several examples of current business philosophy that can serve to set the tone for consumer-oriented care:

- The winners are companies that have learned that the best way to become externally focused and internally aligned is to focus their organizations on the customer . . . The externally focused, internally aligned organization will dominate the future. Put even stronger, this is the only kind of organization that will survive the future.
- Everyone has to be linked to our customer one way or another . . . A customer

driven point of view ensures the survival of the corporation. Those who do will prosper and grow. Those who don't will die. [p. 5]

WHY A CONSUMER SATISFACTION SURVEY?

In his article on how to assess quality of care, Donabedian (1988) stated, "Patient satisfaction may be considered to be one of the desired outcomes of care, even an element in health status itself. It is futile to argue about the validity of patient satisfaction as a measure of quality. Whatever its strengths and limitations as an indicator of quality, information about patient satisfaction should be as indispensable to assessments of quality as to the design and management of health care systems" (p. 743). As has been argued in the prior section, service excellence, regardless of work setting, requires a client-first philosophy. In the domain of health care, Rao and Goldsmith (1991) identified at least seven factors in the professional literature that compel providers to adopt a satisfaction survey as an integral part of an information management system:

- Standards of accreditation bodies (e.g., CARF... The Rehabilitation Accreditation Commission [CARF], Joint Commission on Accreditation of Health Care Organizations [JCAHO], and ASHA Professional Services Board [ASHA PSB])
- Industry dictate (e.g., consumer lobby, case managers)
- Component of risk management programs
- Component of institutional marketing programs
- Component of program/service evaluation
- Research on consumer needs/patient care perspective
- Component of quality improvement processes

In the education arena, federal and state statutes require a management system that tracks educational attainment and other variables that may affect learning. Similarly, ASHA's PSB and Educational Standards Board both list explicit standards that relate to client satisfaction, and university accrediting bodies require course evaluations which by definition is a type of client satisfaction tool.

Without consumer data, you have only impressions. Scientific and systematic methods can provide constructive and reliable answers to the question "How am I doing?," thereby providing information that can be used to support or change technical or interpersonal behaviors. The "Why survey?" question that the clinician may ask should be obvious to the speech-language pathologist (SLP) who views each intervention as a mini experiment—proposing and testing hypotheses, learning from the results of the testing, and then revising one's behavioral strategies to achieve even better results. Without measurement, the effectiveness of these "mini experiments" is left to subjective impressions. A management principle is that people do what you inspect, not necessarily what you expect. A survey inspects "how I'm doing."

Consumer-Oriented Dimensions of Quality

Evidence abounds that consumer satisfaction and its ties to improving quality are the subject of heightened interest within the current service delivery system. According to Packer-Tursman (1994), major initiatives in health care include the following:

- At the federal level, the Agency for Health Care Policy and Research (AHCPR) is likely to play a major role in its efforts to support the design, field testing, and dissemination of a standardized core consumer survey instrument nationwide.

- At the state level, the Minnesota Health Data Institute (MHDI) plans to distribute, on a statewide basis, one million copies of a report outlining the results of its 1995 consumer survey.

- Within the managed care industry, the National Committee for Quality Assurance (NCQA), issued a standardized Annual Member Health Care Survey targeting enrollees of managed care organizations. The survey includes information on health status and incorporates questions from existing questionnaires.

- In the broader health care community, the Picker Institute, located at Beth Israel Hospital in Boston, was created in 1987 to examine the fact and fiction of consumer satisfaction. The Picker Institute plans to release a continuity of care instrument in the near future. This is in addition to the Institute's current patient-based instruments, including one for inpatient care, ambulatory care, and pediatric care.

- Among employer-purchaser efforts, the work of Xerox Corp., GTE Corp., and Digital Equipment Corp. has resulted in an instrument called the Consumer Health Plan Value Survey.

In addition, the American Group Practice Association (AGPA) is working to heighten the science of patient satisfaction surveys (in American Medical News, 1996).

- The effort allows groups to use a standardized satisfaction measure and then "benchmark" their ratings against groups of similar size and makeup. Already the AGPA database contains survey results from over 12,000 patients visiting 328 physicians in 30 specialties.

Finally, the University Health System Consortium (UHC), an alliance of 70 academic health centers and affiliated institutions across the United States, report on the 5-year history of patient satisfaction data sent to each hospital participating in the project (Drachman,1996). The UHC project is intended to help member organizations

- identify peers with high satisfaction ratings;
- pinpoint the best practices responsible for highest ratings; and
- adapt these best practices to their own patient care settings.

The consortium has attempted to establish benchmarks of best practices across the hospitals for each key aspect of care targeted in the survey.

In the early 1980s, Linder-Petz (1982) established a theory of patient satisfaction and identified 10 dimensions that reflect quality of care:

- Accessibility/convenience
- Availability of resources
- Continuity of care
- Efficacy of care
- User-friendly explanations of costs/financial services

- Humaneness
- Professionalism and respect for privacy of information gathering
- Information giving/patient education
- Pleasantness of surroundings
- Quality of care/competence of providers

The uniqueness of the above quality dimensions is that this comprehensive list includes categories that include amenities of care typically noted in guest relations of a hotel culture with several queries regarding quality of care and clinical competence noted in a health care milieu. By the mid-1980s, most U.S. health care providers had begun surveying patients to estimate their level of satisfaction. The surveying process became more sophisticated when providers realized that such tools could help to meet new standards of provider accountability as well as assist providers in improving processes of service delivery. Patient feedback eventually became a powerful barometer of how well providers were rendering what consumers "expected."

In the late 1980s, many health care organizations were conducting satisfaction surveys with positive results, yet anecdotal evidence suggested otherwise. According to Packer-Tursman (1994), the Picker Commonwealth Program for Patient-Centered Care was created in 1987 to account for the discrepancy. In the early course of their work, researchers determined that consumer satisfaction measures, while containing useful information, also contained the following flaws:

- Invariably high scores for health care providers from most patients (perhaps due to low expectations or gratitude for recovery);
- Information from low satisfaction scores that was usually not actionable (data indicating dissatisfaction that provided no information on what needed to be changed or improved).

As a result, these researchers set out in 1987 to explore patients' needs and concerns, as defined by the patients themselves. The researchers conducted focus groups with patients and their family members, reviewed the pertinent literature, and consulted with other health professionals. They found that patients did not focus on the amenities of care, but instead focused on issues of clinical relevance. They categorized their concerns in the following dimensions of care:

- Access
- Physical care, comfort, and alleviation of pain
- Emotional support
- Coordination of care and integration of services
- Involvement of family and friends
- Respect for patients' values, preferences, and expressed needs
- Transition and continuity
- Communication between patients and providers

The literature on patient satisfaction surveys and development of standardized questionnaires has burgeoned in this decade (McDaniel & Nash, 1990). High levels of resources (e.g., consultation, staff time, data analysis, materials, and postage) are now devoted to surveying patients in health care. Yet the same study that praised the widespread use of patient satisfaction surveys (McDaniel & Nash, 1990) also reported that only two of ten health care organizations were using survey data regularly as feedback to administrative and clinical departments.

Universities have also targeted consumer satisfaction as a primary goal. Higher education in the United States is a major service provider consisting of 2,200 four-year colleges and universities that now enroll 8.8 million students, including 5.2 million full-time undergraduates (*Newsweek,* 1996). As the cost of providing education continues to escalate, higher education will be the most expensive service most families will ever buy, thus creating a "buyer beware" situation. Commercially available college guides compare universities by region on such variables as cost, acceptance rate of new students, the average scores on admission tests, the grade point average of admitted students, the percentage of admitted students who complete a degree program, student-teacher ratio/class size, disciplines taught, research dollars awarded, percentage of students accepted into graduate programs, percentage of students achieving a doctorate, percentage of doctoral-level faculty, and amount of scholarship money granted in a given year to a percentage of students. Universities are compared and ranked regionally and nationally, and universities that stay in the top ten tout the results to prospective parents and students. Once students are admitted into a university program, the "consumer criteria "change dramatically from "Do I want to go?" to "Do I want to stay?" or "How well are students' needs being met?". Many student evaluation instruments rate teaching on a 5-point scale from strongly agree to strongly disagree, which is similar in design to the consumer satisfaction surveys found in health care. The education survey instruments may include the following common dimensions of a standard college course:

- Clarity of objectives
- Agreement of objectives with assignments
- Class management
- Presentation of course content
- Preparation of course content
- Mastery of content
- Interest and enthusiasm
- Respect and concern for students
- Availability for consultation
- Ability to encourage discussion, questions, and participation
- Fairness of grading
- Effectiveness of teaching

In addition, students are often afforded the opportunity to provide commentary on strengths and weaknesses of the course, and any suggestions to improve the course. Today, most college and university students are asked to rate the class and teacher at the end of each term's semester.

Methods for Measuring Consumer Satisfaction

To advance service delivery, the SLP needs to regularly identify discrepancies between current reality and the ideal and take appropriate actions to bridge the gap. To assess and improve service delivery at every level of the organization, one must know what sources of information to tap from each of the key consumer groups. In health care, these groups include patients, families/caregivers, physicians, employees, and payers. In education, they include students, principals/deans, employees, regulators, and parents.

According to Leebov and Scott (1994), the success with which your organization assesses the satisfaction of these key consumers depends on how well you can answer these questions:

- What are your current assessment methods, both formal and informal?
- How effective are your current methods in promoting corrective actions?
- To what extent are results effectively shared with people who can act on them to improve service both at job function levels and across function lines?
- To improve your systems for assessing satisfaction, do you focus on identifying priorities? Identifying customer groups? Identifying which evaluation systems or methods work best?
- How effective are your methods for measuring performance at critical points in service processes?
- Which processes have the greatest impact on patient satisfaction?
- What are critical control points in those processes?
- What methods need to be installed to monitor these processes so that you have the data needed to identify improvement priorities and monitor progress?

Once you have targeted service improvements within your organization and the dimensions of service that are to be measured, you can begin to address measurement of consumer satisfaction. Measurement activities must focus on consumers' criteria for judging service excellence, and there are numerous methods for assessment. Service quality, like beauty, often is in the eye of the beholder. Even when your data tells you that you have 98% on-time service delivery, if the patient does not perceive your service as timely, it is not! A key strategy, then, should be to improve consumer perceptions of quality of care. Note the emphasis on *expectations* and *perceptions*. If you have ever been to a Disney park and waited in line for an amusement ride, you were immediately aware of Disney's emphasis on expectations and perceptions. The cartoon character tells you that the wait for this ride will be 25 minutes. However, the process is designed to exceed your expectations. Most likely, you got on the ride in 20 minutes, which was shorter than you expected. To monitor consumer perceptions in your organization, surveys, face-to-face or telephone interviews, and focus groups work well.

Surveys

Health care setting. Rao and Goldsmith (1991) summarized various methods for surveying consumer satisfaction in health care (Table 4–1).

Table 4–1. Methods of Surveying Consumer Satisfaction

QUESTIONNAIRE FORMAT	ADMINISTRATION
Multiple Choice Questions	Mail
Yes/No Questions	Telephone
Rating Scales	Manual Distribution and Immediate Return
Open-Ended Questions	Manual Distribution and Mail Return
	Face-to-Face Interview
TIME FRAMES	
Retrospective	PATIENT TRACKING
Concurrent	Anonymous
Prospective	Identified by Name
	Coded
FREQUENCY OF USE	Identified by Program
Continuous	
Monthly	RESPONSIBILITY FOR GATHERING DATA
Quarterly	Administration
Intermittent/Sporadic	Communications/Media Relations
	Outcomes Management/Program Evaluation
SUBJECT SAMPLE	Consumer Affairs
All discharged patients	Quality Improvement
All patients receiving × visits	Separate clinical department
Random Sample	
Stratified Random Sample	

The instrument used, the *ASHA Consumer Satisfaction Measure* (CSM; 1989) (Appendix 4-A) uses a 5-point rating scale ranging from strongly agree (rating of 5) to strongly disagree (rating of 1). The *CSM* was mailed to all discharged patients who had received at least a minimum of 5 visits per week. The measure was coded with the patient's medical record number to track rate of return and pair results with the patient's diagnosis, length of stay, functional outcomes, and associated costs of care.

Table 4–2 summarizes SLP departmental data captured over a 5-year period. On a 5-point scale, the responses on the *ASHA Consumer Satisfaction Measure* (1989) that were either a 4 or a 5 (i.e., "agree" or "strongly agree") ranged from 75% (SLP planned ahead and the program was well managed) to 95% (the SLP was prepared and organized). In the unsatisfactory area (i.e., scores of 1 [strongly disagree] or 2 [disagree]) the range was from 0 (n = 4 items) to 5% (length & frequency of services). The comment section was usually not completed; however, when comments were added, 95% were complimentary. Negative comments, though infrequent, were given due consideration, and when deemed appropriate, acted upon. For example, comments received regarding patient privacy and confidentiality were investigated. It was found that visitors noted that SLP staff had occasionally been talking about other patients in the SLP office and reception area. Staff were counseled and the policy at present is that no patient discussion is to be conducted in the SLP reception area. Favorable comments were always shared with staff and exceptional service recognized via the performance appraisal process and the organization's employee recognition program. An interesting phenomenon was consistently observed via the comments from former patients over the 5-year period. The most positive comments about particular SLPs pertained to post-discharge follow-up (a quality improvement monitor requiring telephone follow-up with former

Table 4–2. National Rehabilitation Hospital SLP Service Customer Satisfaction:1990–1994*

CONSUMER SATISFACTION MEASURE ITEM	STRONGLY AGREE (5)	= AGREE (4)	NEUTRAL (3)	DISAGREE (2)	STRONGLY DISAGREE (1)	N/A
1a. Timely scheduling	55%	37%	2%	.5%	1 %	4.5%
b. Seen on time	49	41	3	2	.5	4.5
2a. I am better	53	33	7	1	.5	5.5
b. I have benefited	54	35	5	1	.5	4.5
3a. Support staff courtesy	59	34	3	.5	0	3.5
b. SLP courteous and pleasant	68	27	2	0	0	3
c. Considered my special needs	55	34	4	.5	0	16.5
d. Included my family	51	29	5	1	.5	13.5
4a. SLP prepared and organized	64	31		0	0	4
b. Services explained	60	34	3	0	0	3
c. Experienced and knowledgeable	66	26	3	0	0	5
5a. Health and safety precautions	55	34	3	.5	0	7.5
b. Environment clean and pleasant	56	37	3	.5	0	3.5
c. Environment quiet and distraction free	49	40	3	.5	.5	
d. Building easy to get to	54	32	4	1	.5	8.5
6a. Length and frequency of service	47	40	6	4	1	2
b. SLP planned ahead	45	31	9	2	0	3
c. Program well managed	45	31	9	2	0	3
7a. Services were satisfactory	62	32	2	0	.5	3.5
b. Would seek services again	62	30	4	1	.5	2.5
c. Would recommend to others	62	27	3	.5	.5	7

* Number of surveys mailed—1893; number of surveys returned—733; return rate—39%.

patients 30 days after discharge to ascertain communication status, follow-through in treatment tasks, and evidence of satisfactory community reentry). Patients and families uniformly extolled the concern of the SLP for staying in touch after the patient was no longer in his/her care. From year to year over the 5-year period all items except the "length and frequency of service" yielded consistent results. Not surprisingly, as care became more "managed," patients *perceived* their therapy regime as insufficient, stating for example, that they had not recovered as much as they had *expected*.

As described above, the person responsible for the survey's dissemination, retrieval, and analysis of the data must also assure that the following actions routinely and systematically occur:

- Display and/or highlight patient satisfaction results in multiple forums
- Hold SLP staff meetings and document minutes

- Capture and document comments in staff performance appraisals
- Display in SLP reception area or other area open to consumers
- Submit annual SLP review to administration
- Include in employee newsletter
- Communicate results in state speech-language-hearing association newsletter
- Circulate in organization's marketing and media materials
- Merge SLP patient satisfaction data with organization's aggregated clinical outcomes data
- Document follow-up on feedback as part of continuous quality improvement and risk management efforts
- Use data to improve existing programs and to identify new programs
- Use data by year, by SLP, or by program to compare results and identify trends

Consumers of SLP services are asking, "Will I get the services I want?" According to recent data collected by ASHA's Task Force on Treatment Outcome and Cost Effectiveness, the answer is a resounding "Yes" (*ASHA*, 1995). Using the *ASHA Consumer Satisfaction Measure* (*CSM;* 1989), the Task Force contacted 102 purchasers of the ASHA instrument. Thirteen SLP organizations (11 hospitals and 2 universities) provided 1993–1994 data on 538 consumers. Similar to the National Rehabilitation's Hospital experience, the results showed an extremely high level of consumer satisfaction for almost every aspect of their clinical experience. At least 90% of consumers agreed or strongly agreed with 18 of the 21 satisfaction parameters. Most encouragingly, 98% of respondents agreed that, overall, program services were satisfactory.

In an earlier study, Rao, Goldsmith, Wilkerson, and Hildebrandt (1992) asked the question: How does consumer satisfaction as measured by the *ASHA CSM* (1989) compare to clinical outcomes (e.g., "communication") as measured by the *Functional Independence Measure* (*FIM;* Research Foundation, SUNY, 1993). The authors hypothesized that the most satisfied patients with the SLP services would be those who had gained the most from the rehabilitation process in terms of communication skills. Rao et al. (1992) found that ASHA CSM ratings did not correlate with FIM ratings. Even when a patient is discharged from a rehabilitation facility with a severe disability, the perception that the SLP was well prepared, friendly, and professional speaks to quality care and an overall favorable impression of the organization in general and the profession of speech-language pathology in particular.

Dull, Lansky, and Davis (1994) conducted a study to evaluate a patient satisfaction survey to determine its usefulness. Over the course of 18 months, the research staff of the Legacy Health System in Portland, Oregon was charged with evaluating how well the patient satisfaction survey was meeting the needs of its hospital staff, and if needed, redesigning the patient survey process. The study addressed several questions:

1. Who currently uses the results of patient satisfaction surveys (key stakeholders)?
2. What are their objectives for carrying out such a project (goals)?
3. What aspects of the survey process are essential to its success (requirements)?
4. What survey results are useful (results of interest)?
5. Once the results are reviewed, how are they used (intervention)?

Table 4–3. Key Consumer Groups: Goals, Requirements, Results of Interest, and Interventions

	HOSPITAL ADMINISTRATORS	RESEARCHERS	PRACTITIONERS	PATIENTS
Goals	Marketing Public relations Risk management Employee morale General patient satisfaction	Rigorous methods Increased knowledge Validation of other studies Measure change	Salary increases Promotions Satisfied patients Creative problem solving	Improved future care Improved community resource Community pride
Requirements	Inexpensive Informative Effective uses Timely	Sensitive Unbiased Valid Reliable	Timely Relevant Informative Effective	Easy to complete Comprehensible
Results of Interest	Survey comments Highlighted results	Research methods Statistical results	Positive/ negative comments Satisfaction with health service	Completed questionnaire Changes in care due to response
Interventions	Design institution-al changes Respond to indi-vidual negative comments	Evaluate services Incorporate ser-vices	Design solutions Implement	Provide opinion via focus groups

SOURCE: Adapted with permission, Dull. V.T., Lansky, D., & Davis, D. (1994). Evaluating a patient satisfaction survey for maximum benefit. *Journal of Quality Improvement.* 20(8), 444–453.

Table 4.3 summarizes the goals, requirements, results of interest, and interventions for four stakeholder groups. Each cell in the table illustrates the varying needs of these stakeholders. With a redesigned survey to answer each of the above questions for each stakeholder group, Dull et al. (1994) reported a number of changes. Because the majority of administrators and managers voiced concerns about lag time between questionnaire receipt and reporting, an infrared optical mark reader and bar code reader were purchased. This allowed administrators and managers to generate reports in days or weeks rather than months, and to perform major analyses by patient group, disease, clinical procedure, physician, or utilization attributes. In addition, they also streamlined the report to include a graphical display to summarize all mean results with confidence levels on one page. Finally, they created different versions of the patient satisfaction questionnaire for different diagnostic categories. The following are examples of patient care and process changes that occurred over a 16-month period:

- Positive comments are published in the employee newsletter, recognizing services or employees.
- A hospital-wide campaign was begun to decrease unnecessary noise and measure subsequent changes in ratings by patient floor.
- Housekeeping staff began introducing themselves to patients before cleaning

rooms and now leave calling cards when a patient is out of the room to let them know that their room has been cleaned in their absence.

- Responding to patient requests, phlebotomists now wash their hands in clear view of patients before drawing blood to demonstrate concern with hygiene. (Previously, they had washed their hands after drawing blood from patients, so their practices were never seen by the next patient.)

- Staff nurses now give detailed and exact instructions to on-call nurses to clearly state the department's quality expectations so that patient satisfaction is maintained.

- Some nursing units instituted follow-up phone calls to patients' homes 2 days after discharge to check on any problems or concerns about taking medications or managing pain levels.

Face-To-Face or Telephone Interviews

Post-discharge interviews, yielding both quantitative and qualitative data, can involve talking to randomly selected patients or to all former patients within a given period of time. This is an increasingly common practice in the health care industry and not only nets valuable feedback but also enhances consumer loyalty. Acute care facilities typically conduct a follow-up telephone interview within 2 weeks of discharge with queries also regarding health status, compliance with instructions, and overall satisfaction with the hospital stay. Rehabilitation facilities typically conduct a follow-up telephone interview within 90 days of discharge with specific queries regarding functional status, satisfaction, evidence of community reentry, and use of equipment. An acute rehabilitation survey of a random sample of patients discharged from specific programs (e.g., stroke and brain injury) has been in use for 5 years at the National Rehabilitation Hospital in Washington, D.C. (NRH, 1991). Table 4–4 details the questions that constituted the survey.

Results related to question #3 (involvement in treatment decisions) in fiscal year 1994 reflected a 92% satisfaction level, whereas the fiscal year 1995 results of 77% were markedly below the expectation. A number of reasons might have accounted for this change, such as decreased length of stay or reduced staffing. As a result, the hospital

---

Table 4–4. Consumer Satisfaction Survey Following Acute Rehabilitation Stay

---

1. Overall, were you satisfied with your stay at NRH?
2. Did the rehabilitation services and training you received at NRH prepare you for your return to the community?
3. Were you (and/or your family) involved in decisions about your rehabilitation treatment?
4. Are your current living arrangements in line with your discharge plan?
5. Have you received and been able to use satisfactorily the equipment recommended or ordered by your rehabilitation team?
6. Are you satisfied with your present level of participation in activities outside your home (e.g., work, social and leisure activities, school, community activities)?
7. How many days per week do you leave home for an activity not related to medical needs (e.g., work, social and leisure activities, school, community activities)?

SOURCE: National Rehabilitation Hospital. Ninety Day Post-Discharge Follow-up Form (1991). Washington DC. Reprinted with permission.

implemented a new policy that every patient was to be scheduled to attend both the initial and intermediate team conference. Six months after the policy became effective, post-discharge satisfaction data revealed a 98% patient satisfaction with involvement in decisions about rehabilitation.

Focus Groups

Focus groups provide an excellent forum for gathering information from a variety of consumers. Focus groups are carefully designed and facilitated group discussions intended to assess perceptions held by a particular consumer group and test responses to new ideas and approaches. As a patient feedback device, focus groups can be used to learn about consumers' experiences with an organization and their suggestions for improvement. Patient focus groups can also be used to explore what is important to consumers so that the organization can develop appropriate survey questions. A sample focus group query is to determine the consumer weight placed on a given service and then to elicit feedback on how well the organization has delivered on that service:

- How important is this question to you: "When I called to make an appointment, phones were answered promptly."?
- How good are we at answering the phone promptly when you call to make an appointment?

When you measure perceptions of service excellence, you are measuring service attributes that are important to your consumers. Figure 4–1 shows the relationship between the importance of a given service attribute and the satisfaction rating of that attribute as perceived by the consumer (Leebov & Scott, 1994).

Using this grid, the SLP is able to plot the data received from surveys, face-to-face interviews, and focus groups and examine the results to help identify improvement priorities. For example;

- Quadrant #1 (high importance/low performance): Patients may really want to be seen in a timely manner, yet SLP staff usually start sessions late. This is a competitive weakness and should be a high priority in changing staff behavior.
- Quadrant #2 (high importance/high performance): Patients may expect your staff to be polite and friendly and they especially value the fact that these traits are always present in your staff. This is your competitive strength.
- Quadrant #3 (low importance/high performance): The SLP staff may spend significant time, effort, and money to ensure that the surroundings and ambiance in the waiting room are fashionable when your data demonstrate that patients actually want the environment to be safe and comfortable. In fact, patients may feel uncomfortable in surroundings that appear more decorative than functional. Here your performance is superior, but it is also irrelevant.
- Quadrant #4 (low importance/low performance): Although the data suggests that your performance is not high, patients also do not have high expectations or place much importance on these items. Your observational data have found that even though this is a JCAHO requirement, your staff may not always wear name badges. Your patients, however, already familiar with their SLP, really do not care about the name badge requirement.

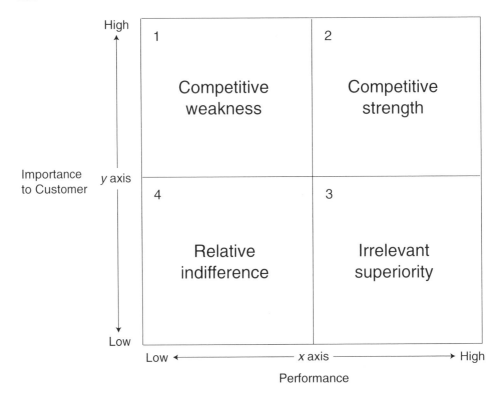

Figure 4–1. Importance-performance (satisfaction) matrix of service factors

SOURCE: Leebov, W., & Scott, G. (1994). *Service Quality Improvement: The Customer Satisfaction Strategy for Health Care.* American Hospital Publishing, Inc., Chicago, IL.

Clearly, management must focus first on those attributes that are considered important to customers, but are rated low in satisfaction.

University setting. Evaluation of SLP graduates also is an essential aspect of measuring satisfaction. In fact, the Educational Standards Board (ESB) of the American Speech-Language-Hearing Association (ASHA, 1994) requires implementation of a comprehensive evaluation plan of the quality and effectiveness of the professional performance of a training program's graduates for at least a 5-year period.

Blosser (1996) describes a tripronged evaluation process to assess students' performance during the externship experience in graduate school. In the first aspect of evaluation, the on-site clinical supervisor evaluates the student's performance at mid-term and at the end of the semester. The supervisor's perceptions of the student's strengths and weaknesses are documented. The midterm evaluation is used to recalibrate the student's externship experience for the remainder of the semester. If problems are noted or if the student's performance exceeds expectations, objectives can be established for modifying assignments, altering instructional approaches, or providing additional supports or resources. It is at this point that interventions from the university/liaison can be implemented, if indicated. The results of the end-of-semester evaluations are collated and shared with faculty prior to the beginning of the next semester in both oral and written format. Results are used to determine curricular modifications, timing the presentation of information, planning on-campus clinical experiences, and placing students at sites in the future.

The second and third aspects of the consumer satisfaction assessment process involve obtaining students' evaluations of the quality of the extern experience and the quality of supervision by the site supervisor. Two different instruments are used because the results are used in different ways. Students complete a computerized, open-ended questionnaire consisting of the following questions:

1. What type of cases did you work with at this site?
2. Did you feel your academic training prepared you for this work?
3. What academic/clinical program changes do you suggest to better prepare students for externing at this site in the future?
4. Did you feel adequately supervised by your on-site supervisor?
5. What indirect service did you provide (e.g., staffings, family conferences)?
6. Were these indirect experiences valuable?
7. What is your overall evaluation of this experience?
8. How might this experience have been more valuable to you?
9. Should the university continue to use this extern site?
10. Would you accept a position at this site if it were offered?

This information is reviewed by the clinic director and made available for students who are seeking information for future extern site placements. Information is also shared with faculty at two critical time periods: when faculty are asked to approve student placements to specific sites, and when curricular revisions are being discussed.

The third aspect of the evaluation process is students' evaluation of the on-site supervisors and the quality of supervision. Students rate supervisors on 13 items using a 7-point rating scale. The information gained about the supervisors' strengths and needs are shared with the supervisors and in discussions with the program director. Most importantly, information is also used to determine if the site supervisors need resources, materials, or inservice instruction to support or develop skills in the area of clinical supervision. It is also used to determine informally if students' personalities might be better suited to working with one supervisor versus another at a setting and is often used to negotiate future placements.

Employer evaluation of graduate students offers a different view that is seldom sought or reported in the professional literature. Pannbacker and Lass (1996) contend that, "In this era of focus on accountability in Speech-Language Pathology and Audiology, training programs should have an evaluation plan to assess the professional performance of its graduates in the workplace. An important component of this plan is evaluation of graduates by their employers" (p. 1). Employers can provide feedback on the individual Clinical Fellow and comparative data of that individual post-graduate with SLPs in the workplace from other training programs (Ryan & Hodson, 1992). According to Pannbacker and Lass (1996), this feedback is necessary to make appropriate changes to improve the curriculum.

Employer feedback is also important because of the apparent schism between academic training programs and clinical service delivery programs. A survey by Henri (1994) of directors and supervisors of community speech and hearing clinics indicates that preparation of recent SLP graduates is falling short of expectations in the workplace. For example, "many employers believed today's graduates have considerable difficulty moving from theory to practice" (p. 45). Sanger, Hux, and Griess (1995) surveyed educators about their opinions of SLP services in the schools. The results indicated that educators have positive opinions about SLP services, although there was some uncertainty about the SLP's roles with certain student groups (e.g., high school students with attention difficulties) and the adequacy of the SLP's training in behavior management, reading, multicultural issues, and teaching English as a second language. Finally, in a survey of ASHA ESB-accredited programs, Allen (1995) found that on-site supervisors believed that second-year graduate students were more ready and capable of entering the work force than did off-site supervisors, who felt that the students needed greater levels of assistance in nearly every skill area. Henri (1994) suggested, "to ensure that programs continue to adjust to the changes and requests of different work environments, surveys concerning the quality of graduate student preparedness should be conducted at specified intervals by graduate programs. Employees, as well as former students, should be surveyed regularly" (p. 46).

Public school setting. The public school setting is another important venue for surveying consumer satisfaction in Speech-Language Pathology. School districts use a number of provider options for SLP services. Most have their own employees and depending on the size of the district, there could be as little as one SLP providing districtwide services, to as many as hundreds of SLPs working in a variety of districtwide buildings and programs. Some school districts' contract with intermediate agencies, such as boards of cooperative educational services for their services, and still others may contract with private practices.

The notions of "customer" and "consumer satisfaction" in schools is difficult and unfamiliar to many SLPs; thus, there is resistance to viewing work in these terms. Traditionally, the student is seen as the one and only customer . . . and in fact most often referred to as the "client" and not the "customer." However, when one is forced into the customer/provider framework of thinking, there is expanded awareness of the cadre of "customers" whose satisfaction is critical to the work of school SLPs.

- taxpayers
- parents
- the school board
- administrators
- teachers
- students
- reimbursement/funding agencies (e.g., Education Departments, Medicaid)

The following scenario published in *Phi Delta Kappan,* an educational journal widely read by administrators and teachers, gives us an idea of measures of consumer satisfaction that school SLPs should be conducting. Raynes, Snell, and Sailor (1991), in their article titled "A Fresh Look at Categorical Programs for Children with Special Needs," discuss a speech service provided to a student every Tuesday and Thursday at

"Customer"	Areas of Satisfaction to be Measured
Teachers	Scheduling of services Understanding of the therapeutic service: What is therapy? Expectations: "As a result of SLP services, what do I expect the student to do in my classroom?" Service delivery model: should services be push-in, pull-out, consultation, etc.? Competence and conduct of SLP
Student	Goal identification: "Was I a partner in developing goals and objectives?" Expectation: "How will I know I am successful?" "When will I be dismissed?"
Administrator	Scheduling of services Service delivery model Participation of SLP on building level teams Timeliness of evaluation and progress reports Competence and conduct of SLPs
Parent	Understanding of child's SLP disorder Expectations of the service Competence and conduct of SLP

Table 4–5. Consumers and Areas of Satisfaction to Be Measured

10:20 A.M. The student is working on specific speech objectives such as "object identification, articulation, and blowing" as directed by the Individualized Education Plan (IEP). According to teachers, the student was making no progress in her ability to send and receive verbal information—crucial skills in middle school. Further, the student's lack of communication interfered significantly with her ability to maintain friendships with peers. In the above vignette, the consumers and the consequent areas of satisfaction to be measured are illustrated in Table 4–5.

Consumer satisfaction instruments can be very simple, such as this open-ended questionnaire developed by a building level SLP to determine teachers' understanding of SLP services and teachers' satisfaction with service models (Ryan, 1995):

1. This year, did you feel as if you knew why your students were receiving "speech"? Y/N

   If no, would you like to know? Y/N

   How can I best provide you with this information?

2. Do you feel your students knew why they needed to come to "speech"? Y/N

3. When a screening or an evaluation took place, did you feel you knew the results in a timely manner? Y/N

   If no, what would be the best way to get that information to you?

   _____written

   _____verbal

   _____conference

   _____other ideas?

4. When we conferenced with parents, did you feel that the information I gave them was in a manner that they were able to understand? Y/N

Do you have any suggestions for the future?

5. Next year, if there are children in your classroom who will be receiving support for "language needs," would you be interested in a "push-in" service delivery model where I would provide service within the classroom (e.g., I would come in during language arts, social studies, etc. and create my service around the academics.)? Y/N

If "push-in" is not your style, would you like me to coordinate treatment in my room with the academics (concepts, vocabulary, etc.) that you are working on at that time? Y/N

Or do you prefer that your children come to my room and just do my things? Y/N

6. Is there anything else you would like to comment on?

Some school districts design districtwide surveys to measure teacher/staff, parent/guardian, or student satisfaction. They may use their own resources for survey design or may choose to contract with consultants who design and pilot surveys and opinion polls prior to releasing them for district use. Most school district-designed surveys seek input on a wide range of topics such as transportation, facilities, home-school communication, and curriculum. Questions dealing with speech-language pathology may appear in a more general context, as specified in Table 4–6.

Measuring consumer satisfaction of SLP services in the schools is still in its infancy. While many school district SLP programs have collected data pertaining to numbers of students served, frequency of service, duration of service, disorder categories addressed, number of students dismissed, and service delivery model(s) used, few have formally addressed consumer satisfaction. As discussed earlier, Sanger et al. (1995) surveyed 628 educators in four states on various attributes of SLPs and SLP services, including service delivery models, role(s) of SLPs in the schools, academic preparation, participation on teams, and perceived effectiveness of services. While the survey itself has not been standardized, it presents itself as a model for targeting various consumer groups in local school districts.

Other Opportunities for Measuring Consumer Satisfaction

The question, "Will I get the services I want?" is increasingly being heard by SLPs and as a consequence being asked routinely as part of outcomes measurement activities. An illustration of a state-based SLP effort in outcomes measurement can be found in Harrison's discussion of state-based initiatives (Chapter 23 of this text). In 1993 the Florida Speech-Language-Hearing Association (FLASHA) embarked on an aggressive statewide campaign to gather outcomes data for a range of diagnostic categories across various clinical settings in the state. On its data collection form, two queries relate to client satisfaction:

Table 4–6. "How Would You Rate the Level of Support From . . ."		
	ADEQUATE	INADEQUATE
1. Resource room teachers		
2. Social workers		
3. Para-educators		
4. Audiologists		
5. Speech-language pathologists		
6. Occupational therapists		
7. Physical therapists		
8. Deaf educators		
9. Orientation and mobility instructors		
10. School psychologists		

Please give an overall rating of Support Staff by CIRCLING one of the letter grades, A–F below:

A   A–   B+   B   B–   C+   C   C–   D+   D   D–   F

- Do you feel you benefited from this therapy?
- Were you satisfied with the outcome of this therapy?

Both FLASHA and the state health care agency will benefit from learning about consumer satisfaction with SLP services and may begin to mutually analyze the data in terms of cost/benefit analysis and quality care. Frazier (1995), in applying a combined "patient satisfaction survey" and "follow-up survey" approach to analyzing voice outcomes (Appendix 4-B), reported that 32 of 55 (58%) of her patients with voice disorders completed the survey that was mailed 2 months post-discharge. Results related to "satisfaction" queries were as follows:

#5 Did you find the therapy valuable to you? **All of the time?** *69%* **Some of the time** *31%*

#6 Were you satisfied with the service? **Yes** *100%*

#7 Was your appointment time convenient for you? **Yes** *100%*

#8 Was your first visit scheduled in a timely fashion? **Yes** *97%* **No** *3%*

In an innovative approach to coping with the rationing and reengineering of SLP services within the United States, Johnson (1996) described one acute care SLP program's attempt to gather meaningful data regarding the cost effectiveness and quality of SLP services as perceived by a major consumer . . . the referring physician. The SLP staff at Henry Ford Hospital in Detroit, Michigan developed focused surveys for three medical specialty groups: neurologists who might refer persons with communication and swallowing problems due to stroke, pediatricians who might refer children with communication and or swallowing problems, and otolaryngologists who might refer persons with voice or swallowing problems. The results were striking. In essence, the SLP staff posed the question by how the person served would be affected if SLP services were not available as part of the physician's armamentarium of preventative and restorative options. Physicians were asked to rate their degree of satisfaction based on their prior experience with SLP services and then rate the relative weight placed on SLP services. Based on historical data, the SLP staff was able to estimate how many patients per medical specialty would be affected by a reduction in SLP services. Further, Johnson provided conservative estimates of outcomes with and without SLP treatment and obtained physician estimates of a cost/benefit analysis of SLP services. The results of the preliminary study demonstrated extremely high physician satisfaction with SLP services and suggested dramatic savings of health care dollars for each of the three patient populations managed by the three physician specialties. For example, if dysphagia services provided by an SLP in an acute care hospital reduce complications and length of stay by at least 1 day for even 10% of persons with stroke admitted to the facility, the estimated ratio of resource savings versus SLP resources expended was $12 to $1 in the stroke population. Comparable satisfaction and cost-savings data were reported for the voice disordered and pediatric populations as well. If SLP services were rationed at Henry Ford Hospital, physicians would clearly be dissatisfied, patients could be ill-served, costs could escalate, and outcomes could deteriorate.

CONCLUSION

SLPs in every practice setting are increasingly taking an interest in what the various consumers have to say about cost, quality, and various other facets of SLP service delivery. Today, administrators, principals, deans, and other administrative oversight authorities of SLP practice are viewing consumer satisfaction as one of the key "outcome measures" with which to evaluate the benefits, effectiveness, and efficiency of the services we provide. Our stakeholders will continue to seek the "gold standard" in order to benchmark our services. They are seeking answers to a variety of questions such as: "How do we compare to physical therapy?"; "How do we compare to SLPs in similar facilities?"; "How do we compare to other SLPs in the same facility?". In short, our administrative support network is increasingly requiring consumer satisfaction data in order to justify expenditures of staff and resources to retain current budgetary levels.

Educational and health care accrediting bodies such as ASHA's ESB and PSB, CARF, and JCAHO require providers to obtain feedback on the quality of care from patients as well as practitioners. Peters (1996) calls the 1990s the decade of the consumer and elaborates as follows: "There are three ways to build customer loyalty: quality product, excitement, and customer service. The first two are largely short-term, but there is tremendous potential for improvement in the area of customer service." Hence, in this highly competitive, reengineered "show me" decade, the SLP is driven to provide service excellence and at the same time required to measure the continuous pursuit of same with an abandon heretofore exercised in measuring productivity. From a business and marketing perspective, consumer satisfaction takes on added import. In such a competitive marketplace, a happy customer leads to an increased market share. Weisman and Koch (1989) aptly conclude:

> It stands to reason, then, that providers who actively seek and respond to patient opinion will enjoy not only healthier and more satisfied patients, but a more favorable position in today's competitive health care marketplace. Clearly, good quality is good business. [p. 167]

REFERENCES

American Medical News. (1996). *The science of measuring satisfaction.* Chicago, IL: May 20: Author.

Allen, R. (1995). Measuring up to expectancy: Employers rate competencies of new clinicians. *Advance* April 24, 6.

American Speech-Language-Hearing Association. (1989). *ASHA consumer satisfaction measure.* Rockville, MD: Author.

American Speech-Language-Hearing Association. (1994). *Accreditation manual: Educational standards board.* Rockville, MD: Author.

ASHA. (1995, May). Treatment outcome: Our consumers are satisfied. *37*(5), 23–24.

Deming, W.E. (1982). *Out of the crisis.* Cambridge, MA: Massachusetts of Technology, Center for Advanced Engineering Study.

Donabedian, A. (1988). The quality of care: How it can be assessed. *JAMA, 260*:1, 743–748.

Drachman, D. A. (1996). Benchmarking patient satisfaction at academic health centers. *The Joint Commission Journal on Quality Improvement, 22*(5), 359–367.

Dull, V.T, Lansky, D., & Davis, N. (1994). Evaluating a patient satisfaction survey for maximum benefit. *The Joint Commission Journal on Quality Improvement, 20*(8), 444–453.

Forum Corporation. (1992). *Leading the customer focused company: Lessons learned from listening to the voices of leaders.* Forum Corporation, Boston, MA.

Frazier, J. (1995). Outcome study of voice patients. Poster session presented to the annual convention of the American Speech-Language-Hearing Association, Orlando, FL.

Harrison, M. (In Press). State Initiatives. In C. Frattali (Ed.), *Outcomes Measurement in Speech Language Pathology.* New York: Thieme Medical Publishers, Inc.

Henri, B.P. (1994). Graduate student preparation: Tomorrow's challenge. *ASHA, 36*(1), 43–46.

Johnson, A. (1996). SLP outcomes in acute care. Paper presented at the ASHA Leadership Conference, Chicago, IL.

Leebov, W., & Scott, G. (1994). *Service Quality Improvement: The Customer Satisfaction Strategy for Health Care,* American Hospital Publishing, Inc., Chicago, IL.

Linder-Petz, A. (1982). Towards a theory of patient satisfaction. *Social Science and Medicine, 16*(5), 577–582.

McDaniel, C., & Nash, J.G. (1990). Compendium of instruments measuring patient satisfaction with nursing care. *Quality Research Bulletin, 16,* 182–188.

National Rehabilitation Hospital. (1991). Ninety Day Post Discharge Follow-up Form, Washington, DC: Author.

Newsweek. (1996). Those scary college costs. April 29, 52–68.

Packer-Tursman, J. (1994). A report card on quality accountability. *HMO Magazine, 34*(3), 47–53.

Pannbacker, M., & Lass, N. (1996). Ivory tower to the workplace: Employer evaluation of graduates. Paper presented to the annual convention of the American Speech-Language-Hearing Association, Seattle, WA.

Raynes, M., Snell, M., & Sailor, W. (1991). A fresh look at categorical programs for children with special needs. *Phi Delta Kappan, 73*(4), 326–331.

Rao, P., & Goldsmith, T. (1991). How to keep your customer satisfied: Consumer satisfaction measure, Poster session presented to the American Congress of Rehabilitation Medicine, Washington, DC.

Rao, P., Goldsmith, T., Wilkerson, D., & Hildebrandt, L. (1992). How to keep your customer satisfied: Consumer satisfaction survey. *HearSay, 7*(1), 34–44.

Research Foundation, State University of New York. (1993). *Guide for the use of the uniform data set for medical rehabilitation: Version 4.0.* Uniform Data System for Medical Rehabilitation and the Center for Functional Assessment Research.

Ryan, M.E., & Hodson, K.E. (1992). Employer evaluations of nurse graduates: A critical program assessment element. *Journal of Nursing Education, 31*(5), 198–202.

Sanger, D.D., Hux, K., & Griess, K. (1995). Educators opinions about speech language pathology services in schools. *Language, Speech, and Hearing Services in Schools, 26*(1), 75–86.

Weisman, E., & Koch, N. (1989). Progress notes: Special patient satisfaction issue. *Quality Review Bulletin, 15*, June, 166, 167.

FIGURE 2

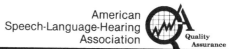

American
Speech-Language-Hearing
Association
Quality
Assurance

Consumer Satisfaction Measure

After answering all items, detach here and return

READ each item carefully and CIRCLE the one answer that is best for you.

SA – Strongly Agree	**N** – Neutral	**SD** – Strongly Disagree
A – Agree	**D** – Disagree	**NA** – Not Applicable

1. **It is important that we see you in a timely manner.**
   A. My appointments were scheduled in a reasonable period of time. SA A N D SD NA
   B. I was seen on time for my scheduled appointments. SA A N D SD NA

2. **It is important that you benefit from Speech-Language Pathology and/or Audiology Services.**
   A. I am better because I received these services. SA A N D SD NA
   B. I feel that I have benefited from speech-language pathology and/or audiology services. SA A N D SD NA

3. **You are important to us; we are here to work with you.**
   A. The support staff (e.g., secretary, transporter, receptionist, assistant) who served me was courteous and pleasant. SA A N D SD NA
   B. The clinician who served me was courteous and pleasant. SA A N D SD NA
   C. Staff considered my special needs (age, culture, education, handicapping condition, eyesight and hearing). SA A N D SD NA
   D. Staff included my family or other persons important to me in the services provided. SA A N D SD NA

4. **Our Speech-Language Pathology and Audiology staff is highly trained and qualified to serve you.**
   A. The clinician was prepared and organized. SA A N D SD NA
   B. The services were explained to me in a way that I could understand. SA A N D SD NA
   C. My clinician was experienced and knowledgeable. SA A N D SD NA

5. **It is important that our environment is secure, comfortable, attractive, distraction free, and easy to reach.**
   A. Health and safety precautions were taken when serving me. SA A N D SD NA
   B. The environment was clean and pleasant. SA A N D SD NA
   C. The environment was quiet and distraction free. SA A N D SD NA
   D. The building and speech-language pathology services were easy to get to. SA A N D SD NA

6. **It is important that we provide you with efficient and comprehensive services.**
   A. I feel that the length and frequency of my service program were appropriate. SA A N D SD NA
   B. My clinician planned ahead and provided sufficient instruction and education to help me retain my skills after my program ended. SA A N D SD NA
   C. I feel that my program was well-managed, involving other services when needed (e.g., teachers, dentist, doctor). SA A N D SD NA

7. **We respect and value your comments.**
   A. Overall, the program services were satisfactory. SA A N D SD NA
   B. I would seek your services again if needed. SA A N D SD NA
   C. I would recommend your services to others. SA A N D SD NA
   D. Check the services you received.
      Speech-Language Pathology [ ]   Audiology [ ]

Comments: _____

Thank you for your time.
CODE [   ] Please staple/seal the questionnaire so that the Center's address is on the outside and return it to us.   © 1989

Source: From *ASHA Consumer Satisfaction Measure,* American Speech-Language-Hearing Association, 1989, Rockville, MD: Author. Reprinted with permission.

MERITER

VOICE THERAPY
Survey

1. Please rate how much your ability to do the following activities has changed **compared to before you started** voice therapy. (circle response)

Activity	Much Worse	Worse	No Change	Better	Much Better	Not Applicable
Talking at home or work	1	2	3	4	5	6
Talking at end of day	1	2	3	4	5	6
Talking in a noisy environment	1	2	3	4	5	6
Singing	1	2	3	4	5	6
Leisure activities	1	2	3	4	5	6
Other (list):	1	2	3	4	5	6

2. Please rate how the **frequency** of your symptoms (voice loss, hoarseness, vocal fatigue, etc.) has changed **compared to before you started** voice therapy. (circle response)

Much More Frequent	More Frequent	No Change	Less Frequent	Much Less Frequent

3. Please rate how the **intensity** of your symptoms (voice loss, hoarseness, vocal fatigue, etc.) has changed **compared to before you started** voice therapy.

Much More Intense	More Intense	No Change	Less Intense	Much Less Intense

4. Please rate how you have followed the instructions and techniques taught by your therapist.

All of the time	Some of the time	None of the time

5. Did you find this therapy valuable to you?

All of the time	Some of the time	None of the time

6. Were you satisfied with our service? ☐Yes ☐No

7. Was your appointment time convenient for you? ☐Yes ☐No

8. Was your first visit scheduled in a timely fashion? ☐Yes ☐No

9. Approximately how many voice therapy sessions did you attend?

1-5	5-10	10-15	15-20	greater than 20

Please list any additional comments: _____

_____

_____

Please feel free to replicate this survey. If you choose to do so, it would be interesting to compare results. Contact Julie Frazier at (608) 267-6174.

CHAPTER 5

Collecting, Analyzing, and Reporting Financial Outcome Data

MICHAEL I. ROLNICK
AND RICHARD M. MERSON

INTRODUCTION

While an understanding of *clinical* outcome data is critical to the delivery of services to individuals with communication and related disorders (Darley, 1982; Frattali, 1992; Frattali, 1993; Goldberg, 1993; Trace, 1995; Wertz, 1993), an analysis of *financial* outcome data may be mandatory for the survival of the profession (Boston, 1994; Colan, 1994; Keatley, Miller, & Mann, 1995; Rolnick, 1996). Health care costs in the past 12 years have escalated from $158 billion dollars in 1980 to well over $473 billion dollars in 1991, or an average increase of 10.5% per year (Statistical Abstracts of the United States, 1994). This has occurred in a fiscal environment in which uncompensated health care costs, health care cost shifting to private insurers, and the uninsured population have increased dramatically. These increases have met with dramatic decreases in potential health care revenues (Statistical Abstracts of the United States, 1994). The clinical services delivered to some 42 million Americans with communication and related disorders will continue to be seriously affected by these fiscal circumstances (Bello, 1994).

It is with considerable concern that we note from the American Speech-Language-Hearing Association Omnibus Survey that only 42% of reporting speech-language pathologists and 29% of audiologists are collecting and reporting treatment or financial outcome data (Slater, 1995). Both clinical and financial outcome data should be collected and integrated using a common tool to answer the financial questions of those who challenge our profession's cost effectiveness and value. It is not enough to know how much improvement occurred or whether our services made a difference; we must also be cost effective and demonstrate the value of our interventions.

In today's health care environment as well as other delivery systems, we are being asked a number of important questions. Boston (1994) summarizes:

The debate on health care reform can be summed up in a single frustratingly complex question: "Who provides what services, to whom, in what settings, for how long, at what cost, to produce what benefit?" [p. 35]

Without aggregate data that reflects case-by-case information, we cannot answer these questions in a meaningful way. For instance, it is important to know the average length of treatment for particular client populations. We should be able to determine the average number of treatments needed to achieve optimal (or acceptable) benefit from treatment. The average cost for our treatment should also be known in a particular service environment. When certain individuals (outliers) exceed the mean values referred to above, we need to have the ability to determine and analyze the reasons for these exceptions.

These pieces of financial information should then be linked to our clients by diagnostic categories. By doing so we can observe and report the differences that exist in our clinical practice patterns as they affect financial outcomes. It is reasonable to expect that the length of stay for one communication disorder will be different from another. Subsequently, the varying costs per case for the treatment of different speech, voice, fluency, language, cognitive-communication, and swallowing disorders will be both identifiable and justified.

This chapter addresses the different aspects of financial data collection, analysis, and reporting. We will familiarize you with the basic terminology and concepts involved in financial outcome analysis as they relate to outcomes data collection and the management of that data in the speech-language pathology environment. Representative examples of financial outcome data are presented and their implications discussed.

DIFFERENTIATING OUTCOMES DATA

In general, outcomes data can be categorized into clinical data and financial data. In this way you can separate two very different but related aspects of a clinical program. Clinical outcomes can be considered in relation to type of client, site of service, type of treatment, differing clinicians, or severity of the presenting disorder. Financial outcomes can also relate to the above variables but with respect to the actual costs involved in obtaining specific clinical outcomes.

Clinical outcome is determined, for example, by comparing an individual's admission severity status with their discharge severity status using a functional outcome measure. The difference between these two values is a functional assessment (Frattali, 1993; Frattali, 1995; Sederer & Dickey, 1996; Seligman, 1995) of improvement or *clinical outcome*. This aspect of change over time in relation to specific variables should not be confused with *clinical efficacy* (Darley, 1982; McReynolds, 1990; Olswang et al., 1990; Pientranton, 1995a; Wertz, 1993), which is a measurement of the effectiveness, efficiency, or effects of a *controlled* treatment or intervention modality in a controlled environment (see Chapter 6 by Olswang).

Financial outcome data relates to the concept of *cost* in relation to the clinical data that has been obtained for the same client or group of clients. Financial outcome includes information on the length of treatment or stay, number of procedures provided, cost per procedure, and subsequent cost per case.

The *length of stay* (LOS) refers to the amount of time a client remains within your treatment program beginning with the first visit and ending with the final contact for which a charge has been generated. The LOS will usually be different for each diagnostic category within your clinical program. The *number of procedures* or treatments provided is the total number of billable contacts generated during the LOS. This number should also differ by diagnosis. *Cost per procedure,* at this point in our discussion, is the actual charge generated for a procedure provided within the LOS. Finally, the *cost per case* is determined by multiplying the cost per procedure by the total number of procedures provided during the length of stay for a particular client.

Assume that Mr. Jones has been referred to your facility for treatment and that you have established an outcomes management system. Your plan is to collect both clinical as well as financial outcome data for the period of time he is under your care. You will first determine his admission status using a clinical outcome measure. When Mr. Jones is discharged you will then use the same measure for discharge assessment. The difference between the two scores will yield a clinical outcome. The amount of time he actually spends in treatment will be his length of stay. The total number of evaluations and treatments will be added to determine the number of procedures provided. Your charges for each of these procedures will then be added to determine the cost per case (the total revenue or charges). Eventually, Mr. Jones 's data will be combined with those of other clients as you develop your data base for aggregate outcome analysis.

Both clinical as well as financial outcome data can be collected and reported as aggregate data to analyze treatment-cost relationships for a comprehensive picture of outcome analysis. In this way, both types of outcome data can serve as invaluable tools in program evaluation and design, and can answer important questions posed by the service delivery industry (Boston, 1994; Eisenberg, 1995; Goldberg, 1993; Sederer & Dickey 1996; Weil, 1995).

COST VERSUS CHARGES

As the service delivery environment have changed, financial terms have been redefined. Traditionally, speech-language pathologists have considered the cost of services to be the amount actually billed to the payer. If, for example, a clinician treated a client with a diagnosis of stuttering for 10 sessions at $50 per session, then the cost was determined to be $500 for that period of intervention. Actually, the $500 would only be a cost to the client or a payer who reimbursed the clinician for that amount. Correctly, the $500 is the amount of gross revenue or charges generated and is not a reflection of the actual costs incurred for providing those services. Furthermore, the revenue charged is very different from the revenue actually collected, as many payers only reimburse a portion of the charges (e.g., usual, customary, or reasonable charges).

Actual cost should be considered as the sum total of financial factors for provision of services, including salary, supplies, rent, and other direct expenses associated with treatment. This category of *direct expenses* is different from those *indirect expenses* incurred when the clinician is working within a business or corporate structure that involves other costs. Administrative and operating expenses that are peripherally related to treatment are examples of indirect expenses. These costs are also considered in determining the actual cost per procedure, which can then be used to calculate the cost per case for a particular diagnosis.

With changes in reimbursement methodologies, many speech-language pathology programs have become *cost centers* rather than *revenue centers*. This is especially true under capitation programs and for services reimbursed by Medicare's prospective payments associated with diagnosis-related groups (DRGs). Under capitation, an agreed-upon fixed dollar amount is given to the provider per enrollee for any and all services that may be provided. Under a prospective payment arrangement, a predetermined fixed payment is made for all clinical services provided to a client for, in the case of Medicare, a particular diagnosis. Regardless of the reimbursement arrangement, the difference between the payment and the costs of providing the services becomes the profit (or loss). If costs exceed the payment, no profit is realized. Even in a fee-for-service payment structure, revenue deductions or contractual allowances may be imposed. This occurs when the payers reimburse at a lower rate than the charges being billed. This shortfall reduces the anticipated gross revenue and interacts with the costs affecting the net income. As a cost center, we must be aware of our direct and indirect costs as they affect our ability to demonstrate a positive "bottom line" or net income in order to remain a viable part of the provision of clinical care within the corporate structure.

Consider a speech-language pathology program that treats a high proportion of Medicare beneficiaries, participates in managed care capitation contracts, services referrals from various fee-for-service indemnity insurance companies, accepts Medicaid recipients, and also treats individuals who can pay out-of-pocket. This *case mix* is typical of many clinical programs in the United States. Increasingly, the charges for treatment become less important than the actual costs of providing that treatment. The program that can track and control direct and indirect costs is able to adjust to a changing case mix as it affects reimbursement.

The continual and systematic collection of financial outcome data relating to costs allows a clinical program to determine the average cost per case for all diagnostic categories. It is important to link these cost data with clinical data to determine *value*. This information, when coupled with clinical outcomes data, can, for example, be analyzed to show the results of cost-cutting initiatives, reengineering, or other attempts to modify clinical service delivery. This approach is threatening to many clinicians (Eisenberg, 1995) who fear that clinical outcome and, therefore, quality of care can be compromised by decreasing costs of providing services. But, collecting both carefully defined financial data, as well as monitoring quality clinical outcomes data, will allow us to obtain the necessary objective information to make appropriate decisions, and to protect the quality of our services to individuals with communication and related disorders.

OUTLIER ANALYSIS

If collecting the average number of treatments provided, length of stay within your program, and actual cost per case are important, you must be able to analyze and account for the individual variations that will occur. Recently the concept of *outlier analysis* has been employed to look at these variances. Any clients who fall outside the parameters of preestablished financial criteria become *outliers*.

For example, if the mean length of stay for 50 clients with vocal fold nodules is 90 days, and 7 of those individuals had a length of stay of 150 days, they are considered to be outliers. The financial component of your outcomes management system should be able to identify specific outliers so that the reasons for their outlier status can be analyzed. There may be appropriate clinical reasons for an extended length of stay. There may also be problems within your program that resulted in these 7 outliers. Your system should be capable of conducting this individual client analysis by diagnostic category, treatment site, and individual clinician. These and other possible factors that could contribute to an individual client's outlier status can then be investigated. If problems are detected, steps can be taken to correct them and thus improve cost effectiveness.

If financial outlier analysis procedures are initiated on an interdisciplinary basis, then speech-language pathologists should link financial data to their clients' clinical outcomes. This linkage may help explain any variances and justify an appropriate intensity of treatment within that interdisciplinary team. Many hospitals are starting to use *service-line management teams* to look at the process of care in specific inpatient populations. These teams of professionals and administrators try to identify duplicative and unnecessary work. They will then eliminate the costs associated with that work. For example, they will scrutinize rehabilitation for dysphagia and other acute-care speech-language pathology services, along with all other hospital services. Your program must have the supporting data to justify the service when this type of outlier analysis begins.

VALUE ANALYSIS

Two types of value analyses are used frequently to influence decision making. These techniques can be employed when a provider or payer seeks to maximize the return on those moneys spent for treatment. *Cost-benefit* and *cost-effectiveness* analyses are two financial techniques commonly used (Boston, 1994; Keatley et al., 1995; Granger et al., 1995).

When both costs (dollars spent) and benefits (dollars saved) are analyzed, a *cost-benefit* analysis is being employed. Either direct costs, indirect costs or both can be factored into the formula. You can also perform this analysis with charges. Using charge per procedure, if a client with dysarthria following a stroke received 10 treatments at $120.00 per treatment, the "cost" would be $1200.00. If this client was able to return to work 3 weeks earlier than expected as a result of her speech improvement, the cost of treatment would be balanced against the economic benefit of an early return to full employment. This type of benefit analysis might be used on a national scale to demonstrate the value of rehabilitative services to a particular client population, such as stroke survivors. In such an example, the total rehabilitation costs would be compared to cost savings involving return to work for the patient or their spouse. You are exposed to a cost-benefit analysis when you propose payment for a specific treatment regimen to a vocational rehabilitation counselor who then looks at the budget, determines the likelihood of the client's return to work, and either approves or denies your request.

When performing a *cost-effectiveness* analysis, the outcomes are reported differently. While cost will be expressed in monetary units, effectiveness may be reported as improvement on a standardized or nonstandardized test, a reduction in observed clinical symptoms, or client satisfaction. This is the type of outcome analysis speech-language pathology is discussing nationally and on an individual facility basis. We are interested in linking costs with clinical outcomes to demonstrate the value of our interventions in obtaining meaningful and functional results in a cost-effective manner.

CRITICAL PATHWAYS AS AN EXPRESSION OF FINANCIAL OUTCOME

The concept of a *critical pathway* is another method of looking at clinical outcome as it relates to a financial outcome. Critical pathway analysis is a method of *graphing* a multidisciplinary staff's treatment activities against a timeline. Critical pathways cover all of the multidisciplinary interventions involved in client care from the time of admission through discharge, including only those vital elements that have been proved to effect client outcomes.

Because the complete interdisciplinary process of treatment is considered in a critical pathway, any variances in that process may affect cost. Indeed, a major motivation for developing critical pathways is to ensure that the cost of care rendered does not exceed the payment. Outlier analysis is an important part of this process. Those cases who required a more intensive level of care over a longer period of time will be looked at carefully during this analysis. The goal is to develop a critical pathway in which all treatments are appropriate, nonduplicative, timely, and effective. Thus, both length and intensity of treatment can be controlled and cost can be contained.

The process of critical pathway development, however, can result in adverse effects on client care. Any decrease in length of stay or reduction in services should never prevent a positive client result. As emphasized by Wilkerson (in Breske, 1995), the interest is ultimately in quality outcomes, efficient processes and lower costs.

USES OF FINANCIAL OUTCOME DATA

In order to make informed decisions, meaningful data about your program should provide the basis for your actions. Appropriate data constitute a powerful tool when presented to support your professional judgments. Financial outcome data can be used in *program evaluation, marketing,* addressing *administrative concerns,* and managing *managed care.*

As pressures mount in service environments, clinical programs need to look closely at their practice patterns to ensure both quality of care and cost effectiveness. This process of *program evaluation* requires the collection, analysis, and reporting of data to take actions that are both appropriate and necessary. Financial outcome data linked to clinical outcome data are extremely helpful.

For example, in reviewing the cost per case for various clinicians working within a particular service line, you note that one clinician has consistent outliers. Her clients have longer lengths of stay and a higher average number of treatments when compared to clients of the other clinicians within the group. After discussions with the supervisor you learn that this clinician has been assigned more complex, severely involved cases. Furthermore, job dissatisfaction, related to these caseload characteristics, has been expressed by this individual. A solution would be to reassign all cases by distributing levels of complexity and severity on an equal basis. You might also discover that this same clinician is unable to discharge clients on a timely basis. A second solution would be to counsel the clinician and ask her to change her practice patterns to coincide with discharge policies. These scenarios are representative of program evaluation and exemplify the benefits of ongoing outcomes data collection and analysis.

Marketing your services to referral sources requires specific data reporting considerations. Consider the case of a number of physicians who have started a group practice within an HMO. The physicians are "at risk" for the total costs of providing care, including the number of referrals for specialty rehabilitative services. The group is seeking a speech-language pathology program that provides high quality, cost-effective treatment. Your program is asked to make a presentation detailing your clinical outcomes and associated lengths of stay, average number of treatments, and total charges per case. Because the physicians are specialists in neurology and otolaryngology, they are interested only in specific diagnoses. By having this type of outcomes data available by clinical diagnosis, your presentation can be both credible and effective.

Administrative concerns can also be addressed using appropriate data. Assume you need to replace a staff member in your acute-care rehabilitation program for dysphagia. The hospital administrators, however, are looking at every staffing request carefully and are requiring full justification. They are especially concerned because a large proportion of patients with dysphagia are covered by Medicare, and any increase in costs may not be covered by its prospective payment structure. Because you have been collecting outcomes data for this diagnosis, you are able to demonstrate a lower number of treatments per case, which is a reduction from the previous year. The clinical outcome remained the same despite the reduced cost of providing service. You could also demonstrate that your program's intervention hastened discharge because patients were swallowing safely. Finally, you could show a lower incidence of rehospitalization for patients with dysphagia who were referred to your service early in their hospital stay compared to patients who were referred late as a result of aspiration. You can provide this type of information with an outcomes management system that links both clinical and financial data.

When *managed care* companies question your request for treatment for a specific diagnosis, you could effectively support the request with data. A data table that lists the average number of treatments required to obtain a specific clinical outcome for a large number of similar clients with the same communication disorder makes it difficult for the managed care organization to deny the request. In the long term these types of data tables may facilitate approvals of future requests without the time-consuming and often futile attempts to justify treatment.

BENCHMARKING

While outcomes data can be used for the above-mentioned purposes, advantages are also found by comparing that data with data obtained from other clinical programs. It may be important to know how your program compares with other similar programs in order to assess your relative effectiveness or position in the marketplace. This process of *benchmarking* is used increasingly throughout the health care environment (e.g., Uniform Data System for Medical Rehabilitation, State University of New York at Buffalo, 1993).

Dictionary definitions commonly describe benchmarking as a standard by which something can be measured or judged. A working definition of benchmarking is the continuous process of measuring our services, or outcomes, against our toughest competitors or those organizations recognized as leaders. Another term often used interchangeably with benchmarking is *competitive benchmarking*. Competitive benchmarking could be as simple as comparing your department's length of stay by diagnosis to that of competing institutions in the same service area. More advanced competitive benchmarking might include comparing the best client outcomes for each service site to client satisfaction measures, social patterns, or levels of economic status within facilities throughout the nation.

In your facility, it would be helpful to know how your program's lengths of stay, average number of treatments, or total charges compare with other local providers for a particular diagnosis. If you find that your outcomes data are far from the benchmark, you may decide to investigate the reasons for this discrepancy. When becoming involved in benchmarking activities, you must be certain that your program is being compared to "peer" organizations with comparable attributes (e.g., American Speech-Language-Hearing Association, National Treatment Outcome Data Collection Project, Williams, Baum, & Stein, 1995).

DATA COLLECTION MECHANISMS

Most organizations collect financial data regarding their clinical service programs. Financial officers and accountants are responsible for establishing cost accounting systems that meet the needs of a particular corporation, university, school district, or private practice. While these systems address many of the financial concerns of an organization, it is the clinical program that is usually most concerned with outcome. Because of managed care pressures and internal cost containment efforts, each speech-language pathology program will have to decide how to establish an outcomes measurement system as a first line of defense for the future. Advances in computer technology, the availability of software programs, and national systems may make the job easier than ever before (Pientranton, 1995b; Ryan, 1995; Trace, 1995). If there is no active outcomes measurement system in place within your organization, if you have no input into what is being measured, or if meaningful cost data are not being linked to pertinent clinical information, it may be time to implement such a system. It has recently been announced that the Joint Commission on Accreditation of Healthcare Organizations approved a plan (Oryx, the Next Evolution in Accreditation, 1997) to formally integrate performance measures into the accreditation process. "The plan requires accredited hospital and long-term care organizations to choose a performance measurement system that has met initial screening requirements by December 31, 1997." (Loeb, personal correspondence).

AVAILABLE OUTCOMES MEASUREMENT SYSTEMS

A variety of computerized systems are now in use to collect and analyze outcomes data. These include commercially available as well as locally developed programs with a variety of features. In nearly all instances, financial data collection is a major component of the system. The following are just a few examples of such systems and how they incorporate financial outcomes.

The most widely used data collection system in rehabilitation in the United States is the UDSMR℠, which contains the Functional Independence Measure (FIM) (State University of New York at Buffalo, 1993). The FIM is being used in over 720 facilities in the United States, Canada, and Australia, and the data base generated currently includes over 800,000 patient records. This is a national and international data base that has been dedicated exclusively to inpatient rehabilitation programs and makes use of a standardized set of 18 multidisciplinary functional scales. The FIM links its 7-point rating scales to both demographic and financial data. Data are collected locally and sent to a central location for computer analysis. Reports are returned to each participating facility on a quarterly basis. Each institution's data are benchmarked against nationwide patterns.

In addition to a summary of FIM data, UDSMR uses several integrated financial formulae. For example, *charge efficiency* is defined as the average gain in overall FIM score per dollar (calculated as total FIM gain divided by charges times 1000 to reflect gain per $1000.00). Further, *LOS efficiency* is the average FIM gain per day or week (calculated as the total FIM gain divided by the length of stay or by seven to reflect gain per week). Finally, UDSmr provides an analysis system (FIM-FRG or *Function Related Group*) that allows the facility to identify which patients are exceeding the expected length of stay per impairment and severity.

Whereas the FIM exemplifies a national system, the *Beaumont Outcome Software System* (BOSS) exemplifies an in-house or facility-specific system (Merson, Rolnick, & Weiner, 1995). Developed at William Beaumont Hospital, Royal Oak, Michigan, the BOSS allows each user to set up specific clinical and outcome data collection parameters and control the collection and analysis functions within the user's facility. Designed as a Windows© based program, it can be used on a personal computer to create tables, charts, and graphs that link clinical and financial outcomes data, as well as client satisfaction, by different service sites. Analysis by specific clinical diagnosis in speech-language pathology is incorporated. Length of stay, average number of treatments, and cost per case are integrated with clinical outcome data. Outlier analysis reports can also be generated with the user determining the outlier parameters to be analyzed. Diagnosis-specific 7-point clinical outcome scales for a variety of inpatient and outpatient speech-language pathology services are provided.

The American Speech-Language-Hearing Association (ASHA) has launched the *ASHA National Treatment Outcome Data Collection Project* (Williams et al., 1995). Both clinical and financial outcome data are being collected from speech-language pathology programs across the nation to develop a national data base. The ASHA project allows local programs to collect admission, discharge, financial, client satisfaction, and demographic data on each client. Computer forms available for data entry are sent to a national site for analysis. Comprehensive reports will be generated and sent to each participating program. This system is collecting information on charges per client by diagnosis, as well as information related to capitated payment structures. The ASHA system currently contains a series of 7-point functional communication scales (Larkins, 1987). Clinical and financial outcomes will be integrated and reported.

Many clinical facilities have developed their own data base systems (Johnson, 1994; Johnson, 1995; Shelton & Bianchi, 1996). Using existing spreadsheet software, database software, or procedures of their own financial departments, these facilities have created innovative tools that are meeting the present needs of clinicians and administrators

Table 5–1. Selected Computerized Systems that Collect, Analyze, and Report Clinical and Financial Outcomes in Speech-Language Pathology

OUTCOMES MEASUREMENT SYSTEM FEATURES	UDSMR	ASHA/NTODCP	BOSS©	OUTCOMES TODAY™	FORMATIONS©	OUTCOME™	R-COM PLUS
Financial Data Linked to Outcome	Yes	Yes	Yes	Yes	Yes	Yes	Yes
Creates Financial Reports	Yes	Yes	Yes	Yes	Yes	Yes	Yes
Creates Tables and Graphs	Yes	Yes	Yes	No	Yes	Yes	Yes
Outlier Analysis	Yes	No	Yes	No	No	No	No
Local or National Database	Both	National	Local	Local	National	Local	Local
Purchase or Subscribe	Subscribe Annually	Undetermined; project is in research phase	Purchase	Purchase	Subscribe Annually	Purchase contract service	Purchase contract service

UDSmr   Uniform Data System for Medical Rehabilitation, State Univ. of New York at Buffalo.
ASHA/NTODCP American Speech-Language-Hearing Association, Rockville, Maryland; The National Treatment Outcome Data Collection Project.
BOSS©   Beaumont Outcome Software System, Parrot Software Inc. BOSS—a software system for local PC installation.
OUTCOMES TODAY© Focus On Therapeutic Outcomes, Inc., Knoxville, Tennessee, an independent data collection service.
FORMATIONS© Formations National Outcome Systems, Chicago, Illinois, an independent data collection service.
OUTCOME™   Evaluation Systems International Inc, Boulder, CO.
R-COM Plus   R-COM Plus, Medical Rehabilitation Facility Software, Resource & Management, Seattle, WA.

alike. There also are a number of consulting firms available to assist speech-language pathology programs in developing or purchasing an outcomes measurement system that would be appropriate to their environment (Evaluation Systems International Inc., 1995; Focus on Therapeutic Outcomes, Inc., 1995; Formations in Health care, Inc., 1995; & R/Com Inc.: Ryan, 1996). Table 5–1 lists some commercially available outcomes measurement systems that integrate financial with clinical data.

INTEGRATED FINANCIAL OUTCOME ANALYSIS

Assume now that you have committed your program to the concept of outcomes measurement and have selected a system to collect data. As the clinical and financial outcomes data become available, it is clear that you must be able to link or integrate those data in such a way that critical questions can be both asked and answered. For instance, it is not enough to know the average cost (or charges) for a large heterogeneous population of individuals with communication disorders. It would more beneficial to look at cost in the following manner:

- Cost by Diagnosis
- Cost by Admission Severity
- Cost by Clinical Outcome
- Cost by Gender or Age
- Cost by Clinician
- Cost by Clinical Site

It would also be helpful to combine any number of these variables so that your program could look at costs by admission severity and age, diagnosis and severity, age, diagnosis and severity, and so on.

Figure 5–1 illustrates four cost-per-case analyses by severity, age, gender, and diagnosis for a pediatric clinic using the Beaumont Outcome Software System (BOSS) (1995). For this population of children with communication disorders, treatment costs tend to diminish with decreasing admission severity, increase with age (in months), remain virtually the same for both males and females, and show higher relative costs for treating apraxia of speech and language disorders than articulation disorders or stuttering. These types of analyses give clinical programs a base from which to continue evaluation. Further analysis, using a combination of variables, should also be performed if one wants to exhaust all the possible causes of variance.

Although we have been aware of the need to report financial data, we have not had an effective means to do so. By integrating our costs with clinical outcomes we can begin to respond to payers who ask "how much?" or "how long?" and to facility administrators who ask "what are the comparative costs of providing services in different environments?"

A cost or charge analysis by severity of condition would be particularly important. Many patients in need of speech-language pathology services in hospitals are referred with more complex medical diagnoses and severe communicative disorders than ever before. Schools are seeing more children who have medical and social histories that include congenital problems, addiction, abuse, and severe injury. Clinical as well as

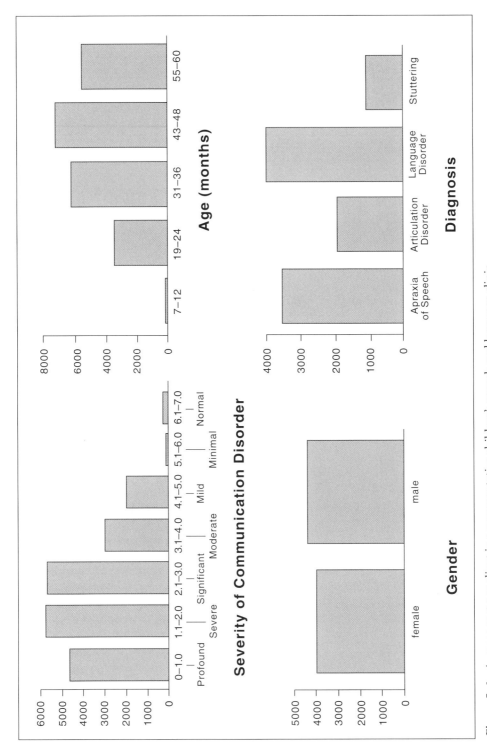

Figure 5–1. Average cost per client in a representative children's speech and language clinic. Cost variations are illustrated for severity of communication disorder, age, gender, and communication disorder diagnosis.

124

financial outcomes will be affected by the severity of disorders being treated. Without the ability to analyze both clinical and financial outcomes data by severity of condition, data may be meaningless.

Consider also the need to know your costs by clinical site of service. For example, your data may show that the costs of providing rehabilitation within an off-site pediatric program are higher than payer expectations. There may be administrative pressure to reduce costs because of a poor net profit in comparison to other sites staffed by your department. Using an outcomes measurement system, you discover that while costs are high, the clinical outcomes exceed those of your other sites. In fact, many families whom you serve are actively seeking referrals to your facility's clinics, physicians, and other services because of their satisfaction with the improvement in their children's speech and language. The value of your pediatric program might now be regarded in a different light. This scenario exemplifies how integration of different outcome parameters can support programs and justify variations in cost by clinical site.

Many professions are looking at practice patterns within the context of critical pathways. By looking at certain aspects of an individual practitioner's manner of treating clients, a "report card" can be generated. That is, practice patterns are analyzed for that individual in relation to his or her peers. In many cases, length of stay, intensity of treatments, and subsequent cost or charges generated per case are aspects that are graded on these report cards. Needless to say, many professionals dislike this concept. However, using financial outcome data that is sensitive to individual clinician performance can have an influence on those practice patterns that do not serve the client or the clinical facility in an appropriate manner.

If a particular speech-language pathologist demonstrates costs far in excess of others providing the same services, an evaluation of the circumstances should be performed. An outcome system that allows for this type of analysis can be a valuable tool.

ANALYSIS OF REPRESENTATIVE OUTCOMES DATA

In Table 5–2 we have displayed representative outcomes data for four different clinical sites in a hospital using BOSS. Both clinical and financial outcomes are presented allowing comparisons of outcomes by site. This type of data begins the process of analyzing each site based on the particular questions being asked. It might be interesting to ask at what functional level clients are discharged. One can see that all sites discharge at about a 5.0 or better on the 7-point scales used. When looking at number of procedures, length of stay and charges per case, however, there is variation. This would be expected based on the differing diagnostic conditions seen at different sites.

Table 5–3 provides a breakdown, by specific clinical diagnosis, of the same outcome parameters. Again, discharge occurs at about the same level of function even though different clinical outcome scales are used for each diagnosis in this particular hospital program. As would be expected, the average number of procedures to attain a comparable clinical outcome is very different. This number of procedures drives the higher charge levels for certain diagnoses. One can begin to see how linking financial data to clinical data would enable clinicians to "predict" the average length of stay, average number of visits, or average charges for a particular diagnosis. This information can be useful when answering relevant questions from clients, families, and payers.

Table 5–2. Sample Outcomes Data by *Clinical Site* and Admission Status, Discharge Status, Clinical Outcome, Procedures, Length of Stay, and Average Charges per Case*

OUTCOME VARIABLES	SITE I N = 253	SITE II N = 293	SITE III N = 136	SITE IV N = 262
Admission Status Average scale value, 1 is profound and 7 is normal.	2.97	2.73	3.97	4.00
Discharge Status Average scale value, 1 is profound and 7 is normal.	5.61	4.90	5.21	4.90
Clinical Outcome Average gain in points on 7-point scale.	2.65	2.17	1.24	.89
Length of Stay Average number of days.	50	400	76	19
Procedures Average number of evaluations and treatments.	4.5	74	28	18
Charges Average "cost" per case.	$ 463	$ 4,312	$ 3,754	$ 2,179

Site I = Outpatient Voice Clinic   Site II = Outpatient Children's Clinic

Site III = Outpatient Adult Rehabilitation   Site IV = Inpatient Adult Rehabilitation

*NOTE: This table does not contain accurate charges or costs. The financial figures are used for illustrative purposes only and cannot be interpreted as average charges or costs for speech-language pathology services.

Table 5–3. Sample Outcomes Data by Communication Diagnosis*

OUTCOME VARIABLES	ADULT APHASIA N = 54	STUTTERING N = 17	DYSPHAGIA N = 41	VOCAL NODULES N = 46	CHILDHOOD LANGUAGE DISORDER N = 43
Admission Status	4.0	3.8	1.9	3.1	2.7
Discharge Status	5.1	5.4	5.1	5.7	4.9
Clinical Outcome (Gain in points on a 7-point scale)	1.1	1.6	3.2	2.6	2.3
Length of Stay (Average number of days)	78	87	20	40	509
Procedures (Average number of evaluations and treatments)	32.5	6.5	4	4	87
Charges (Average "cost" per case)	$ 4,439	$ 563	$ 799	$ 386	$ 5,221

*NOTE: This table does not contain accurate charges or costs. The financial figures are used for illustrative purposes only and cannot be interpreted as average charges or costs for speech-language pathology services.

Table 5–4. Sample Outcomes Data of Adult Clients with Aphasia and Dysarthria Treated in an Outpatient Rehabilitation Program. Outcome Variables Examined Across Age, Gender, and Severity*

OUTCOME VARIABLES	AGE 56–95 YRS. N = 75	AGE 21–55 YRS. N = 23	MALE N = 49	FEMALE N = 49	MILD TO MODERATE N = 41	SEVERE N = 57
Admission Status	3.9	4.1	3.9	4.1	4.8	3.5
Discharge Status	5.1	5.4	5.3	5.1	5.8	5.0
Clinical Outcome (Gain in points on a 7-point scale)	1.1	1.2	1.3	1.0	.93	1.5
Length of Stay (Average number of days)	80	99	98	68	72	53
Procedures (Average number of evaluations and treatments)	36	36	43	27	25	111
Charges (Average "cost" per case)	$ 4,873	$ 4,895	$ 5,871	$ 3,670	$ 3,421	$ 7,095

*NOTE: This table does not necessarily contains accurate charges of costs. The financial figures are used for illustrative purposes only and cannot be interpreted as average charges or costs for speech-language pathology services.

Table 5–4 compares by age, gender, and severity. By using outcomes data in this manner, one can look at the possible effects these variables can have on financial outcome data. As can be seen in this hypothetical example, age appeared to have a potential effect on both the discharge status and length of stay, but the number of procedures and charges remained essentially the same. Males, on the other hand, while showing more improvement, required more procedures, a longer length of stay, and more dollars expended. As might be expected, the more severe the condition, the greater the charges, length of stay, and number of procedures required; however, more change appeared to occur. These data suggest what is seen in many rehabilitation environments; that more severely involved clients tend to carry a greater cost burden. While the reasons for these outcomes are not always clear, differences do exist and require additional investigation. Further data analysis will begin to explain the differences found.

In Table 5–5, the results of an *Outlier Analysis* are presented for the clients seen at four clinical sites. In this example, the average number of procedures per case is analyzed. Four outlier criteria are compared within each site using the same client list at that site. Each outlier criteria (50, 75, 100, 200%) relates to the average number of procedures per case. For example, a 50% criterion equals the average number of procedures per case plus half that number, and a 100% criterion is twice the average. In Site I, at a 50% criterion, 27 of the 253 clients exceeded the mean of 4.50 procedures. By using the 100% criterion, only five outliers were identified. At a criterion of 200%, no outliers were found. One can see how the other sites compared at each established criterion. This use of outlier analysis can help in program evaluation when it becomes clear that too many clients fall outside the average values expected for a defined population. Sys-

Table 5–5. Outlier Analysis by Clinical Site for Mean Number of Procedures

OUTLIER CRITERIA	SITE I N = 253	SITE II N = 292	SITE III N = 136	SITE IV N = 262
Mean (Average number of procedures)	4.50	74.16	27.93	18.05
*50% (Number of clients 50% above the mean)	*27	26	28	45
75% (Number of clients 75% above the mean)	14	20	22	15
**100% (Number of clients 100% above the mean)	**5	16	15	7
200% (Number of clients 200% above the mean)	0	6	8	1

* 27 individuals had 6.75 procedures or 50% more procedures (2.25) than the mean (4.50).

** 5 individuals had 9 procedures or 100% more procedures (4.50) than the mean (4.50).

Site I = Outpatient voice clinic   Site II = Outpatient children's clinic

Site III = Outpatient adult rehabilitation   Site IV = Inpatient adult rehabilitation

tems that perform outlier analysis will enable you to identify which cases fall outside a norm. These cases can then be reviewed to determine the possible and often legitimate reasons for outlier status.

Table 5–6 presents outlier information for length of stay by communication disorder. Each diagnosis was analyzed by the four different outlier criteria used in the example above. As would be expected, the number of outliers decreased as the outlier criteria increased. A close look at the clients with dysphagia might cause a department director some initial concern. Because this diagnosis involved an inpatient condition with a relatively short length of stay, and because most of these patients were covered by Medicare under DRG payment schedules, the number of outliers needed further analysis. These patients were found to have developed secondary medical conditions that increased the total hospital length of stay as well as speech-language pathology. Because the patients required additional treatment due to their medical complications, the clinical staff provided that treatment. In this case, the full outlier analysis demonstrated that quality patient care decisions preempted efficiency concerns.

USING OUTCOMES DATA TO GENERATE FINANCIAL FORMULAE

It is possible to use the above-described data to generate descriptive *outcome formulae*. While one must exercise caution in accepting these formulae and interpreting the results of applying them, their use can be a beneficial exercise in synthesizing data for purposes of financial analysis. With this caution in mind, we present two formulae:

- Cost Effectiveness
- Cost Conformity

Table 5–6. Outlier Analysis by Clinical Diagnosis for Mean Length of Stay (days)

OUTLIER CRITERIA	VOCAL NODULES N = 70	CHILDHOOD LANGUAGE DISORDER N = 72	DYSPHAGIA N = 189	PUBESCENT FALSETTO DISORDER N = 7
Mean (Average length of stay in days)	22	38	14	7
50% (Number of clients 50% above the mean)	*9	17	31	2
75% (Number of clients 75% above the mean)	7	12	22	2
100% (Number of clients 100% above the mean)	**5	11	17	1
200% (Number of clients 200% above the mean)	1	4	9	1

* 9 of 70 individuals had a Length of Stay of 33 days or 50% more days (11) than the mean (22).

** 5 of 70 individuals had a Length of Stay of 44 days or 100% more days (22) than the mean (22).

Cost Effectiveness

Cost effectiveness is commonly referred to as the average cost of care per unit of clinical progress. This is calculated by dividing the average cost (or charges) per client by the gain on a clinical outcome scale (e.g., measured in points on a 7-point scale), which is attained by that individual at the end of treatment.

Cost Effectiveness = Average Per Client Charges ÷ Clinical Outcome Scale Gain

The UDSMR system (1993) incorporates a cost formula that is referred to as *charge efficiency.* It is calculated by dividing the change in functional independence measure (FIM) (i.e., FIM discharge score minus the FIM admission score) by the total charges. The UDSmr also utilizes the *LOS* (length of stay) *efficiency* formula which can be calculated by dividing the FIM charge by the length of stay. The higher the number, the greater the efficiency or the greater gain per unit of time.

Table 5–7 is an example of a *cost effectiveness analysis* involving two groups of clients with dysphonia secondary to unilateral vocal paralysis treated by two different clinicians. Clinician A achieved a cost effectiveness value of $82.51 while that of Clinician B was $148.37. While it may seem that Clinician A did a better job, reporting this type of data in isolation can be misleading unless you also account for those clinical variables that may influence the result. In this scenario, the average severity levels of the clients treated by Clinician A were higher (profound) than those treated by Clinician B (severe). Therefore, in this example, clients who enter treatment with higher severity levels demonstrated greater gain. It is not unusual, for this diagnosis, that clients with higher admission severity levels attain relatively higher gains because they have more potential gain to achieve, as occurred in this scenario. Cost effectiveness, therefore,

Table 5–7. Cost Effectiveness of Treating Clients with Vocal Paralysis Dysphonia by Two Different Clinicians

OUTCOME VARIABLES	CLINICIAN A	CLINICIAN B
Admission Status	1.44 (Profound)	2.34 (Severe)
Discharge Status	5.85 (Minimal)	5.11 (Mild)
Clinical Outcome (Gain in points on a 7-point scale)	4.41	2.77
Length of Stay (Average number of days)	22 (days)	38 (days)
Procedures (Average number of evaluations and treatments)	3.63	4.14
Charges (Average "cost" per case)	$ 363.88	$ 411.00
Cost Effectiveness (Cost ÷ Outcome)	$ 363.88 ÷ 4.41 = $ 82.51	$ 411.00 ÷ 2.77 = $148.37

should be analyzed by differing severity levels. Further, it would appear that these severity levels influenced the mean length of stay and average number of procedures, thereby increasing the total charges.

Cost Conformity

One might also consider a formula for *cost conformity* to describe how a subgroup of clients' outcomes conforms to the actual mean value of some other financial data of a larger group of clients. This concept focuses on comparison of a subset with the group mean. As an example of this, the formula below expresses cost conformity as a percentage of the actual cost effectiveness mean value.

Cost Conformity = Subgroup Cost ÷ *Cost Effectiveness* Mean Value

In Table 5–8 the mean cost effectiveness for treating clients with the same impairment (dysphonia secondary to vocal nodules) and severity is *$167.04* per unit of clinical outcome gain. When we look at a subgroup of the oldest clients with the same diagnosis and severity, the average cost effectiveness is only *$140.48* per unit of clinical outcome. By using the above formula, the cost conformity can be expressed as 84%. This value suggests that the treatment of the oldest clients in the group was in good cost conformity, or equal to or less than 100% of the mean cost effectiveness. In contrast, the youngest clients had a cost effectiveness value of *$185.00* (above the mean) with a subsequent cost conformity of *110% (or 10% greater than the expected value)*. When comparing the two clinicians, it can be seen that Clinician A has a better cost conformity than his colleague. As with all such manipulations of data, the actual reasons for the reported differences are of much interest in the management of a clinical program.

Table 5–8. Cost Conformity of Treatment for Clients
with Vocal Nodules, Examined by Age, Gender, and Clinician.
(Average Cost = $ 167.04)

VARIABLES	CLINICAL OUTCOME	CHARGES (AVERAGE "COST" PER CASE)	COST EFFECTIVENESS	COST CONFORMITY (PERCENT OF AVERAGE COST EFFECTIVENESS)
Male	2.5	$394	$157	94%
Female	2.6	$389	$148	88%
Age: 6–25 years	2.0	$370	$185	110%
Age: 41–65 years	2.8	$397	$140	84%
Clinician A	2.8	$392	$139	*83%
Clinician B	1.6	$379	$231	**138%

* This best cost conformity is 17% less than average cost effectiveness.

** This worst cost conformity is 38% higher than the average cost effectiveness.

CONCLUSION

The use of financial outcome formulae to reduce complex integrated data into a manageable body of information should be approached with caution. Dr. Dennis Burkitt, a well-known medical epidemiologist, would often forewarn his colleagues that "Not everything that counts can be counted, and not everything that can be counted counts." (personal communication, Lauter, 1996). Some of us also remember Wendell Johnson's admonition "The map is not the territory" (Johnson, 1946). No synthesis or condensation of such data to answer financially related questions can portray the clinical realities that face the client, family, and clinician in coping with a communication or related disorder. In fact, financial and clinical outcome measures should be understood for what they are *not*. These measures cannot account for all the direct or indirect costs of delivering services, nor can they account for all the costs to the client undergoing rehabilitation. Financial outcome data, when linked to clinical outcome data, is best regarded as a *shorthand* of the financial implications of clinical care.

Teisberg, Porter, and Brown (1994) remind us that "Health care reform in the United States is on a collision course with economic reality. . . . In industry after industry, the underlying dynamic is the same: competition compels companies to deliver increasing value to customers. The fundamental driver of this continuous quality improvement and cost reduction is innovation" (p. 131).

Integrating financial and clinical outcome data, while indispensable to clinic managers in developing and evaluating new and innovative treatment programs, will demand careful inferences about the value of our services. This activity, however, is critical if we are to sustain our programs in the presence of rapid and unpredictable change. Outcomes management systems must be chosen, and data must be examined from multiple perspectives. This should cause our profession to adopt new terminology and data analysis in helping us achieve the best clinical outcomes while expending the fewest dollars.

REFERENCES

Bello, J. (1994). *Communication facts.* Rockville, MD: American Speech-Language-Hearing Association, Research Information Section.

Boston, B. (1994). Destiny is in the data. *American Speech-Language-Hearing Association, 34,* 35–37.

Breske, S. (1995). Forging Critical Paths for Outcomes Management. *ADVANCE for Speech-Language Pathologists & Audiologists, 5,* 19.

Darley, F.L. (1982). The effect of treatment. In F.L. Darley, *Aphasia* (pp. 144–184). Philadelphia, PA: W.B. Saunders.

Eisenberg, L. (1995). Medicine-molecular, monetary, or more than both? *Journal of the American Medical Association, 274,* 331–334.

Evaluation Systems International Inc. (1995). *Outcome™.* Boulder, CO: Author.

Focus on Therapeutic Outcomes Inc. (1995), *Outcomes Today.* Knoxville, TN: Author.

Formations in Health Care Inc. (1995). *Formations National Outcomes Systems.* Chicago, IL: Author.

Frattali, C.M., Thompson, C.K., Holland, A.L., Wohl, C.B., & Ferketic, M.M. (1995). *Functional Assessment of Communication Skills for Adults (ASHA FACS).* Rockville, MD: American Speech-Language Hearing Association.

Frattali, C.M. (1993). Perspectives on functional assessment: Its use for policy making. *Disability and Rehabilitation, 15,* 1–9.

Frattali, C.M. (1992). Functional assessment of communication: Merging public policy with clinical views. *Aphasiology, 6,* 63–83.

Goldberg, B. (1993). Translating data into practice. *ASHA, 35,* 45–47.

Granger, C.V., Ottenbacher, K.J., & Fiedler, R.C. (1995). The Uniform Data System for Medical Rehabilitation. Report of first admissions for 1993. *American Journal of Physical Medicine & Rehabilitation, 74,* 62–66.

Johnson, A.F. (1994). Creating and Applying Data Base Technology for Outcome Measurement. Conference presentation, *"Outcomes, Reform and Efficacy"* at Department of Speech-Language Sciences & Disorders. Detroit, MI: Henry Ford Hospital Medical Center.

Johnson, D.R. (1995, January). Integrated computer software helps manage information: A better way to prove outcomes and track costs. *Rehabilitation Outcomes Review in HOSPITAL REHAB™.* Atlanta, GA: 119–122.

Johnson, W. (1946). People in quandaries: the semantics of personal adjustment. New York, NY: Harper & Row Publishers.

Joint Commission on Accreditation of Healthcare Organizations (1997). *Oryx: The Next Evolution in Accreditation.* Oakbrook Terrace, Il: Author.

Keatley, M.A., Miller, T.I., & Mann, A. (1995). Treatment Planning Using Outcome Data. *ASHA, 37,* 49–52.

Larkins, P.G. (1987). Program Evaluation System (PES): Determining quality of speech-language and hearing services. *ASHA, 24,* 21–25.

Lauter, C. (1996). Personal Communication. Royal Oak, MI: William Beaumont Hospital.

Loeb, J.M. (1997, February 12). Personal correspondence.

Merson, R.M., Rolnick, M.R., & Weiner, F. (1995). *The Beaumont Outcome Software System (BOSS).* West Bloomfield, MI: Parrot Software Inc.

McReynolds, L. (1990). Historical perspective of treatment efficacy research. In L.B. Olswang, C.K. Thompson, S.F. Warren, N.J. Minghetti (Eds.), *Treatment efficacy research in communication disorders* (pp. 5–14). Rockville, MD: American Speech-Language Hearing Foundation.

Olswang, L.B., Thomson, C.K., Warren, S.F., & Minghetti, N.J. (1990). *Treatment Efficacy Research in Communication Disorders.* Rockville, MD: American Speech-Language Hearing Foundation.

Pietranton, A. (1995a). *Treatment efficacy bibliography.* Rockville Pike, MD: American Speech-Language and Hearing Association, Health Services Division.

Pietranton, A. (1995b). Collecting Outcome Data: Existing Tools, Preliminary Data, Future Directions. Rockville, MD: *ASHA, 37,* 36–38.

Ryan, C. R. (1996). *R/Com Plus Resource Management and Program Evaluation Modules.* Seattle, WA: R/Com Inc.

Rolnick, M.I., & Merson, R.M. (1996, March). User Friendly Computer System tracks speech outcomes. *Rehabilitation Outcomes Review in HOSPITAL REHAB™.* Atlanta, GA: 35–38.

Ryan, C.R. (1995). Creating specialized information systems. *Transitions, 2*(1), 18–21.

Sederer, L.I., & Dickey, B. (1996) *Outcomes Assessment in Clinical Practice.* Baltimore, MD: Williams & Wilkins Press.

Seligman, M.E.P. (1995). The Effectiveness of Psychotherapy. *American Psychologist, 50,* 965–974.

Shelton, R., & Bianchi, B. (1996, January). Patient tracking system helps manage outcomes, costs. *Rehabilitation Outcomes Review in HOSPITAL REHAB™.* Atlanta, GA: 7–10.

Slater, S. (1995). *Omnibus survey results.* Rockville, MD: American Speech-Language Hearing Association, Science and Research Department.

State University of New York at Buffalo, School of Medicine and Biomedical Sciences, The Center for Functional Assessment Research (1993). *Guide for the uniform data set for medical rehabilitation.* Version 4.0. Buffalo, NY: UB Foundation, Inc.

Statistical Abstracts of the United States (1994). U.S. Department of Commerce, Bureau of the Census. Lanham, MD: Bernan Press.

Teisberg, E.O., Porter, M.E., & Brown, G.B. (1994, July–August). Making Competition in Healthcare Work. *Harvard Business Review,* Vol., 131–141.

Trace, R. (1995). Outcomes Measures Lead to Increased Accountability. *ADVANCE for Speech-Language Pathologists & Audiologists,* 6–7.

Weil, T. (1995). How Do Canadian Hospitals Do It? *Hospital Topics, 73,* 10–22.

Wertz, R.T. (1993). Issues in Treatment Efficacy: Adult-Onset Disorders. *ASHA, 35,* 38–39.

Williams, P.S., Baum, H.M., & Stein, M.E. (1995). *ASHA Data Collection Instruments for Measurement of Treatment Outcomes.* Orlando, FL: American Speech-Language Hearing Association Annual Conference.

SUGGESTED READING LIST

Crane, M. (1995). What you charge versus what you're paid. *Medical Economics, 72,* 156–178.

Drucker, P.F. (1995). Really Reinventing Government. *The Atlantic Monthly, 275,* 49–61.

Johnsson, J. (1996). HMO's dominate, shape the market. *American Medical Association, 39,* 4–7.

Robinson, J.C., & Casalino, L.P. (1995). The Growth of Medical Groups Paid Through Capitation in California. *The New England Journal of Medicine, 333,* 1684–1687.

Swigert, N.B. (1994). *ASHA Task Force on Treatment Outcomes and Cost Effectiveness: Reports of the task force.* Rockville, MD: American Speech-Language Hearing Association.

Wilkerson, D.L., Batavia, A.I., & Dejong, G. (1992). Use of functional status measures for payment of medical rehabilitation services. *Archives of Physical Medicine and Rehabilitation, 73,* 111–120.

CHAPTER 6

Treatment Efficacy Research

LESLEY B. OLSWANG

INTRODUCTION

The topic of "treatment efficacy research" has gained considerable attention during the last decade. Like most topics that achieve rapidly growing interest and scrutiny, the increased focus has created an ensemble of ever-changing opinions and ideas, many of which work well together, many of which do not. Writing a chapter puts one in a rare position of defining a perspective; this I do with great enthusiasm, for "treatment efficacy research" has captured my attention for years. The process of writing this chapter has allowed me to reexamine many ideas, to grapple with and redefine many terms, and ultimately, to create a package that reflects a perspective. To that end, the purpose of this chapter is to define "treatment efficacy research," clarifying what it is and what it is not, and to describe the working components of this type of research. The reader should come away with a view of *treatment efficacy research* that places it, along with *treatment outcome research*, as a subcategory of *clinical research*. The differences and similarities between treatment *efficacy* versus *outcome* research will be explored. The reader will also be challenged to consider the components of research (i.e., *research questions, research designs, independent variables, dependent variables, data analysis* and *interpretation*) from a treatment efficacy perspective. The ultimate goal will be to capture the essence of treatment efficacy research. The chapter is not meant as a tutorial for conducting efficacy research, but rather as an introduction for better understanding and appreciating it, and for guiding future research endeavors in the profession and the discipline.

TREATMENT EFFICACY RESEARCH: WHAT IS IT?

Clinical Research

A definition of treatment efficacy research must begin with its superordinate, *clinical research*. Clinical research (or applied research) is that type of research that follows guidelines and principles of science to provide an understanding of human experience and behavior change. Clinical research becomes more narrowly defined as it is viewed as being undertaken to solve some problem of immediate social or economic consequence (Ventry & Schiavetti, 1986). In the discipline of communication sciences and disorders, clinical research is designed to yield a better understanding of the nature of communication and related disorders and the clinical processes of assessment and treatment associated with disorders. The essence of clinical research is that it brings together scientific/methodological rigor and ecological validity; that is, it is clinically relevant science.

Most discussions of clinical research include some debate about the relationship between research and practice, pitting the researcher against the practitioner, and experimental control against informed clinical judgments. In recent years accountability, health care, and education reform have forced practice to become more rigorous and structured. Although clinicians may scrupulously and conscientiously collect data to make informed clinical decisions and to demonstrate accountable service delivery, they are not conducting clinical research. Collection of data does not mean research. A controlled therapeutic condition does not mean research. Research entails using valid scientific methodology to document trends via data collection; accountable clinical work is about making informed clinical decisions via data collection. The two are different.

Efficacy versus Outcome Research

A particular kind of clinical research investigates treatment. During the past several years research regarding treatment has gone in two directions, one documenting efficacy, the other, outcomes. *Efficacy research* and *outcome research* will be differentiated in this chapter and described as though they are separate entities. More accurately, they exist on a continuum where at some point in the middle, they overlap. At their extreme, purest forms, they represent different approaches to examining the influence of treatment on individuals with communication and related disorders. Most often, the lines separating them are blurred; this no doubt reflects the fact that they both embody clinical research principles. In an effort to clarify terminology that has recently become confusing, this chapter will force the research perspectives to their extremes. Simply stated, treatment efficacy research *proves* treatment benefits; treatment outcome research *identifies* treatment benefits.

Efficacy research provides evidence that treatment works by ruling out possible alternative explanations for client change. It also examines the various ways that treatment alters behavior. "Efficacy research documents that changes in performance are directly attributable to the treatment administered" (Campbell, 1995). The proof comes about via well-controlled conditions and data collection beyond standard clinical practice. Typically efficacy research has focused on impairment (versus disability or handicap), but it need not (and should not) maintain its focus here; a point to be discussed later. In fact, recent efficacy research has expanded its emphasis, primarily because of the demands of health care and education reform.

Treatment outcome research, on the other hand, *identifies* treatment benefits. It demonstrates that treatment made a difference to a client by examining changes related to clinical variables. Outcome research measures changes during or after the treatment process and addresses a variety of questions—for example, cost of treatment, quality of care, and achievement of functional change in the client (Campbell, 1995). The outcomes (or benefits of treatment) are documented via clinical, "real world" conditions and data collection of standard clinical practice. Outcome research, because of its focus on accountability, has primarily measured the disability and handicap of individuals with communication and related disorders.

Recent interest in health care reform has pushed health-related professionals to demonstrate their worth. Demands for data that show significant, cost-effective changes in client behavior following intervention have resulted in an increase in outcome research. The interest is *less* on exploring how a treatment alters behavior, but rather that treatment is associated with important changes in the client's life. The essence of the difference between efficacy and outcome research is "proof"; the former attempts to prove a relationship between treatment and client change, and the latter attempts to identify and document a relationship. Both contribute to accountability; both constitute research; both advance the profession.

Components of Treatment Efficacy Research

The *proof* demanded by treatment efficacy research is probably most clearly understood by appreciating the structure of the research. The major components of the research create that structure; they are the research questions, the designs, the independent variables, the dependent variables and the data analysis and interpretation.

Research Questions

The research questions lie at the heart of the structure. Anyone who has ever taken a research course knows that the questions define and determine the nature of the research and the methodology. Efficacy research questions are by definition clinical and attempt to prove some relationship between the implementation of treatment and change in client behavior. I would like to borrow from Salomon (1991), and suggest that there are two broad views of treatment efficacy research, and thus two major types of questions that may be asked—*analytic* and *systemic* questions. Both address clinical issues and both attempt to prove a relationship between treatment and client change, but they each approach the task slightly differently. One is not better, or no more scientific than the other; they merely ask different types of research questions.

One type of treatment efficacy research question takes an *analytic perspective* (Salomon, 1991). This perspective addresses how specific treatment techniques affect specific behavioral changes for individual clients. The analytic perspective primarily, yet not exclusively, focuses on behaviors at the impairment level of a disorder and examines specific circumstances that influence the change of these behaviors. The interest is on narrowly defining treatment strategies and behaviors, "the highly discrete behaviors that observers are trained to discriminate from the ongoing flow of events" (Meyer & Evans, 1993, p. 227). The assumption behind this type of research question is that behaviors can be isolated from their context, and that data are being gathered to support a hypothesis regarding the description and control of a specific behavior (Morris, 1992). By and large, one can use quantitative data for these types of research questions, a point to be discussed later in this chapter.

A second perspective to treatment efficacy research is *systemic* (Salomon, 1991). These questions do not address specific, isolated behaviors per se, but rather behaviors meshed in the context. This perspective primarily, but not exclusively, focuses on behaviors at the disability and handicap level, examining changes due to treatment from a more comprehensive, "in context" perspective. The interest is on more broadly defined functional or life-style changes, such as communication interest, general comfort and well-being, success with peers, "the kinds of behaviors that we seek for ourselves, know when we see them, and would generally regard as universally good" (Meyer & Evans, 1993, p. 227). The assumption behind this type of research question is that the data reflect behaviors that cannot be separated from context; no single hypothesis is being tested, but rather a socially constructed reality is being explained. This perspective would argue that treatment must result in socially valid (i.e., important and meaningful) changes in client lives, using strategies that are socially valid (i.e., acceptable and sustainable) in the real world (Schwartz & Baer, 1991). Systemic treatment efficacy research will most closely resemble treatment outcome research (this is where the blur in the distinction emerges and the continuum of treatment research is best appreciated). Again the difference will be in the proof offered by the efficacy research. Knowing/proving the relationship between the treatment and the "real-world" changes for the client is critical as we attempt to understand the nature of communication and the ways in which intervention can alter the effects of disorders.

Analytic and systemic questions ask about the relationship between a treatment and the change that is observed in the client. The nature of the relationship can be examined in several ways. Appreciating the complexity of the relationship is key to completely understanding how treatment influences client change. One framework, borrowed from Kendall and Norton-Ford (1982), suggests that treatment efficacy questions should examine the *effectiveness* of treatment, the *effects* of treatment, and the *efficiency* of treatment. Keep in mind that effectiveness, effects, and efficiency can be examined from both an analytic and systemic perspective, and further, that these three categories are *not* mutually exclusive. Questions about treatment effectiveness refer to issues of validity, specifically addressing whether a particular treatment works or not. Treatment effectiveness questions investigate a particular treatment, documenting that the treatment and not some other cause is responsible for behavior change (i.e., threats to validity, Ventry & Schiavetti, 1986). Questions about treatment effects refer to issues of multiple behavior change as a result of treatment. Questions concerning treatment effects explore the phenomenon of change in communication, asking in what ways the treatment alters behavior, specifically examining which aspects of treatment differentially influence which behaviors. These questions focus on generalization issues, exploring ways in which behaviors change in relationship to each other as a product of treatment. Treatment efficiency questions address the relative effectiveness of treatment, examining rate and magnitude of change over time. These questions explore the relative effectiveness of two or more treatments. They also examine rate and degree of change by examining the components of a treatment package. These three categories of course overlap. When addressing a question about a treatment's effectiveness, effects and efficiency are examined. The taxonomy is meant to allow researchers the opportunity to view the variety of questions that can be asked and to focus his or her interests and methodology in specified directions.

The framework and terminology offered by Salomon (analytic versus systemic) and Kendall and Norton-Ford (effectiveness, effects, efficiency) captures the complexity of treatment efficacy research, but also provides a sense of organization for constructing research questions. The more we sort through the complexity and raise a variety of questions, the more we will learn about how treatment can alter the communication disorders exhibited by our clients. The research questions serve to pare down the task and focus our examination. The structure offered by frameworks, such as the ones proposed, allow for focusing attention, isolating primary areas of investigation, and guiding methodology.

Designs

Treatment efficacy research can, and should, employ many types of designs. This, of course, reflects the fact that treatment efficacy research asks many types of questions. Systemic questions lend themselves to descriptive, ethnographic studies; here, the focus is on describing the individual within context, with few, if any, manipulations by the examiner. In contrast, analytic questions lend themselves to between-group and within-subject designs, because these questions address how particular manipulations affect change in particular behaviors. Tight experimental control is at the heart of these questions. An array of designs should be considered the tools of the efficacy researcher. The research question will drive the design choice, but because the emphasis is on "proof, " the designs must provide that capability.

Questions that ask whether a group of individuals, on average, changed more often than not with the implementation of treatment lend themselves to between-group designs. Here the focus, and challenge, is on gathering homogenous groups of individuals, treating some and not others, or providing one treatment to one group and another treatment to another, similar group. The minimum number of groups is always two, and groups are formed on the basis of either randomization or matching. Group differences are examined to determine the effectiveness of treatment, or the effectiveness and efficiency of one treatment versus another. Between-group designs are important for determining whether individuals with similar characteristics will respond to treatment and to what degree. Proof is demonstrated by differences in group performances on pre- and posttest measures as documented by statistical procedures. These designs become more powerful with larger groups of individuals, but they often become difficult to implement because homogeneity among subjects is frequently difficult to achieve. Between-group designs are considered important when generality of findings is a target—that is, when attempting to suggest that the findings apply to a large proportion of a population. While this is the case, the trade-off is that these designs do not provide information about individual variation in performance. This trade-off is important in the clinical world.

Questions that ask how particular contextual variables influence behavior are most often addressed by descriptive, ethnographic designs. This approach to research, often termed "qualitative, " explores the natural relationship between client performance and contextual influences, such as setting, persons, activities, and so forth. The word "natural" should not be interpreted as contradicting "proof, " which unfortunately is often the case in some circles. Rather "proof" is demonstrated via tools for documenting credibility and plausibility (Lincoln & Guba, 1985), a point to be discussed later in this chapter.

Questions that ask about the "incidence" and "prevalence" of treatment effects are addressed through epidemiological designs. This approach to research attempts to explore treatment efficacy from the perspective of the population. Large samples, reflecting the population, are used to show trends in treatment benefits. The emphasis of proof here is the unmistakable occurrence of a trend as documented by powerful statistical analyses.

Questions that ask about how a particular manipulation (i.e., treatment) alters behavior over time are best addressed through within subject/time series designs. This approach to research attempts to explore treatment efficacy (effects, effectiveness, and efficiency) by studying one individual at a time and documenting the ways in which a treatment changes performance. At the heart of within-subject methodology is applied behavioral analysis; the environment is manipulated by the experimenter in systematic, predetermined ways (i.e., treatment) and critical behaviors are measured repeatedly over time. Proof is demonstrated by systematic change in subjects' performances as treatment is introduced, altered, and/or withdrawn. At the heart of proof is replication, either within or across subjects. The more replications, the more powerful the proof. Replication across subjects, particularly replications that are yoked in time, provide increased experimental control and allow for greater generalizability of results. Case studies are ones in which a single subject is observed independently from other subjects; they can employ within subject/time series design features to increase their validity, but a case study by itself has little generalizability to a larger sample, and has limited experimental control. The beauty of time series research is the opportunity to examine the unfolding nature of change. The approach allows the researcher to document how treatment changes an individual over time. The power of this observation is that it yields extraordinary insight into the therapeutic process, by revealing how treatment interfaces with particular disorders and subject/client characteristics.

All of these designs allow an opportunity to observe human behavior in the context of treatment and/or no treatment. They all allow for an examination of breadth of change in communication as treatment is introduced. Systematic, controlled manipulation of the environment can be accomplished in all of these designs, but the type of design will determine how it is done. All of the designs can provide powerful information to our knowledge base about communication and related disorders and the role of treatment. Each design poses a different research question and these questions in turn shape the methodology.

Independent Variables

The independent variable of a study refers to the conditions that are manipulated to produce change, or more generally, differences among conditions that are likely to influence subject performance. As such, independent variables include subject/participant characteristics and the treatment(s) attributes. Efficacy research demands that the independent variables be tightly described. The experimenter must know and clearly describe which variables he or she wishes to manipulate and which he or she wishes to control. This applies to both the subject characteristics and the treatment attributes.

Subject characteristics need to accurately and completely describe the participants in every respect that might be critical to the outcome of a study. The researcher needs to specify criteria that will be used to include and exclude an individual as a subject. This means knowing which characteristics all of the subjects must share to be included in the study (inclusionary criteria), and which characteristics none of the subjects must exhibit (exclusionary criteria). Typically, certain characteristics are key and will need to be controlled across participants, while others are less important and can vary. In efficacy research the subjects are very often systematically manipulated to determine how different subject characteristics might interact with the treatment. Subject characteristics, such as language level, age, educational background, severity of disorder, site of lesion, and so on may be altered while the treatment is held constant to determine how efficacy might change. When subjects with particular characteristics respond differently to a treatment than other subjects with varying characteristics, the clinical researcher can begin to gain some insight into how the treatment might be working. Manipulating the subject characteristics, as is often done in within subject/time series designs, becomes an excellent strategy for gaining insight into the nature of disorders.

The independent variable is most often thought of in terms of the treatment itself, and the manipulation of it. Treatments can be manipulated in many ways, including its strength and integrity (Yeaton & Sechrest, 1981). Strength refers to how often a treatment is given and the intensity of a treatment (length of session, number of exposures to teaching items, etc.). Integrity refers to identifying and manipulating the various components of the treatment, including the steps/phases, the instructions (i.e., prompts, cues, consequences, reinforcements), the person implementing the treatment, the setting, the activities, and materials. All aspects of treatment that are important to the research questions must be identified and controlled. Some questions address the efficacy of treatment packages; others examine treatment components. Some questions will explore how much change a client exhibits in a set amount of time and exposure to treatment; others will ask how much treatment is necessary to bring about a particular change in performance. Keep in mind that the research question will determine the kind of manipulation that is allowed and the level of control that is involved in treatment implementation.

Because the focus of efficacy research is on the treatment of disordered populations, an important part of the methodology requires that testing of subjects and implementation of treatment be reliable. This form of reliability is known in the literature as procedural reliability or fidelity. It demonstrates to the reader that the procedures for including subjects and implementing treatment can be trusted and replicated. (See Billingsley, White, & Munson, 1980; Kearns, 1990; LeLaurin & Wolery, 1992.) Conducting procedural reliability is essential in treatment efficacy research.

Dependent Variables

The dependent variables of a study refer to what to measure, how to measure, and when to measure.[1] As necessary for determining the independent variables, the researcher must again refer to the research questions and determine what data are needed to answer them. The efficacy researcher should always be thinking "multiple measures" in an attempt to satisfy issues regarding effectiveness, effects, and efficiency, and to address the complexities of human communication and its disorders. Depen-

---

[1]Measures associated with dependent variables have conventionally been termed "outcome measures." They encompass measures of impairment, disability, and handicap. Recently the term "outcomes" has become associated almost exclusively with "outcome research." This seems an unfortunate drift. To avoid any confusion in this chapter, I will limit my terminology to "measures," and will define the various types of measures that should be considered and utilized in efficacy research.

dent measures are selected because they reflect the construct of interest for the researcher, and they are sensitive to the type and magnitude of change that is expected. The measures can be, and are most often, *behavioral;* these include overt, observable behaviors produced by the subjects. Measures may also be *self reports, inventories, questionnaires,* or *scales,* which allow for the examination of change that is more subjective and not necessarily observable. Finally, measures may be *psychophysiological.* These are measures that allow for the examination of biological events as they reflect psychological states (e.g., cardiovascular, aerodynamic, or neurological measures). The discussion that follows will focus on the need for multiple measures reflecting the complexities inherent in communication and human behavior. Regardless of the focus of the research, the bottom line will always be the same: dependent variables must include data and measures that are needed to measure change and to prove that the change is related to the treatment manipulation.

At first glance, "change" in behavior seems like a relatively simple concept; we want to know if treatment alters communication in some way. The simplicity vanishes quickly when entering the clinical world. Anyone who has worked with an individual with communication disorders knows that "change" can take many forms; it occurs at different times during the treatment process and at different levels of communication. Therefore, examining change must be multidimensional. In this chapter two dimensions will be suggested for viewing and measuring change: levels of change and temporal aspects of change.

Change can and should be examined in terms of levels of performance. For this discussion, the framework provided by the WHO (1980) proves helpful. Accordingly, three levels of change can be documented; these correspond to the three primary levels of a disorder: impairment, disability, and handicap. In measuring change, the researcher would wish to be cognizant of behaviors that reflect these three levels. Measures of impairment will describe behaviors of structure and function (psychological, physiological, anatomical), including linguistic forms, phonological features, airflow, and so on. These are typically overt behaviors that describe the symptoms or topology of a communication impairment, and the processes of language comprehension and production. Disability corresponds to behaviors of functional communication. Handicap refers to behaviors that reflect quality of life and well-being. Efficacy research has typically examined impairment. This is the case because impairment corresponds to "signs of the disorder," and efficacy research has its origins in examining the relationship between treatment and the nature of disorders (Rosenbek, 1995). As our understanding of communication disorders has increased, we have become better able to diagnose by recognizing the impairments ("signs") associated with disorders. Accordingly, we have altered our treatments to better address the nature of the disorders by targeting change in impairments. With increased interest in the disability and handicap associated with disorders, efficacy research has expanded its goals. Primary measures of treatment probably still remain at the impairment level, with secondary measures being made at the disability and handicap level, but this priority is under discussion (see Rosenbek's discussion of dysphagia, 1995). Some might argue that the focus on impairment is as it should be, for this is how we will best advance the profession and the discipline. Others might argue that the focus should shift to disability and handicap, for this is where the ecological impact of treatment will be felt. Certainly the latter orientation corresponds to real-world, consumer priorities, but does it correspond to scientific priorities? An argument might also be made that outcome research grew out of the need to better examine disability and handicap, and that efficacy research should continue its examination of impairment. Of course, there is a middle position that suggests efficacy research must maintain a focus on impairment, while at the same time examining the relationship between impairment, disability, and handicap in controlled, experimental ways, always with an eye on learning more about the nature of disorders. This position is taken in the remainder of our discussion on dependent variables/measures.

Change can also be examined along a time dimension. Temporal aspects of change refer to how and when the treatment shows its effect. A framework that has proven useful in examining temporal aspects of change is borrowed from Rosen and Proctor (1978, 1981), which differentiates intermediate, instrumental, and ultimate change. *Intermediate change* is the change that occurs session-to-session, as an immediate consequence of the treatment process. Intermediate change presumes to contribute to a facilitative climate for continued intervention with the prescribed treatment strategies and techniques. Intermediate change refers to the accomplishments a client shows from session to session; that is, the acquisition of skills, knowledge, and beliefs that move him or her forward in the therapeutic process. *Instrumental change* is the change that occurs with treatment, that leads to other change without further treatment. That is, once attained, these changes serve as the instruments for the attainment of other change. Instrumental change, if linked to the desired target of treatment, can become a criterion for treatment success. Instrumental change becomes a short-term behavioral objective that leads to a longer-term goal. These changes have often been thought of as the triggers for automaticity and generalization of the desired target. Finally, *ultimate change* is the final success, the final objective of treatment. Ultimate change describes the behavior that is desired from the therapeutic process. It either reflects normalized performance, or socially appropriate performance. Measures of ultimate change take into consideration those behaviors that the researcher and the subject hopefully wish to achieve. Measures of social validity typically are used to measure ultimate change. They document change in a subject compared to relevant peers (social comparison) and/or as measured by subjective evaluation by the subject him or herself or significant others. The researcher may be interested in one type of change more than another, or perhaps the relationship between the different temporal aspects of change. The research questions will guide the selection of the dependent measures.

Given the complexity of the task of measuring change, including the levels of measurement and the temporal aspects, this discussion continues by offering further ways to view data and dependent measures. An important consideration is regarding the kind of data that should be collected. One distinction to be made is between quantitative and qualitative data; the distinction is important as they become choices for answering analytic versus systemic research questions. *Quantitative data* refer primarily to observable, countable, behavioral data, yet also include data that are not observable and are sampled via inventories or scales. Quantifiable data are numeric data. Their origin, in applied behavior analysis and quantitative research, is bound in a perspective of objectively gathering facts to prove or disprove a hypothesis. Behaviors are described sufficiently such that they can be counted, yielding frequency and duration measures. Quantitative data are used primarily for addressing analytic research questions. *Qualitative data* reflect interpretation. They form a description of the subject in context, as such reflect a socially constructed reality, a view of the subject and treatment process from an insider's point of view (i.e., the insider being the subject, the researcher, relevant others, etc.). Gathering qualitative data acknowledges that the variables surrounding particular behaviors are complex, interwoven, and difficult to measure, and thus quantitative data alone are inappropriate or insufficient. The complexity of communication is not only acknowledged, but appreciated. As such, data collection involves immersing oneself in the setting and lives of the subject and his or her significant others, and using multiple means to gather data. Participant observation and field notes, interviews, and diaries all become tools for data collection. Qualitative data are used primarily for addressing systemic research questions.

Another way to differentiate data is to distinguish measures obtained during the actual implementation of treatment *(treatment data)* versus data collected apart from treatment in a probe situation *(probe data)*. Treatment data allow for the examination of change within an optimum learning environment; probe data allow for the examination of generalization, or learning beyond the teaching paradigm. Treatment data are collected during the treatment session with all aspects of the treatment paradigm being engaged. This means the subject is receiving prompts, cues, accuracy feedback, reinforcement, and so on as the treatment dictates. Accordingly, treatment data are useful for addressing questions that relate to intermediate change—the change that reflects accomplishments from session to session. Treatment data may also have its place in addressing questions regarding instrumental change. Research no doubt should be investigating how performance during treatment serves as a trigger for the acquisition of the desired treatment target. Probe data are collected outside of treatment. These data are evoked in a variety of settings, with a variety of people, with a variety of materials, and with varying amounts of structure. On one hand, probe data can closely resemble the treatment paradigm, by taking place in the clinic room, with the clinician, clinical materials, and a high degree of structure, but no accuracy feedback. On the other hand, probe data can also be very distant from the treatment paradigm, and more closely resemble a naturalistic environment. As such, probe data may be collected in a nonclinical environment (as the home) by other people (as the spouse or parent) in a natural situation (as mealtime). Probe data serve to measure learning beyond the treatment paradigm, and thus may be tapping near and far transfer. As such, probe data will serve to measure both instrumental and ultimate change, with of course an emphasis on the latter. As researchers examine the ecological/social validity of treatments, which corresponds to ultimate change, probe measures must tap behaviors of disability and handicap, and these are certainly best measured in a nontreatment, naturalistic probe situation.

Treatment data and probe data must also be discussed in terms of *target measures* and *control measures,* yet another important distinction in measures. Target measures are those measures that are somehow related to the treatment target and are expected to change. There are three categories of target measures, as follows:

1. Behaviors and measures that are directly reflected by or tied to manipulations of the independent variables. They can be the treatment data themselves, or probe data. The latter would be most commonly referred to as stimulus generalization data.

2. Behaviors and measures that are not directly reflected by or tied to manipulations of the independent variables, but related to them. They cannot, by defini-

tion, be treatment data. As probe data they are most commonly referred to as response generalization data.

3. Behaviors and measures that are not directly reflected by or tied to manipulations of the independent variables, nor apparently related to them, but they are important to the diagnosis of the client, and may perhaps change as a result of treatment.

An example might help clarify these three categories. If a researcher were investigating a treatment for dysarthria of speech, where the focus was on breathing and spacing, the following measures might be selected: Category (1) Rate of production and intelligibility of a single word list, structured sentences, and reading of the Rainbow Passage. Category (2) Ratings of intelligibility and comprehensibility of conversational speech, and client satisfaction with treatment. Category (3) Measure of nasal air flow. Multiple target measures allow for an investigation of treatment effects, and provide important information regarding the breadth of change that has resulted from the treatment.

Control measures are those measures that are *not* related to the treatment target and are *not* expected to change. They must, however, be behaviors that are related to the problem, be communicatively and developmentally appropriate, but far enough away from the problem that they are not expected to change as a result of treatment, but may change due to other causes (e.g., maturation, spontaneous recovery). These are the behaviors and measures that are used to help demonstrate the effectiveness of treatment. The assumption is that if target behaviors change and control behaviors do not, then the change is more likely to be due to the treatment than some other cause. A control behavior for the dysarthric client might be intraoral air pressure, since this is related to the problem, but not a part of the treatment. While quantitative data might most readily come to mind when discussing target and control measures, that need not be the case. Qualitative data are useful in completely describing the phenomenon of change, and should always be considered when selecting measures.

With all of this discussion about types of data and measures, a key element is the researcher's (and consumer's) confidence in the *truthfulness* and *trustworthiness* of the data. Truthfulness refers to the *validity* of the data, or how accurately the data measure the phenomenon of interest. To ensure valid data, the researcher must observe behaviors that will representatively reflect change. Using multiple measures, considering temporal aspects and levels of change, data will appropriately address questions of effectiveness, effects, and efficiency. The research must maintain a broad perspective in attempting to document change due to treatment and not other external or internal forces. Both qualitative and quantitative data must be valid. To ensure validity, we must have adequate amounts of data, adequate variety of data, and adequate confirming and disconfirming evidence to demonstrate plausibility. The bottom line is that the data must reflect what we know and believe to be true about the communication development and disorders.

Reliability refers to the trustworthiness of our data. This means that the data must be amenable to collection over time without concern for variability in performance other than what is "true" for the client, versus being in the "mind of the beholder." The research must be able to trust the data to be credible over time, truly fluctuating as a result of the subject's changing abilities. For quantitative data, reliability is ensured in part by having independent observers sample the collection of the same data. For qualitative data, credibility is ensured by having different sources of data yield the same conclusions (Lincoln & Guba, 1985). The bottom line for reliability and credibility is that the data do not purely reflect what is in the researcher's mind, but rather that others can trust in the way the data have been collected.

Data Analysis and Interpretation

Persuasive evidence for documenting the efficacy of treatment will come in many forms, depending upon the research question, the research design, and data. The evidence may be statistical or clinical, but in either case the goal is to document significant change; change that is neither random nor unimportant (Bain & Dollaghan, 1991; Kazdin, 1980).

Statistical procedures examine whether the changes in the dependent measures likely occurred by "chance." Typically a level of confidence (.05 or .01) is selected as the criterion for determining statistical significance. The changes in performance are examined with a statistical test that yields a probability value. Statistical significance is judged by whether the probability level is equal to or below the level of confidence selected. To find that a relationship in an experiment (i.e., a relationship between the introduction of treatment and behavior change) is statistically significant does not mean that there is necessarily a genuine relationship between the two. The statistical analysis only indicates the probability; chance is never completely eliminated. Other causes, as sampling error, could have caused the results; however, convention and logic argue that when a probability level is as low as .05 or .01, one can assume that the relationship between the variables of interest are real. Statistical analyses require careful selection of procedures; this is not a simple task. While the goal, and underlying assumption, of statistical forms of evaluation is to conduct a relatively bias-free and consistent method of data analysis and interpretation, bias can slip into the picture. Selection of tests, criteria for significance, and even more basic, a flaw in the design (e.g., sample size, heterogeneity of subjects, heterogeneity in procedures), may yield invalid results. The use of statistics to analyze data is not the end-all in efficacy research, particularly if interests lie in determining how subjects change and whether change is important in real life.

Clinical forms of data analysis also attempt to document that change is significant and not due to chance or other threats to validity. While this form of data analysis is nonstatistical, it is not necessarily nonnumerical. A valuable nonstatistical, yet numerical, procedure for evaluating quantitative data is visual inspection. Visual inspection is commonly used in within-subject/time series designs, where repeated, continuous data are available for individual subjects. The examiner views the data for each subject separately, and then in comparison to other subjects, to determine trends in the rate and degree/magnitude of change with the introduction and withdrawal of different types of manipulations. The researcher looks for trends during the initial phase in which no treatment is provided (baseline), changes in the trends when treatment is introduced, how the trends change as the treatment unfolds and/or other manipulations are introduced, and changes and trends in the data when treatment is withdrawn. Replication of trends within and across subjects lends credence to the validity of the findings. The availability of repeated, continuous data makes examination of data through visual inspection less arbitrary than one might expect. The unfolding nature of treatment benefits can be observed and analyzed with these data, where pre- and posttest data make such an analysis difficult, if not impossible. As with statistical procedures, nonstatistical, visual inspection requires criteria for suggesting significance. Changes in performance need to be robust and immediately apparent, making statistical procedures oftentimes seem redundant. Well-constructed designs and clear trends in the data increase the validity of interpretation. On top of this, replication across subjects powerfully increases the generalizability of results. This latter point can best be appreciated by clinical researchers (and practitioners) who know only too well about individual variation among even the most homogeneous subjects. When robust, clear trends in change are replicated over and over across subjects, the validity of the phenomenon is enhanced and the ability to generalize the findings increases.

Visual inspection speaks directly to quantitative data. Nonstatistical means of analyzing qualitative data also exist. For a complete discussion of this topic, the reader is referred to Lincoln and Guba (1985), Bogdan and Biklen, (1992), and Glesne and Peshkin (1992) as beginning references. Data analysis of qualitative data is the process of systematically searching and arranging the data that have been collected to better understand the phenomenon of interest. This entails working closely with the data, "organizing them, breaking them into manageable units, synthesizing them, searching for patterns, discovering what is important and what is to be learned" (Bogdan & Biklen, 1992, p. 153). Patterns and trends in the data lead to conclusions. Conclusions become more credible and plausible in a number of ways. First, the researcher must have adequate amounts of data. Prolonged engagement in a setting, yielding numerous examples of patterns and trends, contribute importantly to the strength of the interpretation. Second, the researcher must have adequate variety of evidence; this is known as "triangulation." Credibility increases when data come from different sources, methods, and investigators. Different sources can mean multiple copies of one type of source (e.g., interview respondents—parent, siblings, teacher), or different sources of the same information (e.g., verifying an interview with field notes). Different methods means different data collection modes or types of data (e.g., interview, questionnaire, observation, behavioral measurement). Different investigators means using data from another study or working on a team with different questions but overlapping data. Third, the researcher must recognize and utilize concordance and discrepancy in the data. Disconfirming or negative evidence often sheds light on a particular trend or helps reach a particular conclusion. The researcher needs to look for such evidence, and if found, it needs to be analyzed in light of the patterns. Fourth, and finally, credibility and plausibility are enhanced with dramatic data that are so noteworthy as to be difficult to ignore. However, a caution must be made; "whiz bang" effects must never stand alone. Recently, the success of Facilitated Communication as a treatment for children with autism was documented by reports of "whiz bang" effects. Observations of extraordinary communication breakthroughs in communication via computers were used as proof of treatment efficacy. These claims, unfortunately, were bold and misleading. Extraordinary, "whiz bang" effects must always be viewed in light of other confirming and disconfirming evidence, and must be accompanied by triangulation. Qualitative data has a place in efficacy research. These type of data afford researchers a unique look at how treatment alters subjects' behaviors in context. As with quantitative data, analysis must proceed in line with the assumptions of the data. No doubt, someday clinical researchers will become better equipped to utilize quantitative and qualitative data as complementary sources of valid information.

Clinically, significant change also addresses whether or not changes in performance are important, and whether or not the results are real to the subject (or relevant others). Many years ago Wolf (1978) introduced the notion of social validity or social acceptability of treatment. "The acceptability of treatment includes several areas, such as whether the focus of treatment, the procedures used, and the results of treatment are acceptable to the client or those in contact with the client . . . Essentially social validation of clinical importance of behavior change can be determined in two ways, which have been referred to as the social comparison and subjective evaluation methods" (Kazdin, 1980, pp. 365, 366). *Social comparison* compares behavior of the subject before and after treatment with the behavior of "nondeviant peers." The question asks whether the subject's behavior following treatment is distinguishable from relevant peers. The emphasis here must be on relevant peers. For example, subjects with developmental disabilities would be compared to others with this diagnosis, but for whom the "treatment target" is *not* of concern. *Subjective evaluation* examines the importance of behavior change by assessing the opinions of the client and individuals who are likely to have contact with the client about the benefits of treatment; this type of evaluation has recently been termed "consumer satisfaction" (Baer, 1988; Baer & Schwartz, 1991; Schwartz & Baer, 1991). Subjective evaluations most appropriately examine whether changes are important in terms of communication function (disability) and quality of life (handicap). Social validity has become increasingly important in clinical research, and appropriately, the science and technology for examining social validity has improved (Schwartz & Baer, 1991). Clinical significance is no longer the pale sidekick of statistical analysis. Its place in research, and the advancement of science, has been proven and adopted.

CONCLUSION

Why bother to conduct efficacy research? The current need goes beyond calls for accountability for our profession. Certainly accountability is important, yet the appeal of efficacy research is that it goes beyond practice and embraces theory as well (Olswang, 1993). The process of conducting efficacy research, and the results obtained, can contribute to the discipline of communication sciences and disorders in critical ways. By examining how manipulations of the environment (i.e., treatment) alters communication behaviors in individuals with disorders, we have much to gain in our understanding about communication itself and about the nature of disorders. Treatment efficacy research is an investigatory tool for examining the effects of environmental variables (treatment) on organismic variables (communication and related behaviors). As such, efficacy research is not limited to being solely a category of research designed to answer clinical questions regarding whether or not a treatment is effective. Rather, efficacy research should be viewed as part of an armament of tools for the discipline, for furthering scientific knowledge, and for investigating phenomena with both theoretical and clinical application. The beauty of efficacy research truly is that it naturally addresses both theoretical and clinical questions simultaneously (see Olswang, 1993). Basic and applied researchers need to appreciate this perspective and appreciate the findings that such research generates. Our gains in theory will ultimately advance our efforts to demonstrate accountability; similarly, our gains in accountability should ultimately advance our knowledge in theory.

So why isn't more efficacy research being conducted? Several reasons contribute to the paucity of treatment efficacy research. First, research training, doctoral training, still primarily focuses on basic research, or applied research with an emphasis on studying nature of disorders or assessment. Research training also primarily embraces group designs, which as discussed above is only one design used in efficacy research, and it can be very limiting. Second, and related, few mentors exist for training new researchers in this type of research. Research is certainly most often associated with the discipline rather than the profession, and basic scientists are often the major contributors to the discipline's research base. Basic scientists, while perhaps appreciating that efficacy research can contribute to the discipline, will not be conducting this type of clinical research. This creates a limited number of research mentors for future clinical researchers.

Third, efficacy research is time consuming and difficult in ways basic research and clinical research examining assessment are not. Efficacy research most often requires large commitments of time in implementing treatment and monitoring change. Very often long-term benefits, as well as short-term benefits, are examined, stretching out the time frame even further. Efficacy research also obligates the researcher to major involvement with the client and family that other forms of research do not, particularly basic research, but clinical research as well. Researchers cannot bring in families for treatment and ignore all of the other related issues that emerge. Similarly, treatment typically uncovers characteristics about the client, the family, and the disorder that complicate the design in unexpected ways. This occurs in part because of the time frame involved, but also because the treatment process itself often triggers the discovery of unexpected variables, which need to be controlled or somehow managed.

Fourth, treatment efficacy research is expensive. Costs are high because of materials, personnel, and technology used in data collection and analysis. Well-controlled experiments typically require external funding, which is getting harder and harder to obtain. This is particularly true in recent years with federal and state funding being cut in health care and education. While basic science is also experiencing economic belt-tightening, it appears somewhat less threatened for now. Clinical research often falls in the cracks for funding. The basic science sources do not view this research as a priority, and the health care, education sources view practice rather than research as a priority. Economic reform has made this problem increasingly obvious. All of these causes contribute to efficacy research being conducted less often than it should be.

Advancements in the discipline and the profession demand more clinical research. Treatment efficacy research, in fact, is at the core of the discipline and the profession. Efficacy research can address theory and practice simultaneously; it can lead to a better understanding of disorders and the therapeutic process. In the current climate of health care and education reform, administrators are pushing our profession to define standards for treatment success. If the profession does not respond, most assuredly administrators will respond for us. They will provide the definitions for successful treatments and for failures. Clinical researchers must take charge and build the knowledge base for the discipline and the profession. This can be done by recognizing the importance of clinical science for both the advancement of theory and the advancement of practice. Treatment efficacy research is at the heart of our future.

REFERENCES

Baer, D. (1988). If you know why you're changing a behavior, you'll know when you've changed it enough. *Behavioral Assessment, 10,* 219–223.

Bain, B., & Dollaghan, C. (1991). Treatment efficacy: the notion of clinically significant change. *Language, Speech, and Hearing Services in Schools, 22,* 264–270.

Billingsley, F., White, O., & Munson, R. (1980). Procedural reliability: a rationale and an example. *Behavioral Assessment, 2,* 229–241.

Bogdan, R., & Biklen, S. (1992). *Qualitative research for education: an introduction to theory and methods.* Boston: Allyn and Bacon.

Campbell, T. (December, 1995). Functional treatment outcomes for young children with communication disorders. Presentation to the Academy of Neurogenic Communication Disorders and Sciences, Orlando, FL.

Glesne, C., & Peshkin, A. (1992). *Becoming qualitative researchers: an introduction.* White Plains, NY: Longman.

Kazdin, A. (1980). *Research design in clinical psychology.* New York: Harper & Row.

Kearns, K. (1990). Reliability of procedures and measures. In L. Olswang, C. Thompson, S. Warren, & N. Minghetti (Eds.), *Treatment efficacy research in communication disorders* (pp. 79–90).

Kendall, P., & Norton-Ford, J. (1982). Therapy outcome research methods. In P. Kendall & J. Butcher (eds.), *Handbook of research methods in clinical psychology* (pp. 429–460). New York: John Wiley and Sons.

LeLaurin, K., & Wolery, M. (1992). Research standards in early intervention: defining, describing, and measuring the independent variable. *Journal of Early Intervention, 16*(3), 275–287.

Lincoln, Y., & Guba, E. (1985). *Naturalistic inquiry.* Beverly Hills, CA: Sage Publications.

Meyer, L., & Evans, I. (1993). Science and practice in behavioral intervention: meaningful outcomes, research validity, and usable knowledge. *The Journal of the Associations for Persons with Severe Handicaps, 18,* 224–234.

Morris, E. (1992). ABA Presidential Address: the aim, progress, and evolution of behavior analysis. *The Behavior Analyst, 15,* 3–29.

Olswang, L. (1993). Treatment efficacy research: a paradigm for investigating clinical practice and theory. *Journal of Fluency Disorders, 18*(283), 125–131.

Rosen, A., & Proctor, E. (1978). Specifying the treatment process: the basis for effectiveness research. *Journal of Social Service Research, 2,* 25–43.

Rosen, A., & Proctor, E. (1981). Distinctions between treatment outcomes and their implications for treatment evaluation. *Journal of Consulting and Clinical Psychology, 49,* 418–425.

Rosenbek, J. (1995). Efficacy in dysphagia. *Dysphagia, 10,* 263–267.

Salomon, G. (1991). Transcending the qualitative-quantitative debate: the analytic and systemic approaches to educational research. *Educational Researcher, 20*(6), 10–18.

Schwartz, I., & Baer, D. (1991). Social validity assessments: Is current practice state of the art? *Journal of Applied Behavior Analysis, 24*(2), 189–204.

Schwartz, I. (1991). The study of consumer behavior and social validity: an essential partnership for applied behavior analysis. *Journal of Applied Behavior Analysis, 24*(2), 241–244.

Strand, E. (October, 1995). Ethical issues related to progressive disease. *Special Interest Division-2, Neurophysiology and Neurogenic Speech and Language Disorders, 5,* 3–8.

Ventry, I., & Schiavetti, N. (1986). Evaluating research in speech pathology and audiology. New York: Macmillan Publishing Co.

Wolf, M. (1978). Social validity: the case for subjective measurement, or how behavior analysis is finding its heart. *Journal of Applied Behavior Analysis, 11,* 203–214.

World Health Organization. (1980). International Classification of Impairments, Disabilities and Handicaps. Geneva, Switzerland: Author.

Yeaton, W., & Sechrest, L. (1981). Critical dimensions in the choice and maintenance of successful treatments: strength, integrity, and effectiveness. *Journal of Consulting and Clinical Psychology, 49*(2), 156–167.

CHAPTER 7

Program Evaluation

DEBORAH L. WILKERSON

INTRODUCTION

Service delivery has now taken on characteristics of a product more than ever, with product lines, marketing efforts, competitive forces, consumer input, and cost-containment initiatives as much a part of the lingo as client care. Program evaluation, an analytic approach used traditionally and widely in education, social services, and health care, can be viewed anew as a mechanism to facilitate an organization's internal review of its programs' (product's) effectiveness and efficiency, and to build evidence for external communications about the programs.

Program evaluation here refers to an enterprise that depends on aggregations of data collected about individuals receiving services. Certainly, at the core of the program is the individual person served, and the basic unit of information for program evaluation is the individual. It is the individual consumer's rights, values, goals, outcomes, and satisfaction that are of concern, not the clinician's or the program manager's. But in program evaluation we are not focusing on analysis of the achievement of outcome or quality of care for an individual, but on the outcomes and their correlates at various levels of aggregation (see Figure 7–1). At the program level, data for groups of individuals served by the "program" of interest—for example, a traumatic brain injury program, or augmentative communication program—are aggregated to describe inputs, processes, and outcomes for the group. Several programs may be aggregated to study patterns for an organization; studies of outcome across organizations for the field—or subfields—of rehabilitation may also be conducted. As those active in health care during the 1990s can attest, outcomes and health care effectiveness as a whole are also issues for much debate. However, it is crucial that at each level of aggregation, legitimate groupings of variables be made. Risk and/or severity adjustment will also be important (Iezzoni, 1994).

This chapter addresses definitions pertinent to program evaluation, the kinds of questions such an approach is designed to answer, basic components of a program evaluation system, comparative data and report card concepts, and reporting for decision making.

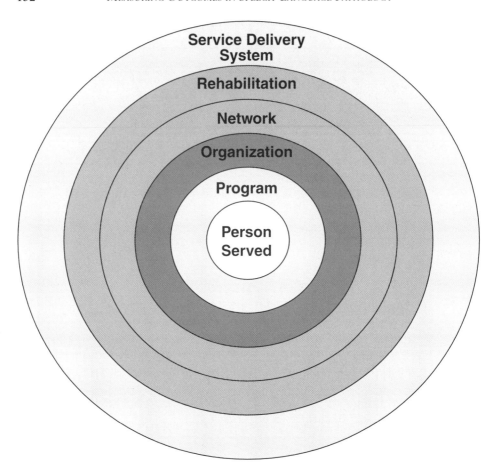

Figure 7–1. Levels of Aggregation and Analysis

What Is Program Evaluation?

Traditional evaluation literature (Knutson, 1969; Weiss, 1972) cites two major types of evaluation. First, *formative evaluation* is used while a program is ongoing, and can serve to inform corrections in program direction, or improvements in service. CARF... The Rehabilitation Accreditation Commission, has for more than 3 decades required an ongoing outcome-based program evaluation system, which fits into this category. As the concepts of outcomes management (Ellwood, 1988) and quality improvement (Deming, 1982) have evolved, the distinction between these concepts and formative evaluation has become blurred (Wilkerson & Johnston, 1997). The purposes are the same, and reflect key steps in program evaluation, outcomes management, and quality improvement:

- establish program goals, clarifying what outcomes are really important;
- specify quantifiable objectives to meet those goals;
- select measures which indicate progress toward objectives;

- measure program performance on those measures;
- compare performance to desired objectives;
- identify potential changes in the program likely to enhance performance toward desired objectives;
- implement program changes;
- measure program performance once again, comparing to the objective;
- reenter the cycle.

A second model of program evaluation, *summative evaluation,* can be used to determine whether a completed program was successful. This model, though perhaps less prevalent in rehabilitation and other service delivery environments, can be useful in determining whether to replicate new delivery system configurations. Conceptually, summative evaluation sets an end point objective, implements and carries out the program, then assesses whether the goal was met, and if not, why not.

Integrating Evaluative Functions—Relationship of Program Evaluation to Outcomes Management and Quality Improvement

In a cost-conscious environment, it is unwise to maintain overlapping functions in different parts of the organizational structure. The functions just summarized describe a continuous process of assessing client and program needs and objectives, ensuring that appropriate and sufficient care is given, and using information to improve the individual's and the program's performance. While organizations may continue to operate separate departments in utilization review, program evaluation, and quality improvement, this should not be necessary if thought is given to a model for implementing these systems. Breaking down old boundaries and territoriality may be admittedly a difficult challenge and an issue that will require some rethinking and reorganization of players within an organization.

The concepts of outcomes measurement, outcomes management, program evaluation, and quality improvement are closely related, and the interchange of terms is often confusing. Distinctions have been drawn between the concepts (Forer, 1996) that separate outcomes evaluation (outcomes only) from program evaluation (outcomes and related costs/processes) and quality improvement (broader inclusion of processes, including nonclinical areas). However, there is risk in attempting to compartmentalize these activities, rather than to view a singular evaluative system with multiple components.

DEFINITIONS AND CONCEPTS

As noted in Chapter 1, definitions, and even nuances within definitions, can vary, and language used to describe similar concepts may vary. An often confusing example is the use of the word "disability" as defined by the WHO (1980) (person-level function affected), compared with the model summarized by the Institute of Medicine (Pope & Tarlov, 1991) (societal-level function affected). Following are definitions adopted for the discussion that follows for this chapter.

The Disablement Framework

In 1980, the World Health Organization (WHO) published the International Classification of Impairments, Disabilities and Handicaps (ICIDH), a scheme designed to reflect the consequences of disease (WHO, 1980; Wood & Badley, 1981). The ICIDH contains both a conceptual model and definitions of the key terms, as well as a numerical classification scheme that can be used to code an individual's experiences with respect to the overall concept of disablement. As a reminder of the discussion presented in Chapter 1, paraphrasing from the WHO (1980) definitions:

> Impairment = organ system level loss of structure or function (e.g., interpretation of specific speech functions);
>
> Disability = person level loss of the ability to function in ways considered normal for a human being (e.g., inability to communicate);
>
> Handicap = societal level disadvantage for the person created by the intersection of the impairment or disability with the environment and that person's roles (e.g., trouble performing a job because of communication difficulties).

It is important to understand that the process of disablement is not necessarily linear. Though a disability does typically arise from an impairment, a handicap may arise from either an impairment or disability, but need not result at all if the environment is accessible and reasonably accommodating to persons with impairments or disabilities. It is especially important to using the WHO framework in defining outcomes that handicap be recognized as a function of the person in the social and physical environment. This recognition has implications for the types of goals set for persons and programs, the types of measures and measurement points selected for a program evaluation system, and ultimately, the types of services provided.

A Comment on the Controversy over "Handicap"

The ICIDH is used worldwide for many program definition, census, and public disability policy purposes. However, the word "handicap" has fallen into some disfavor in the United States, probably because of its misuse in being applied to persons. People in the disability community object to being labeled "handicapped," and rightly so. The term denotes a negative picture of disadvantage. The activist U.S. disability community of the 1970s and 1980s worked hard to clarify that the word "disability" refers to a neutral trait, and a person with a disability need not be handicapped (Heumann, 1977). Ironically, this interpretation follows exactly what this author sees as the intent of the WHO framework, but the disfavor in use of the word "handicap" in this country has sometimes resulted in rejection of the WHO framework. The Institute of Medicine (Pope & Tarlov, 1991) proposed a solution: to adopt a substitute language that places "disability" in the position of societal-level disadvantage. The person-level concept then becomes "functional limitations." Adoption of the substitute framework will simply perpetuate the negative portrayal of persons with disabilities (functional limitations), only using a new word.

This chapter will continue to refer to the WHO framework without apology, understanding that the term "handicap" is meant to refer to an environmental and societal disadvantage. Handicap *is* a negative concept, and reducing or eliminating it should be the ultimate goal (or outcome) of speech-language pathology services, of rehabilitation, and of health care and education in general, whether accomplished through curing pathology, avoiding impairment, reducing disability, or fixing the social and physical environment.

This is not to say that impairment- or disability-related goals are not relevant to program evaluation. Organizations or therapists establishing outcome goals, whether for individuals or for programs, can think in terms of immediate, intermediate, and ultimate outcome goals. For example, reduction of disability (improving communication skills) should be measured as appropriate. Programs can look at their effectiveness as measured by increase in communication function scores, for example (reduction in disability). However, programs may also wish to examine the degree to which persons served return to prior role (reduction in handicap), or the degree to which augmentative communication tools facilitate communication with family members (fix the environment, reduce handicap).

Using a Systems Approach: Input—Process—Outcome

Program evaluation involves not just the description of effectiveness (outcome) of which we are all so aware, but begs the relationship between parts of a systems model—input, process, and outcome. CARF standards (CARF, 1997) require the utilization of program evaluation or outcomes management data in the decision making at all levels of an organization. To be most useful in decision making, outcomes data must be related to knowledge about inputs and processes used to produce the desired outcome: If outcomes are less than projected or desired, what must be changed to make outcomes better? If efficiency is low due to high cost, and costs are brought down, are outcomes preserved, or do they suffer? Which costs can be brought down without ruining outcomes?

Answering such questions requires information about all three legs of the system stool, yet many program evaluation data systems lack information important to explain the variation in outcome and costs, especially information about processes of care. Table 7–1 provides examples of common elements of a systems model to be included in a program evaluation system.

Table 7–1. Examples of Data Elements for Program Evaluation Using a Systems Model

INPUT	PROCESS	OUTCOME
Referral source	Type of assessment procedure(s)	Discharge functional status
Beginning status	Type of treatment(s)	Living arrangements at discharge
Client characteristics	Nonclinical services for clients	Follow-up functional status
	Team approach to client	Follow-up living arrangement
	Amount of treatment	Quality of life
	Units of service	Consumer satisfaction with care
	Cost of care to provider	Community integration
	Price of care to payer	[Cost of care to provider]*
		[Price of care to payer]*

*Cost and price (charges, amount reimbursed) are measures of resource utilization, but are frequently considered as outcome variables (cost outcomes as opposed to clinical or client outcomes).

KEY QUESTIONS TO BE
ANSWERED BY PROGRAM EVALUATION

A program evaluation system that cannot or does not answer questions important to its various audiences is virtually doomed to failure from incomplete or inaccurate data, or undermining actions by those who are being asked to collect information. Specific questions to be addressed must be developed by the organization, preferably with substantial input from those who must collect and who will receive and use the resulting data. In program evaluation, we are seeking primarily to address real-world questions of effectiveness and efficiency, rather than the question of treatment efficacy addressed in controlled research (see Table 7–2). Several broad categories of questions are suggested.

Have We Set the Right Goals?

Program evaluation begins with a definition of goals and objectives. As scrutiny of services and cost have become more prominent, and as managed care has touched the health care service environment, it is increasingly important for a program evaluation effort to examine the outcome goals that are to be the focus of subsequent measurement assessment. The program should review goals to ensure that:

- goals and objectives specified for the program evaluation system match the desires of consumers and their sponsors (payers), the design of the program, and the philosophy of what benefits should accrue to persons served;

- measures in the program evaluation system reflect the ultimate goals of the program, not solely intermediate steps or ancillary outcomes;

- the goals, objectives and measures reflect a conceptual framework consistent with the mission of the program.

The ICIDH (WHO, 1980) and other conceptual frameworks of disablement and disability are candidates to provide a foundation for the evaluation system. A program that has as its ultimate goal to return people to work (a reduction in handicap) through, for example, provision of augmentative communication devices and training must at least measure rates of return to work. Since an intermediate program goal is to supply and train in use of augmentative communication devices, rates of device use and communication skills (disability reduction) would be appropriate intermediate outcome measures as well.

Level of Function Framework

Another way of viewing the framework for evaluation is to consider a hierarchy of function, or level-of-function framework (Wilkerson, 1992). Using a simple hierarchi-

Table 7–2. The Three Es: Efficacy, Effectiveness, and Efficiency

Efficacy	Can it work for a carefully defined and controlled group?
Effectiveness	Does it work in a real-world setting?
Efficiency	What resources are used relative to the outcome achieved?

Table 7–3. Level of Function

MICRO

Range of motion
Memory
Endurance
Strength
Cognition
Speech and language processes

MESO

Activities of daily living
Walking
Wheelchair propulsion
Communicating
Operating equipment
Interacting with people

MACRO

Working
Learning
Parenting
Recreation
Homemaking
Social life
Community participation
Creating

SOURCE: Wilkerson, 1997.

cal structure, such a framework is based on micro-, meso-, and macro-levels of function. At the micro-level of function are the basic building blocks of function at the organ system and person units of analysis—strength, range of motion, speech, language, and memory, for example. These micro-level functions must be packaged to form meso-level functions such as maneuvering a wheelchair, walking, eating, communicating, and a host of other daily activities at the person unit of analysis. For example, strength, range of motion, and cognition must be assembled to use a wheelchair for locomotion. Meso-level functions must be packaged, in turn, to form macro-level functions at the person unit of analysis and interface with a social and physical environment—work, attend school, parenting, participating in leisure activities (see Table 7–3). For example, one must package together locomotion, eating, dressing, getting and using transportation, communicating, and other meso-level functions all in order to perform the macro-level function of work.

The level-of-function framework is not inconsistent with the WHO framework, except that the ICIDH concepts are not necessarily hierarchical, and the micro-meso-macro levels are precisely hierarchical. What is significant about the hierarchy is the fact that the emphasis on a level of function changes with one's perspective. While the speech-language pathologist must focus in the treatment setting on micro-level functions (e.g., motor skills for speech production; swallowing; memory), the client, family, employer, payer, and society-at-large are most concerned with the macro-level functions (return to work; maintenance of health to avoid future expense).

We must understand the fit of micro-level functions into the meso- and macro-level functions of concern. For program evaluation purposes, the true goals and objectives for clients and the programs serving them must be specified, and corresponding measures selected. If the macro-level goal function is return to work, then attendant micro- or meso-level goals may be measured (especially for clinician comfort and explanatory value). However, eliminating the macro-level functions from the program objectives will omit from the evaluation those goals likely to be most important to consumers, payers, employers, and managed care organizations.

Are We Reaching the Goals We Have Set?

A most basic question to be answered through program evaluation is "Are we reaching the goals we have set?" Assuming that goals and attendant measures are constructed to reflect the values of the consumer, the payer, and the program, answering this question tells us the degree to which our customers will have their expectations met—a notion entirely consistent with a quality improvement paradigm. Determining whether goals are met requires that:

- goals are measurable
- performance is measured
- performance-to-goal comparisons are tracked over time.

Because we cannot always express program goals in quantifiable terms, we must choose indicators with valid and reliable measures. Moreover, a program may have specific goals, especially intermediate goals, too numerous to measure completely. In these cases, we should choose performance indicators that the program managers, staff, and target audiences can agree upon. For example, many specific functions may form the target for client outcomes—speech production, reading and writing skills, language comprehension and expression, use of augmentative and alternative communication (AAC) devices/systems, social interaction, swallowing function, locomotion and mobility, and so forth. The program may choose to focus on one or two indicators, most likely at the macro-level of function.

We must also express a target goal for the aggregation of persons served, based on either prior experience of the program, or benchmark information, if available. For example, a program may develop over time the expectation that 85% of persons served in the AAC group achieve, by the time of program discharge, a level of communication function that is either independent with devices/systems, or requires only minimal assistance from another person. We can obtain this expectation by compiling baseline data for a time, by inquiring of similar programs what their outcomes show, or by setting internal goals based on values, beliefs, and determination of the program staff. Assessing performance against this goal is then a fairly straightforward matter of assessing each client's functional level on a scale of communication function, and calculating what proportion of clients reach minimal assistance level or better at discharge. This exercise is then repeated across all measurable goals expressed in the program evaluation system.

Are We Worth It?

The question that is perhaps of most urgency to programs in a competitive environment is: "Are we worth it?", that is, worth the price of the program, worth the choice of setting or service approach, or worth the involvement in speech-language pathology services at all. This question gets to the central point of evaluating the *value* of a program. It involves not only effectiveness assessment, but a comparison of effectiveness to resources utilized (efficiency), and a comparison of program results to expectations of the program's consumers and their sponsors (consumer satisfaction).

The value assessment can range from simple—as in comparison of the organization's efficiency measure to that of a regional or national aggregation, to complex—as in a program evaluation model that balances multiple indicators in a weighted model comparing an organization to a comparison base. Program evaluation models may compare an organization's performance to its own goals, or the performance of external comparison groups. CARF (1997) standards require that organizations rank or weight evaluation objectives, and a program evaluation model is a useful framework for conforming. The UDSmr[SM] program evaluation model reported to data management subscribers incorporates several competing goals (e.g., minimize length of stay, maximize functional gain), weights each goal differently (e.g., maximize discharge to community is higher than minimize charges), computes a performance index which compares the organization to regional or national groups, and arrives at a summary index (UDS, 1993; Granger et al., 1996). This kind of model is an excellent way to concisely summarize program value and highlight broad areas for more investigation.

Consumer Satisfaction as an Indicator of Value

Consumer satisfaction is an important component of an organization's evaluation system. Satisfaction can be viewed as one outcome variable, but is also crucial in goal-setting for the program. Principles of quality improvement rest on assessing consumers' desires for service, and consumers' satisfaction with services provided. CARF standards require that programs use input from persons served in program planning (consumer-based planning) (CARF, 1997).

Domains of interest include satisfaction with the care environment and service delivery process; with the degree to which consumer is involved with the team in care planning; with the relationships developed with team members; or with the outcome of clinical care (reduction in impairment, disability or handicap). Since there are no global standardized measures of consumer satisfaction for rehabilitation, it is common for programs to develop their own list of consumer satisfaction questions to be addressed to persons served and/or their families either during the service period, at the end of services, or at a point following services.

Depending on the domains addressed in a consumer satisfaction survey, either process or outcome components can be evaluated. If consumers' responses are identifiable (i.e., can be added to a computer record for the individual), satisfaction results can be analyzed in relation to clinical outcome and care process variables (e.g., impairment, functional gain, team, program, referral source) for even more insight into program successes and needs for improvement (See Rao, Goldsmith, Wilkerson, & Hildebrandt, 1992) (see Chapter 4 by Rao, Blosser, & Huffman for additional information).

Where Do We Need to Improve?

This question forms the critical link between program evaluation and quality improvement—a link which, while not a traditional one, should be forged in order to create a cost-effective system of information use. In the model proposed here, findings from the program evaluation and outcomes management system are used to trigger process improvement efforts typical of quality or performance improvement paradigms (Deming, 1982; JCAHO, 1997) (see Chapter 8 by Frattali for additional information).

The concept of improvement implies a comparison of performance to a target, whether for outcome, process, or structural aspects of quality. Improvement also implies a temporal aspect—change toward a target over time. The target against which improvement is measured may be internal (e.g., compared to last year's performance for our program, or to the organization's strategic plan goals) or external (e.g., compared to the regional average, or to the best practice or a facility identified as a benchmark). A program evaluation model which sets quantitative targets based on either internal or external comparisons, and which routinely tracks actual performance against those quantitative targets, forms a foundation for review. Where the review of data shows performance falling short of target expectations, more in-depth review is warranted, and a continuous quality improvement (CQI)-type process improvement effort swings into place. During the CQI effort, additional data and a more focused study approach are employed to identify just where processes can be changed to improve outcomes. Once processes are modified, and potentially, revised goals or performance targets are in place, the overall system is reentered, and the data collection and performance comparisons are begun again.

How Do We Compare?

Traditional program evaluation efforts have been conducted primarily for the benefit of the organization for its internal use. CARF standards have for many years required that accredited organizations not only have an outcome-based program evaluation system in place, but also that the information gained be used throughout all levels of the organization in decision making (CARF, 1997).

It is increasingly important to consumers, payers, and providers to know how a program's effectiveness and efficiency compare to other programs. A program may be an extraordinary value and still not be competitive in a given "marketplace" for services. For example, a fine luxury automobile may last 20 years, perform very well across many quality indicators, and be considered of high value, even at a high price; however, most car buyers simply do not possess the resources to purchase a luxury vehicle. Similarly, as health care cost containment efforts have increased, it is often the price itself, in addition to value, that guides selection of services. Knowledge of how one program compares to other similar programs can help programs (a) improve where necessary to excel in value, and (b) understand where the program is positioned within the health care marketplace.

Comparison data may be available from multiple sources, or may be difficult to impossible to obtain, depending on the specific indicators one wishes to compare, and on the program's organizational setting. The business environment of health care in the 1990s and the attendant concerns about program confidentiality prevent most organization-specific comparisons. Exceptions can be found where national networks involving many rehabilitation organizations may compare performance across programs within the network. Also, some entities may force public disclosure of data that allow comparisons to be made by consumers, payers, and other providers. For example, a number of states make hospital discharge data available. In addition, the NCQA, which accredits managed care organizations, plans to make available to the public data from health care plans reporting on the Health Plan Employer Data and Information Set (HEDIS) performance data set (NCQA, 1996). While public disclosure requirements do not, as of 1996, include rehabilitation- or speech-language service-specific outcomes measures, this trend may well change with anticipated continued consumer choice in health care (DeJong & Sutton, 1996).

Comparison of an organization's performance to an aggregation of regional or national organizations is commonly available, but usually requires joining a group and contributing data to a pooled data system. Subscribers to pooled data systems in medical rehabilitation receive reports that show service population characteristics, outcomes, and resource utilization (usually length of stay or visits, and charges) for specified patient groupings (commonly diagnostic groups such as orthopedic injuries, stroke, brain injury, spinal cord injury, arthritis, etc.) (Formations in Healthcare, 1993; UDS, 1993). Limited data are published in the open literature (Fiedler, Granger, & Ottenbacher, 1996) and can be used as a comparison base in the absence of participation in a pooled data system.

Drawing valid comparisons of effectiveness or efficiency across groups of clients requires that comparison groups be similar, especially in the factors that are most related to determining outcome (Iezzoni, 1994). This means, at a minimum, that the groups be of the same diagnostic group (e.g., stroke, traumatic brain injury) and be served by similar programs. More accurate comparisons require also that groups be similar in severity of impairment and/or disability, or whatever other risk factors are related to the dependent variable of interest. Admission functional status is a strong predictor of discharge functional status (Heinemann, Linacre, Wright, Hamilton, & Granger, 1994). A simple severity-adjustment method, therefore, would entail grouping clients within a diagnostic group by high, medium, and low admission functional status before comparisons are made. This kind of severity adjustment may not be available for regional and national comparison groups from a pooled data system, but can be used within an organization's program evaluation system to compare trends over time for program decision making.

Significant work has been done using function-related groups (FRGs) based on the Functional Independence Measure (FIM[sm]-FRGs) to classify rehabilitation inpatients with respect to predicted length of stay (Stineman, Escarce, Goin, Hamilton, Granger, & Williams, 1994) for purposes of reimbursement. Stineman and colleagues (1996) have also begun to look at using FIM-FRGs to adjust for outcome comparisons as well. However, definitive disability severity adjustment methodologies for rehabilitation have yet to come into widespread use for program evaluation systems. This is, however, one of the next major topics likely to contribute to advances in this field.

Programs also should be aware that those who have time, resources, and clout (e.g., payers, consumers) can request data from individual organizations and conduct their own comparisons of effectiveness and efficiency.

Issues in Using Comparative Data

When identifying a comparison base (usually through selection of a pooled data system to join) it is important to understand to what your organization will be compared. Since access to the most detailed comparison information is available only through such subscriptions, the organization will most likely be limited to comparisons with other subscribers to the same service. Exceptions are comparisons to published data, e.g. UDSMR^{SM} annual data (Fiedler et al., 1996) or to members of the organization's corporate network. It is therefore imperative that some knowledge be gained about the other programs included in the comparison base:

- *General program type and characteristics* (inpatient/subacute/outpatient, free-standing/unit, public/private, size, geographic distribution, urban/rural, diversity of affiliation with corporate networks, etc.). How similar or different is your organization from the others in the aggregation?

- *Numbers of organizations in comparison groups.* Is the sample size sufficient to moderate influence of extreme values from one or two organizations in the comparison base (including yours!).

- *Client grouping variables.* What client characteristics are used to form comparison groups, and how finely are the groups defined (e.g., all stroke or right- versus left-hemisphere stroke)? Are severity adjustments included in the groupings (e.g., for admission functional status)?

- *Other information on which to judge representativeness.* Is there sufficient information available about the comparison base and the specific client groupings reported so that you can assess the degree to which your program or population is representative of the comparison base? If your group is very different from the comparison base in key aspects, users of the information will not be inclined to take seriously any comparisons or implications for program change.

On Report Cards

The concept of a report card is relatively new to the health care field, but reflects the same intent as a report card from education or consumer products circles. Key quantitative indicators of quality performance are chosen for display in a uniform and concise format so that the performance of the "reportee" can be assessed across all indicators, and so that comparisons can be made from one "reportee" to another. Report cards can be generated by either external reviewers (if they have access to the data for indicators), or by the "reportee," or organization whose performance is being summarized. As with education and consumer products, it is natural to be skeptical of a self-generated report card; yet it is in 1996 unlikely that external reviewers would have access to sufficient information on effectiveness and efficiency of organizations to produce an independently generated report card.

Two factors for generating report cards are missing currently. First, there currently is no standardized template of performance indicators in rehabilitation on which to generate report cards. While individual organizations may use a report-card format to publicize their own performance, indicators must be chosen by the organization, and are therefore not uniform from organization to organization. Second, no independent entity has established a requirement or incentive for uniform report card generation in rehabilitation. NCQA, with its HEDIS data set, provides such an incentive and performance indicator set for managed care organizations, but this system is not specific to, nor appropriate for, speech-language pathology services or rehabilitation programs. Until state health planning agencies or accrediting bodies, for example, introduce a similar incentive and define a uniform template of performance indicators, report cards will remain organizationally generated, and subject to the self-generated report card suspicion. Nonetheless, the managers of those programs who are willing to share their performance should be applauded, and their report cards evaluated with a dose of caution and a review of evidence that data are accurate, complete, and unbiased.

BASIC COMPONENTS OF A PROGRAM EVALUATION SYSTEM

Implementing a new program evaluation system can be a daunting task for an organization, whether involving a pooled data system or developed entirely by the organization. There are resources in the literature to help guide the many choices a program will need to make (CARF, 1997; JCAHO, 1997; Fuhrer, 1987; Johnston & Granger, 1994; Johnston, Wilkerson, & Maney, 1992; Johnston & Wilkerson, 1992; Forer, 1996; Weiss, 1972). A common set of components for a program evaluation system—themes common to many of the resources cited—can provide a template for system development. Table 7–4 provides a brief sample of these elements in a tabular format.

1. Select or Describe a Framework for Program Goals

Identifying a conceptual framework for the program helps clarify that the right goals for the particular program have been identified and has implications for which measures are selected. Are there short-range or long-range goals; are micro-level, meso-level or macro-level functions the focus; are consumer goals typically reduction in impairment, disability, or handicap? What is the balance of effectiveness (outcome) and efficiency (cost/outcome) goals? Are goals internally referenced (in comparison to one's own organizational trends) or externally referenced (in comparison to regional or national norms or benchmarks)?

2. Establish Program Goals within the Framework

The aggregation of individual consumers' goals form the basis for program goals related to clinical outcomes. It is not the case that clinicians should establish goals *for* their consumers, but with consumer input. Once baseline clinical outcomes are reflected (e.g., 86% of persons who have sustained stroke achieve modified independence in communication skills), the program's goals in communication disability outcome can be established. The 86% figure should reflect the degree to which individual consumers both desire and achieve modified independence in communication.

The array of goals and specific measurable objectives chosen by the program constitute a program evaluation model reflecting the values and ranking of goals for the program. They should include effectiveness, efficiency, and satisfaction goals; they may include outcome as well as process goals.

Table 7–4. Sample Program Evaluation Management Report
& Program Evaluation Model
Acme Rehab Stroke Program Calendar Year 1996

Objective	Measure	Population	Performance Goal	CY95 Actual Performance	CY95 Performance Index (Actual Goal)	CY96 Actual Performance	CY96 Performance Index	Target for Action? Referred to:
Maximize communication skills outcomes	Percent of clients who are discharged at level 6+ on expression (independent; may use assistive tech)	Clients in high, medium and low function at admission groups	High 95% Med 80% Low 65%	96% 85% 58%	1.01 1.06 .89	95% 82% 62%	1.00 1.02 .95	— — SLP
Maximize return to community	Percent of clients responding "agree" or "strongly agree" on survey item: "Participating in community life?"	All clients who participated in stroke program	90%	70%	.78	66%	.73	Case Management Team, QI Council, Program Management Team
Maximize retention of benefits in community	Percent of clients still living in the community at follow-up 90 days post-discharge	All clients who participated in stroke program	87%	83%	.95	77%	.88	Case Management Team

Objective	Measure						Responsibility
Maximize efficiency	Mean functional status change admission-discharge / days LOS (LOS Efficiency)	1.10 (Regional mean)	1.02	.93	1.10	1.00	Program Management Team
Maximize consumer satisfaction	Percent of clients who respond "agree" or "strongly agree" on all seven satisfaction survey questions	All clients served in stroke program who respond to satisfaction survey at follow-up / 100%	72%	.72	74%	.74	QI Council review all "dissatisfied" responses; refer to Prog. Mgmt. and Case Mgmt. Teams

NOTE: This table is for illustrative purposes only; all data are fictitious. Types of objectives and measures as well as quantitative goals and performance levels must be tailored to the type of program (e.g., education, health care), populations served, and meaningful measures and goals.

165

3. Define Measurable Indicators of Performance with Respect to Goals (Select Measurement Tools and Input/Process/Outcome Variables of Interest)

Specific indicators and measures must then be selected to quantify the goals expressed by the program evaluation model. For clinical outcomes, indicators should be based on valid, reliable measurement tools. Indicators may be absolute (e.g., for a percentage of the population to achieve a certain level of function at follow-up) or comparative (e.g., for the program to maintain an efficiency index better than the regional average).

4. Identify the Population for Analysis, Including Severity Adjusters

Those to whom selected measures apply must be specified, and any severity adjuster variables indicated. For example, a program may assess communication function gain separately for (a) clients with low-to-medium admission functional status and (b) those with high admission functional status. Only clients participating in certain aspects of a program may be included, for example, those in AAC programs to assess satisfaction with AAC devices/systems at follow-up.

5. Use Baseline Data to Determine Quantitative Goals for Your Program

Once measures are specified, levels of expected performance should be set for the program and designated subsets of the consumer population. Setting expected performance levels may be based on benchmarks or external comparison data, or on baseline data gathered by the organization during an early data collection period. Establishing quantitative goals is important so that actual performance can be compared. Quantitative goals should not be considered as thresholds, but can be continually increased under a quality improvement model; they do, however, give the program a target for performance and provide another comparative angle for the evaluation.

6. Establish Measurement Points

Time periods for measurement of client-related variables must be established (e.g., admission, discharge, follow-up; periodic); their selection depends upon the nature of the program, the conceptual framework for the program's goals, as well as the program's capacity for data gathering. Multiple measurement points are essential if change in functional status is to be measured; measurement at a point or points following the close of service delivery is crucial to assess the retention of outcomes and the reduction of handicap. Long-term programs (e.g., outpatient, community integration programs) may select arbitrary periodic points of measurement (e.g., every 6 months), especially when service contacts are sporadic and unevenly spaced.

7. Determine Need for and Source of Comparative Information

As discussed earlier, the use of external comparison data is very valuable to a program's understanding of its relative quality and potential opportunities for improvement.

Comparison data sources for specific measurable goals should be identified, and the organizations performance targets expressed in the same terms.

8. Develop a Program Evaluation (PE) Model

A program evaluation model reflects your program's concepts of value, and of the relative ranking/weighting among goals. The model may identify only those limited top-ranked goals for presentation, while other data remains for other analyses or as explanatory variables. Alternatively, weights for each goal can be established, and weighting values multiplied by the performance index. This type of system further clarifies the program's values.

The UDSMR^SM's program evaluation model for inpatient medical rehabilitation is a good example; this model, containing 5 measures, is reported to subscribers with each quarterly report, and allows comparisons of an overall model "score" to that of regional or national comparison groups (Granger, Kelley-Hayes, Johnston, Deutsch, Braun, & Fiedler, 1996). A program may change the weights to reflect its own program values and the relative weights given to competing goals. For example, minimizing charges may be of lower weight than having high percentages of the patient population achieve independent function; another program may value minimizing LOS more highly, and weight it equally with functional gain.

9. Collect Data

Collecting complete, accurate, and reliable data for the evaluation system is no trivial matter. Data collection efforts for the most part now involve computer-based information systems, but not always. Either paper-based or computer-based systems should be structured in such a way as to minimize disruption to the clinical process—ideally, to enhance it. Whatever collection methods are used, data elements needed for the program evaluation model are crucial, and must be complete and accurate if they are to form the basis for decision making a program improvement.

10. Analyze and Report Data on Actual Performance

Actual program performance on specified measures, for specified analysis populations, is reported for specified time periods (e.g., quarterly and annually). Methods for summarizing data vary widely depending on factors such as: (1) whether the organization participates in a pooled data system that summarizes data for the organization, (2) the internal resources available to analyze and report data (e.g., data management personnel, information systems support, software with analysis and reporting capability), and (3) the nature and structure of the information system containing the data (e.g., computer-based or paper-based; simple and accessible versus difficult to access).

11. Compute a Performance Index

Comparing actual performance to performance goals is at the crux of program evaluation. One way to quickly assess the pattern of performance relative to goals is to compute a performance index as the ratio of actual to goal measures. For example, if the goal is for 80% of clients in the stroke program to maintain a level of modified independence at 3-month follow-up, and 85% of clients are found to be at that level, the ratio is .85/.80 or 1.06. In other words, the program achieved 106% of its goal on this measure.

12. Interpret Data and Act on Implications for Program Change

Finally, the organization's decision makers at all levels should review information provided through data analysis and identify implications for further investigation, process improvement studies, or program change. For example, if the program's outcomes in a specified goal area are not as high as expected (e.g., only 55% of clients maintained modified independence levels in communication function at follow-up, yielding a performance index of .69), the program must turn to assessing reasons for such a pattern. While it is always possible to set goals unrealistically high (or low), or to inadequately account for severity, often internal processes are the focus of program change. In this example, the program may hold team discussion about reasons client function is not maintained, and the team may be aware of likely causes (e.g., inavailability of assistive devices; delays in service delivery resulting in insufficient training). If causes are suspected, program changes can be made and performance remeasured over time to determine if program changes improved performance (assuming homogeneous case mix for different groups). If the team does not have ideas about suspected causes for poor program performance, more investigation may be necessary (e.g., a consumer survey of clients whose follow-up function is low to assess the reasons for decline, such as problems in the environment, complications, or new impairments). In essence, the evaluation findings may well—and should—spin off into a quality improvement or process analysis as described in Chapter 8.

REPORTING FOR DECISION MAKING AND CHANGE

One of the most difficult steps in the program evaluation cycle is the final one—gaining useful information from the data collected, and applying that information to decision making and quality improvement changes for the program (CARF, 1995). Several considerations may assist programs in truly utilizing information from the program evaluation system, and avoiding the disastrous scenario of conducting data collection activity without purpose and useful application.

1. Tailor Content to the Audience

Different audiences for the information from a PE system are interested in different levels and aggregations of information. Clinicians want to know about their teams, the populations with whom they work, the functional areas that are targets for improvement for their consumers, and how their clients' outcomes compare to an external comparison base. High-level administrators and board members want the big picture—how does the program compare overall to other programs; in what areas are improvements needed to increase efficiency; how can the information be used to promote the program?

It is crucial to involve the decision makers at all levels of the organization in receiving and interpreting program evaluation results, and to tailor the reporting to each level of decision making. Similar to politics, all quality improvement change is local—the lowest unit of decision making is the one which must have sufficient information to institute process analysis and quality improvement efforts. For example, if TBI survivors receiving speech-language pathology services are not reaching established program goals of better communication and social interaction or return to school and work, then those working directly with the program must (1) know the performance measures and become aware that goals are not being met, and (2) be able to analyze the related program processes in detail to identify where change is needed.

Even though QI change may be "local," policy and resource allocation to support program evaluation and quality improvement decision making emanates from high levels of the organization. It is essential, therefore, that the person in charge (administrator, principal, rehabilitation manager, chief executive officer) be included in the audience for evaluation system findings, at least at a summary level, for example, the PE model conclusions, major comparisons with regional and national indicators (e.g., efficiency measures), and summary of QI changes instituted as a result of program evaluation findings.

2. Produce Accurate, Complete, and Timely Reports

Users of the information from a program evaluation system will not be willing to act on information they consider old, inaccurate, or incomplete. This can present a problem when an information system is cumbersome, or resources are insufficient to analyze and report data in a timely manner, or when the key actors are too busy or inaccessible to commit to studying and interpreting the information. If the data collection system does provide for feasibly gathering complete information (e.g., cases are missing key data elements or have incomplete outcome measure scores), users will not have confidence in the findings and again, will be reluctant, or even refuse, to act.

3. Use Program Evaluation Findings as Clues for Further Investigation

It is important to understand that at times, the information from the program evaluation system is too gross, too blunt an instrument, on which to pinpoint needed program change. However, not meeting established goals or performing poorly with respect to established comparison groups should prompt further examination—either cutting the data more finely to better adjust for severity or to isolate program components ripe for process improvement. The program evaluation effort is not complete until the information is used either to confirm, communicate, and reward excellent performance, or to make process or program changes where performance is less than desired.

CONCLUSION

Program evaluation efforts are likely to continue to be a factor for speech-language pathology programs for the foreseeable future, but the integration with other evaluative systems will increase. The field needs more clarity on the relationship of these efforts to one another, good models of best practice, and more experience in using evaluation information to manage the outcomes and costs of programs. Accountability for the kinds of goals established as well as the success in meeting those goals will be driven by those other than the provider, as they have in the past: by managed care organizations, school systems, other public and private payers of speech-language pathology services, and perhaps eventually—hopefully—by individual consumers. Providers conducting program evaluation efforts need to focus on ways to streamline data collection, integrate data collection with the clinical process so as not to add a layer on a shrinking resource, efficiently analyze the data to turn it into useful information, and look for better ways to utilize the information gained to increase quality of services.

REFERENCES

CARF . . . The Rehabilitation Accreditation Commission [CARF]. (1997). *1997 Standards Manual and Interpretive Guidelines for Medical Rehabilitation.* Tucson: Author.

CARF . . . The Rehabilitation Accreditation Commission [CARF]. (1995). *Operations Analysis of 1994–1995 Survey Activities.* Tucson: Author.

Deming, W. E. (1982). *Out of the Crisis.* Cambridge, MA: Massachusetts Institute of Technology Center for Advanced Engineering Study.

DeJong, G., & Sutton, J. P. (1996). Rehab 2000: The evolution of medical rehabilitation in American health care. In P. K. Landrum, N. D. Schmidt, & A. McLean Jr. (Eds), *Outcome-Oriented Rehabilitation: Principles, Strategies, and Tools for Effective Program Management.* Gaithersburg, MD: Aspen Publishers, Inc.

Ellwood, P. (1988). Outcomes Management: A Technology of Patient Experience. *New England Journal of Medicine, 318,* 1549–1556.

Fiedler, R. C., Granger, C. V., & Ottenbacher, K. J. (1996) The Uniform Data System for Medical Rehabilitation: Report of first admissions for 1994. *American Journal of Physical Medicine and Rehabilitation, 75*(2), 125–129.

Formations in Healthcare, Inc. (1993). *Rehabilitation Outcomes Reports.* Chicago: Author.

Forer, S. (1996). *Outcome Management and Program Evaluation Made Easy: A Toolkit for Occupational Therapy Practitioners.* Bethesda, MD: The American Occupational Therapy Association.

Fuhrer, Marcus J. (Ed.). (1987). *Rehabilitation Outcomes: Analysis and Measurement.* Baltimore: Paul H. Brookes Publishing Co.

Granger, C., Kelley-Hayes, M., Johnston, M., Deutsch, A., Braun, S., & Fiedler, R. (1996). Quality and outcome measures in medical rehabilitation. In Braddom, R. (Ed.), *Physical Medicine and Rehabilitation,* pp. 239–253. Philadelphia: W.B. Saunders.

Heinemann, A. W., Linacre, J. M., Wright, B. D., Hamilton, B. B., & Granger, C. V. (1994). Prediction of rehabilitation outcomes with disability measures. *Archives of Physical Medicine and Rehabilitation, 75*(2), 133–143.

Heumann, J. (1977). Independent living programs. In S. S. Pflueger (Ed.), *Independent Living: Emerging Issues in Rehabilitation.* Washington, DC: Institute for Research Utilization.

Iezzoni, L. (Ed.). (1994). *Risk adjustment for measuring health care outcomes.* Ann Arbor: Health Administration Press.

Johnston, M.V., & Granger, C. V. (1994). Outcomes research in medical rehabilitation: A primer and introduction to a series. *American Journal of Physical Medicine and Rehabilitation, 73*(4), 296–303.

Johnston, M.V., & Wilkerson, D.L. (1992). Program evaluation and quality improvement systems in brain injury rehabilitation. *Journal of Head Trauma Rehabilitation, 7*(4), 68–82.

Johnston, M. V., Wilkerson, D. L., & Maney, M. (1992). Evaluation of the quality and outcomes of medical rehabilitation programs. In J.A. DeLisa, & B. Gans, et al. (Eds.), *Rehabilitation Medicine: Principles and Practice,* 2nd Ed. Philadelphia: Lippincott.

Joint Commission on Accreditation of Healthcare Organizations [JCAHO]. (1997). *Accreditation Manual for Hospitals: Vol. I. Standards.* Oakbrook Terrace, IL: Author.

National Committee for Quality Assurance [NCQA]. (1996). *HEDIS.* NCQA site on the World Wide Web (http:\\www.ncqa.com).

Knutson, A.L. (1969). Evaluation for What? In H.C. Schulberg, A. Sheldon, & F. Baker (Eds.), *Program Evaluation in the Health Fields.* New York: Behavioral Publications, pp. 42–58.

Pope, A. M., & Tarlov, A. R. (1991). *Disability in America: Toward a National Agenda for Prevention.* Report of the Committee on a National Agenda for the Prevention of Disabilities, Division of Health Promotion and Disease Prevention, Institute of Medicine. Washington, DC: National Academy Press.

Rao, P., Goldsmith, T., Wilkerson, D., & Hildebrandt, L. (1992). How to keep your customer satisfied: Customer satisfaction survey. *Hear Say: The Journal of the Ohio Speech and Hearing Association,* Winter.

Stineman, M. G., Escarce, J. J., Goin, J. E., Hamilton, B. B., Granger, C. V., & Williams, S. V. (1994). A case-mix classification system for medical rehabilitation. *Medical Care, 32*(4), 366–379.

Stineman, M. G., Hamilton, B.B., Goin, J. E., Granger, C. V., & Fiedler, R. C. (1996). Functional gain and length of stay for major rehabilitation impairment categories: Patterns revealed by function-related groups. *American Journal of Physical Medicine and Rehabilitation, 75*(1), 68–78.

Uniform Data System for Medical Rehabilitation [UDSmr^SM]. (1993). *Guide for the Uniform Data Set for Medical Rehabilitation (Adult FIM^SM), Version 4.0.* Buffalo, NY: State University of New York at Buffalo.

Weiss, C. H. (1972). Evaluation Research. Englewood Cliffs, NJ: Prentice-Hall, Inc.

Wilkerson, D. (1992). Level of function as an organizing framework for functional assessment applications. *Archives of Physical Medicine and Rehabilitation, 73,* 977. (abstract). Article presented at annual meeting of the American Congress of Rehabilitation Medicine, San Francisco, CA, November 1992.

Wilkerson, D. (1996). Level of function as an organizing framework for functional assessment applications. Manuscript submitted for publication.

Wilkerson, D., & Johnston, M. (1997). Outcomes research and clinical program monitoring systems: Current capability and future directions. In M. J. Fuhrer (Ed.), *Medical Rehabilitation Research.* Baltimore: Paul H. Brookes Publishing Co.

Wilkerson, D. (1996). Program and Outcome Evaluation: Opportunity for the 1990s. *Occupational Therapy Practice, 2*(2), 1–15.

Wilkerson, D. (1996). Quality Improvement. In M. Johnson (Ed.), *Occupational Therapy Manager,* Part 2, Chapter 12, Evaluation of Programs. Rockville, MD: The American Occupational Therapy Association.

Wood, P.H.N, & Badley, E. M. (1981). People with Disabilities—Towards Acquiring Information Which Reflects More Sensitively Their Problems and Needs. Monograph No. 12: International Exchange of Information in Rehabilitation Project. World Rehabilitation Fund, National Institute of Handicapped Research. Washington, DC: U.S. Department of Education.

World Health Organization. (1980). *International classification of impairments, disabilities, and handicaps.* Geneva: Author.

CHAPTER 8

Quality Improvement

CAROL M. FRATTALI

INTRODUCTION

Aggressive reforms, driven by public pressures to cap spending, have changed dramatically the ways in which health care and education services are financed and delivered. While 20 years is not an unusually long time, I have, during my career, witnessed a total transformation of service delivery philosophy from "the best regardless of the means," "to the most for the least." It has thrown the system into a frenzy of cost-cutting activities, which have given rise to the unregulated use of support personnel and multiskilled practitioners, the systematic flattening of the organizational chart with elimination of the middle manager, the merging of multidisciplinary rehabilitation at the expense of discipline-specific autonomy and exclusive scopes of practice, and creation of lower-cost alternatives of care. The most serious accusation leveled at policymakers who have supported such sweeping systemic change is that quality of care has suffered. Admonitions abound: Hospital patients are being discharged quicker and sicker; managed care neither manages nor cares; the only outcome of interest is the dollar saved. But, the reported declines in quality routinely are countered with demands to "prove it," thus deflating the strength of the argument.

Can we prove that quality of care has suffered? Can we capture, in an objective and systematic way, quality of care at all? In the rush to compete on the basis of cost in a human service system turned business, does quality even matter to the decision makers? The latter question is both disturbing and short-sighted. Competition on the basis of cost eventually will stabilize. There is only so much funding that can be cut or care that can be pared before the result is rendered unacceptable by even the lowest standard. Thus, the distinguishing feature of competition over the long term will not be cost but quality.

My purposes here are to describe the basic principles of quality measurement, describe the linkage of processes to clinical outcomes, suggest a model for improvement, introduce some quality process tools, and offer an example of how the model can be applied to clinical practice.

THE BASICS

Improving quality is regarded widely as a soft concept in the human services. How can one capture quality when, in fact, quality is in the eye of the beholder? To what beholder do we pay the most attention? Quality to one may not be considered quality to another. Consider the perspectives of the practitioner and the payer. While the practitioner may uphold the technical aspects of care and consequent micro-level behavioral changes as important indicators of quality of care, the payer may care only about the cost efficiency of care and consequent macro-level of independence achieved by the client (independence being equated with dollars saved). Another perspective is introduced by the client and/or family. They may care mostly that care has strong interpersonal features (e.g., an empathetic clinician who explains procedures and expected results with patience and in lay terms) and results in functional improvement or resumption of premorbid work and leisure activities. The varying perspectives of stakeholders, then, span a range of desirable outcomes. But, rather than enter the exhaustive discussion of what *outcomes* to target in efforts to improve quality, my intention here is to turn your attention to *process* as a link to outcomes and, thus, improvements in quality of care.

Defining Quality Improvement

Quality improvement is the effort to improve the level of performance of *key processes*. It suggests a systematic method of studying work processes to improve their outcomes. These work processes can be clinical (e.g., assessment procedures, treatment procedures), administrative (e.g., staffing, continuity of care, referral procedures), financial (e.g., billing, costs, resource use), and technical (e.g., equipment maintenance and use). Quality improvement involves a three-step process of

- measuring the current level of performance,
- finding ways to improve that performance, and
- instituting new and better methods (Berwick, Godfrey, & Roessner, 1990).

Quality improvement, according to Berwick and colleagues (1990), is but one aspect of quality management. The other two aspects are quality planning and quality control. *Quality planning* involves developing a definition of quality as it applies to consumers, developing measures of quality, designing products and services that coincide with consumer needs, designing processes capable of providing those products and services, and transferring those processes into routine operations of the organization.

Quality control involves developing and maintaining operational methods for ensuring that processes work as they are designed to work and that target levels of performance (or outcomes) are being achieved. Quality control, too, requires a definition of quality, knowledge of expected performance or targets, measurements of actual performance, a way to compare expected to actual performance, and a way to take action when measured results fall short of expected results. Quality improvement, which begins with measuring the current level of performance, often is where organizations start first in quality management.

Basic Principles of Quality Improvement

Berwick and colleagues (1990) have condensed an expansive body of knowledge from the professional literature into a set of basic principles of quality improvement. They are expanded here from an earlier publication (Frattali, Blosser, Eiten, et al., 1996):

1. Productive Work Is Accomplished through Work Processes.

Clinicians receive various kinds of inputs (e.g., school reports, laboratory findings, family accounts) that, in turn, are used in performing clinical tasks (e.g., assessment methods, treatment methods, staff/family education) to effect targeted outcomes (e.g., correct diagnoses, functional communication, community reintegration). The linkage of inputs to specific tasks constitutes a work process. The first step of improving quality is to understand these work processes. Second, these processes must be studied to determine where they break down. Third, by understanding the needs of consumers and defining them carefully, the quality of these work processes can be improved.

While often pursued, it usually is not enough to improve our own individual work processes. This is because our work typically depends on and influences the work of others. For example, a treatment procedure may involve the work of suppliers who manufacture devices (e.g., augmentative communication systems, oral prostheses) used in treatment, of laboratory technicians or engineers who conduct tests to determine the effectiveness or appropriateness of the procedure, and of professional staff who transfer use of the procedure to other clinical situations or interventions. Thus, our work is interdependent. In order to improve a work process, then, others must be involved in the effort. This effort gives rise to teamwork.

2. Sound Consumer-Supplier Relationships Are Essential to Improving Quality.

Modern-day theory about quality improvement focuses foremost on consumers and their needs or expectations. Thus, improving quality means striving to improve the capability and reliability of processes to meet or even exceed the needs of those served by the processes. In clinical service delivery, consumers include not only clients but their sponsors (e.g., families, caregivers, payers, administrators, teachers, the community at large). Thus, the first step to improving quality is to identify various consumers' needs and select work processes for improvement that can meet those defined needs. Admittedly, these needs can be diametrically opposed. For example, a payer may want costs controlled, but clients and their families may want access to the most advanced technologies of care. Such trade-offs make quality planning difficult, but they do not change the premise that "the better the organization can understand and meet the needs of its diverse customers, the more successful it will be in the long run" (Berwick et al., 1990, p. 35).

Good consumer-supplier relationships are characterized by clear communication and mutual trust. This is true of both external relationships (i.e., between an organization and its customers) and internal relationships (i.e., between individuals involved within a work process). Indeed, a central concept of quality improvement is that the quality of products and services provided to external consumers are determined largely by the quality of internal consumer-supplier relationships. Consequently, quality improvement efforts invest heavily in forms of interaction, measurement, and clarification of roles that can help internal consumers and suppliers understand and serve each other more effectively.

3. The Main Source of Quality Defects Is Problems in the Process, Not People.

Most work processes are complex. The frequency with which defects occur, then, is not surprising. When processes break down, our inclination is to place blame on people. For example, an incorrect diagnosis suggests an incompetent diagnostician. But, in fact, the source of the problem might have been faulty equipment, medical record mix-ups, or computer breakdowns. Failures in quality usually can be traced to inherent flaws in the processes in which people work, not to the failure of people to do their work as they are instructed. Berwick et al. (1990) state, "The old assumption is that quality fails when people do the right things wrong; the new assumption is that, more often, quality failures arise when people do the wrong things right" (p. 36).

Many individuals who work in flawed systems expend considerable energy to overcome these flaws in order to render quality service. Important improvements in quality are not, however, achieved by these individuals who must compensate repeatedly for flawed processes. They are achieved by improvements in the work processes themselves.

4. Quality Improvement Focuses on the Most Vital Processes.

Those who try to improve everything often find themselves buried in measurements and data and end up taking action on none. It is important, therefore, to select only those processes that are the most critical from a consumer's point of view. A good rule is offered by JCAHO (1997). One should select processes that are high risk (can result in morbidity or mortality), high volume (affect the largest numbers of consumers), or problem prone (have flaws and generate the most consumer complaints).

5. Variability of Work Processes Is a Key to Improving Quality.

In every process, and in every measurement, variability exists. When clinical investigators conduct experimental research to determine treatment efficacy, they design the study to control, as much as possible, the unwanted variability contributed, for example, by differences among subjects or among treatment procedures. The aim of quality improvement is to both understand variation and reduce the causes of variation, which, in turn, increases the likelihood of the desired outcome. Causes of variation that can be reduced or eliminated, for example, can be found in use of clinical measures with no documented reliability and validity, malfunctioning equipment, scientifically unproven treatment methods, and poorly trained staff. Controlling sources of variation can have dramatic effects on quality.

6. New Organizational Structures Can Help the Quality Improvement Effort.

A "guiding arm" is critical to the success of any large-scale or organization-wide quality improvement effort. Often, a steering committee, comprised of executive, managerial, and front-line staff representatives, is formed to strategically plan the quality improvement effort. Sometimes called a "quality council," the steering group is most effective when it consists of the same leaders who operate other key organization functions. These leaders plan training of managers and teams, form the technical infrastructure for improvement, create and maintain procedures for nomination and selection of work processes to be improved, create and maintain forms of recognition of the work of quality improvement teams, and evaluate and improve the quality improvement effort itself.

7. The Approach to Quality Is Statistical Thinking.

Quality improvement began with engineers and statisticians asking the question, "Why does quality fail?" They found that the scientific method held the key to improvement of processes. Clinicians are familiar with this investigative process. Clients come to us with deficits. We conduct diagnostic procedures to find causes, determine the need for treatment, and directions for treatment. We apply treatment procedures. We assess the results of treatment to guide our next steps. A similar method is applied when improving quality. We begin with a failure to meet the needs of consumers. Perhaps procedures are wrong, equipment is broken, or clinicians are improperly trained. The quality improvement team performs diagnostic tests, formulates hypotheses of cause, tests those hypotheses, designs and applies remedies, and assesses the effect of the remedies. They plan. They do. They study. If the remedy works, they act (institute the change).

A scientific approach to quality improvement is based on data. It includes measurement of

- consumer needs
- inputs
- characteristics of work processes
- results (outcomes).

Measurement is used to gain knowledge of work processes so that they can be understood, and thus improved.

OPTIMIZING CLINICAL OUTCOMES: THE LINK TO PROCESS

Quality of clinical care can be improved only if its processes are understood, defined, and employed consistently and appropriately to reduce their variances and the unpredictability of the outcome. The fear, however, is that "cookbook care" will result. Ideally, a combination of the science and art of clinical practice should prevail. But explicit protocols of care are taking precedence in a clinical environment aimed at managed care and cost savings. Thus, the process of care has growing appeal both to administrators and payers. These processes offer a yardstick of performance that, if applied, can optimize targeted outcomes.

JCAHO (1997) details dimensions of performance that it considers worthy of quality measurement and improvement (Table 8–1). These dimensions involve doing the right thing (i.e., clinical procedures that are efficacious and appropriate to the client's

---

Table 8–1. Dimensions of Performance.

I. DOING THE RIGHT THING

The *efficacy* of the procedure or treatment in relation to the patient's condition
    The degree to which the care/intervention for the patient has been shown to accomplish
    the desired/projected outcome(s).
The *appropriateness* of a specific test, procedure, or service to meet the patient's needs
    The degree to which the care/intervention provided is relevant to the patient's clinical
    needs, given the current state of knowledge.

II. DOING THE RIGHT THING WELL

The *availability* of a needed test, procedure, treatment, or service to the patient who needs it.
    The degree to which appropriate care/intervention is available to meet the patient's needs.
The *timeliness* with which a needed test, procedure, treatment, or service is provided to the
patient.
    The degree to which the care/intervention is provided to the patient at the most beneficial
    or necessary time.
The *effectiveness* with which tests, procedures, treatment, and services are provided.
    The degree to which the care/intervention is provided in the correct manner, given the cur-
    rent state of knowledge, in order to achieve the desired/projected outcome for the patient.
The *continuity* of the services provided to the patient with respect to other services, practition-
ers, and providers and over time.
    The degree to which the care/intervention for the patient is coordinated among practition-
    ers, among organizations, and over time.
The *safety* of the patient (and others) to whom the services are provided.
    The degree to which the risk of an intervention and the risk in the care environment are
    reduced for the patient and others, including the health care provider.
The *efficiency* with which services are provided.
    The relationship between the outcomes (results of care) and the resources used to deliver
    patient care.
The *respect* and *caring* with which services are provided.
    The degree to which the patient or a designee is involved in his or her own care decisions
    and to which those providing services do so with sensitivity and respect for the patient's
    needs, expectations, and individual differences.

Reprinted by permission of the Joint Commission on Accreditation of Healthcare Organizations. From *Accredita-tion manual for hospitals* (1997, pp. 130–131). Oakbrook Terrace, IL: Joint Commission on Accreditation of Health-care Organizations.

clinical needs) and doing the right thing well (i.e., the availability of the procedure, the timeliness with which it was conducted, its effectiveness, continuity of the services pro-vided, the safety of the client and others when conducting the procedure, the efficiency with which services are provided, and the respect and caring with which services are provided). These dimensions typically are addressed by a profession's standards of practice, otherwise known as preferred practice patterns, practice guidelines, or critical paths (Frattali & Sutherland Cornett, 1994).

Preferred Practice Patterns

Preferred practice patterns, according to ASHA, are "statements that define universally applicable characteristics of activities directed toward individual patients/clients, which address structural requisites of the practice, processes to be carried out, and expected outcomes" (ASHA, 1993a, p. iii). In 1993, a set of 43 preferred practice patterns were approved by ASHA's Legislative Council for the professions of speech-language pathology and audiology. Developed by the ASHA Task Force on Clinical Standards following widespread peer review, they were based primarily on available treatment efficacy data found in the professional literature, and secondarily on expert opinion. The preferred practice patterns specify, among other dimensions, the clinical indications for performing each procedure, basic clinical processes, setting and equipment specifications, and safety and health precautions. A plan is in place to update the practice patterns periodically as more becomes known scientifically about clinical assessment and treatment procedures.

Practice Guidelines

In comparison to preferred practice patterns, practice guidelines offer more detail about the clinical process. According to the Institute of Medicine (in Agency for Health Care Policy and Research, 1990), practice guidelines are defined as "systematically developed statements to assist practitioner and patient decisions about appropriate health care for specific clinical circumstances" (p. 3). ASHA defines practice guidelines as "a recommended set of procedures for a specific area of practice, based on research findings and current practice, that details the knowledge and skills needed to perform the procedures competently (ASHA, 1993a, p. iii). The foundation of the development of practice guidelines, then, is explicitness and available scientific knowledge.

Many practice guidelines have been developed by ASHA, and are updated periodically as new clinical, scientific, and technological knowledge becomes available. They are compiled in the publication, *ASHA Desk Reference* (ASHA, 1996), which includes position statements, practice guidelines, definitions, and technical reports, among other important practice documents.

Critical Paths

The concept of critical paths emerged in health care more than a decade ago as a nursing and case management initiative at Boston's New England Medical Center (Lumsdon & Hagland, 1993). Both the concept and term are borrowed from project management in the field of engineering. Critical paths, and related clinical pathways and care maps, are charts showing the key interventions that typically lead to the successful treatment of clients in a homogeneous population. They are clinical management tools that organize, sequence, and time the major interventions of an interdisciplinary team of practitioners for a particular case type or condition. They usually are organized with length of stay graphed on an axis against an intervention axis.

Despite the interchangeable use of terminology, Kaine (1992) makes a distinction between clinical and critical pathways. Clinical pathways are treatment regimes, agreed upon by consensus, that include all the elements of care, regardless of the effect on client outcomes; critical pathways are treatment regimes that include only those vital elements proven to affect client outcomes. Care maps, too, are distinguishable. According to Zander (1993), care maps show the relationship of sets of interventions to sets of intermediate outcomes along a time line. They show cause and effect relationships across time and are considered superior to clinical or critical pathways.

Regardless of the tool used, all of these treatment regimes represent the care rendered to a majority but not the totality of clients in a given population. Because individual clients respond to interventions in different and often unpredictable ways, there always will be variances from the norm. These measures, then, allow for continual variance analysis and corrective action as needed.

A MODEL FOR IMPROVEMENT

The study of work processes, whether clinical, administrative, financial, or technical, involves its own systematic process that is grounded in the scientific method. If statisticians and engineers began by asking, Why does quality fail?, they logically would proceed by asking a subset of questions to reveal knowledge about specific work processes. These questions would dictate a model for improvement by leading the investigator from an aim, to current knowledge, to a cycle of learning and improvement. Three questions that might be asked are these:

- What are we trying to accomplish? (aim or intended outcome)
- How will we know that a change is an improvement? (current knowledge)
- What changes can we make that will result in improvement? (new knowledge)

These questions form the basis of a model introduced by Associates in Process Improvement, Inc. (API) (Langley, Nolan, & Nolan, 1992) (Figure 8–1). Having an aim (or desired outcome), baseline data that describe the current situation, and criteria with which to measure improvement (e.g., process and outcome measures) constitute what is known as a Plan-Do-Study-Act (PDSA) cycle (Figure 8–2). This cycle, introduced by the late Walter Shewhart (a statistician at Bell Telephone Laboratories credited with bringing industrial processes into statistical control), but sometimes known as the Deming cycle (after the late W. Edwards Deming [1982], a consultant in statistical studies who advanced the philosophy and methods of quality improvement in the manufacturing and service industries worldwide), involves four phases:

1. Plan (a trial is developed)
2. Do (the trial is performed and data are collected)
3. Study (the data are studied and compared to previous knowledge)
4. Act (changes are made based on the new knowledge)

The API Model relies heavily on the continual collection and interpretation of data using agreed-upon measures of quality and is based on building knowledge and taking action based on this knowledge. Langley, Nolan, and Nolan (1992) explain that the use of observation is an important source of learning for improving quality, but observation alone is not enough. Thus, in a clinical context, the collection and use of data help to overcome the subjectivities inherent in observation, provide more objective evidence with which to make clinical decisions, and can lead to better patient outcomes.

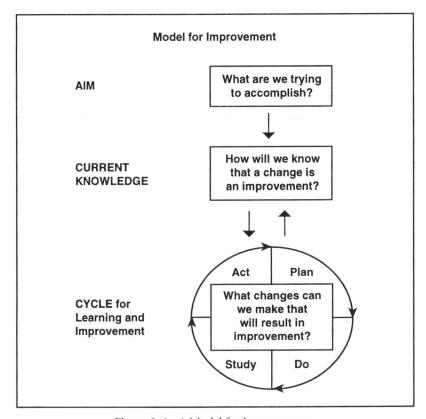

Figure 8–1. A Model for Improvement

SOURCE: Langley, G. J., Nolan, K. M., & Nolan, T. W. (1992). *The foundation for improvement (Part 1)*. Silver Spring, MD: Associates in Process Improvement, Inc. Used by permission.

Tools for Data Collection, Analysis, and Problem Solving

Once a model for improvement is selected, a combination of tools can be used to organize and analyze data, and solve problems inherent in the process. The tools often are called statistical process control tools. Some of these tools, however, are not statistical tools at all but effective ways to organize information or ideas. It is helpful to think of these tools as pictorial means to display and analyze information.

Brassard (1988) calls these tools graphical problem-solving techniques. They identify variations in work processes, the root causes of problems, the relative importance of problems to be solved, and the impact of subsequent changes. Some common graphical tools associated with methods to improve quality (Figure 8–3) are:

Flow charts. Pictorial representations showing sequentially all the steps of a work process. Flow charts identify the actual path a process follows, and helps identify redundancies, inefficiencies, misunderstandings, waiting loops, and inspection steps.

Cause-and-effect diagrams. Also called fishbone diagrams, they show the relationship between an effect (outcome) and all the possible causes influencing it. These diagrams help a team identify and define an outcome or problem, determine causes of a given outcome or problem, or identify causes for variation in a process.

Pareto charts. A special form of vertical bar graphs, showing the frequency of events in descending order to help determine which problems to solve and in what order. Pareto charts allow a team to categorize occurrences and focus on those that are most frequent and most important.

Run charts. Visual representations of data that display points on a graph to show levels of performance over time. Run charts are used to identify trends, analyze performance data, and monitor actions taken to improve performance.

Control charts. Run charts with statistically determined upper and lower control limits, drawn as lines on either side of the process average. They detect movement away from the average and capture variation in a work process.

Histograms. Bar graphs that display the distribution of data or the number of units in each category. Histograms help determine whether variation is normal or suggests areas needing further attention.

Scatter diagrams. Pictorial representations of the possible relationship between two variables (e.g., the effect of room temperature on equipment functioning). They are used when teams want to test a theory about cause and effect, analyze raw data, and monitor action taken to improve performance.

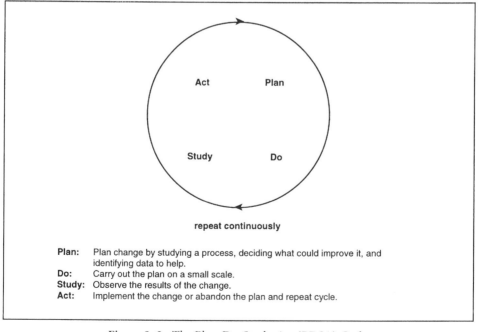

Figure 8–2. The Plan-Do-Study-Act (PDSA) Cycle

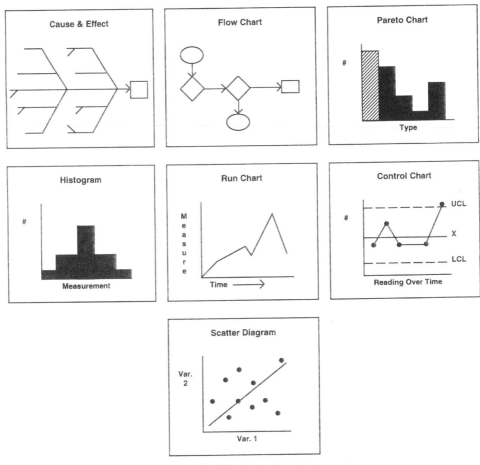

Figure 8–3. Graphical Tools for Quality Improvement

SOURCE: Brassard, M. (1988). *The memory jogger.* Metheun, MA: Goal/QPC. Adapted by permission.

Resources to learn more about these and other tools and their applications include *The Memory Jogger* (Brassard, 1988), *The Team Handbook* (Scholtes, 1988), *A Pocket Guide to Quality Improvement Tools* (JCAHO, 1992), and *Total Quality Management: A Continuous Process for Improvement* (ASHA, 1993b).

A Clinical Example

The questions that constitute API's Model reveal a logical investigative process that is feasible for use by clinicians in their routine practice, and practical in their ability to acquire new knowledge about clinical interventions and their effects.

What Are We Trying to Accomplish?

The first question addresses your clinical aim or desired outcomes for the client. One aim, for example, could be functional communication that allows the client to live independently. The aim involves the client's needs to communicate basic needs, use the telephone, and engage in daily planning—basic skills that would allow him or her to return home without the need for personal assistance. The aim addresses the concerns of the client whose goal is independence, and the payer whose goal is cost savings. Thus, the aim takes into consideration the perspectives of key stakeholders.

How Will We Know a Change Is an Improvement?

The question forces your attention to the current state of knowledge. The process then would involve the need to collect baseline data. If functional communication is your aim, then baseline data would be collected using a functional communication measure that validly and reliably captures information on the ability to communicate basic needs, use the telephone, and engage in daily planning. At this stage in the process, your measure or measures of quality are identified, and operationally defined, in this case, a reliable and valid measure of functional communication.

While the selected measure of quality is an outcome measure, other measures of quality can include process measures. Examples are clinical practice guidelines, treatment protocols, or critical paths, which allow evaluation of the clinician's performance during the clinical process and its link to the outcome of care.

What Changes Can We Make That Will Result in Improvement?

This question activates the PDSA cycle. For example, in the "Plan" stage, process measures (e.g., a critical path, practice guideline) could form the basis of the care plan. Once initiated ("Do"), data are collected to determine compliance with the path, and studied ("Study"). Is there compliance at each step of the critical path? Are there any variances? If so, why? and, What is the client's response to treatment (using the functional communication measure that served as the baseline measure)? Based on these data, you "Act" by continuing treatment as planned, modifying treatment, or discontinuing treatment. The learning that results can lead to improvements in work processes (e.g., refinements in the critical path or practice guideline, development of clinical competencies, formulation of client selection criteria), and in the quality of the treatment rendered. Thus, all decisions are data based and lead to better or more predictable client outcomes.

As a clinician reenters the cycle of learning and improvement, more cost effective methods of treatment can be tried. For example, the clinician could include treatment trials using a combination of professional staff and support personnel, family/staff instruction, computer-assisted treatment, and group treatment. As new methods are tried, outcomes can be monitored for comparisons to more traditional treatment methods to determine effectiveness, while at the same time tracking costs to determine efficiency.

CONCLUSION

Use of a practical and data-driven model for improvement allows us to provide better and perhaps more efficient quality of service. The model can also expand our thinking beyond discipline-specific clinical interventions to clinical, financial, administrative, and technical interventions applied across disciplines that interact systemwide to constitute quality care. Given the reality of current cost constraints in a competitive service delivery system, three recommendations are offered:

1. *Accept current definitions of quality of care.* Quality of care is the degree to which desired client outcomes are achieved using cost-effective means.

2. *Consistently apply a data-driven model for improvement to acquire new knowledge.* Such a model might require us to answer three questions: What are we trying to accomplish? How will we know that a change is an improvement? What changes can we make that will result in improvement?

3. *Share the knowledge acquired with key stakeholders.* Decisions today are made with data. The key to service delivery reforms is to communicate, in the form of objective data, what is known clinically about both the effectiveness and efficiency of interventions.

Currently, methods to improve quality tackle only a few of the difficulties facing service delivery today. The looming pressures resulting from regulation and cost containment alone render quality improvement a diversion to many who must meet current fiscal demands (Berwick et al., 1990). But, far from being a diversion, methods to improve quality can lead directly to greater efficiency and cost reduction. And, if predictions are accurate, competition in service delivery will shift from a pure price basis to a combination of price and quality. As a result, the issue of quality will become fundamental to the survival of any service organization, and will become the basis for competition over the next decade and beyond.

ACKNOWLEDGMENT

This chapter is dedicated to Marni Hope Reisberg, M.S., CCC/SLP, a colleague and friend, who died on May 25, 1996. Her knowledge about quality improvement, which she so generously shared, is conveyed throughout its pages.

REFERENCES

Agency for Health Care Policy and Research. (1990, August). Clinical guideline development. *AHCPR Program Note.* Rockville, MD: Author.

American Speech-Language-Hearing Association. (1993a, March). Preferred practice patterns for the professions of speech-language pathology and audiology. *Asha (Suppl. 11)*, 1–97.

American Speech-Language-Hearing Association. (1993b). *Total quality management: A continuous process for improvement.* Rockville, MD: Ad Hoc Committee on Quality Improvement.

American Speech-Language-Hearing Association. (1996). *ASHA desk reference.* Rockville, MD: Author.

Berwick, D.M., Godfrey, A.B., & Roessner, J. (1990). *Curing health care.* San Francisco, CA: Jossey-Bass Publishers.

Brassard, M. (1988). *The memory jogger.* Methuen, MA: GOAL/QPC.

Deming, W. E. (1982). *Out of the crisis.* Cambridge, MA: Massachusetts Institute of Technology, Center for Advanced Engineering Study.

Frattali, C.M., Blosser, J., Eiten, L., Huffman, N., Kimbarow, M. et. al. (1996, Summer). Quality improvement: The basics. *Newsletter of ASHA Special Interest Division 11: Administration and supervision.* Rockville, MD: ASHA.

Frattali, C.M., & Sutherland Cornett, B. (1994). Improving quality in the context of managed care. *In Managing managed care: A practical guide for audiologists and speech-language pathologists.* Rockville, MD: Ad Hoc Committee on Managed Care of the American Speech-Language-Hearing Association.

Joint Commission on Accreditation of Healthcare Organizations. (1992). *A pocket guide to quality improvement tools.* Oakbrook Terrace, IL: Author.

Joint Commission on Accreditation of Healthcare Organizations. (1997). *Accreditation manual for hospitals.* Oakbrook Terrace, IL: Author.

Kaine, R. (1992). Practice protocols by a different name are not quite the same. *Hospital Rehabilitation, 2,* 124.

Langley, G.J., Nolan, K.M., & Nolan, T.W. (1992). The foundation of improvement. Silver Spring, MD: Associates in Process Improvement, Inc.

Lumsdon, K., & Hagland, M. (1993). Mapping care. *Hospital & Health Networks, 67,* 34–40.

Scholtes, P. R. (1988). *The team handbook.* Madison, WI: Joiner.

Zander, K. (1993). Critical pathways. In M.M. Melum & M.K. Finioris (Eds.), *Total quality management: the health care pioneers* (pp. 305–314). Chicago, IL: American Hospital Association.

CHAPTER 9

Designing Automated Outcomes Management Systems

MARY ANN KEATLEY, THOMAS I. MILLER,
AND ALEX JOHNSON

INTRODUCTION

A key consideration in the development or acquisition of any outcomes information system is automation. The quantity of data involved makes it virtually impossible to collect, analyze, and report results in a "paper-and-pencil" environment. Thus, the issue faced by many managers becomes what type of automated system to use. Although an array of automated systems exist in the marketplace, there are few, if any, references to them in the professional literature, nor have any passed the test of time to determine their usefulness. Most commercially available systems contain a specific set of variables, including functional outcomes or level of functional communication independence measured on a specific scale; length of stay/number of treatment sessions; and the average cost of treatment. More sophisticated software programs allow users to configure the software to meet their needs (e.g., choose specific variables and measurement scales), permit the user to include client satisfaction measures, quality-of-life scales, and perform statistical analyses for critical pathways of care.

The purposes of this chapter are to outline the basic steps in developing an automated system, define the purposes for use of the system, identify end-user considerations, and specify the members of the development team. Considerations for developing the components of an automated system and the functional reports that can be generated are discussed. Finally, lessons learned over the years by those who have completed the process of automation are presented. These lessons can perhaps save you time and money by avoiding common pitfalls.

DESIGNING A FRAMEWORK FOR AUTOMATION

Before automating a system, a conceptual model and strategic plan must be developed on an organizationwide basis. The success with which this is accomplished can be expedited by following systematic steps. All are at least considered in developing an automated system:

1. Convene an outcomes management team comprised of individuals within your program as well as any necessary consultants or experts. (See section on Development Team for Purpose and Team Composition.)

2. Determine the investigative and technical questions to be addressed by your outcomes model. These questions should reveal the extent to which you can accomplish your primary goal of improving the overall communication and related skills of clients seen in your program. Questions for example, may include:

   a. What do we want to know about program effectiveness that this set of data elements can answer?

   b. What amount of time and personnel costs are required for data collection? Will the information yielded by the data be worth the cost? Is there a less expensive way?

   c. How can we ensure that the data collected are accurate and reliable?

   d. Where will the data be stored?

   e. At what intervals are the data collected?

   f. Who is responsible for collecting the data?

   g. Who is responsible for aggregating, analyzing, and summarizing the data?

   h. What types of analyses and summaries are best for your program?

   i. To whom are the summaries distributed?

   j. Who is responsible for making decisions based on the summaries?

   k. What actions will be taken as a result of these decisions?

3. Define and codify all major diagnostic groups to be studied (e.g., cleft palate, dysfluency, neurogenic populations [e.g., aphasia, apraxia, dysarthria], cognitive-communication impairments, dysphagia, developmental articulation and/or language disorders, deaf and/or hearing impaired). Diagnostic groupings can be the same as those used by other data bases, such as the American Speech-Language-Hearing Association's National Outcomes Measures (NOMS) (ASHA, 1995), the Uniform Data System for Medical Rehabilitation (State University of New York at Buffalo, 1993) or the International Classification of Disease (ICD) (Jones, et al., 1994). The value of a common nomenclature to define diagnostic groups is found in the ability to aggregate data from different data bases, thus creating a more powerful data base. The ICD classification system is the most common coding system used; however, it pertains exclusively to medical diagnoses. Therefore, many of the communication and related disorder diagnoses are not classified (e.g., developmental articulation and language disorders, dysphagia) thus potentially complicating matters for billing purposes.

4. Clearly define variables (e.g., demographic data elements, assessment and treatment codes, measurement scales, client satisfaction variables, quality-of-life measures), desired outcomes, and critical pathways for specific diagnostic groups. For example:

   a. Improvements in communication based upon statistically valid and reliable measurement scales.

   b. Correlations of clinical improvements with functional gains and the costs associated with those gains.

   c. Quality-of-life ratings in relationship to specific speech, language, cognitive, or swallowing improvements.

   d. Client satisfaction with services and service providers.

   e. Achievement of clinical goals.

   f. Length of stay or number of outpatient visits necessary to achieve goals.

   g. Cost effectiveness for various treatment methodologies, and service providers.

   h. Points of diminishing return for specific treatment methods and diagnoses.

   i. Critical pathways based on sound clinical judgments and proven outcomes.

5. Establish appropriate measurement tools (e.g., communication rating scales, quality-of-life questionnaires, specific measures of voice, fluency).

6. Define data collection procedures to ensure validity, reliability, and reproducibility of data.

7. Define confounding variables (e.g., multiple diagnoses; barriers to treatment, such as premorbid factors, irregular attendance), and decide how each will be treated in your outcomes measurement protocol.

8. Pilot test the system by collecting data retrospectively or prospectively over a predetermined time span or for a specific number of clients to refine and debug the automated system.

9. Define the proper statistical analyses (e.g., t-tests, chi square, regression analyses) for data interpretation.

10. Analyze data. Depending on the automated system used, data may be sent to local, regional, or national repositories for comparative analysis. We recommend monitoring your own results initially prior to comparing your outcomes to other groups. While normative data can help you compare the performance of your facility to other similar facilities, it is first necessary to have data and trends in performance in your own setting.

11. Disseminate outcomes reports to data contributors, clinical service providers and key decision makers, such as clinicians, facility administrators, financial analysts, and payers.

12. Reconvene the design team to discuss results and make decisions about actions to be taken based on results (e.g., alter treatment protocols related to frequency, duration, sequence, or actual therapeutic techniques).

13. Automate your system to coincide with the needs of your program and allow for

Table 9–1. Flowchart of Designing an Automated System

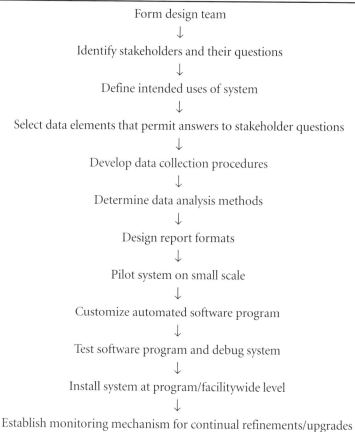

Form design team
↓
Identify stakeholders and their questions
↓
Define intended uses of system
↓
Select data elements that permit answers to stakeholder questions
↓
Develop data collection procedures
↓
Determine data analysis methods
↓
Design report formats
↓
Pilot system on small scale
↓
Customize automated software program
↓
Test software program and debug system
↓
Install system at program/facilitywide level
↓
Establish monitoring mechanism for continual refinements/upgrades

the integration of data with the overall mission of your facility. For example, the primary goal of your facility may be to provide the most cost-effective service in your area, while another center may want to have the highest client satisfaction. Table 9–1 summarizes the basic steps in designing an automated system.

Intended Uses of the System

Clear and detailed specification of your purposes is essential for the success of any outcomes management system. A statement of intended uses should be articulated clearly before any plans are developed, funding is allocated, software is chosen, and/or data are collected. Ambiguous statements, such as "the system will be used for quality improvement or management purposes," provide little guidance.

In order to specify your purposes, you might describe the uses of the system in two steps. Step one is the ultimate purpose—for example, a system that provides evidence of clients' improvements in functional abilities will be used to improve care, secure managed care contracts, allocate resources, reward staff, and market services to the public. Step two is a description of the method to achieve the ultimate purpose—for example, the system is designed to quantify clients' improvements in functional abilities from admission to discharge, and at 3 months follow-up. These steps are followed by identification of diagnostic groups to be monitored, types of decisions to be made, actions to be taken, and development of specific protocols for the collection, analysis, and reporting of data.

Too many organizations, rushing headlong in the push to measure outcomes, design systems without first defining their purposes. For example, one administrator asked department heads to complete a lengthy questionnaire specifying the outcome questions they believed needed to be answered. Good questions emerged: "What are our clinical outcomes?" "How can we evaluate the treatment we provide?" "What does it cost to provide these services?" But, without taking the time to reformulate the questions into a clear statement of purpose, the administrator proceeded too quickly to program initiation. He spent the next 6 months identifying or developing the outcome measures and data collection protocols needed to answer the 50 or more questions identified by department heads. At the end of the 6 months, many of the instruments were identified or developed but the intended uses of the data once collected remained unclear. Which stakeholders could benefit from the findings? How often were the findings needed? What kinds of decisions depended on the findings? What actions would be based on the findings, and who would be charged to take action? Once these issues were addressed, some of the work completed over the last 6 months was found to be premature.

Attention to specific research questions requires research designs that may or may not have been considered when establishing data collection protocols. For example, if the director of the speech-language pathology program was interested in comparing the effectiveness of 10 treatment sessions for right-hemisphere stroke patients scheduled once a week for 10 weeks to the same number of sessions scheduled in two intensive weeks of five sessions per week, a research design would need to be incorporated into the data collection plan. This design would, for example, need to specify the characteristics of patients who could participate as subjects in the study, standards of improvement in functional status made by clinicians unbiased to the patients' course of treatment, and the appropriate time and conditions for retesting (e.g., at the end of each session, each week, treatment completion). None of these considerations could be anticipated if the purposes for data collection were not determined initially. If the primary purpose of outcomes data collection is marketing, then a system for sampling client satisfaction might be employed that would yield enough data for the biennial hospital newsletter.

Identifying Stakeholders

Clarifying the intended uses of the outcomes management system requires that stakeholders in the care rendered be identified. By identifying the stakeholders, you can appropriately choose the methods for communicating results and the actions that are likely to be taken as a consequence of those results.

Typical stakeholder groups include the general public, clients and families, payers and managed care organizations, administrators/governing boards, clinicians, and researchers. Because each group needs outcomes information in a format tailored to its needs, data reporting formats must also be designed.

Examples of stakeholder needs and possible data reporting options follow:

For The General Public

Purpose. General outcomes information pertaining to quality of care.

Report format. Presented in lay terms with measures that are meaningful. Bar graphs of client satisfaction with care and the care environment, as well as the perceived effectiveness of the clinician. Graphs of results can be accompanied with journalistic reports of case studies or monthly monitoring of outcomes. Of special interest to consumers will be costs and outcomes for various treatments adjusted for severity and compared to a normative group.

For Clients and Families

Purpose. Outcomes information for shared decision making.

Report format. Pie charts showing the percentage of clients treated for the same condition, adjusted for severity and other risk factors (e.g., age, diagnosis), whose outcomes were full functional recovery, recovery to 75% of normal; 50% of normal; 25% of normal, no recovery, or regression). Use different pie charts for each of several treatment options.

For Managed Care Organizations (MCOs)

Purpose. To share objective evidence of cost effectiveness.

Report format. Tables and graphs of means and frequency distributions showing lengths of stay (LOS) and improvement per inpatient day or number of outpatient sessions. Outcome results will show overall costs and costs per unit of improvement, as well as comparisons across clinicians and clinical settings.

For Administrators

Purpose. To allocate human and/or finanical resources.

Report format. From statistical models, outcome results will contain predictions of client recovery times and costs for a variety of diagnoses for contract negotiations with MCOs. Outcome results will also provide comparisons of service delivery alterations, including staffing patterns, specific procedures, or services to identify those that are the least expensive while achieving the best outcomes.

For Clinicians

Purpose. To develop or modify treatment protocols.

Report format. Results track outcomes of individual clients or client groups over time to permit comparisons of costs, number of sessions, LOS, client satisfaction, and clinical outcomes. Clinicians can then utilize the information to monitor care and make changes as necessary. Comparisons between clinicians must be confidential (i.e., identities stripped from the data) so that clinicians will receive their own reports but will be unable to identify any other clinicians in the comparative data.

For Researchers

Purpose. To determine statistically relevant information regarding outcome variables that could be used to change treatment protocols, costs for service, or candidacy for treatment.

Report format. Statistical models can show significant effects of treatment methods, use of technology, and so on. By displaying information in tables and graphs, important results can be easily interpreted.

FORMING A DESIGN TEAM

Members of the design team are chosen to both set and accomplish the goals of the outcomes management project. Automation of an outcomes system should begin with a plan, which is adopted by the design team, based on detailed guidelines or treatment protocols, measurement scales, and so on, from all participants affected by outcomes monitoring, or those individuals whose job functions might be altered by the results. The team frequently is representative of all personnel within your facility whose work influences the outcomes of care. The team also includes primary decision makers in the facility who use outcomes data as a management tool. Often consultative experts in outcomes measurement and management are retained to expedite the process. A carefully selected team can lead to efficient and accurate accomplishment of goals.

Team Purpose and Composition

The purpose of the design team is to develop guidelines for selecting data elements, collecting data, analyzing data, and using data in the context of the mission of the program or organization. In all cases the team should ask, "How will these data help us to understand or explain the extent to which we are accomplishing our goals?". Members of a design team, depending on the work setting, can include a combination of the following individuals:

- *Administrator* with primary decision-making power to initiate and implement the process.
- *Management Information Systems Representative* who is familiar with the integration of automated information systems throughout the facility.
- *Financial Officer* who can determine the necessary resources for the project and the cost data elements that should be incorporated into the system.

- *Service Providers* may include speech-language pathologists or audiologists, each of whom represent a clinical area or population (e.g., neurogenics, pediatrics, adults, dysphagia). Other service providers include, for example, physical therapists, occupational therapists, physicians, nurses, case managers, teachers, counselors, and school psychologists.

- *Quality Improvement & Utilization Review Representative* who assists in defining data elements to measure the quality and utilization of care.

- *Medical Records Representative* who has knowledge of documentation in client records that can be captured by/or downloaded into an automated system. This can save considerable time in collecting basic demographic information.

- *Managed Care Agents* who are key members in today's health care market and work in medical settings or consult with private practitioners. The agents will often be the individuals most likely to use outcomes information to market MCOs, or insurance adjustors, regarding the need for specific services for individual clients. As part of the team they are able to define the necessary outcomes information that will enhance their communication with payers.

- *Public Relations/Marketing Representative* may want to serve on the outcomes development team as the purveyor of success stories originating from the data.

- *Outcomes Manager* who is the organizer and communications link among team members. The coordinator is frequently an individual with experience in developing outcomes systems who has an overall picture of the key components necessary for putting the system in place, as well as a timeline for project initiation and completion. Many outcomes coordinators work with outside consultants to help design and execute the plan for development and automation of the system.

Because staff time represents resource utilization, it is critical to streamline the teamwork process by determining which members are essential participants, and at what points during the project their expertise is needed. Buy-in is essential to the success of the outcomes process; all stakeholders should be included at the outset of the project and at key points thereafter. By understanding the usefulness of outcomes the information for each of the key players, the system can be designed to answer their questions while allowing for the integration of data from all areas affecting client care. Experience has shown that scrutinizing performance through outcomes may be threatening to various individuals when, in fact, the primary purpose is to increase efficiency and improve quality.

DESIRED FEATURES OF AN AUTOMATED SYSTEM

An automated system should be sufficiently comprehensive yet flexible. It should run on personal computers that allow each department administrator, clinician, or researcher to enter or access data. Administrators may have different report needs than clinicians. For example, the administrator may want a management snapshot report that quantifies and summarizes all relevant data; whereas the clinician may want to track the progress of individual clients. In order to satisfy the differing needs of key stakeholders, automated systems should have the following components:

1. The capability of documenting demographic variables (e.g., age, diagnosis), LOS, number of sessions, clinical results, financial variables (costs, charges, reimbursement), client satisfaction, and quality of life.

2. The ability to perform descriptive statistical analyses (e.g., means, medians, frequency distributions, standard deviations) and inferential statistical analyses (e.g., t-tests, chi-squares, confidence intervals, Analysis of Variance).

3. The ability to perform prediction models from client data stored in the data base. This feature allows the user to predict certain variables (e.g., the extent of client improvement based upon diagnosis, severity, age, gender; or the extent of treatment required to obtain a targeted outcome).

4. The ability to store regional or national data to allow you to compare your data with other similar programs.

5. Software flexibility that allows for the reconfiguration or alteration of data elements as new questions arise that require entry of new data elements.

6. The ability to produce numerous report formats from the data that can be altered based on the questions to be answered.

7. A filter or type of software feature that allows the user to examine specific client populations, providers of care, payers, or treatment sites, based on the information to be analyzed. By setting specific parameters in the software, the program will scan the entire data base and analyze only those data that are pertinent to the information requested (e.g., males, 55 years and older, with a diagnosis of left-hemisphere stroke).

8. The ability to generate presentation graphics such as bar graphs, pie charts, or scatter plots that are comprehensible to key stakeholders.

9. Password protection to control access to data.

10. Compatibility with other computer systems to allow for interfacing and downloading of information. For example, the system could allow client records, admissions, and financial information to be downloaded into the outcomes program for analysis.

11. Research capabilities to compare specific treatment techniques and systematically evaluate critical pathways of care.

12. The ability to handle multiple outcome measures (e.g., tests of clinical improvement, scales of client satisfaction, functional communication measures).

13. The capability to provide on-line information (i.e., computer-generated data that are current day by day or hour by hour) rather than reports that are generated only monthly, quarterly, or annually.

Report Generation Features

Once the intended uses of an automated outcomes management system are defined, the data elements needed to answer stakeholders' questions are selected, data collection procedures are developed, and methods of analyzing data are determined, formats for reporting results can be designed. As described above, it is essential to present information in formats useful to key stakeholders. Thus, several formats may be warranted. While the researcher may want sophisticated statistical analyses illustrated, consumers or payers may want simple universally understood graphic displays of data. Automated systems that provide a range of report display features, therefore, are more desirable.

The ideal software provides considerable flexibility in the way graphics and reports are generated. It allows the results to be presented in a variety of graphic formats, such as pie charts and bar graphs (see Figs. 9–1 and 9–2). Thus, it permits latitude in customizing reports. The ideal software also offers utilities that allow users to develop their own reporting styles. If such utilities are not included in the software, off-the-shelf software packages may be utilized to permit users to link outcomes data to a separate presentation package designed solely for producing reports or graphs. This linkage, however, can require considerable "tinkering" to interface the two programs.

Software can be programmed to permit the reports to be produced at any time or "upon demand." This provides for the timely reporting of data, and avoids the delays inherent in relying upon a data bank to produce, for example, quarterly reports. Software also can be programmed to allow for the same report formats to be generated at any time. This means saving report templates or the commands that generate them. Boilerplate text also can accompany reports into which quantitative findings are automatically inserted. For example, a report may always begin, "The client was admitted with a rating of _____ on the scale of functional communication." The "_____" is filled in by the software. Reports should always specify how data were selected from the data base so that there is no ambiguity about how the results were derived. In addition, selection criteria, should always be designated, such as date or date ranges, age, gender, diagnosis, and severity at admission.

Reporting features should, at a minimum, permit not only summary information about a single client, but changes in the client's status during and after treatment. At the same time, the software should permit reports about groups of clients, which allows

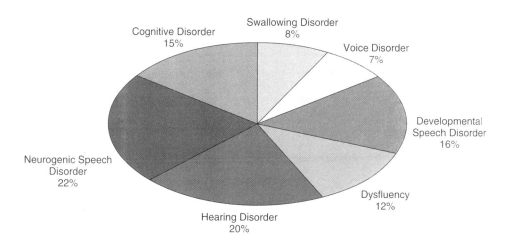

Figure 9–1. Diagnostic Categories

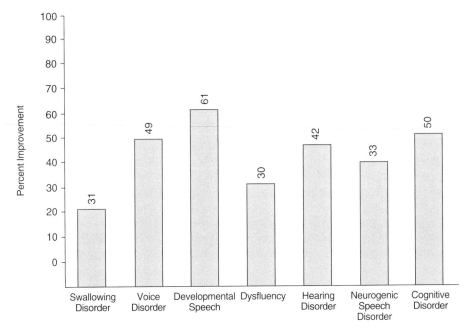

Figure 9–2. Percent Improvement by Diagnostic Category

investigation of trends and can be used for the purposes of managed care contract negotiations, marketing, and clinical management.

The software should provide a range of predesigned report templates. Reporting features that include data from a variety of domains—clinical, financial, client demographics—are likely to be helpful to facility administrators by providing a summary of facility performance at that time or during the same quarter as the previous year. Table 9–1 provides an example of a Management Snapshot Report summarizing annual data regarding client census, financial information, treatment sessions for various diagnoses, client outcomes, and percent of clients representing each diagnostic category. In-depth analyses that compare one variable (e.g., client improvement) to another (e.g., number of treatment sessions) help clinicians and researchers to gain new knowledge about the effects of clinical care. For example, the frequency distribution of discharge scores cross-tabulated by categories of admission severity helps to explain improvement by allowing the clinician to predict how a client may respond to treatment based on their initial severity level.

Software Considerations

The true test of any automated system is the ability to access data and manipulate the data base with statistical tools in order to generate meaningful information. While the best software will transform raw data into results, skill is required for accurate and valid interpretations.

Outcomes managers must not only understand principles of research, research methods, and statistics, but also must be familiar with how the data are collected and entered into the data base, how and when the data can be modified, and the intended uses of the data. An efficient system requires interpretation of results in the context of the mission of the program and the needs of the stakeholders. Thus, outcomes managers must be in regular contact with the stakeholders for whom the data are being analyzed to ensure that the generated reports are both accurate and meaningful.

Hardware Considerations

With the amount of data to be analyzed and the speed with which the user must access these data, hardware requirements are an important consideration. For example, several of the commercially available systems (such as FIMware (SUNY, 1993) and Polaris Outcome System (Warren, 1995) require, at a minimum, a 486 personal computer; whereas other systems, such as the Beaumont Outcome Software System (Merson, Rolnick, & Weiner, 1995), require a 386 personal computer or higher. If many stakeholders want simultaneous access to data, then computer networking capabilities are essential. Otherwise, only one user may access the system at a time. However, too often, purchasers of software anticipate that many stakeholders will want access to the actual data base in order to manipulate the data and generate their own reports. But this often does not occur in actual practice. Many individuals will want the results of the analyses conducted, but few will go through the process of generating them. Consequently, stand-alone systems (e.g., small personal computers) can be quite adequate for software purchasers. The most efficient method of report generation is to designate an outcomes manager who can generate specific reports for the staff and administrators.

Individual computer terminals will be essential if users from remote sites are to access the same data base. However, the kind of system that allows many users access may also create many more hardware and software problems than your facility may want to solve. Wherever the data base is stored, capacity for many billions of bytes of data are likely to be required over many years for a large clinic. If your clinic has satellite facilities, then the advantage of networks is that everyone can access and enter data in a timely manner. However, additional costs are involved and, frequently, there is need for an additional staff member to manage the network.

Commercially Available Systems

With advances in computer technology, a growing number of automated outcomes management systems are becoming commercially available. Two of the systems—the Beaumont Outcome Software System (BOSS; Merson, Rolnick, & Weiner, 1995), and OUTCOME™ (Keatley & Miller, 1993)—provide outcome information specifically for speech-language pathology services. FIMWARE® Clinical Profiles in Medical Rehab (SUNY, 1993), Polaris Outcome System (Warren, 1995) and Rehabilitation Outcome Reporting System with PECS© (Harvey & Jellinek, 1979) include communication outcome systems as part of the overall rehabilitation outcomes management package. In lieu of providing software, Formations National Outcomes System (Formations in Health Care, Inc., 1991) uses bubble sheets that the facility completes and

Table 9–2. Management Snapshot Report:
Speech-Language Pathology and Audiology*
Time Period: 1995

CENSUS

Number of clients treated	620.0
Number of evaluations in speech-language pathology	312.0
Number of evaluations in audiology	180.0
Number of treatment sessions	6250.0

FINANCES

Average total charge per session	$80.00
Average total cost per session	$57.00
Averagetotal reimbursement per session	$64.00
Total annual charges	$500,000.00
Total Annual costs	$356,000.00
Total annual reimbursements	$400.000.00

TREATMENT

Number of sessions speech therapy	1420.0
Number of sessions language therapy	1500.0
Number of sessions voice therapy	550.0
Number of sessions dysfluency therapy	400.0
Number of sessions dysphagia therapy	325.0
Number of sessions cognitive therapy	1050.0
Number of sessions auditory treatment	1005.0

CLIENT OUTCOMES

Average quality of life (1–100)	76.4
Average overall communication improvement (1–10)	3.8
Average functional speech-language improvement (1-10)	3.2
Average functional hearing improvement (1–10)	4.4
% of clients returned to gainful employment	36.1
% of clients gaining functional feeding/swallowing	77.2

CLIENT CHARACTERISTICS

% with developmental speech-language disorders	16.2
% with neurogenic speech disorders	22.7
% with dysfluency	12.1
% with voice disorders	7.3
% with cognitive disorders	15.0
% with swallowing disorders	8.4
% with hearing disorders	20.6

FILTER: All clients seen in 1995.

INTERPRETATION: Six hundred and twenty clients were treated in 1995 for an average charge of $80.00 per session and a reimbursement of $64.00, and a total revenue of $43,750.00. Speech and language therapy accounted for the greatest number of sessions, and dysphagia treatment the least. Overall communication improvement was 3.8 points on a 10-point scale with functional gains noted in both speech-language pathology and audiology services. Over three-fourths (76%) of the dysphagia clients regained functional feeding and swallowing skills, and 36% of all clients returned to gainful employment.

*NOTE: This table does not contain accurate charges or costs. The financial figures are used for illustrative purposes only and cannot be interpreted as average charges or costs for speech-language pathology services.

sends to a central location for analysis. Table 9–3 describes each software program for quick reference.

DESIGNING AN AUTOMATED SYSTEM: A CASE EXAMPLE

One approach to enhancing the understanding of complex processes is via the case example. We present here an example of an automated outcomes management system that Henry Ford Health System (HFHS) in Detroit, Michigan has developed and used over the past 3 years. Rather than review all aspects of the system that has been developed, we highlight and briefly describe the key features of the system, and discuss the processes that were used in design, implementation, and application of the system. Finally, we critique the system using some of the steps outlined earlier in this chapter.

Description of the HFHS Speech-Language Pathology Outcomes System

The system under consideration in this example was developed by one of the chapter authors (Johnson, 1995 a, b, c) for use in the Division of Speech-Language Sciences & Disorders in the Department of Neurology at HFHS in Detroit. Briefly, the Division consists of 15 speech-language pathologists who provide care to children and adults in acute care and outpatient settings. Division staff are assigned to either the inpatient hospital, main outpatient clinic, voice laboratory, or one of several satellite locations. Clinicians from the division see approximately 5,000 patients annually. Clinicians are specialized in one or more of several clinical areas: dysphagia, adult neurogenic disorders, voice disorders, or pediatric communication disorders.

In late 1991, members of the division staff expressed an interest in developing a coordinated data base that would facilitate tracking of patients through programs, allow for identification of patients according to several key variables, track productivity, and analyze clinical outcomes on subgroups of the total patient population. The demand for such information came from many sources, internal and external, and it was increasingly clear that an organized central source of basic demographic, clinical, and productivity information would be useful for a variety of purposes.

The remainder of this section will be devoted to a critical analysis of the Henry Ford project with regard to the step-by-step approach outlined earlier in this chapter.

Convene a Design Team

Now, several years after the conceptualization of the project, it seems that this would have been such an obvious strategy for beginning the project and insuring that the activities being carried out were strategic and moved the project forward. The group that was designing the project began with some naiveté, and underestimated the amount of time, energy, and effort needed to accomplish the final product. There was a team of sorts, but roles were informal and not well delineated, and this caused a lack of smoothness that might have been achieved had more deliberate delineation of responsibilities been achieved early in the process. Key members of the planning group includ-

TABLE 9–3. Features of Selected Automated Outcomes Management Systems

SOFTWARE	CLASS	DEVELOPER	FEATURES	CLIENT GROUPS	HARDWARE REQUIREMENTS
Beaumont Outcome Software System (BOSS) (Merson, Rolnick, & Weiner, 1995)	Speech-language pathology	Parrot Software	Reports clinical and financial outcomes. Uses 7-point clinical scales only. Outcome variables include: admission status, discharge status, treatment outcome, total procedures, length of stay, total charges per case. Data can be reported in tables and bar graphs. Demo disk available.	Adult and pediatric population. Multiple speech/language diagnoses.	386 PC compatible system. Microsoft WINDOWS™, VGA graphics, 4 megabytes of RAM, 3 megabytes of memory.
FIMware® Clinical Profiles in Medical Rehab (SUNY, 1993)	Multidisciplinary rehabilitation	Uniform Data System for Medical Rehabilitation℠	Enables UDSMR℠ subscribers to document and track Functional Independence Measure (FIM), and WeeFIM®) for pediatrics. Uses 7-point scale only. Rates locomotion, self-care, sphincter control, transfers, communication, and social cognition. Produces chart-ready patient profiles. Exports data for other applications. Demo disk available.	Adult and pediatric populations. Multiple diagnoses.	486 PC, 200 megabyte hardrive, 8 megabytes RAM memory, VGA graphics, laser printer, WINDOWS™ 3.1 or higher.
Formations National Outcomes Systems* (Formations in Health Care, Inc., 1991)	Multidisciplinary rehabilitation	Formations in Health Care, Inc., A Medirisk Company	Includes the following scales: Functional Independence Measure, Level of Rehabilitation Scale-III, Medical Outcomes Scales, occupational and orthopedic outcomes	Adult population only. Impairment codes and ICD-9 codes are used to categorize patient populations.	Software not available. Opscan bubble sheets used to gather data that is analyzed onsite.

OUTCOME™ (Keatley & Miller, 1993)	Speech-language pathology and multidisciplinary rehabilitation	Evaluation Systems International, Inc.	for outpatient and patient satisfaction. Generates information on length of stay, net charges, functional outcomes, medical improvement, decrease in pain, return to community, and return to work. Accepts any scale and variables user prefers. Programmed for ASHA's Functional Communication Measures (7-point scale). Analyzes functional outcome data for patient improvement financial variables, critical pathways, length of stay/number of sessions, effectiveness of treatment techniques, and patient demographics. Adjusts for severity and predicts outcomes for similar patient populations. Exports data for other applications. Produces multiple reports, color graphics. Demo disk available.	Adult and pediatric population. Multiple diagnoses can be evaluated.	386 or higher IBM PC compatible. Microsoft WINDOWS™, 8 megabytes of RAM, 2.5 megabytes of memory, VGA color monitor, mouse driver (optional).
Polaris Outcome System (Warren, 1995)	Multidisciplinary rehabilitation	Polaris Group™ (A subsidiary of NOVA Care Inc.)	Uses 7-point scale. Analyzes functional outcome data for patient improvement, length of stay, financial variables, and demographics. Produces multiple reports, graphics	Program developed for geriatric population. Multiple diagnoses can be evaluated.	486 PC, 10 megabytes RAM, Windows™ 3.1 or higher, mouse driven.

(continued)

TABLE 9–3. Features of Selected Automated Outcomes Management Systems (*continued*)

SOFTWARE	CLASS	DEVELOPER	FEATURES	CLIENT GROUPS	HARDWARE REQUIREMENTS
			available. Based on 16 impairment categories of UDS. Demo disk available.		
Rehabilitation Outcome Reporting System with PECS© (Harvey, & Jellinek, 1979)	Multidisciplinary rehabilitation	Marianjoy Rehabilitation Hospital	6-interval LifeScales™ with graphic reporting for each. Tracks multiple outcomes including functional patient outcomes, demographics, goals and status, and discharge status. Includes six domains (medical severity, applied self-care, motor skills, cognition, community reintegration and pain). Produces multiple reports and physician letters.	Adult and pediatric population. All levels of care and medical diagnoses.	386 PC compatible, 2 megabytes RAM, DOS 3.3 or higher, VGA color monitor, 200 megabytes hard drive.

*Automated outcome system not available, but bubble sheets are used for analysis.

Table 9–4. HFHS Speech-Language Data Base:
Key Questions to Be Answered by Outcomes Data

---

1. What is the average amount of change on the ASHA FCMs that a patient with X diagnosis makes as he or she moves through the treatment continuum?
2. How many (and what type) of clinical and human resources are used to achieve functional changes in patients enrolled in HFHS Speech-Language Programs?
3. How do routinely obtained clinical data predict functional outcomes?

---

ed the division director, a computer programming consultant from within the institution, and an outside data management specialist.

Define the Various Questions to Be Addressed by the Outcomes Model

In the preliminary stages of the project the planning group, in concert with the clinical staff, identified two sets of outcomes data that would be of general interest for program evaluation and planning purposes within the division. The primary outcome instrument to be used was the Functional Communication Measures (ASHA, 1987), developed by the American Speech-Language-Hearing Association in an attempt to provide systematic ratings of communication (and swallowing) performance along a continuum of independence. The clinical staff in the division were already using these measures as part of their regular reporting system and were familiar with the scoring methodology. Based on input from the division staff, it was determined that there was a desire to also track consistent test data on patients. This desire was based in part on the fact that considerable test data were being collected on patients enrolled in various treatment programs, and there was interest in determining if any of these "objective" data were predictive of functional clinical outcomes.

Table 9–4 presents typical questions addressed by the outcomes measurement system being used in this example.

Other questions for consideration at this step are articulated earlier in this chapter. These considerations include the *process* of data collection and management. Table 9–5 summarizes these important issues for purposes of this discussion. In this case, the responsibilities for completion of necessary data forms were assigned to the speech-language pathologists. Data are recorded on scannable sheets to facilitate data

---

Table 9–5. Process of Data Collection Management: HFHS Speech-Language Data Base

---

Intervals for Data Collection: Admission and Discharge

Responsibility for Collection of Data: Primary clinician on each case

Responsibility for Data Preparation: Division receptionist

Responsibility for Data Processing: Director, Outside Consultant

Responsibility for Reporting Results: Director

Frequency of Reports: Quarterly

---

entry. Use of scannable sheets has the advantage of facilitating data processing, because the need for manual entry of data is eliminated. There are, however, some disadvantages. There is an obvious initial expense for the purchase or lease of a scanner that interfaces with the computer system. In addition, professional and support staff have to be educated to complete the forms properly. At HFHS, the Division receptionist collects the data forms and then periodically scans them into the Division computer network.

Define All Major Diagnostic Groups
to Be Evaluated and Clearly Define Variables
and Outcomes of Interest

At the surface, it seems obvious that diagnostic coding would be important for purposes of outcomes measurement. However, what became apparent in this situation was that the coding model used by the clinical program (i.e., ICD-9 codes) did not serve the analysis well. For example, using the code for aphasia (i.e., 784.3) would generate a list of patients who met the criteria for the specific population of interest (stroke patients with left-hemisphere involvement). However, it would also introduce some patients with "aphasia" who represented different etiologic categories (i.e., traumatic brain injury, dementia). While this is not a major problem on a case-by-case basis, it becomes obvious that as data are aggregated, treatment gains and losses may be obscured if patients from different etiologic categories are combined. Members of the division are in the process of considering a variety of classification models, which might allow for more useful differentiation of various patient groups.

Establish Appropriate Measurement Tools
and Define Data Collection Procedures
to Insure Reliability and Reproducibility

Identification of appropriate measurement tools was a challenge for the authors of the HFHS program. There were few published instruments at the time that the data base was being developed, and those available for specific speech and language applications had minimal validity and reliability data. The staff decided to use the ASHA Functional Communication Measures (FCMs), as they were originally developed through a consensus panel of ASHA members and were comprehensive in addressing the many areas (e.g., voice, swallowing, language) that deserve attention in measuring outcomes. Ongoing assessment and measurement of reliability has been essential to the use of the FCMs in the HFHS program. Training tapes for each FCM were developed and presented to the staff at monthly staff meetings. Initially reliability scores across clinicians were in the 60% range. With ongoing training over the past 12 months, scores have improved to the desired 85 to 90% range. It was somewhat surprising to the speech-language staff at Henry Ford that their reliability scores were initially low. This observation suggests careful attention to reliability of clinical judgments as an essential ingredient of any outcomes measurement program. As a result of the attention paid to determining reliability, a training program for new staff members has been instituted that requires reliability in FCM ratings prior to using the scales to rate patients and enter information into the data base.

Consider Reporting Characteristics That Are Desirable and Essential

The most challenging aspect of the HFHS outcome system has been the integration of the large volume of information being acquired into a reasonable reporting structure. Some of the preassembled outcomes measurement systems are highly flexible in that they aggregate and compare data from various patients and patient groups. In most "home-grown" systems this particular facet of data management and reporting requires the assistance of someone who has extensive knowledge of the software package that has been developed. In some data base software programs it is relatively easy to perform a query of the data, which generates a list of individual patients who meet specific characteristics. Examples of the "query" process are as follows:

1. Generate a list of patients whose age is under 6 years, who had a diagnostic code of language disorder, and who failed the initial hearing screening; and for each case listed, show their change in communication on the FCMs over a 3-month period of treatment.

2. Generate a list of patients who were seen during the acute phase of recovery from stroke, had a diagnosis of aphasia, and went to an inpatient rehabilitation setting. Show their change in communication on the FCMs from admission to discharge.

Characteristics common to these examples include selection of specific patient groups and resultant communication measures.

This is a useful way to answer specific questions that are addressed frequently in our clinical practice. The preparation of standard reports requires extensive organization and software knowledge if meaningful and useful information is to be generated.

There are numerous advantages to the development of a data base for use by speech-language pathologists in their specific settings. Data base developments and outcomes measurement systems can be customized to fit the specific needs, case mix, and clinical philosophies of the organization. The obvious disadvantage to such a system is that it requires constant attention, as programs grow and change. In addition, the time requirements of a busy clinical practice may not allow for the resources in time and energy that may be necessary for design of the overall structure, implementation of a data collection and analysis system, and generation of reports. In packaged programs available on the market, it is, of course, feasible to deal with these issues in a more timely way. On the other hand, preassembled programs may not provide the necessary flexibility required or be adaptable to a specific program. Most important, it is essential that those interested in the development of a data base and outcomes measurement system understand that regardless of the source of the package, considerable attention will need to be given to the selection of items to include in the content of the program. Because there is currently no outcomes measurement scale that is suited to meet the needs of all programs, clinicians and administrators must ensure that issues of validity of the content of the program and reliability of the judgments being made are satisfactory.

LESSONS LEARNED

Although automation is the wave of the future in human service delivery, and those who have data to support treatment- and cost-effectiveness will most likely survive, it is not a panacea. Automating a system, whether you work in a school, clinic, hospital, or in private practice, requires diligence. It may involve development of specific measurement scales appropriate to your caseload, evaluation of the various client characteristics to be measured, and interpretation of results by individuals who can expertly evaluate whether the data are reasonable. Experience in developing outcomes management systems has taught us some valuable lessons:

1. It is more effective to measure a limited set of variables rather than include all possible variables in your data base. Too many variables will make the program run slowly and may complicate data interpretation.

2. The tools that are used to measure client outcomes should be valid and reliable before programming them into your system.

3. The variables chosen for your program should allow you to answer the important questions posed by key stakeholders.

4. If you decide to design your own software program, you must define your variables, measurement scales, and outcome domains (e.g., functional improvement, client satisfaction, and quality of life), before starting to program the software. It is very costly to add or change features once programming begins.

5. Software that is purchased "off-the-shelf" should give the user the option to change or delete variables as they become outdated. For example, you may want to evaluate which of several treatment techniques is most effective; but once that is determined, you can delete that variable and insert a different one.

6. Preprogrammed software packages should include various measures of client outcomes, including financial information, LOS/number of sessions, functional status, client satisfaction, and quality of life. The packages that limit evaluation of client outcomes make it difficult to generate complete pictures of the effects of care.

7. Software programs should include the capability to perform analyses using both descriptive and inferential statistics. Otherwise, important data interpretations may be lost.

8. Programs should be capable of viewing individual client information as well as aggregate data, because the needs of the various stakeholders will be different.

9. Once data are generated, they should be interpreted with an "expert eye." Computer programs are only as good as the developers and users, and flaws may be present until the software is thoroughly debugged.

10. Involve all individuals who will use the program or will be affected by the results to insure "buy-in."

CONCLUSION

Automation of an outcomes management system is essential for organizing and analyzing, in a meaningful format, the large quantity of data that are generated in clinical settings. The beauty of automation is its ability to integrate multiple variables and analyze them statistically to increase knowledge, which leads to better practice patterns. The importance of developing, at the outset, a specification of purposes through a strategic plan cannot be overstated. The initial identification of stakeholders and end-users, their involvement in the development of the system, and their diverse needs dramatically increases the likelihood of organizational acceptance and the effectiveness of the system. By choosing the most appropriate automated system, clinicians can focus on what is important to consumers—increased access to treatment and cost effectiveness. As we move farther into the competitive 1990s, automated outcomes management systems will become a necessity, not a luxury.

REFERENCES

American Speech-Language-Hearing Association. (1987). *Functional Communication Measures*. Rockville, MD: Author.

Formations in Health Care, Inc. (1991). *Level of Rehabilitation Scale-III*. Chicago, IL: Formations in Health Care, Inc.

Granger, C.V. and Hamilton, B.B. (1993). Uniform Data System for Medical Rehabilitation. *FIMware Implementation and User Guide (Adult FIM)*. Version 4.0. Buffalo, NY: State University of New York at Buffalo.

Harvey, R.F., & Jellinek, H.M. (1979). *PECS: Patient Evaluation and Conference System*. Wheaton, IL: Marianjoy Rehabilitation Center.

Johnson, A.F. (1995a). A new clinical data base for medical speech-language pathology. *Special Interest Division 2: Neurogenic Communication Disorders Newsletter*. Rockville, MD: American Speech-Language Hearing Association.

Johnson, A.F. (1995b). Development utilization of data base technology: Measuring clinical outcomes. Annual meeting of the American Speech-Language Association, Orlando, FL.

Johnson, A.F. (1995c). Utilizing clinical data for outcomes measurement. *Teias: Journal of the Texas Speech-Language-Hearing Association*.

Jones, M.D., Brough, K.L., Hall. D.C., & Aarons, W.S. (1994). *St. Anthony's Compact ICD-9-CM Code Book for Physician Payment*. Reston, VA: St. Anthony Publishing Co.

Keatley, M.A., & Miller, T.I. (1993). *OUTCOME*. Boulder, CO: Evaluation Systems International, Inc.

Merson, R., Rolnick, M., & Weiner, F. (1995). *Beaumont Outcome Software System*. Bloomfield, MI: Parrot Software.

St. Anthony's Compact ICD-9-CM Code Book for Physician Payment. (1994). Reston, VA:

Warren, R. (1995). *Polaris Outcome System*. Hingham, MA: Polaris Group.

ADDITIONAL SOURCES OF INFORMATION

Bunch, W.H., & Dvonch, V.M. (1994). The "value" of functional independence measure scores. *American Journal of Physical Medicine and Rehabilitation, 73*, 40–43.

Donabedian, A. (1992). The role of outcomes in quality assessment and assurance. *Quality Review Bulletin 18,* 356–360.

Frattali, C.M. (1993). Perspectives on functional assessment: Its use for policy making. *Disability and Rehabilitation, 15,* 1–9.

Iezzoni, L.I. (1994) (Ed.). *Risk adjustment for measuring health care outcomes.* Ann Arbor, MI: Health Administration Press.

Keatley, M.A., Miller, T.I., & Mann, A. (1995). Treatment planning using outcome data. *ASHA, 37,* 49–52.

Keatley, M.A. (1994). Managing patient care through outcomes analysis. *Inside Case Management, 1,* 7–8.

Keatley, M.A., Lemmon, J., Miller, T.I., & Miller, M. (1995). Using 'normative data' for outcomes comparisons. *Behavioral Health Management, 15,* 20, 21.

U.S. Office of Technology Assessment. (June 1988). *The Quality of Medical Care: Information for Consumers.* OTA-H-386 (Washington, DC: U.S. Government Printing Office)

Wiley, G. (1992). Outcomes and the future of rehab. *Rehab Management 5,* 123–125.

CHAPTER 10

Overcoming Barriers to Outcomes Measurement

REG WARREN

INTRODUCTION

Naumann (1994) states "value is achieved when the expected benefits are much greater than the expected sacrifice" (p. 8). In today's rehabilitation industry, creating value for outcomes measurement remains a challenge. Most services are paid for by Medicare, a predominantly cost-based system, which does not require the formal measurement of patient outcomes. Accreditation standards of The Rehabiliation Accreditation Commission (CARF) and The Joint Commission on Accreditation of Healthcare Organizations (JCAHO) contain outcomes measurement requirements, but these primarily have been applied in the hospital setting[1]. While managed care provides increasing incentive for measurement and benchmarking, the challenges of maintaining data integrity and providing on-demand access to information remain as potential barriers to creating value (Burgess, 1996). Given these constraints, clinical organizations are often challenged by a mentality of compliance regarding outcomes measurement. As a result, they often struggle to link outcomes measurement with the values of the organization.

This chapter, which focuses on activities in rehabilitation, provides a practical review of the factors and challenges related to integrating outcomes measurement into the priorities of your organization or setting. However, before continuing, review the list of "Assumptions about Outcomes Measurements " in Table 10–1.

If you are confident that most or all of these assumptions are true in your work setting, move on to another chapter. If you are not sure, this chapter may be helpful in removing barriers commonly encountered when developing or improving systems for outcomes measurement. Thus, it is considered a companion chapter to the preceding chapter by Keatley, Miller, and Johnson. Suggestions are provided for each of the following stages of outcomes measurement:

Table 10–1. Assumptions about Outcome Measurement

Health care providers understand why outcomes are important.
Clinical providers believe computer-based technology enhances their level of practice.
The clinician's role is to collect data; we, the managers, will use the information.
Train and the data will be produced.
Traditionally, quarterly outcome reports have been of significant value to health care organizations.

- Creating value in your culture
- Defining objectives
- Preparing to measure
- Implementation

CREATING VALUE IN YOUR CULTURE

Outcomes measurement may be important to you, but it is essential to understand the factors that motivate the organization in which you work or with whom you are consulting. External and internal marketplace factors, current and future, have a lot to do with the day-to-day priorities of those who potentially use outcomes information.

External Factors

Payer influences loom large in today's rehabilitation industry. For example, when similar groups of clients are grouped by payer, managed care enrollees in a subacute, skilled nursing facility (SNF) setting typically present with shorter lengths of rehabilitation stay yet similar functional gains when compared to non-HMO Medicare beneficiaries. Such differences tend to be more dramatic in aggressive managed care markets (Warren, 1996).

Looking ahead to a new health care infrastructure, patient triage and LOS in settings of integrated health care networks will be influenced by the number and type of levels of care available and marketing objectives of the organization. These factors trickle down to case management practices and have a direct influence on how rehabilitation teams function. Unfortunately, clinical teams often perceive themselves as downstream recipients of constraints passed on by others.

Today, payer demands present a more immediate incentive for measurement than accreditation, consumer-driven, or quality improvement activities. Tomorrow, consumer demand for a balance of quality (outcomes to standards, access to services and satisfaction) with cost efficiency will become much more relevant to operators/owners.

Internal Factors

Traditionally, setting has been predictive of type of client, level of care, and anticipated outcome. Today, competition and pressures of health care and education reform have created considerable variability in the nature of rehabilitation practice in all settings

(DeJong, in press). For instance, if you practice in an acute medical rehabilitation hospital, LOS is becoming shorter for more acute patients, case management utilizes increasing integration with outpatient and home health services, and there is a striking reduction in orthopedic admissions.

Acute medical settings (acute hospital unit or freestanding) have been the traditional location for the provision of rehabilitation services. Typically, analysis of outcomes was performed quarterly by external data bases such as the UDSMR^{SM} (Fiedler Granger, 1997). Today, competition with the SNF subacute setting, managed care capitation, and risk-sharing in contract arrangements render external, quarterly benchmarking to other hospital providers inadequate. Facility-based, on-demand analysis of outcomes, often at the level of a specific medical or treatment diagnosis, is now necessary to remain competitive.

In the SNF setting, variation in practice is at an all-time high (Lewin, 1995; Wolk & Blair, 1994). At one end of the continuum there are slow-paced, multidisciplinary programs coalescing to the incentives of retrospective, cost-based reimbursement, treating patients for long periods of time. Here, outcomes measurement has little value and is considered redundant to required assessments such as the Minimum Data Set (MDS) (Morris, 1991). Conversely, there are a growing number of sophisticated, transdisciplinary subacutes where LOS is aggressively managed, yet functional outcomes and discharge to community match rehabilitation hospital performance at 30% less charges (Sherman & Meyer, 1995). At this end of the SNF continuum, the value of outcomes is clearly understood.

Outpatient care is shifting its traditional role from a "continuation of inpatient rehabilitation." Today, outpatient services are restricted to short-term, attainable goals. In outpatient programs, a managed care payer mix of 50 to 60% is not uncommon. Capitation, consumer satisfaction, and risk-sharing are the routine. Primarily due to perceived savings in cost, home health is emerging as the post-acute discharge setting of choice. However, limited information is available on outcomes in this environment (Kramer, in press).

What, if anything, provides incentive to collect and use outcomes information in the setting where you work?

Large Corporate Environments

Similar to the restructuring of the banking industry in the last 10 years, health care entities are gradually being acquired by large corporations who see profitability in the economies of scale of nationally based service delivery systems (de La Fiente, 1993). In the corporate culture, business priorities can shift rapidly, and thus incentives for outcomes and measurement may shift. Publicly owned businesses tend to focus on short-term, quarterly return. Motivation to measure patient outcomes will vary according to the perceived association of outcomes with financial incentives in the short-term, and strategic advantage over the long-term.

Recently, a nationally based contract service organization trained over 4500 clinicians on an outcomes measurement system, yet has realized only 10% use and reporting. Why? Most of this corporation's current business was still geared to retrospective cost-based Medicare reimbursement, where formal measurement of outcomes is not required. Management understood the longer-term strategic value of outcomes; however, the field operators viewed outcomes as having little to do with day-to-day priorities. As health care resources lessen, operators support only what is necessary to compete and remain profitable.

What strategies are driving your organization's objectives? How are these strategies shaping incentives for outcomes measurement? Are corporate and field perspectives about outcomes measurement aligned?

Take a close look at payer, marketplace, and your company's incentives before you set objectives for starting, maintaining, or rebuilding an outcomes measurement program. Specifically,

- Understand whether the culture places value on measurement and why.

- Explain relevant external and internal incentives to all clinical staff; if you don't, outcomes measurement may be perceived as another administrative mandate.

DEFINING OBJECTIVES

Now that you have identified the relative value of measurement for your organization, the objectives of your outcomes program can be identified. Objectives should be associated with: utilization of data, scope of measurement, systems support, and integration with external data bases.

Utilization of Data

How are you going to use the information you collect?

- Establish an initial clinical data base for your organization?
- Subscribe to an external data base?
- Develop marketing materials?
- Negotiate payer contracts?
- Develop clinical pathways?
- Develop customized reporting for customers?

The more you plan to do, the more time, cooperation, and money you will need. As described in the previous chapter, the basic outcomes data set, including client demographics, outcome measures, and financial elements, will fulfill some but not all of the above uses.

Who is going to use the information you collect?

Identify the audience or customer who will be using outcomes data. Potential users include clinicians, clients and families, managers, owners, payers, professional and consumer organizations. Conduct focus groups to identify what data elements provide the most value to your key customers. Then, identify the minimal data set which meets their needs. The challenge is to provide users with the ability to obtain and understand outcomes information that has practical application to their set of values.

Scope of Measurement

Review of numerous outcome systems reveals that measuring pre/post and follow-up outcomes and related client demographics and financial variables can be accomplished with approximately 50 different data elements, including a disability measure. This is a minimum data set. As you add capability for clinical pathways, medical impairment measures, and/or cost analysis, data requirements increase dramatically. Using outcome measures on an interim basis (e.g., weekly) also increases data collection and entry time.

The need for information should be balanced with available or planned human and financial resources. It is not unusual for organizations to have compliance problems when data collection requirements from clinical providers are increased. While data entry may take only 10-15 minutes per patient, gathering the information from various sources may take considerably more time. The need for information must be balanced with available or planned resources.

Start with a minimum set of data by determining what you are going to do with the information you derive. Then, collect it yourself from client records, files, and information systems. Note how long it takes and how many different sources have to be accessed.

Systems Support

Redundancy of data entry and lack of integrated reporting systems often frustrate clinicians and rehabilitation managers. The ideal is to have single-step data entry, no redundancy, and integrated reporting. More typically though, multiple information systems for billing, outcomes measurement, and documentation are already in place. As a result, clinicians are constantly reentering items like client name, social security number, and historical data.

While review of data input and reporting systems is beyond the scope of this chapter, it is relevant to point out that there is a clear trade-off in using a system for outcomes that is not integrated with your other business systems. If you wait until an integrated system is developed or purchased, you will have lost considerable time and momentum. Conversely, starting prior to system integration will necessitate duplicate entry of data. Both situations are problematic; the former delays the collection of data, the latter creates duplication of effort.

If you are just getting a system off the ground, initiate a "minimal cost," stand-alone system (either paper and pencil or basic software) and concurrently work toward integrated business systems.

External Data Bases

Benchmarking to industry standards is important. The requirements of external data bases such as Medirisk, Inc. (Medirisk, 1996) or UDSMR[SM] (Fiedler & Granger, 1997), should be considered. Recently a major subacute provider decided to include requirements of an external data base even though it had collected over 20,000 outcomes on an in-house data set. This provider's strategy was clear: obtain the capability to compare performance to national standards via analysis of objective, third-party review. A recent review of existing data on subacute outcomes (Haffy, in press) underscores the difficulty of incompatible data sets. Even if you do not completely agree with the scales being used by an external data base, providing your organization with the opportunity to benchmark its services against those of others will increase the level of motivation to measure outcomes.

Conduct a focus group to review existing scales, data requirements, and systems. Obtain as much consensus as possible concerning trade-offs with scope of measurement, systems support, and external data bases.

PREPARING TO MEASURE: TRAINING

Now that you have analyzed incentives and identified objectives, you are ready to begin the most important phase of the process: training the people who will collect and use outcomes information. Whether you work in a traditional setting with on-site services (e.g., medical records, administrative and quality improvement staff) or in a contract service environment with centralized but limited local support, it is necessary to enlist cooperation from key players on setting objectives and harnessing necessary support for training, data collection, analysis, and data utilization. Getting clinicians and support staff to "buy in" becomes even more challenging when you are working with multiple contractors and owners.

The first time outcomes measurement becomes a reality for an organization is when training is started. How much time will it take? Will it interfere with my other duties? Is training really necessary? I have to take a test? Loss of productivity? Training won't be off-site, will it?

There are two critical components in training individuals to participate in an outcomes measurement program:

- Teaching the big picture
- Outcome measures, training, and reliability testing

Here are some barriers and solutions for each training component.

Teaching the Big Picture

Barrier Often, training is squeezed into a busy clinical schedule and the time allotted is insufficient. As a result, rationale as to why measurement is important is considered nonessential and is not provided. The management assumption is that compliance provides sufficient incentive.

Solution. Spending even a half-hour discussing health care or education reform, reimbursement trends, marketing, or whatever is most relevant to the incentives you have identified will significantly improve the response of those asked to measure. For large organizations in particular, mere compliance to an outcomes protocol produces poor follow-through by those who are trained, and results in unplanned management costs in order to elicit cooperation and compliance. Teaching value motivates those trained and provides for consistent and maintained participation.

Outcomes Measures, Training, and Reliability Testing

Barrier. Training clinicians how to measure without reliability assessment makes your data vulnerable to claims that it may be biased or slanted to reflect positively on your practice. Reliability testing can be achieved using a variety of sampling techniques (Barlow et al., 1984). Sometimes reliability testing is not conducted due to cost or time constraints. In addition, some clinicians may be sensitive to being tested for the sake of reliability.

Solution. Explain the need to ensure reliability. Most reliability standards are set between 70 and 90% for a reason; rating outcomes (e.g., disability) is not a perfect science. Provide rapid feedback to clinicians about reliability results. If a clinician is having difficulty, arrange follow-up training and keep results confidential.

Barrier. Expect your organization to underestimate the time to conduct and follow-up on training. Whether you purchase the training from a database group or develop a train-the-trainer model for larger organizations, there is considerable expense associated with outcomes training.

Solution. Identify the cost (both expenses and lost revenue) associated with training. Review with your organization before going forward. When funding is limited, choose to thoroughly train a smaller number of clinicians.

IMPLEMENTATION

Whether you are introducing outcomes measurement to your organization or are augmenting an existing system, there are some definite strategies to assure integration with your culture and its values. These are described below during the following phases of implementation:

- testing your system
- audit and integrity procedures
- distribution and reporting of outcomes information
- using outcomes information
- revisiting your plan to create value for the organization

Testing Your System

There are two phases in testing an outcomes measurement system: beta testing and piloting. Beta testing is designed to work out initial bugs in the system; piloting is used to test the system on a representative user sample in your organization.

Select your beta facilities, unit, or personnel carefully. Revisit internal and external incentives and choose a site which will ensure cooperation throughout all phases of training, data collection, analysis, and utilization. Conducting a beta test means "trying it out." Be sure that the site knows that adjustments to protocol, data requirements, new releases of software, and so on occur as a result of its feedback; often this means protocol updates, additional training sessions, and slowing of the learning curve. Don't let these activities come as a surprise; otherwise they will be perceived as problems with the system.

Once you have worked out the bugs in the most ideal setting, spread the process to a larger group of pilot facilities more typical of your portfolio to test the feasibility of the system. Do this after you have elicited a positive response from the beta group. Provide an opportunity for the beta group to talk about the value it received during the process to targeted pilot facilities. The strategy here is to create a positive introduction of outcomes measurement to your organization.

AUDIT AND INTEGRITY PROCEDURES

There is a definite learning curve to providing accurate, complete, and reliable data. Paper and pencil systems are most labor intensive from a data clean-up standpoint, but are the least expensive to initiate. Most software systems have closed data entry fields so that errors are minimized but not eliminated. For instance, a system may require a medical diagnosis at admission, and may provide a correct list of codes as a resource, but cannot ascertain if the clinician chose the correct code. In general, data collection will take three to four times longer in the initial stages of implementation than it will later on. That is, a basic prepost protocol with approximately 50 different data elements will require about 10 minutes to enter once all of the necessary information is at hand and efficiencies of system input have been reached.

Provide a written protocol on how the system will work in your setting. Data base groups provide manuals related to data entry requirements and reporting, but these procedures need to be integrated into the logistics of your setting. For example, how will comorbidity information be obtained and ranked? Who will determine the accuracy of information entered? How will financial data be obtained? Who will coordinate data collection at a given facility?

Personnel that audit data and provide follow-up regarding compliance of clinical teams should use a teaching rather than corrective approach. If the audit process is used as a teaching opportunity, future data input will be more accurate and complete. If clinicians emerge from the audit feeling punished, have a talk with the audit personnel. In general, most people become uncomfortable when someone is checking their work. Inform clinical teams that audits are an important phase of data integrity and that, like data collection, data audit is part of their responsibility.

Distribution and Reporting of Outcomes Data

First and foremost, the value of outcomes measurement occurs only when information of interest is provided to users in formats that meet their needs. Traditionally, outcomes data has been sent to an external source for analysis and reporting on a quarterly basis. Often, clinicians and other personnel submitting the data would never see the reports, or would see the information 4 to 5 months after the fact. Most managers will not sift through reams of paper. They want key points, identification of outliers, and recommendations on what to do next.

Today, information technology and software systems provide on-demand access to outcomes data and provide for the reinforcing experience of seeing results immediately after the work has been done. Often the question is posed: "How many client outcomes do I need before I can produce a meaningful report?" While there is a fairly straightforward answer from a statistical standpoint, the logistical answer is "run a report as soon as you have your first five to ten outcomes." The reason for this is that there are three stages in providing value to the user with outcomes information:

- understanding the structure and capability of the of the reporting system
- interpretation
- using the information derived from the report.

Understanding Report Structure and Capability

Even after the most thorough training, legitimate interest may not occur until users see their own data in contrast to a benchmark or standard. Usually, identification with data that represents one's own performance produces considerable attention.

- Provide a thorough explanation of the variables in the report.
- Point out the usefulness of the information for case management, marketing, family education, and establishing thresholds for evaluating parameters of program function.
- Explain that outcomes information will help establish a common platform from which providers, managers, and payers can communicate and make decisions regarding client care and program function.

Interpretation

Often, voluminous outcome reports do not provide value except to those who have the time and the interest to dissect all of the detail; such individuals are usually in the minority. The key is to provide the user with a path to understanding the data. The path should begin with an overview of performance on key outcome benchmarks, such as those shown in Figure 10–1.

Here, data are collapsed across key factors such as diagnosis and payer. However, your first goal is to provide the user with a baseline for overall performance based on average or median measures. Figure 10–1 illustrates that, compared to the larger data base, Business X is providing services to a population of comparable age and disability; however, Business X patients begin their rehabilitation at 15 days post onset of the primary medical diagnosis versus 31 days post onset for the larger data base. Compared to the data base, Business X provided rehabilitation in 6 less days (LOS), with comparable gains and discharge to community and 28% less overall charges per case. Note a 41% managed care payer mix for Business X. This level of information provides an overall view of provider performance.

The next step along the path is to review each of the benchmarks individually as they are analyzed, for example—by factors of interest (e.g., diagnosis and payer). At this stage, "interactions or outliers" can be identified. For example, in Figure 10–2 it is clear

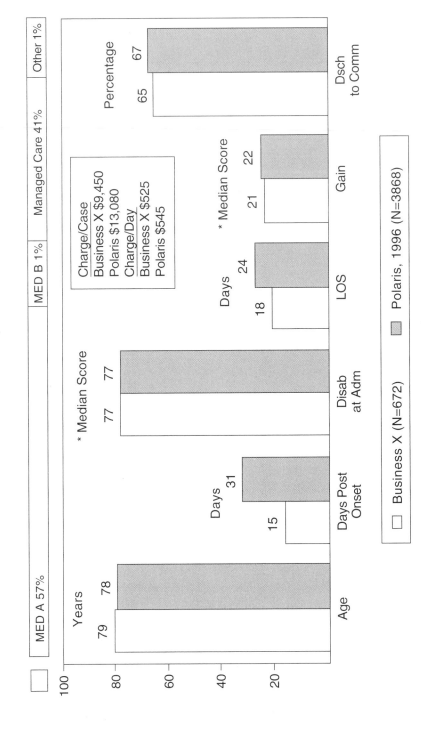

Figure 10–1. Benchmark: Business X Subacute and Polaris Subacute Outcomes

* Functional Independence Measure

SOURCE: The Polaris Group, Inc., Outcomes Research, 3/95–7/96 (Printed 08/30/96).

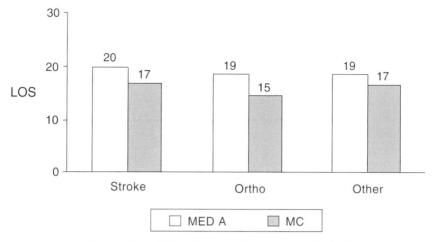

Figure 10–2. LOS × Payer and Impairment (Stable)

that the Business X average of 18 days for length of stay (LOS) is reasonably stable across three major patient groups (stroke, orthopedics, and other) and two payers (Med A and Managed Care) and MC LOS is consistently less than MedA LOS.

As a result, the user can use the overall facility average with some confidence. In contrast, Figure 10–3 shows that, although the Business X average LOS is of 18 days, two outlier groups (stroke Med A and orthopedic, managed care) vary significantly from the average, yet did not skew the average because they cancel out one another. Here, the facility average is variable across patient type and payer, such that the "outliers" should be mentioned when reporting overall facility length of stay.

The relationship among report factors and levels must systematically be explained to the user. To assist you in meeting this objective, purchase or develop a reporting system that provides well organized, graphic representation of information. *Provide a path for the interpretation process.*

Using Outcomes Information

Creating value with outcomes reporting essentially means to turn data into information that the user groups consider critical to their business or primary area of responsibility. Primary user groups include clinicians, rehabilitation managers, clients and families, and payers. For each group, value is enhanced when data can be aggregated at a level meaningful to the group's interest. Let's consider some examples, which build on those in the previous chapter:

Clinicians and Rehabilitation Managers

There are multiple opportunites for creating opportunity with providers:

- on-demand access to trended data for case management and client advocacy
- creating marketing position

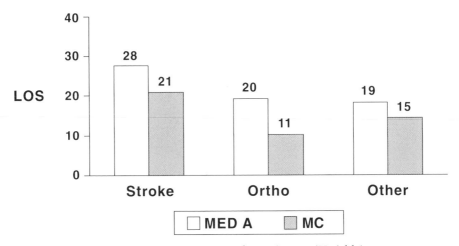

Figure 10–3. LOS × Payer and Impairment (Variable)

- negotiating contract rates
- managing program structure
- benchmarking their facility or region of facilities against other groups within their organization or to national standards
- managing shift to managed care models

The facility depicted in Figure 10–3 is in a competitive, managed care market they may wish to determine whether outcomes are different for stroke patients on a capitated plan versus traditional Medicare. Analysis of reducing length of stay on gain and discharge to community helps create a threshold for clinical teams who are reticent to reduce utilization of therapies for fear that outcomes will be compromised. For the rehabilitation manager, outcomes provide a barometer for balancing cost-efficiency with client care. While standard reporting formats would become too lengthy to break down such an analysis beyond a statement of variability such as standard deviation or confidence intervals, ad-hoc query can be helpful.

User-friendly "query" tools such as the one depicted in Figure 10–4 provide such flexibility. Here carrier, impairment group (stroke), gain, LOS, and percent discharge to community have been selected.

Clinicians plan treatment around assessment, prognosis, and anticipated disposition at discharge. However, they must provide appropriate services within the constraints of the payer. For example, Medicare regulations require that rehabilitation in a SNF environment be provided only on a one-to-one basis and only by a skilled clinician; that is, no group treatment and no rehabilitation aides or extenders can be used. Managed care, on the other hand, is limiting utilization via per diem caps or case caps, and promoting the use of group treatment and support personnel.

Outcomes, combined with results of the query described in Figure 10–4, can be useful as a barometer to track the impact of reducing care on the results of rehabilitation.

Figure 10–5 provides the results of the query described earlier.

Clearly, length of stay for the managed care group is much shorter than the

Medicare group, yet gain and discharge to community were not compromised. Showing this type of analysis to clinicians eases their reevaluation of practice standards and assures them that management will be able to ascertain when and if further reduction of length of stay would endanger client outcomes. Conversely, if the results had demonstrated comprimised gains for the MC groups, clinicians can use such information to advocate for services beyond limits set by payers.

Query Tool

Patient Characteristic

- ☒ Carrier
- ☐ Clinical Level of Care
- ☐ Education
- ☐ Ethnicity
- ☐ Gender
- ☒ Impairment Group
- ☐ Living Setting at Admission
- ☐ Living Setting at Discharge
- ☐ Major Surgical Procedure
- ☐ Martial Status
- ☐ Medical Complexity Status
- ☐ Other Referring Party
- ☐ Patient Home Zip Code
- ☐ Patient Satisfaction
- ☐ Payer

Patient Characteristics

- ☐ Carrier
- ☐ Impairment Group

Outcomes Variable

- ☐ Length of Stay
- ☐ Gain
- ☐ Discharge to community

Patient Characteristics

- ☐ English Language
- ☐ Primary Medical Diagnosis
- ☐ Referral Zip
- ☐ Referring Facility
- ☐ Referring Physician
- ☐ Rehabilitation Status
- ☐ Rehabilitation Setting
- ☐ Treatment Medical Diagnosis
- ☐ Vocational Status at Admission

Outcome Variable

- ☐ Age
- ☐ Days Post Onset
- ☐ Admission Assessment
- ☐ Discharge Assessment
- ☒ Gain

Outcome Variable

- ☒ Length of Stay
- ☐ % Living in Comm Prior to Onset of Prim Dx
- ☐ % Living in Comm Immed Prior to Rehab
- ☒ % Discharged to Community
- ☐ Charge per Case
- ☐ Charge per Day

Figure 10–4. Query Tool

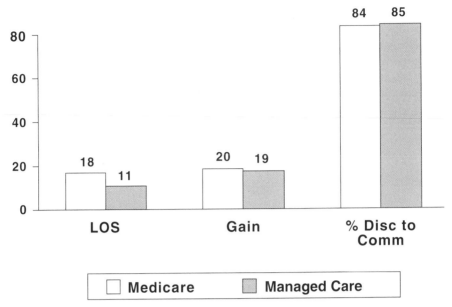

Figure 10–5. Stroke Matched

Client/Family

Graphic portrayal of progress is reinforcing to clients and provides meaningful information to families. When progress is less than anticipated, access to trended data on outcomes of clients with similar profiles, including comorbildity and medical complexity (relationship of comorbidity to targeted functional skills) is effective in providing a framework for shaping expectations. While a universally accepted measure of medical complexity for rehabilitation has yet to be identified (Stineman, 1994), scales are commercially available (e.g., Medirisk, 1996; The Polaris Group, 1996). Another approach is to match patients on diagnosis, age, and disability (Warren, 1995).

Payer

An industry survey by Foster Higgins (Hale, 1994) polled 350 managed care providers about the relative value of outcomes information. Less than 9% viewed outcomes as the primary factor for assuring success in their marketplace. As you would expect, over 75% identified price as the key success factor. However, as certain managed care marketplaces mature and variability in price is minimized, outcomes are gaining momentum as a method of differentiating quality of care, especially when combined with pricing, access to service, and satisfaction data. In the future, Medicare is likely to institute a prospective payment mechanism for rehabilitation, which incorporates levels of patient disability and case-mix (Wilkerson et al., 1992). All of these factors point to the notion that providers, payers, and consumers increasingly are being asked to "share risk." Trended outcomes information has considerable value as a basis for risk sharing for all participants in the rehabilitation process (McMillan, 1993).

CONCLUSION

The role of outcomes measurement and its relationship to the perceived value of rehabilitation is evolving. Traditionally, *provider-driven* expectations viewed outcomes as a proxy of quality, but not directly related to reimbursement. Satisfactory outcomes were identified by the professional opinion of the provider. At present we are experiencing a transition in which the emergence of managed care and diminishing health care resources have created a *payer-driven* environment in which value is clearly defined as the relationship between the result of the care and the cost of the care. Here, emphasis is placed on uniformity of measurement so that providers can be compared to benchmarks. In the future we envision *consumer-driven* health care wherein performance, compared to benchmarks on client-centered measures not bound by episode or setting, will be dominant in a privatized health care marketplace.

Barriers to preparing your organization for the evolving role of outcomes measurement can be overcome if you recognize the incentives for measurement within your organization, create value by providing users of outcomes information with a clear path through the data, and provide access to the data with flexibility to query levels of the data of specific interest to the user.

REFERENCES

Barlow, D. H., Hayes, S. C., & Nelson, R. O. (1984). *The Scientist Practioner.* New York: Pergamon Press.

Burgess, C. (1996). Outcomes Survey. Lakewood, CA: Connie Burgess and Associates.

De Jong, G. (in press). Rehab 2000: The evolution of medical rehabilitation in American health care. In P. K. Landrum (Ed.), *Outcome Oriented Rehabilitation Principles, Strategies and tools for Effective Program Management.* Gaithersburg, MD: Aspen Publishers, Inc.

de LaFiente, D. (1993). For-profit chains' growth helps boost rehab industry. *Modern Healthcare, 23,* 58–62.

Fiedler, R.C., & Granger, C.V., (1997). Uniform Data System for Medical Rehabilitation: Report of first admissions for 1995. *American Journal of Physical Medicine and Rehabilitation, 76,* 76–81.

Haffy, W. (in press). Subacute rehabilitation outcomes. *Journal of Subacute Care.*

Hale, J. (1994). *National Survey of Employer Sponsored Health Plans.* Princeton, NJ: Foster Higgins.

Kramer, M. (in press). Comments on "rehabilitation care and outcomes from the patients perspective". In H. Palmer & R. Warren (Eds), Proceedings of the working group on improving health care outcomes through geriatric rehabilitation. *The Boston Working Group.* Medical Care.

Lewin-VHI: (1995). Subacute care: policy synthesis and market area analysis. A Report submitted to DMHS, office of the Assistant Secretary for Planning and Evaluation.

McMillan, A. (1993). Trends in medicare health maintenance organization enrollment: 1986–93. *Health Care Financing Review, 15,* 135–146.

Medirisk, Inc. (1996). Chicago, IL.

Morris, J. (1991). Resident assessment instrument training manual and resource guide. Natick, MA, Eliot Press.

Naumann, E. (1994). Delivering value. *Executive Excellence, Sept.*

Polaris Group, Inc. (1996). Hingham, MA.

Sherman, D., & Meyer, S. (1995). Rehabilitation outcomes by site of service: a comparison of hospitals to subacute units of freestanding skilled nursing facilities. Washington, DC: American Health Care Association.

Stineman, M., Escarce, J., Goin, J., Hamilton, B., Granger, C., & Williams, S. (1994). A case-mix classification system for medical rehabilitation. *Medical Care, 32,* 306.

Warren, R.L. (1995). Form and functions of subacute rehabilitation. Invited presentation at medical rehabilitation: Form and function under managed care. Buffalo, NY: Uniform Data System.

Warren, R.L. (1996). Value of rehabilitation in the managed care marketplace. Paper presented to the Washington State Health Care Association, Seattle, WA.

Wilkerson, D., Batavia, A., & De Jong, G. (1992). Use of functional status measure for payment of medical rehabiliation services. *Archives of Physical Medicine and Rehabilitation, 73,* 111–120.

Wolk, S., & Blair, D. (1994). Trends in medical rehabilitation. Reston, VA: American Rehabilitation Association.

CHAPTER 11

Outcomes Measurement in Culturally and Linguistically Diverse Populations

HORTENCIA KAYSER

INTRODUCTION

Over sixty million individuals of color are residing in the United States (Battle, 1993). As we near the twenty-first century, the numbers of Hispanics will have increased by an estimated 21%, the Asian population by 22%, and African Americans by 12%, but the mainstream white population will have increased only by 2%. Battle (1993) states that the minority will become the majority by the year 2030.

It is estimated that 10% or 6 million persons from culturally and linguistically diverse backgrounds are communicatively impaired (Boone & Plante, 1993). This figure may be higher because these populations are more affected than the white population by poverty, environment, teratogens, traumatic brain injury, and other diseases that occur frequently among African Americans, Native Americans, and Hispanics (Battle, 1993; Harris, 1993; Reyes, 1995; Wallace, 1993).

When an individual from a linguistically diverse background is determined to have an impairment, disability, or handicap, we assume that the client will concur. But disability and handicap especially are determined largely by the group's cultural beliefs. Taylor (1987) states that each culture will define for itself what is deviant and what is normal. Speech-language pathologists (SLPs) cannot assume that mainstream definitions of communication and related disorders are universal. Culturally and linguistically diverse populations will vary in their understanding and beliefs of how impairments, disabilities, and handicaps occur, how they will be perceived by their community, and how they will affect the member's interactions and productivity in that society. Thus, what may be a disability for the mainstream culture may not be viewed as a disability for another cultural group. Additionally, what may be a handicapping condition for one group may be accepted and nurtured within the community for another group.

The standardization of outcome measures becomes problematic because there are inter- and intravariations for culturally and linguistically diverse populations. What and how the SLP uses to measure treatment outcomes will depend upon that professional's understanding and acceptance of the client's culture. For example, the SLP may believe that treatment has improved the client's communicative abilities, but the client and family may believe that the client's ability to function in a specific cultural role has not improved. Definitions, heterogeneity of groups, cultural beliefs, and standardized instruments are important factors that play a distinct role in the accurate and appropriate measurement of client function and treatment outcomes.

This chapter provides an overview of issues and factors that will affect measurement for individuals from culturally and linguistically diverse groups. It begins with a brief discussion of culture, how different cultural groups view impairment, disability, and handicapping conditions, and offers exemplars of these perspectives and their impact on outcomes measurement. Issues related to measurement include standardization of instruments, considerations, and recommendations in the adaptation of instruments, the effects of translation, and how interpreters may assist the SLP. Finally, there will be a discussion concerning research as it relates to cultural sensitivity.

CULTURE

Taylor (1987) defines culture as the set of perceptions, technologies, and survival systems used by members of a specified group to ensure the acquisition and perpetuation of what they consider to be a high quality of life. Culture is arbitrary, changeable; it has internal variations and overlaps with other cultures. It is learned and exists at different levels of conscious awareness. To say that there is a "Hispanic culture" would be a misconception of what is known about Cuban-American, Puerto Rican, and Mexican-American individuals. Each of these groups has a set of perceptions, technologies, and survival systems that have developed because of each ones different histories and experiences within the United States. These groups also change with exposure to mainstream values and beliefs, which create subgroups of Hispanics (i.e., Cuban American, Puerto Rican, Mexican American). This phenomenon holds true for all of the major cultural and linguistic groups in the United States.

Cultures will vary in their understanding and beliefs concerning disease, treatment, and disease consequences. Religious and other beliefs play a central role in the explanation of disabilities for many of these individuals. Physicians, for example, differ in their notions about the practice of medicine. We assume that medicine is a constant and rigorous science, but physicians around the world disagree on the diagnosis and treatment of diseases. Payer (1988) reports that physicians in Europe will disagree on the treatment of disease depending upon the country and culture in which the physician practices and resides. The diagnosis will be influenced by culture in which what the doctor learned in medical school, what is known, what other doctors say, and what the doctor knows will reassure the patient. Payer (1988) sites a World Health Organization (WHO) study that found that doctors from different countries diagnosed different causes of death even when shown identical information from the same death certificates. While the practice of medicine is influenced by a certain amount of scientific input, culture can intervene considerably in diagnosis and treatment.

Culturally and linguistically diverse individuals do have different views of medicine, illness, impairment, disability, and handicap. What they believe is the cause of their difficulties and how these are treated, or whether the impairment *should* be treated, is influenced in large part by culture and the belief system within that culture. African, Asian, Hispanic, and Native Americans have cultural roots that have influenced their perceptions and definitions of impairments, disabilities, and handicaps. The following section reviews some of the ideologies, beliefs, and concerns of these major cultural groups in the United States. The reader is cautioned not to generalize these characteristics to all members of a particular group because culturally and linguistically diverse populations have great intragroup heterogeneity.

DIFFERING VIEWS OF IMPAIRMENT, DISABILITY, AND HANDICAP

The Hispanic Perspective

Hispanics are a heterogenous people. Those of Mexican decent have a mixture of European and Indian ideology and practices; those from the Caribbean have a mixture of Indian, European, and African influences. The common basis for many Hispanics' belief system is Catholic ideology. Mexican Catholic ideology includes Indian practices, but Cuban and Puerto Rican Catholicism may include African religious beliefs (e.g., Yoruba), sometimes called Santerismo or Espiritismo (Harry, 1992). The greater the influence of African tradition, the more the perspective reflects an animistic view, that is, a belief that spiritual influences abound throughout the universe (Harry, 1992). These spirits can have a negative influence (e.g., illness) as well as positive influence (e.g., wellness).

Among Mexican Americans, there is a belief that an "evil eye" or "mal ojo," which is obtained by admiring an individual or envying the person, will cause that person illness. Curanderos, or medicine women, are called to perform rituals, prayers, and provide herbal medicinal teas to counteract the evil that affected the afflicted individual. There are beliefs that explain speech disorders, such as "susto," a severe fright that might cause a child to stutter. If a pregnant woman views a full moon or an eclipse, the event will cause a cleft palate in the unborn child (Langdon, 1992; Maestas & Erickson, 1992). Table 11–1 summarizes those beliefs concerning illness and its consequences, which are reported for Hispanic populations, as well as for the other populations addressed throughout this chapter.

Children who are born with birth defects and adults who have suffered strokes may be viewed as gifts from God or as punishment for sins committed by the mother or individual, respectively (Langdon, 1992). These views of how a disability was obtained, then affect what is believed, should be done to correct or not correct the disorder. Harry (1992) and Teller (1988) describe Hispanics as having a fatalistic view of life. Reyes (1995) describes this as an external locus of control. That is, one does not and cannot change what has happened to them. Treatment, then, may be affected by the client's

Table 11–1. Reported beliefs about disease and its consequences by culturally and linguistically diverse populations.

HISPANIC	AFRICAN AMERICAN	NATIVE AMERICAN	ASIAN AMERICAN	PACIFIC ISLANDER
Families may believe in "curanderismo" (e.g., folk medicine using herbs, prayers, and rituals).	Approaches to health vary depending on income and educational level of families.	Healing and purification ceremonies are common in tribes.	Asian parents may believe children who are "disabled" have only visible/physical symptoms.	Families may call upon faith healers or use folk medicine.
Families may resist institutionalization (i.e., individuals with disabilities may be cared for at home.)	Some African-Americans believe that handicapping conditions are due to evil spirits, the devil, punishment for disobeying God, and/or bad luck.	Some accept a disabled child as the Great Spirit's gift.	Only physical disabilities are worthy of treatment.	Massage and use of fruits, roots, and leaves as treatment are common.
A visible disability may be attributed to external causes (e.g., witchcraft, the moon).	African-American families are often able to accept children who have disabilities, in part due to extended family support and strong ties to the church.	Some believe that handicapping condition resulted from witchcraft or moral transgressions.	Invisible deficits such as stuttering, learning disability, are believed to result from "not trying hard enough."	Some families protect disabled children and do not expect them to be independent.
Parents may believe that they are being punished for wrongdoing.		Some accept handicapped individuals because of a strong belief that these individuals still have a role to play in the community.	Some believe that handicapping conditions occur as one's "fate" and nothing can or should be done to interfere.	Some Hawaiian families attribute physical disabilities to spiritual causes.
Families differ in their reactions to disabilities and may receive social support.		Some believe that a child was born with a disability because that child made a choice prenatally to be disabled.	Some believe that birth defects and disabilities result from sins committed by parents or ancestors.	The disabilities may be viewed as beyond the control of human beings.
Catholic parents may accept disabilities stoically (i.e., a larger divine plan not comprehensible to humans).			If a child's defects represents a punishment for sins, he or she will be looked upon as an object of shame and isolated from society.	Some believe that spirits can cause disabilities in children.
Some families may hide a disabled child if the family takes pride in themselves for health and vitality.			To "save face" some families are hesitant to seek medical.	Some view a handicap as a gift from God; thus the individual is to be protected and sheltered.
				Among Samoans there is tendency toward intolerance for disabilities. Families may conceal the disability.

Children with disabilities may be indulged by family and friends.

Children with disabilities may not be expected to participate in treatment and their own care.

Families may not accept invisible disabling conditions (e.g., learning disabilities).

Some families may use spiritualists to seek healing and dispel evil spirits.

care for children with disabilities.

Many believe that caring for disabled individuals is the responsibility of the family, not the school.

Health practices may involve acupuncture, herbs, massage, and baths in hot springs.

Some may visit religious shrines or temples to seek healing.

Some Samoans believe that the birth of a disabled child is a sign of God's displeasure with the family.

SOURCES FOR HISPANIC POPULATIONS: Anderson & Fenichel (1989); Hanline & Daley (1992); Langdon (1992); Maestas & Erickson (1992); Meyerson (1983); and Roseberry-McKibben (1995).

SOURCES FOR AFRICAN-AMERICAN POPULATIONS: Willis (1992); Hanline & Daley (1992); and Roseberry-McKibben, (1995).

SOURCES FOR NATIVE AMERICAN POPULATIONS: Anderson & Fenichel (1989); Harris (1986, 1993); Joe & Malach (1992); and Roseberry-McKibben, (1995).

SOURCES FOR ASIAN AMERICAN POPULATIONS: Allen, et al (1992); Anderson & Fenichel (1989); Bebout & Arthur (1992); Chan (1992); Ethridge (1990); Matsuda (1989); Lewis & Vang (1987); Long (1992); and Roseberry-McKibben (1994, 1995).

SOURCES FOR PACIFIC ISLANDER POPULATIONS: Barker (1993); Blaisdell (1989); Cheng & Hammer (1992); Fiatoa & Palafox (1980); Fitzgerald & Hammer (1994); Mokuau & Tauili'ili (1992); Roseberry-McKibben (1995); and Stewart (1986).

229

attitude. Thus, the client may not be an active participant in the treatment program (Wallace, 1995).

The practice of traditional folk medicine may be sought first, in addition to treatment, or sought after treatment if the client perceives that the treatment is not effective. These practices may also depend upon the availability of curanderos or yerberos. Marin, Marin, Padilla, and de la Rocha (1983) reported that in East Los Angeles only a small percentage of respondents to their questionnaire on health services stated that they could find a curandero (7%), a yerbero (15%), or a partera (midwife, 2%). Marin and colleagues suggest that the use of folk medicine may actually be limited. Teller (1988) states that the belief and use of folk medicine for diseases and disabilities is probably used in conjunction with Western medicine rather than instead of medicine. The use of folk medicine will vary depending upon the assimilation of the individual into mainstream views of disease and disability.

Two important aspects of Hispanic cultures that may influence treatment outcomes and satisfaction with services from an agency include: (1) the importance of people, individuals, their qualities as a person, and inner importance; and (2) the importance of relationships. There are specific concepts that influence Hispanic relationships with the outside world. These include respeto (respect), dignidad (dignity), personalismo (personalism), honor (honor), and confianza (trust) (Harry, 1992). These qualities transcend social class, therefore, a person who has a low income, is an individual, and has fulfilled obligations to family and community is respected. The mainstream belief that a professional should be respected because of skill rather than personal disposition is not always accepted by Hispanics. The person and his or her qualities cannot be separated from the professional. It becomes important to respect the *person* who provides the professional services.

Relationships are important. Networking among community members and extended families make up the community's system of trustworthy individuals. Hispanics trust people and rely on people. The agency or clinic is not a person and not an entity that can be trusted and relied upon. Thus, a Hispanic family will respect the individual whom they can trust and who also happens to be a professional, but may not understand or trust the agency or organization. Therefore, it is frequently observed that a Hispanic family will depend upon the one SLP to whom they can talk or call upon, but may not rate highly or value the agency where the clinican is employed.

The African-American Perspective

The African-American perception of illness and its consequences has not been fully studied. Like all of the culturally and linguistically diverse groups, African Americans are a heterogeneous population that includes individuals from all socioeconomic and educational levels. African-Americans did have a different beginning in this country through a forced slavery system that treated them as property and investments that needed to be protected. Harrison and Harrison (1971) reported that slave owners provided health care, especially for pregnant women and children, primarily as a function of protecting one's property. Infant mortality rates for African Americans during the slavery era were the same as that for whites. During the post-Emancipation period, health care for women and children plummeted and depended upon the actions of benevolent white people. Roseberry-McKibben (1995) reports that African Americans continue to have a higher mortality rate than other groups, higher infant mortality rate than whites (20:10.5 per 1000), 10 times higher death from nutritional deficiencies in infancy than whites, and poverty that affects 1 of every 2 African-American children. Health status and the quality of services have been found to be tied to the economic status of African Americans (Harrison & Harrison, 1971; Roseberry-McKibben, 1995).

Harrison and Harrison (1971) state that slave owners would not allow African Americans to settle their own disputes and arguments because of the possibility that a slave might be injured. The result was increased use of witchcraft as a means of revenge among the slaves. Witchcraft was a means of causing harm to others and also healing illness. Rural African Americans were described as more likely than urban African Americans to continue to use folk remedies, magical thought, and have feelings of fatalism about disease and death. Roseberry-McKibben (1995) describes African Americans as attributing handicapping conditions to evil spirits, the work of the devil, and punishment for disobeying God. Terrell and Terrell (1993) and Payne-Johnson (1992) state that religion is important in the lives of African Americans. These explanations of illness and disability must be viewed with caution, since African Americans do come from a variety of educational and socioeconomic levels, which in turn will affect their understanding of disabilities and their motivation and resources for seeking treatment.

A result of the injustices that African Americans have experienced is mistrust of whites and institutions (Harry, 1992; Harrison & Harrison, 1971; Terrell & Terrell, 1993). Terrell and Terrell (1993) suggest that this mistrust affects the measurement of performance. Individuals with higher levels of mistrust of whites perform worse on measurements than individuals with lower levels of mistrust. They describe the pattern of response in African Americans as *silence*. Harry (1992) states that this mistrust extends to the schools with the overidentification of African American students as disabled or mentally challenged. Harrison & Harrison (1971) stated that African Americans' suspicion and anxiety of medical facilities that are managed by white professionals will result in two types of behaviors: testing and avoidance. *Testing* involves observation of a facility or professionals to determine whether the staff are friendly, helpful, and genuinely interested in African Americans. They report that some individuals may visit a waiting room and observe for a number of minutes and then walk out. The results of the observation, positive or negative, will be reported to family and friends. *Avoidance* is an attempt to preserve the African American's self-esteem by staying away from agencies so that the individual does not experience rejection or harm when interacting with whites. The results of avoidance can only result in serious delays of treatment or no treatment.

Effective outcome measurements among African Americans must begin with an understanding of the African American experience and acknowledgment of the serious injustices that have affected many African American's perception of measurement, poor treatment in agencies, and continued inequities in health care, education, and employment. Trust is the foundation of the client-clinician relationship. Developing trust will be paramount in effective and appropriate outcome measurements and treatment efficacy.

Asian/Pacific Islander Perspective

Asian/Pacific Islanders, too, come from a variety of backgrounds and cultures. Their immigration into this country began in the 1800s and has increased dramatically with the refugee populations from Southeast Asian wars. In the United States, the Asian/Pacific Islander cultures will vary in education, socioeconomic status, and assimilation to Western values. For example, the reliance on Western medicine will depend upon assimilation and education. Kraut (1990) states that traditional Asian cultures from China, Vietnam, Indonesia, and Korea turn to Asian herb shops for treatment rather than medical facilities for a variety of health problems. He reports mistrust of Western medicine and states that Chinese immigrants will rely on herbalists, acupuncturists, and pharmacies using traditional Chinese medicine. Kraut's report provides insight for speech-language pathologists who attempt to serve these populations. But mistrust of Western ways is only part of the difficulty in providing services to the culturally and linguistically diverse group. Religion and communication style also will influence treatment outcomes and their measurement.

Cheng (1987) states that all of the Asian/Pacific Islander cultures have been influenced by the Chinese culture and are rooted in three major religions; Buddhism, Taoism, and Confucianism. Harry (1992) describes these religions as having similar values, which include social and personal harmony. She further states that the common features for these religions promote social order, rules of propriety, filial piety, benevolence, loyalty, cooperation, reciprocity, and obligation. Cheng (1993) describes these cultures as valuing harmony, humility, education and respect. Cheng (1993) reports that Christianity has also had an influence on these cultures, (e.g., 19% of Koreans are Buddhist) and that the assimilation of the various groups will range from great difficulty to none. The reader is referred to Cheng (1993) for a detailed description of the history, family, language, education, and religion of 11 Asian/Pacific Islander cultures.

Harry (1992) and Roseberry-McKibben (1995) report that for many of these cultures there is a common belief that the family is to be honored through education or excellence in a profession. This builds cohesiveness, status, and the reputation of the family; thus, to "save face" becomes paramount for families and communities. Disabilities are then viewed as a reflection of the family. Harry (1992) states that there is much stigma related to disability. Families may feel shame because of the disability present in a family member and may express this shame through stoic behavior. Cheng (1993) describes these behaviors as based on the belief that the disability is "karma" or fate. Families may believe that nothing should be done to remediate the disability or the family may be reluctant to seek assistance. The parents of children with severe disabilities may be protective and tolerant of deviant behaviors. Milder disabilities are not acknowledged by the parents and may be referred to as laziness or a reluctance to try.

The social interactions between the SLP and client is crucial for accurate outcomes assessment. SLPs must be aware that Asian/Pacific Island cultures do have different norms from American standards for social interactions. Harry (1992) and Cheng (1993) state that harmony is important for these groups during social interactions. The results will be a reluctance to engage in confrontation or to promote oneself before a group. Indirectness and silence may be valued. The nonverbal interaction, such as subtle gestures, posture, positioning, facial expressions, and eye contact, are used to convey messages more frequently than English-speaking mainstream Americans. Among the Japanese, personal space is greater than among Americans, thus touch is not appropriate. For many Asian/Pacific Island populations, honorifics (i.e., speech style dependent upon rank and respect) and formalities are the norm.

Cheng (1993) emphasizes that the Asian/Pacific Islanders are numerous and heterogeneous in cultures, languages, and beliefs. SLPs must individualize treatment, as well as measurement of its outcome, on the basis of the specific culture of the client. Generalizations should be avoided from one group to another.

Native American Perspective

There are two important concepts that will influence the interactions between mainstream SLPs and Native Americans. The first concept is related to religious beliefs, and the second is concerned with the Native American perception of the individual and his or her interactions with others. The former concept will affect the individual's perception of disability, while both may affect treatment.

Among Native American peoples, there is a belief in the continuity of life of the spirit and inseparable interaction among mind, body, and spirit. Harris (1993) states that there is no word for *religion* in most American Indian languages because spirituality is an important aspect of day-to-day life. Harry (1992) discusses the traditional interpretations of healing and illness as tied to the idea of harmony or disharmony between these three aspects of the individual. Natural and unnatural illness is interpreted as caused by the violation of a sacred taboo or evil powers, respectively. The Indian belief system, then, encourages staying away from situations perceived to be negative and thus keeping oneself strong. Thus, the medical or biological explanation of disabilities may be problematic for clients who have traditional beliefs. Harry (1992) and Harris (1993) explain the common belief that a spirit chooses a body to inhabit and the disabled body is the physical manifestation of the spirit. They state that most traditional Indian languages do not have terms for retarded, disabled, or handicapped. Thus, individuals with disabilities are given names that describe the disability, for example, One-Who-Walks-With-A-Limp. These individuals are allowed to integrate into the community without absolute comformity to all standards.

The second concept discussed by Harry (1992) and Harris (1993) relates to interactions. Among Native Americans, there is a preference for a low-key and slower-paced style of discourse. Individuals do not attempt to dominate others, give directions to others, ask for information on personal or family matters, and draw attention to oneself or to others. Acquaintances are not addressed in a familiar manner and gaze is not too direct. These discourse rules will ultimately affect assessment and treatment. The questions requested by SLPs may be perceived as inappropriate and the response may be silence. Treatment outcomes can only be framed within these people's perceptions of disability as it is within their society. The religious beliefs concerning the cause and treatment of a disability combined with discourse interactional rules will pose a formidable challenge for the clinician.

Vining (personal communication, 1996), for example, states that a mother who has a child with Down syndrome will explain that the disorder was a result of her viewing an upsetting circumstance or event during the pregnancy, and this occurrence upset the harmony within the child. The mother will first attempt to resolve this disharmony through visits with the Medicine Man. The ceremony will bring the mother and child back into harmony with the spiritual and physical world. These beliefs will affect treatment, because the mother will believe that it does not matter what is done by the clinician or herself; there will not be a change in the child. There is a belief of a lack of control. Vining suggests that for this mother, there must be a support system to educate and assure the mother that change is possible, and thereby, she would feel confident that something can be achieved to improve the child's status.

The perceptions of disease and its consequences by various culturally and linguistically diverse groups are ingrained into the belief system of the culture. The interaction of religious beliefs, causes of disabilities, impairments, and handicaps, and how these are explained and treated are not easily changed by a SLP's Western explanation and a packet of handouts. Culturally and linguistically diverse individuals maintain their belief systems to varying degrees and will only consider Western explanations and treatment procedures with time, trust in the professional, and culturally sensitive education.

CLINICAL PRACTICE AND OUTCOMES MEASUREMENT

Outcome measures are important for the accurate and objective assessment of an individual's impairment, disability, and/or handicap. Norms for these instruments, however (particularly our standardized tests of impairment), have historically been developed from a population that is primarily middle class, English speaking, and of European background. Culturally and linguistically diverse populations often are not reflected in the norms developed for the various classes of outcome measures. Thus, clinicians may be forced to change the instrument or its administration procedures to "fit" the diverse populations served within an agency. This section focuses on the difficulties in standardizing outcome measures for culturally and linguistically diverse populations and the *usual* practice in attempting to meet their needs. These include translating and adapting outcome measures, and using an interpreter for the collection of data. It should be noted at the outset of this discussion, however, that any changes to a measure will threaten its reliability and validity. Clinician interpretations therefore must be made with caution.

STANDARDIZED INSTRUMENTS

For the past 30 years, speech-language pathologists have attempted to assess individuals from culturally and linguistically diverse populations with speech and language impairments by using standardized instruments that were developed for monolingual mainstream English speakers. Over these years of practice, research, and reflection, speech-language pathologists have recognized this as a biased practice unlikely to capture a representative sample of the client's abilities. Criticisms of tests and their use with diverse populations abound. Kayser (1995) lists a number of these criticisms in Table 11–2.

A single standardized outcome measure for many culturally and linguistically diverse populations in the United States is not possible. The demographics for the different cultural populations, census within a region, generational shifts in cultural ideologies, language, levels of bilingualism, education, and other variables all contribute to invalidating the process of standardizing a measure for clients from any specific group. Speech-language pathologists must still account for the client's progress and satisfaction with clinical services. Therefore, outcome measures may need to be modified

---

Table 11–2. Potential Limitations of Outcome Measures from the Perspective of Cultural/Linguistic Diversity

---

1. Lack of validity (Does not measure what it is intended to measure). The test does not have:
   a. *face validity* (appears sound).
   b. *content validity* (tasks on tests are representative of larger sample of behavior).
   c. *predictive validity* (predicts some later success).
   d. *concurrent validity* (gives results similar to existing tests).
   e. *construct validity* (reflects a valid theory of nature of language and language learning).
2. Lack of reliability (does not consistently give same results). The test does not have:
   a. split-half correlations.
   b. parallel forms.
   c. Reliable retesting within and across examiners using the same test.
   d. explicit ratings criteria.
3. Standardization and norms do not include all groups to be tested.
4. Test is not well developed.
5. Content of test is biased by:
   a. author(s) of test.
   b. standardization group.
   c. dialect and language group.
   d. items not reflective of cultural and linguistic background.
6. Tests are biased due to:
   a. use of middle-class mainstream values and experiences.
   b. Lack of consideration of other cultural groups' experiences
7. Test fosters low expectancy for culturally and linguistically diverse individuals.
8. Test shapes curriculum and does not lead to meaningful instruction.
9. Test evaluates only a segment of individual's communicative abilities.
10. Test is perceived as accurate.
11. Test is not objective.
12. Test lacks linguistic realism and authenticity.

SOURCES: Adapted from: On some dimensions of language proficiency by M. Canale, 1983. In J. W. Oller (Ed)., *Issues in language testing research.* Rowley, MA: Newbury House. *Speech and language assessment for the bilingual handicapped* (2nd Ed.). by L. J. Mattes & D. R. Omark, 1991. Oceanside, CA: Academic Communication Associates. *Assessing bilingual exceptional children: In-service manual.* by D. R. Omark & D. L. Watson, 1983. San Diego, CA: Los Amigos Research Associates. Adapted with permission.

through translation, adaptation, and/or an interpreter. The following are brief discussions and suggestions for each of these areas.

Translating and Adapting Instruments

Test instruments written in English are frequently translated by SLPs and their agencies. The purpose of this activity is to measure the client's speech and language abilities by using the standardized instrument's theoretical and language framework. Merely translating the test does not equate to an appropriate assessment instrument (Erickson & Iglesias, 1986; Kayser, 1989). A translated test used for describing an impairment does not take into consideration differences in languages in areas such as honorifics, gender markers, semantics, structural rules, registers, dialectal variations, and cultural norms for who speaks what to whom and when. If these language areas are not addressed in the translation, it is possible to have a client respond incorrectly to an inappropriately translated item because of any of the above language differences. Thus the measure becomes an unreliable means of measurement (Kayser, 1995).

A second concern is cultural variation. Translations of instruments neglect complex variables such as cultural norms, beliefs, life expectations and experiences, roles, and acceptable and unacceptable inter- and intragroup relationships. A direct translation of an outcome measure will need to be adapted so that a true measure of a client's performance can be obtained.

Adapting a test instrument requires that the tasks and content of the original instrument are changed to include culturally appropriate items (Gavillan-Torres,1984; Kayser, 1989) and are therefore less biased for the client from a culturally and linguistically different background. The content is reviewed and revised to reflect the needs of the population served. For example, the vocabulary may be altered to reflect dialectal variations. The functional assessment of an adult may require additional roles that may not be included in the original form (e.g., directing the decision making process of family plans). It may mean omitting items that are not considered appropriate by the cultural group (e.g., does he or she make his own breakfast). These changes may be made through group discussions with focus groups from the community, who could act as the informants of acceptable and unacceptable questions concerning the development of the outcome measure.

Discussions surrounding the instrument adaptation among team members may be frustrating because of the overt and covert issues surrounding culture. There are conscious as well as subconscious behaviors and norms related to the culture that team discussion may not immediately recognize. Continued observation, discussion, and verification from cultural informants will produce a cultural and sensitivity awareness to the population on the part of professionals and also produce a measure that is reflective of the group of interest.

Using Interpreters

Frequently, speech-language pathologists use the terms *interpreter* and *translator* interchangeably, but they have different meanings and functions. An interpreter is one who conveys information from one language to the other in the oral modality. A translator is one who conveys information in the written modality (Langdon, 1992). This discussion is limited to the term interpreter because speech-language pathologists are more likely to depend on interpreters in clinical practice.

Interpreters are an important link between the professional and the client. Their skills in interpreting information conveyed by the SLP is crucial for accurate assessment of client outcomes. To maintain high quality of service, there should be educational, clinical, and linguistic competencies for interpreters in all clinical settings. Langdon (1992) suggests that interpreters should have a minimum of a high school diploma with communication skills that are adequate for the tasks assigned by the speech-language pathologist. They should have oral and written abilities in English and the minority language. Langdon (1992) states that the role of the interpreter requires an ability to stay emotionally uninvolved with the discussions and an ability to maintain confidentiality and neutrality. When an untrained individual serves in this role, there may be omitted, misinterpreted, or misunderstood information relayed to the family (Kayser, 1993).

The Special Interest Division 14 (Communication Sciences and Disorders in Culturally and Linguistically Diverse Populations) of the American Speech-Language-Hearing-Association (ASHA) drafted a position statement concerning the competencies of interpreters and SLPs who work with interpreters (ASHA, in progress) (Appendix 11–A). This draft statement, subject to approval by ASHA's Executive Board and Legislative Council, outlines the proposed competencies for interpreters and SLPs who team with an interpreter. According to the statement, the SLP's knowledge base about the clients' backgrounds are important to the interpreting process. Therefore, these professionals should have knowledge of the cultural group, second language acquisition, informal and formal nonbiased assessments, culturally appropriate intervention, and cultural sensitivity that might affect intervention. The team (i.e., SLP and interpreter) is responsible for the well-being of linguistically diverse clients, therefore, the professional must be able to competently direct the activities of the interpreter.

RESEARCH

ASHA Special Interest Division 14 formed a research committee to develop guidelines and a position statement concerning research with diverse populations. The impetus for this committee was concern by ASHA members from culturally and linguistically different groups about the types and results of research that were presented to the membership about diverse populations. The key theme of this draft policy document is that researchers must be culturally sensitive to the group under study. This means that there needs to be culturally sensitive researchers who can develop research questions and designs that are appropriate to groups from diverse backgrounds. Research results cannot be generalized if subject pools are homogeneous and do not present the variety of subgroups within any major group (e.g., Hispanic, African American).

It is important to improve our services to culturally and linguistically diverse groups. We must know what measurement and treatments are effective. Most importantly, we do not want to see these diverse groups subjected to the norms of the current majority mainstream population.

A Research Paradigm Shift

Taylor (1992) and Saville-Troike (1986) have recommended that the study of culturally and linguistically diverse groups include an understanding of culture. The research methodology that encourages the use of the culture's perspective in the research question is called ethnography. *Ethnography,* a branch of anthropology, is the science of describing a group and its culture through observation, interviews, notes in a diary, or a multitude of other data collection techniques (Lutz, 1980). This research methodology is inductive in that few explicit assumptions are made about relationships. Ethnographic research has no set assumptions, and the results and conclusions are interpreted from the perspective of the population under study.

Although this methodology may be viewed as subjective by experimental researchers, the study of culturally and linguistically different populations must include the perspective of the individuals who are studied. An experimental design must take into consideration the culture and its possible influence on the subjects. Adding the culture's perspective provides the framework from which to develop research designs, tasks, and procedures that can measure the target behaviors of interest to the researcher and of importance to the community. Understanding the cultural impact on a variety of variables requires the researcher to become culturally competent. Taylor (cited in Kayser, 1995) (see Appendix 11–B) lists characteristics of the culturally competent researcher.

CONCLUSION

There are numerous factors that will affect outcomes measurement for individuals from culturally and linguistically diverse populations. These include cultural beliefs, culturally and linguistically appropriate measures, translating and adapting instruments, teaming with interpreters, and cultural sensitivity of researchers and research designs. Diverse groups will view impairment, disability, and handicapping conditions differently from mainstream Americans. The use of standardized instruments validated on mainstream populations are inappropriate. Therefore, their adaptation and translation will persist as the usual practice. Interpreters can assist the SLP in the majority of client-clinician interactions, but both the interpreter and the professional must have clinical and educational competencies that will best serve the client. Finally, test development and clinical research practices must include cultural sensitivity, not only of the research questions and designs, but also of the researcher.

REFERENCES

American Speech-Language-Hearing-Association (in progress). Draft position statement on Teaming with Interpreters. Special Interest Division 14, Communication Disorders and Sciences in Culturally and Linguistically Diverse Populations.

Anderson, P.P., & Fenichel, E.S.P. (1989). *Serving culturally diverse families of infants and toddlers with disabilities.* Washington, DC: National Center for Clinical Infant Programs.

Allen, J., McNeill, E., & Schmidt, V. (1992). *Cultural awareness for children.* New York: Addison-Wesley (in progress).

Battle, D. (1993). *Communication disorders in multicultural populations.* Boston, MA: Andover Medical Publishers.

Bebout, L., & Arthur, B. (1992). Cross-cultural attitudes about speech disorders. *Journal of Speech and Hearing Research, 35,* (2) 45-52.

Blaisdell, K. (1989). Historical and cultural aspects of native Hawaiian health. *Social Process in Hawaii, 32,* 1–21.

Boone, D., & Plante, E. (1993). *Human communication and its disorders.* Englewood Cliffs, NJ: Prentice Hall.

Chan, S. (1992). Families with Asian roots. In E.W. Lynch & M.J. Hanson (Eds.), *Developing cross-cultural competence: A guide to working with young children and their families* (pp. 181–257). Baltimore: Paul H. Brookes Publishing Co.

Cheng, L.L. (1987). Cross-cultural and linguistic considerations in working with Asian populations. *Asha (6),* 33–37.

Cheng, L.L. (1993). Asian-American Cultures. In D. Battle (Ed.), *Communication disorders in multicultural populations* (pp. 38–77). Boston, MA: Andover Medical Publications.

Cheng, L.L., & Hammer, C.S. (1992). *Cultural perceptions of disabilities.* San Diego: Los Amigos Research Associates.

Ethridge, J.M. (1990). *China's unfinished revolution.* San Francisco; China Books & Periodicals.

Erickson, J., & Iglesias, A. (1986). Speech and language disorders in Hispanics. In O. Taylor (Ed.), *Nature of communication disorders in culturally and linguistically diverse populations* (pp. 181–218). San Diego, CA: College-Hill Press.

Fiatoa, L., & Palafox, N. (1980). The Samoans. In N. Palafox & A. Warren (Eds.), *Cross-cultural caring* (250–271). Honolulu: The University of Sawaii, School of Medicine.

Fitzgerald, M.H. & Barker, J.C. (1993). Rehabilitation services for the Pacific. *The Western*

Gavillan-Torres, E. (1984). Issues of assessment of limited-English-proficient students and of truly disabled in the United States. In N. Miller (Ed.) *Bilingualism and language disability: Assessment and remediation* (pp. 131–153). San Diego, CA: College-Hill Press.

Giger, J., & Davidhizar, R. (1991). *Transcultural Nursing.* St. Louis: Mosby Year Book.

Hammer, C.S. (1994). Working with families of Chamorro and Carolinian cultures. *American Journal of Speech-Language Pathology, 3* (3), 5–12.

Hanline, M.F., & Dalen, S.E. (1992). Family coping strategies and strengths in Hispanic, African-American, and Caucasian families of young children. *Topics in Early Childhood Special Education, 12* (3), 351–366.

Harris, G. (1986). Barriers to the delivery of speech, language, and hearing services to Native Americans. In O. Taylor (Ed.), *Nature of communication disorders in culturally and linguistically diverse children.* San Diego: College-Hill Press.

Harris, G. (1993). American Indian cultures: A lesson in diversity. In D. Battle (Ed.), *Communication disorders in multicultural populations* (pp. 78–113). Boston, MA: Andover Medical Publishers.

Harrison, I. (1975). Healing status and healing practices: continuations from an African past. *Journal of African Studies, 2* (4) 547–560.

Harrison, I., & Harrison, D.S. (1971). The Black family experience and health behavior. In C.O. Crawford (Ed.), *Health and the family: a Medical-Sociological analysis* (pp. 175–199). New York: Macmillan.

Harry, B. (1992). *Cultural diversity, families, and the special education system: Communication and empowerment.* New York: Teachers College Press.

Hines-Martin, V. (1992). A research review: family caregivers of chronically ill African-American elderly. *Journal Of Gerontological Nursing, 18,* (2), 25–29.

Joe, J.R., & Malach, R.S. (1992). Families with Native American roots. In W.E. Lynch & M.J. Hanson (Eds.), *Developing cross-cultural competence: A guide to working with young children and their families* (pp. 89–119). Baltimore: Paul H. Brookes Publishing Co.

Kayser, H. (1989). Speech and language assessment of Spanish-English speaking children. *Language, Speech, and Hearing Services in Schools, 20,* 226–244.

Kayser, H. (1993). Hispanic cultures. In D. Battle (Ed.), *Communication disorders in multicultural populations* (pp. 114–157). Boston, MA: Andover Medical Publishers.

Kayser, H. (1995). *Bilingual speech language pathology: An Hispanic focus.* San Diego, CA: Singular Publishing Group.

Kraut, A. (1990). Healers and strangers: Immigrant attitudes toward the physician in American. *Journal of the American Medical Association, 263* (13), 1807–1811.

Langdon, H.W. (1992). *Hispanic children and adults with communication disorders: Assessment and intervention.* Gaithersburg, MD: Aspen.

Lewis, J., & Vang, L. (1987). *The Hmong language: Sounds and alphabets.* Indochinese Refugee Education Guide. Arlington, VA: Center for Applied Linguistics.

Long, S. O. (1992). *Japan: A country study.* Washington, DC: Department of Army.

Lutz, F. (1980). Ethnography—The holistic approach to understanding schooling. In J. Green & C. Wallet (Eds.), *Ethnography and language in educational settings* (pp. 5–63). Norwood, NJ: Ablex.

Maestas, A.G., & Erickson, J.G. (1992). Mexican Immigrant mothers' beliefs about disabilities. *American Journal of Speech-Language Pathology, 1* (4), 5–10.

Marin, B.V., Marin, G., Padilla, A.M., & de la Rocha, C. (1983). Utilization of traditional and nontraditional sources of health care among Hispanics. *Hispanic Journal of Behavioral Sciences, 5* (1), 65–80.

Matsuda, M. (1989). Working with Asian parents; Some communication strategies. *Topics in Language Disorders, 9,* 45–53.

Meyerson, M.D. (1983). Genetic counseling for families of Chicano children with birth defects. In D.R. Omark & J.G. Erickson (Eds.), *The bilingual exceptional child.* San Diego, CA: Los Amigos Research Associates.

Mokuau, N. & Tauili'ili, P. (1992). Families with Native Hawaiian and Pacific Island roots. In W.E. Lynch & M.J. Hanson (Eds.), *Developing cross-cultural competence: A guide for working with young children and their families* (pp. 301–318). Baltimore, MD: Paul H. Brookes Publishing Co.

Munoz, E., Tortella, B.J., Sakmyster, M.A., Liversonese, D.S., Mccormac, M., Odom, J.W., & Torres, R. (1992). Traumatic injury in Hispanic Americans: A distinct entity. In A. Furino (Ed.), *Health Policy and the Hispanic* (pp. 126–131). Boulder, Colorado: Westview Press.

Payer, L. (1988). *Medicine and culture: varieties of treatment in the United States, England, West Germany, and France.* New York: Penguin.

Payne-Johnson, J. (1992). An ethnocentric perspective on African American elderly persons and functional communication assessment. *The Howard Journal of Communications, 3,* 3 and 4 (Winter-spring), 194–203.

Perrone, B., Stockel, H.H., & Krueger, V. (1989). *Medicine Women, Curanderas, and Women Doctors.* Norman, OK: University of Oklahoma press.

Reyes, B. (1995). Considerations in the assessment and treatment of neurogenic communication disorders in bilingual adults. In H. Kayser (Ed.) *Bilingual speech language pathology: An Hispanic focus* (pp. 153–182). San Diego, CA: Singular Publishing Group.

Roseberry-McKibbin, C.A. (1994). Assessment and intervention for Limited English Proficient children with language disorders. *American Journal of Speech-Language Pathology, 3 (3),* 77–88.

Roseberry-McKibbin, C.A. (1995). *Multicultural students with special language needs:Practical strategies for assessment and intervention.* Oceanside, CA: Academic Communication Associates.

Saville-Troike, M. (1986). Anthropological considerations in the study of communication. In O. Taylor (Ed.), *Nature of communication disorders in culturally and linguistically diverse populations* (pp. 47–72). San Diego, CA: College-Hill Press.

Smart, J. & Smart, D. (1992). Cultural issues in the rehabilitation of Hispanics. *Journal of Rehabilitation, 58,* 29–37.

Solis, J., Marks, G., and Garcia, M. (1990). Acculturation, access to care and use of preventative services by Hispanics. *American Journal of Public Health, 80,* 11–19, suppl.

Stewart, J. L. (1986). Hearing disorders among the indigenous peoples of North America and the Pacific Basin. In O. Taylor (Ed.), *Nature of communication disorders in culturally and linguistically diverse populations* (pp. 237–276). San Diego, CA: College-Hill Press.

Steward, J.L. (1992). Native American populations. *Asha, 34* (5), 40–42.

Taylor, O. (1987). Clinical practice as a social occasion. In Cole, L. & Deal, V. (Eds.), *Communication Disorders in multicultural populations.* Rockville, MD: ASHA.

Taylor, O. (1992, April). *Research designs and methodologies that NIDCD should encourage and support for intramural and extramural research on people of color.* Article presented to the

Working Group: Research and Research Training Needs of Minority Persons and Minority Health Issues, National Institute on Deafness and other Communication Disorders, National Institutes of Health. Bethesda, MD.

Teller, C.A. (1988). Physical health status and health care utilization in the Texas borderlands. In S.R. Ross (Ed.), *Views Across the Border.* Albuquerque, NM: University of New Mexico Press.

Wallace, G. (1993). Adult neurogenic disorders. In D. Battle (Ed.), *Communication disorders in multicultural populations* (pp. 239–255). Boston, MA: Andover Medical Publishers.

Wallace, G. (1995). *Adult aphasia: Clinical management for the practicing clinician.* Reading, MA: Andover Medical Publishers.

Willis, W. (1992). Families with African American roots. In E.W. Lynch and M.J. Hanson (Eds.), *Developing cross-cultural competence: A guide for working with young children and their families* (pp. 121–150). Baltimore: Paul H. Brookes Publishing Co.

Zuniga, M.E. (1992). Families with Latino roots. In E.W. Lynch & M.J. Hanson (Eds.), *Developing cross-cultural competence: A guide to working with young children and their families* (pp. 151–179). Baltimore: Paul H. Brookes Publishing Co.

Draft: *ASHA Position Statement on Interpreters*
(Subject to Approval by the ASHA Executive Board
and Legislative Council)

POSITION STATEMENT

ASHA recognizes that there is a dramatic increase of persons in our nation who speak a language other than English. There is also a paucity of bilingual speech-language pathologists to serve these individuals appropriately. In an attempt to meet the assessment and intervention needs of these persons with communicative impairments, speech, language, and hearing services are provided with the assistance of an interpreter/translator. ASHA recognizes that an interpreter/translator is an individual who must receive training in interpretation (oral modality) and translation (written modality) in order to provide the highest quality of service to linguistically and culturally diverse populations. Therefore, ASHA supports the following statements:

a. Schools, clinics, and hospitals should exhaust all means of obtaining a speech-language pathologist or audiologist who is bilingual before seeking the assistance of an interpreter/translator.

b. When teaming with an interpreter appears to be the only alternative after all other measures have been sought, training should be provided concerning the purpose of the meeting, assessment measures, or intervention program. Training should include the institution's procedures and guidelines. It is also recommended that the professional and the interpreter have briefing and debriefing meetings to discuss the client, interpreter, and professional interactions.

c. Competencies of interpreters must be determined before using their services. Competencies should include, but are not limited to, high proficiency levels in English and the target language; knowledge of cultural and linguistic nuances; and knowledge of cross-cultural and generational differences and expectations.

d. Upon mastery of the competencies, certification or recognition of competencies would assist in ensuring that interpreters possess the skills necessary for providing effective services.

e. It is also the position of the Association that any speech-language pathologist or audiologist who supervises and teams with an interpreter/translator for serving culturally and linguistically diverse populations have knowledge of competencies as stated in the Position Statement on Clinical Management of Minority Language Handicapped Individuals (ASHA, 1985). These include knowledge of :(1) the process of normal speech and language acquisition for both bilingual and monolingual individuals and how those processes are manifested in oral (or manually coded) and written language; (2) formal and informal assessment procedures to distinguish between communication differences and communication disorders in oral (or manually coded) and written language; (3) intervention strategies for treatment of communicative disorders in the client's language; and (4) cultural factors that affect the delivery of speech-language pathology and audiology services to the client's language community.

REFERENCES

American Speech-Language-Hearing Association, Committee on the Status of Racial Minorities (1985). Clinical management of communicatively handicapped minority language populations. *ASHA, 27*(6), 29–32.

American Speech-Language-Hearing Association. (1995, March). Task Force on support personnel. Position statement for training, credentialing, use and supervision of support personnel in speech-language pathology. *ASHA, 37,* (Suppl. 14, pp. 21).

American Speech-Language-Hearing Association. (1996, April). Guidelines for the training, credentialing, use, and supervision of speech language pathology assistants. *ASHA, 38,* (Suppl. 15).

Kayser, H. (1995). Interpreters. In H. Kayser (Ed.), *Bilingual speech language pathology: An Hispanic focus* (pp. 207–221). San Diego: Singular Publishing Group.

Langdon, H. W. (1992). *Interpreter/translator process in the educational setting: A resource manual.* Sacramento, CA: Resources in Special Education.

Matsuda, M., & O'Connor, L. C. (1993). *Creating an effective partnership: Training bilingual communication aides.* Presentation at the annual convention of the California Speech, Language and Hearing Association. Palm Springs.

Attributes of the Culturally Sensitive Researcher

1. Truth is determined by the preceptor's culture. That is, each culture views what is true from its own experiences and beliefs.

2. Culture and cultural diversity should be part of every segment of research in communication sciences and disorders. This should include developmental, cognitive, epidemiological, normative, assessment procedures, and treatment efficacy research.

3. Research topics and what is researchable are culturally determined. What has been researched and may seem appropriate for English-speaking subjects may be inappropriate and offensive for the minority population of interest.

4. Research results are never generalized from one subgroup of minority subjects to a larger group of minorities or to the majority culture. These overgeneralizations are ethnocentric and do not consider variation within a culture.

5. The interpretation of the results by the researcher is culture-bound. Therefore, errors are inevitable without sensitivity and knowledge of differences within and between culturally and linguistically diverse populations.

6. Issues, research designs, and instruments to measure independent variables are culturally driven. A task and its measurement may be appropriate for one group but insignificant for another group.

7. The culture must be taken into consideration when framing research questions, methodologies, and analyses.

8. Cross-cultural comparisons that examine cultural differences should be completed without contamination from variables such as socioeconomic status, gender, education, and geography.

SOURCE: Taylor, O. (1992, April). *Research designs and methodologies that NIDCD should encourage and support for intramural and extramural research on people of color.* Article presented to the Working Group: Research and Research Training Needs of minority persons and Minority Health Issues, National Institute on Deafness and Other Communication Disorders, National Institutes of Health. Bethesda, MD. From H. Kayser (1995). Research and Conclusions. In H. Kayser (Ed.), Bilingual speech language pathology: An Hispanic focus (pp. 291–306). San Diego, CA: Singular Publishing Co. Reprinted with permission.

CHAPTER 12

Outcomes Measurement in Aphasia

AUDREY L. HOLLAND AND CYNTHIA K. THOMPSON

INTRODUCTION

The value of treatment for aphasia has received considerable attention in the past several years. As noted by Holland, Fromm, DeRuyter, and Stein (1996), in the English language alone there are at least 20 studies of aphasia treatment efficacy/effectiveness which report data on 60 or more aphasic individuals, an additional 40 studies conducted with groups of from 10 to 60 individuals, and well over 100 studies that have examined the effects of specific treatments in fewer than 10 aphasic persons. The studies in this latter category include well-controlled single-subject experimental designs and single case studies. Holland et al. (1996) conclude that "findings from these studies indicate that individuals with aphasia meeting specific selection criteria who are treated improve more than those who do not receive treatment. Both the quality and the quantity of their language are better than if they were not treated" (p. S28). This is, no doubt, good news. Speech-language pathologists (SLPs) can go to sleep at night reasonably certain that they are doing something useful for society.

Much of the aforementioned research has been spawned by aphasia researchers who desire to know the answers to questions such as: What are the general outcomes of aphasia treatment? What are the effects of certain variables like severity and age on the outcome of treatment? When, relative to the onset of aphasia, is it most beneficial to begin treatment? What types of treatment are the most effective? What types of treatments are effective for certain aspects of aphasia, such as naming deficits or sentence production deficits? Are some treatments better than others for certain types of aphasic impairments? What aspects or components of treatment are the most effective?

Recently, however, treatment research in aphasia also has been driven by pressure from key players in the health care community, including regulators, payers, and others who are demanding that SLPs (as well as other professionals) document the value of their interventions with aphasic patients. This pressure has stepped up treatment research efforts and has resulted in some refocusing of research goals. Crucial to third party payers, for example, are answers to questions such as: What is the average length of treatment for persons with aphasia? What does it cost to rehabilitate persons with aphasia? Are the services provided by Clinic A more cost effective than those provided by Clinic B? Is Treatment A better than Treatment B, with the "better" treatment defined as the one that results in better clinical outcome, greater patient satisfaction, and is more cost effective (Frattali, personal communication, 1995)?

SOME UNANSWERED QUESTIONS IN THE APHASIA TREATMENT LITERATURE

Given the nature of the times—the changes in reimbursement patterns, the growing necessity of cost containment in the medical arena, and the dictate to measure concrete functional changes—the issue of outcome from aphasia treatment remains before us. The great majority of the 200 or more studies noted above have reported positive changes in performance as a result of treatment. Nevertheless, many questions concerning outcomes in aphasia treatment have not been fully addressed. For example, most treatment studies have strict inclusionary and exclusionary criteria, such as a single-episode left-hemispheric stroke, which leave SLPs ill prepared to talk about clinical efficacy with individuals who have had more than one stroke. In addition, we have not completely answered questions concerning the effects of various patient variables such as overall cognitive status, patient motivation, and psychosocial support on treatment outcome; and we have not completely answered questions pertaining to when is the best time to provide treatment. Indeed, the belief held by many clinical aphasiologists that early treatment is more effective than that which is delayed until spontaneous recovery is complete has recently been challenged. That is, well-controlled studies investigating the effects of specific treatments for aphasia—which are largely conducted on chronically aphasic individuals who are sometimes several years post stroke—have resulted in positive changes in language. In addition, Wertz et al. (1986) showed in a large group treatment study that individuals whose treatment was deferred for 3 months showed gains similar to their earlier-treated cohorts. Thus, the question as to when treatment should be provided in order to achieve the most desirous outcome remains unclear.

We also have not completely answered questions concerning the most effective types of treatment. For example, we do not know if the best approach is one of remediation or compensation (Weniger & Bertoni, 1993) or if one approach or the other is superior for certain patient deficits. Indeed, we will be better able to answer these questions once we learn more about how the brain recovers and what effect(s) treatment might have on that recovery. There is evidence, for example, that reorganizational processes are at work in the damaged human brain (see, for example, Weiller, Isensee, Rijntjes, Huber, Muller, Bier, Durschka, Woods, Noth, & Diener, 1995). This reorganization may reflect modified connectivity, whereby (1) the function of damaged mechanisms is regained; (2) the function of damaged mechanisms is taken over by undamaged cortical areas in the left hemisphere, as suggested by the findings of Heiss and colleagues (1993), or perhaps by remotely located cortical areas such as the nonlanguage-dominate, right hemisphere as suggested by Beeson and colleagues (1993, 1994) and Price and coworkers (1993); or (3) the "function" of damaged mechanisms or compensation for their functions is regained with new connections that bypass the affected mechanism. In any case, the extent to which treatment influences these processes is unknown (Thompson, 1995). For example, remediational procedures that stimulate the language network (or parts of it) may result in better improvement for some patients than compensatory treatments that may bypass networks for language.

What treatments are the most effective for what patients? How do we match appropriate treatments to particular aphasic individuals? What components of treatment are the most essential for optimal outcome? These questions too remain largely unanswered. Indeed, many approaches to treatment for aphasia have been examined in the literature, but researchers have only just begun to examine which ones are better than others or which variables within a treatment package are the most powerful.

Finally, we have yet to critically examine aspects of service delivery. How often should treatment be applied? For how long? The answers to these questions as well as those posed above are important in our current health care climate, and while we continue to gather more and more data about aphasia treatment efficacy/effectiveness, we have much work to do.

Indeed, there are a number of unanswered questions in the aphasia treatment literature. As well, it is important to point out that there are limitations in the existing aphasia treatment research. For example, experimental control has not been demonstrated in all of the studies. That is, either control groups or control phases, required when using single-subject experimental designs, have not always been included. For example, case studies that often describe in detail the intervention provided for a particular patient are not experimentally controlled. Because of this lack of experimental control, one cannot be certain that the improvements documented were a direct result of the treatment provided. Indeed, the effects of other variables—such as family interventions or even spontaneous recovery—cannot be ruled out as possible contributors to the documented treatment effects. Only when the proper controls are included in a study can we confidently conclude that the treatment was effective.

Other limitations in the aphasia treatment data base concern the treatment itself. Some treatment studies in the aphasia literature have not detailed the treatment applied well enough to allow clinicians to replicate it. That is, in well-known group studies examining the effects of treatment (e.g., those by Wertz & colleagues [1981, 1986], Hartman & Landau [1987], Basso, Capitani, & Vignolo [1979], Shewan & Kertesz [1984], and Poeck, Huber, & Willmes [1989]) the treatment(s) provided were not described in detail. For example, in the Wertz et al., (1981) study, two types of treatment were provided for two groups of subjects: "Group A received traditional, individual treatment . . . [and] Group B received group treatment by a speech-language pathologist who stimulated language through social interaction with no direct manipulation of speech and language deficits" (p. 581). Taking another example, consider the treatment applied in the Shewan and Kertesz (1984) study. In this study, general "stimulation" treatment was compared with Language Oriented Therapy (LOT). Neither treatment was described in detail; indeed, even LOT—which provides a wide array of language tasks focused on virtually every language problem that an aphasic individual might present—is only described in general by the authors. While the purpose of these studies was to document the effects of treatment in general, and not to detail the outcome of a particular treatment approach, the lack of detail regarding the treatments that were applied leaves much to the imagination. It is possible (and likely), for example, that the language problems treated and the treatment applied varied across subjects in these studies. The point here is that given the descriptions of treatment provided, clinicians simply could not replicate them in their clinical practice.

Other studies that have focused on the effects of a specific treatment—and are not so concerned with the outcome of treatment in *general*—also sometimes do not adequately describe the treatment applied (see Thompson, 1989, for a review). However, because of the nature of these studies, they are more likely to provide descriptions is of treatment that are useful for clinicians. For example, Simmons, Kearns, and Potechin (1987) examined the effects of training a subject's wife to decrease interruptions and use convergent questions in communicating with her aphasic spouse. The treatment provided was well described and involved recognition training using videotaped conversations between the aphasic patient and his spouse. Results of the study showed that the treatment resulted in changes in the spouse's communication behavior in three untrained conversational conditions. In another series of studies, Thompson and colleagues (Thompson, Shapiro, & Roberts, 1993; Thompson, Shapiro, Tait, Jacobs, & Schneider, 1996; Thompson, Shapiro, Ballard, Jacobs, Schneider, & Tait, in press) investigated the effects of Linguistic-Specific Treatment for sentence production deficits in aphasic patients with agrammatism. This treatment, which is based on aspects of linguistic theory, is highly specified and provides methods for training complex sentences such as *wh*-questions, object relatives, and passives. Thompson and colleagues have shown that this treatment results in improved sentence production in aphasic patients.

OUTCOMES MEASUREMENT IN APHASIA TREATMENT RESEARCH

One of the key aspects of determining the efficacy/effectiveness of treatment concerns outcomes measurement. Indeed, research that attempts to answer the questions posed above will not only need to utilize proper experimental designs, provide clear and replicable descriptions of treatment, and attend to other important aspects of treatment research, but also will need to broaden its dependent measures. That is, the types of measures that are used to document treatment efficacy/effectiveness will need to include measures that directly evaluate how treatment has affected the language deficit that the aphasic patient presents. In addition, measures that evaluate how changes in the language deficit affect the abilities of the aphasic individual to communicate functionally and to reenter social, occupational, and other environments will need to be considered. In the remainder of this chapter we summarize the types of outcome measures that have traditionally been used to document aphasia treatment efficacy/effectiveness, and we discuss how outcome measurement needs to be expanded both in aphasia treatment research and in our clinical practice.

LEVEL OF OUTCOMES MEASUREMENT

Virtually all aphasia treatment studies in the literature—either those examining the effects of treatment in general such as the Wertz et al. (1981, 1986) studies, or those examining the effects of specific treatments such as the Simmons et al. (1987) and the Thompson et al. (1993, 1996, in press) studies discussed above—are limited in terms of the outcome measures used to document the effects of treatment. Wertz and colleagues used standardized tests, such as the PICA (Porch, 1967) to examine the effects of treatment. Similarly, Simmons, Thompson, and their colleagues used standardized aphasia test batteries (i.e., the *Western Aphasia Battery,* Kertesz, 1982), as well as additional probe measures. For example, Simmons tested the spouse's use of specific behaviors in videotaped conversational conditions in which the aphasic subject and spouse were instructed to discuss recently viewed TV sports broadcasts or TV talk shows. Thompson and colleagues too used controlled discourse conditions to examine treatment efficacy. Their subjects were asked to tell the story of Cinderella and Little Red Riding Hood; responses were tape recorded and analyzed linguistically. In addition, production of the specific sentence types of interest in the study were tested prior to treatment and daily throughout the treatment period using a sentence production priming procedure in order to examine patterns of acquisition and generalization of sentence production.

What aspects of outcomes measurement are missing from these studies? In order to answer this question, consider the World Health Organization (WHO) framework for classifying illnesses. As pointed out by Frattali in Chapter 1, ICIDH—the most widely recognized conceptual framework for describing consequential aspects of illness—comes from the WHO (1980). *Impairments* include any loss or abnormality of psychological, physiological, or anatomical structure or function representing deviation from a norm. *Disabilities* are concerned with the functional consequences of an impairment and include any restriction or lack of ability to perform an activity in a manner or within a range considered normal for a human being. Finally, *handicaps* include disadvantages resulting from an impairment or disability that limit or prevent the fulfillment of a role that is normal (depending on age, sex, and social and cultural factors) for that individual. A handicap, then, is the social consequence of an impairment or disability. Table 12–1 presents the WHO framework as it applies to an individual with aphasia. Aphasia is the impairment. The aphasic individual's difficulties in performing daily life communication activities are the resulting disabilities, which include difficulty talking

Table 12–1. The World Health Organization (WHO) Classification Framework (1980).

	IMPAIRMENT	DISABILITY	HANDICAP
DEFINITIONS	Abnormality of structure or function at the organ level	Functional consequence of impairment	Social consequences of an impairment or disability
EXAMPLES	Aphasia	Communication problems in the context of daily life activities	Isolation, joblessness, dependency, role changes
OUTCOME MEASURES	Traditional instrumental and behavioral measures	Functional status measures	Quality of life scales, handicap inventories, wellness measures

SOURCE: World Health Organization (1980). Reprinted with perission.

with friends, understanding news reports, using the telephone, writing letters and notes, understanding written instructions, and so on. The aphasic individual's disabilities then lead to social isolation, loss of job, dependence on others, and other handicapping conditions.

A sample of outcome measures used to evaluate each level of the deficit is listed in Table 12–2. Measures of impairment include traditional instrumental and behavioral measures such as standardized aphasia test batteries and supplementary tests for specific areas of deficit. As well, special probe measures that are used by both clinicians and researchers to test learning and generalization of certain aspects of language also are tests of impairment-level phenomena. For example, in studies in which aphasic subjects have been trained to use gestures as either an alternative or augmentative communication system, regular and systematic testing of gestural use is undertaken (see, for example, Alexander & Loverso, 1993). Similarly, studies concerned with treatment for naming deficits in aphasia have incorporated naming probe tasks (see, for example, Raymer, Thompson, Jacobs, & le Grand, 1993). Another example of specialized probing of impairment-level phenomena is discourse sampling. Using tasks such as picture description or story telling, narrative discourse samples are collected and analyzed for pragmatic, linguistic, or other parameters in order to determine how treatment has affected spontaneous language use (see, for example, Fink, Schwartz, Rochon, Myers, Socolof, & Bluestone, 1995; Schwartz, Saffran, Fink, Myers, & Martin, 1994; Thompson et al., 1993, 1996; in press).

In contrast to tests of impairment are measures of disability which include general rehabilitation measures such as the PECS (Harvey & Jellinek, 1981), the RIC-FAS (Cichowski, 1995), and FIM (State University of New York at Buffalo, 1993). These measures examine functional ability across a number of domains—one of which is communication. Measures that address only communication also are available. These include measures that (1) use rating scales to rate a patient's observed abilities to perform certain functions, and (2) those that directly test functional communication abilities. Those that utilize an observational and rating scale format include the *Communicative Effectiveness Index* (CETI; Lomas, Pickard, Bester, Elbard, Finlayson, & Zoghabib, 1989) and the newly developed ASHA FACS (Frattali, Thompson, Holland, Wohl, & Ferketic, 1995). Tests of functional communication that employ a direct assessment strategy include the CADL (Holland, 1980) and the *Amsterdam-Nijmegan Everyday Language Test* (ANELT; Blomert, Kean, Koster, & Schokker, 1994).

Finally, measures of handicap that include quality of life scales, handicap inventories, and wellness measures are included on Table 12–2. These include psychosocial measures, quality of life measures, and measures of well-being.

The great majority of the 200 or more studies noted above have reported positive change in performance as a result of treatment. Notably, however, these changes were measured primarily by scores derived from measures of impairment. Indeed, as can be seen in Table 12–2, there are many more measures available for examining impairment-level phenomena as compared to disabilities and handicaps. Measures of impairment have as their very legitimate goal describing the extent and severity of the aphasia itself, that is, the impairment. Therefore, they are very appropriate to use as outcome measures in treatment studies for aphasia. Supplementary tests and other probe measures that are concerned more with examining specific aspects of language also are appropriate. These tests, however, were not designed for measuring the func-

Table 12–2. Outcome Measures for Examining the Effects of Aphasia Treatment Using the World Health Organization (WHO) Classification Framework (1980).*

IMPAIRMENT: TRADITIONAL INSTRUMENTAL AND BEHAVIORAL MEASURES	DISABILITY: FUNCTIONAL STATUS MEASURES	HANDICAP: QUALITY OF LIFE SCALES, HANDICAP INVENTORIES, WELLNESS MEASURES
Standardized Aphasia Test Batteries Aphasia Diagnostic Profiles (Helm-Estabrooks, 1993) Boston Diagnostic Aphasia Examination (Goodglass & Kaplan, 1983) Porch Index of Communicative Ability (1967, 1971) Western Aphasia Battery (Kertesz, 1982) *Supplementary Tests for Aphasic Impairments* Auditory Comprehension Test for Sentences (ACTS; Shewan, 1979) Token Test (TT; DeRenzi & Vignolo, 1962) The Boston Naming Test (BNT; Kaplan, Goodglass, & Weintraub, 1983) The Psycholinguistic Assessment of Language Production in Aphasia (PALPA; Kay et al., 1992) New England Pantomime Test (Duffy & Duffy, 1984) *Controlled Probe Tasks* Sentence Production Priming Task (Thompson et al., in press) Naming Probe Tasks (Hillis, 1989; Raymer, Thompson, Jacobs, & leGrand, 1993) Gestural Production Probe Tasks (Alexander & Loverso, 1993; Conlon & McNeil, 1989) *Discourse Sampling* Picture Description (Helm-Estabrooks et al., 1981) Story Telling (Schwartz et al., Thompson et al.) Mealtime conversation (Wambaugh & Thompson, 1989) Conversational Dyads (Simmons et al., 1979; Thompson & Byrne, 1984)	*General Rehabilitation Measures* Patient Evaluation and Conference System (PECS; Harvey & Jellinek, 1981) Rehabilitation Institute of Chicago Functional Assessment Scale (RIC-FAS, Cichowski, 1995) Level of Rehabilitation Scale III (LORS III; Parkside Associates, 1986) Functional Independence Measure Version 4.0 (FIM; State University of New York at Buffalo, 1993) *Measures of Functional Communication—Rating Scales* The Functional Communication Profile (FCP; Sarno, 1969) The Communicative Effectiveness Index (CETI; Lomas et al., 1989) Revised Edinburgh Functional Communication Profile (EFCP; Wirz, 1990) The Communication Profile: A Functional Skills Survey (Payne, 1994) ASHA Functional Assessment of Communication Skills for Adults (ASHA FACS; Frattali et al., 1995) *Direct Assessment of Functional Communication* Communicative Abilities in Daily Living (CADL; Holland, 1980) The Amsterdam-Nijmegen Everyday Language Test (ANELT; Blomert et al., 1994)	*Psychosocial Measures: Depression Scales* Beck Depression Scale (Beck et al., 1961) Center for Epidemiologic Studies-Depression Scale (EDS-D; Radloff, 1977) Structured Assessment of Depression in Brain Damaged Individuals (SADBDI; Hibbard et al., 1993) *Health-Related Quality of Life Measures* Sickness Impact Profile (SIP; Bergner et al., 1981) SF-36 (Ware & Sherbourne, 1992) *Measures of Well-Being* The Ryff Scales (Ryff, 1989) Life History Survey (Records et al., 1992) Affect Balance Scale (ABS; Bradburn, 1969)

*The measures included in this table represent only selected measures of each type that are available.

tional consequences of the aphasic impairment or for assessing the social handicap imposed by aphasia.

In order to fully assess the outcome of our treatment efforts, measures of disability and handicap must be considered. We describe some of these below, beginning with an overview of general rehabilitation measures that are used in settings in which aphasic patients are treated. We then discuss measures of functional communication that have been specially designed for assessing outcome(s) of aphasia treatment. Finally, we discuss some outcome measures that are infrequently used with aphasic patients, but have potentially interesting roles for evaluating chronic aphasia in relation to the social handicaps that may result from the aphasia. We have not attempted to be comprehensive in what follows. Rather, we have chosen to concentrate on those measures that appear to us to be in the widest circulation, or seem to us to have the greatest promise for use both clinically and in our treatment research efforts.

GENERAL REHABILITATION MEASURES

Management of aphasia is squarely situated in the field of stroke rehabilitation, historically the domain of physical medicine and rehabilitation. This domain has long been cognizant of the importance of functional restoration, and has provided leadership in the measurement of functional status. A number of measures designed with the common goal of measuring functional restoration have been developed in the past 15 years. As noted in Table 12–2, among them are the PECS (Harvey & Jellinek, 1981), the RIC-FAS, Chichowski, 1995), the LORS III (Parkside Associates, 1986), and the FIM (State University of New York at Buffalo, 1993). Although all of these measures represent improvements over previous attempts, it is clear that the FIM has become the most widely used. FIM data, along with pertinent demographic and discharge information, are part of the UDS, estimated by Werner (1994) to be used by over 500 rehabilitation sites nationally. Because of its dominance in general rehabilitation, it will be the only measure described here.

The FIM utilizes a 7-point rating scale to rate self-care, sphincter control, mobility, locomotion, communication ("expression-vocal/nonvocal" and "comprehension-auditory/visual"), and social cognition. The scale sets out to measure relative independence, and is anchored at complete dependence (1) and complete independence (7). The general consensus among SLPs seems to be that the process of rating communication in this global way renders the FIM insensitive to meaningful change. Another negative evaluation by SLPs is that it is difficult to anchor "expression" and "comprehension" with the concept of relative dependence/independence. Aware of these concerns, Warren (1995) suggested that it is prudent for SLPs also to rate patients on the three social cognition scales (social interaction, problem solving, memory) using the combined score to characterize pre- and posttreatment change.

Even though the FIM lacks sensitivity to important issues relevant to outcome of speech and language services for aphasic adults, it should be noted that the size of the available (and growing) data base provides some compensation for its lack of sensitivity to many aspects of the impairments and handicaps that result from aphasia. That is to say, small but highly consistent changes from a very large data base may well reflect clinically significant changes.

Before leaving the FIM, it should be noted that "expression" and "comprehension" per se cannot comfortably be accepted as "functional outcomes." These terms are intrinsically intrapersonal; that is, they describe single individuals, alternating these roles as they send and receive information. The functional outcomes of communication deficits generally involve more than one sender and receiver, and are thus interpersonal.

MEASURES OF FUNCTIONAL COMMUNICATION

Speech-language pathologists have long recognized that the results of the formal measurement of an individual's language strengths and weaknesses (i.e., measures of impairment) sometimes do not directly reflect the extent and manner in which that individual uses language in interpersonal contexts. For example, aphasic speakers and their conversational partners often act effectively together to create meaning in a way that is impossible for the aphasic speaker to achieve alone, a process Goodwin (1995) describes as "the co-construction of meaning." Additionally, aphasic speakers can frequently capitalize on the context of their communicative attempts, and through inventive use of nonverbal cues and verbal fragments, are often able to get complex messages across despite their language deficits. This is the crux of the difference between the formal properties of language and language as part of the process of social communication. This distinction is also the crux of the difference between formal language assessment and assessment of what happens to language and its nonverbal supplements or substitutes when in use as communication. For example, auditory comprehension as measured on a formal language test clearly has some relationship to, but is not isomorphic with, the ability to follow a conversation about an exciting topic with a familiar partner in an appropriate context. Similarly, performance on a confrontation naming test is only a kissing cousin of generating self-selected words in the conversational context described above. In both cases, the latter examples are the functional outcomes of language impairments, relating to the disabilities and the social handicaps imposed by the condition.

Despite the richness implicit in defining and measuring language as part of social communication, Elman and Bernstein-Ellis (1995) noted that the term "functional communication" has evolved with two different meanings over the past two decades. On the one hand, "functional communication" is often taken to mean the complex behaviors of using language to communicate, that is, of functioning as a language user. On the other, the word "functional" is used synonymously with "utilitarian", that is, comprising the limited skills needed to communicate basic needs and emotions. Unfortunately, it is this latter sense of "functional" that dominates managed care. Nonetheless, as we describe functional communication measures, it is imperative to remember that the limited definition fails to satisfy the communication needs of most individuals. Further, quality of life issues are far from satisfied by it. The astute clinician must never confuse the "functional" of being able to communicate basic needs with the"functional" of being able to participate freely and fully in the communicating world.

Measures of functional communication have arisen largely from the profession's perception of the need to bridge the chasm between describing the linguistic phenomena of aphasia (measuring the impairment) and its consequences for everyday living (measuring the resulting disability and handicap). Rather than attempting to be comprehensive, we have chosen to discuss those measures that have historical importance or that have relatively strong psychometric properties, or both. Two broad forms of measurement have emerged: (1) the use of rating scales which assess functional communication by having others rate aspects of communicative behavior based on their observations of the aphasic individual's ability to communicate, and (2) techniques of direct observation and assessment, which involve sets of test items that are presented by the examiner to elicit a particular response. The two forms of measurement each have strengths and weaknesses. For example, some authorities in the area of functional assessment assert that performance of communication can only be validly measured if one directly observes the individual in actual communication situations, or gets reports of direct observations made from others (Lomas et al., 1989). On the other side of the coin is the issue of reliability; rating scales based on observations of others sometimes have been criticized because reliability of rating may be low when two raters, for example, estimate an individual's ability to do something based on their subjective impression. Of course the issue of reliability can—and should—be examined during test development; however, some measures fall short on this. The validity of direct testing methods also can—and should—be examined when developing direct tests of functional communication by comparing real world performance with test performance.

One other important difference between the two forms of testing concerns the time required to administer the measures. Rating scale formats tend to be shorter; direct testing tends to take a longer time. Therefore, rating scales—or shortened versions of direct tests—are preferred in the clinical arena where we often cannot completely assess—or treat—our patients because of time constraints imposed by health care policies. In the research arena, however, time constraints usually do not drive our research protocols. Therefore, researchers will need to examine the psychometric properties of the measures available for examining functional communication prior to selecting them for use in their treatment research.

MEASURES OF FUNCTIONAL COMMUNICATION USING RATING SCALES

The Functional Communication Profile (FCP)

Since 1965, when Sarno first extended physical medicine's notions of functional restoration to include recovery from aphasia, there has been consistent interest in rating functional communication. Sarno's contributions to understanding functional communication are many, including the development of *the Functional Communication Profile* (FCP; Sarno, 1969), a 45-item, 9-point rating scale (poor to normal). The FCP is designed to be used by clinicians who have observed communicative behaviors including gesturing, understanding, reading, writing, and calculating (these latter two are grouped as "miscellaneous" on the FCP). The setting in which the FCP was originally used was a rehabilitation unit; behaviors relevant to that setting are, therefore, featured. However, the FCP can certainly be used in other settings as well. Although the FCP's reliability is relatively strong, it is recommended that attention be given to developing sound interrater reliability for coworkers who are using the profile.

THE COMMUNICATIVE EFFECTIVENESS INDEX (CETI)

The CETI (Lomas et al., 1989) rating scale differs markedly from the FCP, primarily because it utilizes the perceptions of significant others. The CETI was derived using a procedure by which a large number of partner-generated statements was reiteratively reduced by group consensus until the final set of 16 items was reached. These items focus on communication of needs and the ability to interact with other people. In using the scale clinically, partners rate the behaviors by placing a pencil mark on a 10-mm line, anchored on a continuum from "not at all able" to "as able as before the stroke." The CETI was carefully developed and has strong psychometric properties, including test-retest and interrater reliability, and good construct validity. The CETI items are shown in Table 12–3. Note that many of them appear to be excellent first approximations to a series of functional outcome statements, which could serve as a focus of intervention.

The CETI is part of the standard evaluation procedure in the Aphasia Clinic at the University of Arizona, where conversation groups are central, and where functional goals for treatment are not unlike many CETI items. It has been our experience that family members of newly aphasic patients are likely to rate behaviors more liberally on this scale than when the aphasia has become more chronic. This experience is independent of scores on formal aphasia tests, which frequently document improvement as the spouse-derived CETI scores fall. We have interpreted this observation as suggesting that

---

Table 12–3. CETI Items

Please Rate _____'s ability at . . .
1. Getting somebody's attention.
2. Getting involved in group conversations that are about him/her.
3. Giving yes and no answers appropriately.
4. Communicating his/her emotions.
5. Indicating that he/she understands what is being said to him/her.
6. Having coffee-time visits and conversations with friends and neighbors (around the bedside or at home.
7. Having a one-to-one conversation with you.
8. Saying the name of someone whose face is in front of him/her.
9. Communicating physical problems such as aches and pains.
10. Having a spontaneous conversation (i.e., starting the conversation and/or changing the subject).
11. Responding to or communicating anything (including yes or no) without words.
12. Starting a conversation with people who are not close family.
13. Understanding writing.
14. Being part of a conversation when it is fast and there are a number of people involved.
15. Participating in a conversatiion with strangers.
16. Describing or discussing something in depth.

SOURCE: Lomas et al. (1989). Reprinted with permission.

spouses develop a more valid perspective of the aphasia as their experience with it grows, rather than a weakness of the instrument itself.

Communication Profile: A Functional Skills Survey

Recently developed by Payne (1994), this instrument is not yet widely used. The Profile utilizes an interview format, in which adults with a variety of communication disorders rate the relative importance of 26 communication skills on a 5-point scale. The measure's focus on "importance" (i.e., a given skill's centrality in a given patient's lifestyle) makes it fundamentally different from the other measures reviewed here. It presents an interesting perspective, nonetheless. Its other strength is its cultural sensitivity. Finally, data using the instrument show differences as a function of living arrangement, type of employment, and income—features which are seldom accounted for in functional outcome measurement for communication disorders.

ASHA Functional Assessment of Communication Skills for Adults (ASHA FACS)

The ASHA FACS (Frattali et al., 1995) was developed primarily to fill the profession's need for a short, sensitive, reliable and valid rating measure for examining functional communication skills. The measure is unique in that it is focused explicitly on evaluating disability rather than impairment. That is, virtually all other rating scales of functional communication include ratings of impairments such as auditory comprehension, as well as ratings of disability such as the ability to follow directions. The ASHA FACS is focused only on the effects of impairments on everyday life activities. the instrument also is unique in that it includes both quantitative and qualitative scales for scoring behaviors, (the former a 7-point scale; the latter a 5-point scale). Quantitative performance is anchored at its low end by "does not do," and at its upper, by "does," with points in between reflecting the relative amount of assistance needed to perform the communicative act. Forty-three behaviors from four domains are assessed, including social communication; communication of basic needs; reading, writing and number concepts; and daily planning. Qualitative scoring is intended to yield information about the nature of the person's communicative attempts, and addresses the dimensions of adequacy, appropriateness, promptness, and ability to take one's appropriate share of the burden of communication. The ASHA FACS requires approximately 20 minutes to complete, and can be quickly scored either by hand or by using a computer program that is part of the test packet.

In addition to its attention to detail and its pertinence, a major strength of ASHA FACS is that it has been well researched and thoroughly standardized. Two pilot tests resulted in extensive revision, based both on statistical considerations, and feedback from pilot testers at geographically representative sites, who used it with a culturally diverse sample of patients. A final version was field tested on 131 aphasic individuals and 54 persons whose cognitive-communicative impairments resulting from traumatic brain injury, again representing both geographic and cultural diversity. For both the second pilot test and the field test, high inter- and intrarater reliability were established, as was external validity, internal consistency, and social validity. On the basis of its extensive standardization, it can be concluded that the ASHA FACS is psychometrically sound. Too, the feedback collected from users during pilot and field testing was influential in making the instrument user-friendly and responsive to measuring outcomes that are relevant to payers. We do not believe it is an exaggeration to suggest that the ASHA FACS can serve as an appropriate model for functional outcomes measurement in Speech-Language Pathology generally.

Table 12–4 presents the four communication domains examined in the ASHA FACS, as well as the test items (behaviors) included within each. As with the CETI, these items may be useful for developing functional treatment goals. Indeed, any treatment for aphasia—even that focused on impairment-level phenomena—should result in changes in functional communication. Treatment focused on improving sentence production, for example, should result in improved functional skills such as the ability to participate in conversations or ability to explain how to do something. If such functional outcomes are not seen as a result of treatment, the treatment may indeed be deemed ineffective.

DIRECT ASSESSMENT OF
FUNCTIONAL COMMUNICATION

Communicative Abilities in Daily Living (CADL)

When the CADL was published (Holland, 1980) it became the first direct measure of communication disability. Its original form was a highly controlled interview. The CADL had 68 context-rich items designed to evoke a variety of speech acts and verbal interchanges, as well as simple reading, writing, and mathematical transactions typical of everyday language use. A 3-point scoring system was utilized to rate the success of each communicative behavior tested. A score of 2 points was given to responses that effectively got a message across; a score of one was assigned to answers that were "in the ballpark," and a score of zero was given to ineffective attempts or wrong answers. Scores were independent of the modality used. For example, if a gesture got a particular message across, it was scored as a 2 and considered to be just as effective as a verbal response that also got the message across. The CADL was validated in a number of ways; most importantly CADL performance was correlated with (1) in situ observations of aphasic persons' actual functional communication in their daily lives, and (2) impairment based measures—the Boston Diagnostic Aphasia Examination (BDAE) and the PICA—as well as ratings on the FCP. The CADL required approximately 35 minutes to administer and both inter- and intrarater reliability were reported to be high. Although the CADL was primarily designed to be used with aphasic patients, it was also validated for use with mentally retarded adults and with experienced hearing aid users (Holland, 1980). The CADL also was used successfully with individuals with Alzheimer's Disease (Fromm, 1988).

In response to criticisms that the CADL was too time consuming and that the role-playing required for part of the test was too difficult, CADL has been shortened and the role playing eliminated (Holland, Frattali, & Fromm, 1996). This 50-item version, CADL 2, takes approximately 25 minutes to administer. It introduces a number of more contemporary formats and contexts for individual items, but CADL-2 retains its scoring format and continues to adhere to measuring speech acts, verbal interchanges, and simple reading, writing, and transactions that involve numbers.

Table 12–4. ASHA FACS Conceptual Framework

Social Communication	Communication of Basic Needs	Reading, Writing Number Concepts	Daily Planning
BEHAVIORS			
Uses names of familiar people	Recognizes familiar faces/voices	Understands simple signs	Tells time
Expresses agreement/disagreement	Makes strong likes/dislikes known	Uses reference materials	Dials telephone numbers
Explains how to do something	Expresses feelings	Follows written directions	Keeps scheduled appointments
Requests information	Requests help	Understands printed material	Uses a calendar
Exchanges information on the telephone	Makes needs/wants known	Prints/writes/types name	Follows a map
Answers yes/no questions	Responds in an emergency	Completes forms	
Follows directions		Writes messages	
Understands facial expressions/tone of voice		Understands signs with numbers	
Understands nonliteral meaning and intent		Makes money transactions	
Understands conversations in noisy surroundings		Understands units of measurement	
Understands TV/radio			
Participates in conversations			
Recognizes/corrects communication errors			

	QUALITATIVE DIMENSIONS		
Adequacy	Appropriateness	Promptness	Communication Sharing
DEFINITIONS			
Frequency with which client understands gist of message *and* gets point across	Frequency with which client's communication is relevant *and* done under the right circumstances	Frequency with which client responds without delay *and* in an efficient manner	Extent to which a client's communication poses a burden to the communication partner

Reprinted with permission from the American Speech-Language-Hearing Association.

The Amsterdam-Nijmegan Everyday Language Test (ANELT)

The ANELT was developed by Blomert as a test for measuring verbal communicative abilities in Dutch-speaking aphasic patients (first described in English by Blomert, 1990). A German language version also has been standardized, and publication of the English standardization is "imminent" (Blomberg et al., 1994). The ANELT, which has two parallel versions of 10 items each, comprises short, context-setting scenarios for which the aphasic individual is required to provide an appropriate verbal response. For example Item 1 is as follows:

You are now at the dry cleaner's. You have come to pick this up and you get it back like this (present shirt with scorch mark). What do you say? (1994, p. 385)

Responses are scored for understandability (defined by these investigators as, "content independent of linguistic form") and for intelligibility (defined as "relating to the perception of the utterance per se, independent of the content or meaning). Thus, if the patient responds to the above scenario by saying "mulluky mulluky," it would be scored as intelligible, but not understandable.

Test-retest and interrater reliability measures have shown the ANELT to be reliable, and criterion and construct validity measures show the ANELT to be sensitive for measuring verbal communication across a variety of aphasic syndromes. Among the problems with the ANELT is that it examines only verbal communicative effectiveness and the aphasic individual must be able to understand the test items in order to respond to them. It could be argued, for example, that an aphasic person's ability to respond to an item like the one presented above may not reflect his or her ability to express concern or disappointment in a similar real life situation. Auditory comprehension ability would not be an issue in the real case and, as we pointed out earlier, the aphasic individual would likely be able to use both verbal and nonverbal means to express his or herself if such a situation arose. Blomert et al. (1994) argue, however, that verbal communicative effectiveness as measured by the ANELT (especially in terms of the "understandability" scoring) reflects the general severity of aphasia (including auditory comprehension deficits) and, therefore, it is a good measure of overall communicative functioning.

PSYCHOSOCIAL OUTCOME AND WELL-BEING MEASURES

The functional rating scales and test instruments just discussed define "functional" slanted in the direction of its utilitarian meaning described earlier in this chapter. This leaves a number of unanswered concerns. For example, to be able to make needs and wants known following clinical intervention might in fact satisfy fiscal intermediaries that a particular aphasic individual has lessened the disability of aphasia. And to some extent this is true. But what if this aphasic person were a lawyer? An actor? A speech-language pathologist? Or what if he were the best joke teller in his local Lion's Club? In order to discuss the other sense of "fully functioning," assessment tools that address the handicap imposed by aphasia must be included.

We believe that the most effective way to address impact of aphasia from the standpoint of its handicap is to move away from measures of language and communication into the larger arena of the ability to function in society. For this reason, the measures described next focus on quality of life. We will first discuss psychosocial outcomes measurement. We will then discuss health-related quality of life scales. Finally we will discuss measures that can be used to study returning to wellness after stroke. In the long run, the closer one gets to the goal of wellness following stroke, the less stroke's handicap, and the higher the probability that one's life is qualitatively improved. This is independent in some ways from the degree of impairment.

QUALITY-OF-LIFE ISSUES

Psychosocial Outcome Measures

Bishop and Pet (1995) list a number of psychobehavioral/psychosocial problems that can occur in the wake of stroke. These include (but certainly are not limited to) anxiety, adjustment disorders, sexual dysfunction, mood changes, and sleep disorders. The major psychosocial sequel to stroke is depression. Many researchers believe that roughly 50% of stroke patients are at risk for depression (Spencer, Tompkins, Schulz, & Rau, 1993; Diller & Bishop, 1995). There is every reason to believe that the presence of depression adversely affects recovery from aphasia, or, more optimistically, that relief from depression can increase the potential for recovery from aphasia. Although it is the case that the so-called "talking therapies" may have limited utility for aphasic people, a variety of approaches to the management of depression poststroke are available, ranging from counseling to pharmacological intervention. Therefore, a particularly important psychosocial outcome for aphasia is the documentation of depression, and of changes in depression and mood following stroke (or following treatment for aphasia).

Depression Scales

A number of scales can be adapted for use with aphasic patients. Holland, Greenhouse, Fromm, and Swindell (1989) used a modified form of the *Beck Depression Scale* (Beck, Ward, Mendelson, Mock, & Erbaugh, 1961) successfully with an unselected sample of poststroke patients, including individuals with aphasia and cognitive deficits following right hemisphere brain damage. Spencer, Tompkins, Schulz and Rau (1993) have effectively used the *Center for Epidemiologic Studies-Depression Scale* (CES-D; Radloff, 1977) with a wide range of stroke survivor and recommend it for use not only with stroke survivors, but also with their support persons as well (Schulz, Tompkins & Rau, 1988). Finally, a modification of the *Schedule of Affective Disorders and Schizophrenia* (SADS; Endicott & Spitzer, 1987), has recently been completed for stroke survivors and is called the *Structured Assessment of Depression in Brain Damaged Individuals* (SADBDI; Hibbard et al., 1993). It takes aphasia, short term memory, and neglect into account, and although not widely known, has potential for being a very useful measure.

Health-Related Quality-of-Life Measures (HQL)

Another series of measures directly relate quality of life to the medical realities that are the fallout of various physical conditions. A recent review of such measures conducted by Tate, Dijkers, and Johnson-Greene (1996) suggests that there are many scales, some geared specifically to specific diseases/disorders, and almost as many unanswered questions about both the concept and ways to measure it appropriately. Nonetheless, they single out a few measures that they believe either have established usage in stroke, or are appropriate measures to consider. Two that are of potential interest to clinical aphasiologists and have been referred to in Chapter 3 are the SIP (Bergner, et al., 1981), which has been used by DeHaan and colleagues (1993a, 1993b) to investigate quality-of-life issues poststroke, and the *SF-36* (Ware & Sherbourne, 1992), which is the short form of an instrument developed for the Medical Outcome Study. Although good reliability and validity have been reported for both measures, it is not clear that they have ever been specifically evaluated with aphasic stroke survivors.

Measures of Well-being

Measuring depression in aphasia, or linking quality of life specifically to an unfortunate physical condition, is perhaps looking pessimistically at psychosocial outcome. It is also possible to look more optimistically by using measures geared to wellness. Many speech-language pathologists have known aphasic individuals who courageously just get on with life, returning with grace and equanimity to living as fully as possible. For still other aphasic people, who have otherwise made excellent recoveries, measures of well-being remove the ceiling effects found in more utilitarian measures, and thus give space for measuring change and improvement. One particularly interesting set of scales has been developed by Ryff (1989). These scales measure aspects of well-being including self-acceptance, positive relations with others, autonomy, environmental mastery, purpose in life, and personal growth. Ryff presents impressive reliability and validity data for the scales, and has developed short forms of each which have good correlations with the parent scales. To our knowledge, the use of the Ryff scales with aphasic adults have not been reported in the literature.

Recently, Elman and Bernstein-Ellis (1996) have reported on the successful use of the *Affect Balance Scale* (ABS: Bradburn, 1969) to measure the effects of their aphasia group treatment approach. This simple 10-item scale is also part of life history survey developed by Records, Tomblin, and Freese (1996) for their study of quality-of-life issues of young adults who were language impaired as children.

CONCLUSION

We have reviewed a number of measures here, but we have focused the review on measures of disability and handicap and, of those, we have focused on measures that seem to us most likely to be attractive to clinicians. In this time of decreased funding for assessment (and for treatment) of aphasic patients, it is somewhat daunting to suggest additional testing for aphasic individuals. Yet measurement of functional outcomes is a clear and growing necessity. We cautiously suggest that issues beyond utilitarian functional communication should be considered in relation to outcome in aphasia. At the very least, enhancing communication measures with measurement using some psychosocial outcome scales is a realistic approach to this complex problem.

Table 12–5. The WHO (1980) Framework as a guide
for Treatment Research and Clinical Management.

	PRETESTING	TREATMENT FOCUS	OUTCOME MEASUREMENT
HANDICAP			
DISABILITY			
IMPAIRMENT			

Adapted from Schwartz & Whyte (1992).

We agree with Schwartz and White (1992) who suggested that in our treatment research and in our clinical practice the WHO (1980) framework can be used as a guideline. That is, both testing and treatment focused at the levels of impairment, disability, and handicap need to be provided. We suggest that clinicians and researchers alike use Table 12–5 in designing their interventions for aphasia by filling in all of the slots on the matrix. We need to continue to use traditional measures of impairment both prior to, during, and at the end of the treatment period. However, as we have emphasized in this chapter, testing needs to be expanded to include measures of disability and handicap. Too, the treatments that we provide need to be focused more explicitly on all aspects of the aphasia. As pointed out by Schwartz (1992), "diverse approaches [to treatment] are needed to adequately address the range of issues posed by aphasia and its rehabilitation" (p. 18).

As the foregoing attests, outcomes measurement in aphasia has been of interest for at least a quarter of a century. However, recent changes in health care delivery and the attendant requirement for health professionals to validate the effects of their interventions have caused a recent extensive furor of activity. For some professionals, this emphasis on functional outcome is viewed with suspicion, if not outright alarm. For others, increased concern with the outcome of aphasia treatment is a refreshing idea. To show that our work makes a difference in everyday life is a very exciting challenge, made a lot easier by the fact that measures for such documentation are available, and more are appearing with regularity. In no way does this push to demonstrate real world effects negate the findings that have derived from past aphasia treatment research, nor does it suggest that all treatment research must examine functional outcomes. Indeed, as we pointed out here, we need more basic research on clinical methods in aphasia. We must continue to examine the efficacy of treatment in our clinical laboratories in order to create more effective management approaches. We must also keep in mind that our dependent measures can and should be expanded to include measures of real world abilities and issues.

For the aphasic individual and his or her family, the overriding issues are not changes in aphasia test scores or in the number of creative treatment strategies that are available. Rather, the issues are firmly grounded in "getting another job," "talking better," "following the Steelers on TV," "being comfortable going out to dinner again," "getting a good laugh out of the grandbaby's new words," that is, moving on with the unfinished business of life. How those things are accomplished is what expanded outcomes measurement will ultimately help us to document.

REFERENCES

Alexander, M. P., & Loverso, F. (1993). A specific treatment for global aphasia. In M. Lemme (Ed.), *Clinical aphasiology,* Vol. 21 (pp. 277–289). Austin, TX: Pro-Ed.

Basso, A., Capitani, E., & Vignolo, L. (1979). Influence of rehabilitation of language skills in aphasic patients: A controlled study. *Archives of Neurology, 36,* 190–196.

Beck, A., Ward, C., Mendelson, M., Mock, J., & Erbaugh, J. (1961). An inventory for measuring depression. *Archives of General Psychiatry, 4,* 461–471.

Beeson, P., Rapcsak, S., & Rubens, A. (1993). Verbal learning and aphasia. *Journal of Clinical and Experimental Neuropsychology, 15,* 91.

Beeson, P., Rapcsak, Rubens, A., & Bayles, K. (1994). Verbal learning and the right hemisphere. *Conference proceedings: Clinical aphasiology, (vol.* 21). Austin, TX: Pro-Ed.

Bergner, M., Bobbitt, R., Carter, W., & Gilson, B. (1981). The sickness impact profile: Development and final revision of a health status measure. *Medical Care, 19,* 787–805.

Bishop, D. & Pet, R. (1995). Psychobehavioral problems other than depression in stroke. *Topics in Stroke Rehabilitation 2,* 56–58.

Blomert, L., (1990). What functional assessment can contribute to setting goals for aphasia therapy. *Aphasiology, 4,* 307–320.

Blomert, L., Kean, M.-L., Koster, C., & Schokker, J. (1994). Amsterdam-Nijmegen Everyday Language Test: Construction, reliability, and validity. *Aphasiology, 8,* 381–407.

Bradburn, N. (1969). *The structure of psychological well-being.* Chicago: Aldine.

Cichowski, K. (1993). *Rehabilitation Institute of Chicago functional assessment scale (Revised).* Chicago: Rehabilitation Institute of Chicago.

Conlon, C. P., & McNeil, M. R. (1989). The efficacy of treatment for two globally aphasic adults using visual action therapy. In T. Prescott (Ed.), *Clinical aphasiology,* Vol. 19 (pp. 185–195). Austin, TX: Pro-Ed.

DeHaan, R., Aronson, N., Limberg, M., Langton-Hwere, R., & van Crevel. (1993a). Measuring quality of life in stroke. *Stroke, 24,* 320–327.

DeHaan, R., Horn, Limburg, M. van der Meulen, & Bossuyt, P. (1993b). A comparison of five stroke scales with measures of disability, handicap, and quality of life. *Stroke, 24,* 178–181.

DeRenzi, E., & Vignolo, L. A. (1962). The Token Test: A sensitive test to detect receptive disturbances in aphasics. *Brain, 85,* 665–678.

Diller, L. & Bishop, D. (1995). Depression and stroke. *Topics in Stroke Rehabilitation, 2,* 44–55.

Duffy, R. and Duffy, J. (1975). Pantomime recognition in aphasics. *Journal of Speech Hearing Research, 18,* 115–132.

Elman, R. & Bernstein-Ellis, E. (1996). *Effectiveness of group communication treatment for individuals with chronic aphasia: Results on communicative and linguistic measures.* Paper presented to the Clinical Aphasiology Conference, Newport, Rhode Island.

Elman, R.,& Bernstein-Ellis, E. (1995). What is functional? *American Journal of Speech-Language Pathology, 4,* 115–117.

Endicott, J., & Spitzer, R. (1978). A diagnostic interview. The schedule for affective disorders and schizophrenia. *Archives of General Psychiatry, 35.* 837–844.

Fink, R. B., Schwartz, M. F., Rochon, E., Myers, J. L., Socolof, G. S., & Bluestone, R. (1995). Syntax stimulation revisited: An analysis of generalization treatment effects. *American Journal of Speech-Language Pathology, 4,* 99–104.

Frattali, C., Thompson, C., Holland, A., Wohl, C, & Ferketic, M. (1995). *American Speech-Language-Hearing Association functional assessment of communication skills for adults.* Rockville, MD.: ASHA.

Goodwin, C. (1995). Co-constructing meaning in conversations with an aphasic man. In Jacoby, S., & Ochs, E. (Eds.), *Research on Language and Social Interaction (Special issue on co-construction)*: 233–260.

Hartman, J., & Landau, W. (1987). Comparison of formal language therapy with supportive counseling for aphasia due to acute vascular accident. *Archives of Neurology, 24* , 646–649.

Harvey, R., & Jellinek, H. (1981). Functional performance assessment: Program approach. *Archives of Physical Medicine and Rehabilitation, 62,* 456–461.

Helm-Estabrooks, N. (1992). *Aphasia Diagnostic Profiles* Chicago: Riverside.

Helm-Estabrooks, N., Fitzpatrick, P., & Barresi, B. (1981). Response of an agrammatic patient to a syntax stimulation program for aphasia. *Journal of Speech and Hearing Disorders, 46,* 422–427.

Hibbard, M., Gordon, W., Stein, P., Grober. S, & Sliwinski, M. (1992). Rehabilitation psychological awareness of disability in patients after stroke. *Rehabilitation Psychology 37,* 103–120.

Hillis, A. E. (1989). Efficacy and generalization of treatment for aphasic naming errors. *Archives of Physical Medicine and Rehabilitation, 70,* 632–636.

Holland, A. (1980). *Communicative abilities in daily living.* Austin TX: Pro-Ed.

Holland, A., Frattali, C., & Fromm, D. (in press) *Communicative abilities in daily living—CADL 2.* Austin TX: Pro-Ed.

Holland, A. L., Fromm, D. S., DeRuyter, F., & Stein, M. (1996). Treatment Efficacy: Aphasia. *Journal of Speech and Hearing Research, 39,* S27–S36.

Kaplan, E., Goodglass, H., & Weintraub, S. (1983). *The Boston Naming Test.* Philadelphia: Lea & Febiger.

Kay, J., Lesser, R., & Coltheart, M. (1992). *Psycholinguistic Assessment of Language Production in Aphasia.* East Sussex, UK: Lawrence Erlbaum, Lt.

Kertesz, A. (1982). *Western aphasia battery.* New York: Grune and Stratton.

Lomas, J., Pickard, L., Bester, S., Elbard, H., Finlayson, A., & Zoghabib. (1989). The Communicative Effectiveness Index: Development and psychometric evaluation of a functional communication measure for adult aphasia. *Journal of Speech and Hearing Disorders, 54,* 113–124.

Parkside Associates. (1986). *LORS American Data System (LADS) data manual.* Parkridge IL: Author.

Payne J., (1994). *Communication profile: A functional skills survey.* San Antonio, TX: Communication Skill Builders.

Poeck, K., Huber, W., & Willmes, K. (1989). Outcome of intensive language treatment in aphasia. *Journal of Speech and Hearing Disorders, 54,* 471–479.

Porch, B. (1967). *Porch index of communicative ability.* Palo Alto CA: Consulting Psychologists Press.

Price, C., Wise, R., Howard, D., Warburton, E., & Frackowiak, R. (1993). The role of the right hemisphere in the recovery of language after stroke. *Journal of Cerebral Blood Flow and Metabolism, 13,* 520.

Radloff, L. (1977). The CES-D Scale: A self-report depression scale for research in the general population. *Applied Psychological Measurement,* 385–401.

Raymer, A. M., Thompson, C. K., Jacobs, B., & Le Grand, H. R. (1993). Phonological treatment of naming deficits in aphasia: model-based generalization analysis. *Aphasiology, 7,* 27–53.

Raymer, A. M., Thompson, C. K., Jacobs, B., & Le Grand, H. R. (1993). Phonlogical treatment of naming deficits in aphasia model-based generalization analysis. *Aphasiology, 7,* 27–53.

Records, N., Tomblin, B., & Buckwalter, P. (1996). *Present life history.* (in preparation.)

Ryff, C. (1989). Scales of psychological well-being (short form). *Journal of Personality and Social Psychology, 57,* 1069–1081.

Saffran, E. M., Berndt, R. S., & Schwartz, M. F. (1989). The quantitative analysis of agrammatic production: Procedure and data. *Brain and Language, 37,* 440–479.

Sarno, M.(1965). A measurement of functional communication in aphasia. *Archives of Physical Medicine & Rehabilitation, 46,* 101–107.

Sarno, M. (1969). *The functional communication profile: Manual of directions.* New York: Institute of Rehabilitation Medicine.

Schulz, R., Tompkins, C., & Rau, M. (1988). A longitudinal study of the psychosocial impact of stroke on primary support persons. *Psychology and Aging, 3,* 131–141.

Schwartz, M. F., & Whyte, J. (1992). Methodological issues in aphasia treatment research: The big picture. In: *Aphasia treatment: Current approaches and research opportunities* (pp. 17–23). Bethesda, MD: U.S. Department of Health and Human Services, NIH Publication No. 93–3424.

Schwartz, M. FF., Saffran, E. M., Fink, R. B., Myers, J. L., & Martin, N. (1994). Mapping therapy: a treatment programme for agrammatism. *Aphasiology, 8,* 19–54.

Shewan, C. (1979). *Auditory comprehension test for sentences.* Chicago: Biolinguistics Clinical Institutes.

Shewan, C., & Kertesz, A. (1984). Effects of speech and language treatment on recovery from aphasia. *Brain and Language, 23,* 272–299.

Simmons, N., Kearns, K. P., & Potechin, G. (1987). Treatment of aphasia through family member training. In R. H. Brookshire (Ed.), *Clinical aphasiology,* Vol. 17. (pp. 106–116). Minneapolis, MN: BRK Publishers.

Skinner, C., Wirz, S., Thompson, I., and Davidson, J. (1984). *Edinburgh functional communication profile.* Winslow: Winslow Press.

Spencer, K., Tompkins, C., Schulz, R., & Rau, M. (1993). The psychosocial outcomes of stroke: A longitudinal study of depression risk. *Clinical Aphasiology Conference Proceedings.* Austin, TX: Pro-Ed.

State University of New York at Buffalo (1993). Guide for the Uniform Da for Medical Rehabilitation (Adult FIM), Version 4.0. Buffalo, N.Y.: Author

Tate, D., Dijkers, M., Johnson-Greene, L. (1996). Outcome measures in quality of life. *Topics in Stroke Rehabilitation, 2,* 1–17.

Thompson, C. K. (1989). Generalization in the treatment of aphasia. In L. V. McReynolds & J. Spradlin (Eds.), *Generalization strategies in the treatment of communication disorders* (pp. 82–115). Philadelphia: B. C. Decker.

Thompson, C. K. (1995). Modern approaches to aphasia treatment. Paper presented at the Behavioral Neurology Conference. Chicago, Illinois.

Thompson, C. K., & Byrne, M. E. (1984). Across setting generalization of social conventions in aphasia: An experimental analysis of "loose training". In R. H. Brookshire (Ed.), Clinical aphasiology conference proceedings (pp. 132–142). Minneapolis, MN: BRK Publishers.

Thompson, C. K., Shapiro, L. P., Ballard, K., Jacobs, B., Schneider, S., & Tait, M. (in press). Training and generalized production of *wh-* and NP-Movement Structures in Agrammatic Speakers. *Journal of Speech and Hearing Research.*

Thompson, C. K., Shapiro, L. P., & Roberts, M. (1993). Treatment of sentence production deficits in aphasia: A linguistic-specific approach to *wh-*interrogative training and generalization. *Aphasiology, 7,* 111–133.

Thompson, C. K., Shapiro, L. P., Tait, M., Jacobs, B., & Schneider, S. (1996). Training *wh-*questions production in agrammatic aphasia: Analysis of argument and adjunct movement. *Brain and Language, 52,* 175–228.

Thompson, C.K., Shapiro, L.P., Tait, M.E., Jacobs, J., & Schneider, L. (1997) Training and generalized production of wh-questions and NP-movement structures in agrammatic aphasia. *Journal of Speech and Hearing Research, 40,* 228–244.

Wambaugh, J., & Thompson, C. K. (1989). Training and generalization of grammatic aphasic adults' *wh-*interrogative productions. *Journal of Speech and Hearing Disorders, 54,* 504–525.

Ware, J., & Sherbourne, C. (1992). The MOS 36-item short-form health survey (SF-36). I: Conceptual framework and item selection. *Medical Care, 30,* 473–483.

Warren, R., (1995). *The role of the Functional Independence Measure (FIM) in aphasia rehabilitation.* Paper presented to the Clinical Aphasiology Conference, Sun River. Oregon.

Weiller, C., Isensee, C., Rijuntjes, M., Huber, W., Muller, S., Bier, D., Dutschka, K., Woods, R.,

North, J., & Diener, H. C. (1995). Recovery from Wernicke's aphasia: A positron emission tomographic study. *Annals of Neurology, 37*(6), 723–732.

Weniger, D., & Bertoni, B. (1993). Which route to aphasia therapy? In Holland, A., & Forbes, M., (Eds.) *Aphasia Treatment: World Perspectives.* San Diego: Singular.

Werner, R., (1994). Functional assessment issues (Forward). *Topics in Stroke Rehabilitation, 1, 3.*

Wertz, R.T., Weiss, D., Aten J., Brookshire, R., Garcia-Bunuel, L., Holland, A., Kurtzke, J., LaPointe, L., Milianti, F., Brannegan, R., Greenbaum, H., Marshall, R., Vogel, D., Carter, J., Barnes, N., & Goodman, R. (1986). Comparison of clinic, home, and deferred language treatment for aphasia: A Veterans Administration cooperative study. *Archives of Neurology, 43,* 653–658.

Wertz, R. T., Collins, M. J., Weiss, D., Kurtzke, J. F., Friden, T., Brookshire, R. H., Pierce, J., Holtzapple, P., Hubbard, D. J., Porch, B. E., West, J. A., Davis, L., Matovitch, V., Morley, G. K., & Resurreccion, E. (1981). Veterans Administration cooperative study on aphasia: A comparison of individual and group treatment. *Journal of Speech and Hearing Research, 24,* 580–594.

World Health Organization. (1980). *International classification of impairments, disabilities and handicaps.* Geneva: Author.

CHAPTER 13

Outcomes Measurement in Cognitive Communication Disorders

SECTION 1 : BRENDA L. B. ADAMOVICH
SECTION 2 : CONNIE A. TOMPKINS AND
MARGARET T. LEHMAN
SECTION 3 : MICHELLE BOURGEOIS

INTRODUCTION

The ability to communicate requires complex interactions among cognitive domains such as language, attention, and memory. Skills in these areas may be impaired as a result of traumatic brain injury (TBI), right-hemisphere brain damage (RBD), and dementia.

Cognitive-communicative impairments have been defined by ASHA (1987) as "those communicative disorders that result from deficits in linguistic and non-linguistic cognitive processes" (p. 4). Language deficits can be outward manifestations of underlying impairments in cognitive processes such as attention, perception, and/or memory; inflexibility, impulsivity, or disorganized thinking; difficulty processing complex information; problems learning new information; inefficient retrieval of stored information; ineffective problem solving or judgment; inappropriate social behavior (pragmatics); and impaired executive functioning.

As described in Chapter 1 of this text, the International Classification of Impairments, Disabilities, and Handicaps (ICIDH), developed by the World Health Organization (WHO) (1980), defines impairment as resultant losses of psychological or physical function; disability as restricted ability to perform everyday life activities; and handicap as a social disadvantage resulting from the impairment and/or disability. The theoretical framework of disablement developed by the WHO provides a good description of how culture, values, and resources modify the impact of neurological disorders. This model provides an appropriate framework for examining the sequelae of neurological damage.

With tightened health care spending due to managed care and other cost-cutting efforts, there is an increased focus on payment for treatment that results in the greatest improvement in functional everyday abilities. Potentially, there will be no third-party coverage of treatment that focuses on impairments alone. Reimbursement would be available for only those treatments that reduce disabilities and/or handicaps in a timely manner. This chapter describes outcome measures and clinical research pertaining to impairments, disabilities, and handicaps of individuals with TBI, RBD, and dementia. Due to the extent of information presented, this chapter is organized into three separate sections, with references appearing at the end of the chapter.

SECTION 1 : TRAUMATIC BRAIN INJURY

Brenda L. B. Adamovich

TBI is the leading cause of death and disability in the United States for individuals aged 40 years and under. The primary cause of TBI is motor vehicle accidents. In the United States, 2 million head injuries result each year, with a cost per year of $25 billion, resulting from medical treatment, rehabilitation, support services, and lost insurance (Bigler, 1990). Memory and other cognitive impairments are the most long-lasting and incapacitating sequelae of TBI. The number of specialized programs for patients with TBI has grown over the past 10 years from a handful to almost 1000 programs across the United States. The quality of care, in general, has improved from lifetime nursing home placements to programs that focus on home and community reentry, with emphasis on metacognitive skills, functional gains, and empowerment.

Outcome Measures

Impairment

Two classes of neurobehavioral sequelae occur following TBI, caused by the occurrence of discrete focal brain lesions and widespread diffuse brain lesions. Focal lesions may cause speech, language, voice, hearing, fluency, and/or swallowing impairments similar to those that occur following stroke. Outcome measures and clinical research specific to these areas have been reviewed elsewhere in this book. Widespread, diffuse brain damage typically occurs following closed head injury (CHI) and results in cognitive-communicative impairments due to impaired attention, information processing, and cognition. Specific cognitive processes that cause impaired communication include perception, discrimination, organization, recall, and reasoning. Perception refers to the integration and interpretation of information received at the sense organs based on an internal or stored representation of the stimulus. Discrimination refers to the ability to differentiate two or more stimuli. Organization refers to the ability to deal with discrete actions or components that must be grouped or sequenced according to the priority of each component, using a learned strategy. General organizational skills include categorization, closure, and sequencing. Memory deficits occur due to ineffective encoding of information, inadequate storage of information, difficulty retrieving information using recognition, cued recall or free recall, and/or a lack of strategies to deal with interferences. Reasoning and problem solving require the generation of responses based on relevant information to formulate a solution to a problem that must then be checked or tested as to appropriateness of the solution.

General measures that have been used to predict outcome relevant to impairment (as well as disability and handicap) include the duration of a coma, coma outcome, post-traumatic amnesia (PTA), and age. The *Glasgow Coma Scale* (*GCS*) (Jennett et al., 1981) is most often used to assess the duration of coma, assigning a number based on ratings of eye opening, motor responses, and verbal responses. The most widely used measure for outcome of coma is the *Glasgow Outcome Scale* (Jennett & Bond, 1975), in which patients are rated on a scale from vegetative to disability ratings of severe to mild. PTA refers to the time between injury and recovery of continuous memory. Retrograde amnesia refers to the period of memory loss prior to injury and is thought to be not as improved in the prediction of outcome (Bond, 1990). The *Galveston Orientation and Amnesia Test* (*GOAT*), (Levin, O'Donnell, & Grossman, 1975) is widely used to measure PTA.

The most commonly used neuropsychological tests that can be used to obtain measurements of cognitive impairments are summarized in Table 13–1. Several tests are often combined to form test batteries; however, if test batteries are too lengthy, fatigue and impaired concentration interfere with performance and may invalidate results (Bond, 1990).

The *Scales of Cognitive Ability for Traumatic Brain Injury* (*SCATBI*) is a diagnostic test for adolescents and adults (Adamovich & Henderson, 1992) that is designed to assess cognitive-linguistic status after CHI and to describe the extent of changes during and following rehabilitation. This test was constructed to measure performance on five scales—perception and discrimination, orientation, organization, recall, and reasoning—each representing a general area of cognitive ability that may be impaired after CHI and is ultimately necessary to function in day-to-day living. Each scale is made up of a series of small tests, or "testlets" (Thissen, Steinberg, & Mooney, 1989). Testlets are collections of similar items designed to measure a common trait or subdomain. In general, individual items within each testlet were designed to exhibit a slight progression in difficulty. The cognitive rehabilitation treatment hierarchy, based on the hierarchy of cognitive processes in the SCATBI, satisfies theories of instruction and general learning as stated by Collins et al. (1989) and Bruner (1966). Collins et al. state that previously trained abilities are used to train new abilities. Bruner advocates that previously learned material should be repeated in an increasing level of detail and difficulty, which he refers to as a spiral curriculum.

Disabilities

Cognitive impairments can cause reduced abilities in social interactions and interpersonal or pragmatic communication, which lead to problems with social adjustment and can result in a handicap. A disability in pragmatic communication can result from cognitive impairments that cause an inability to comprehend subtlety in language, such as in metaphorical and figurative use, and reduced ability to draw conclusions and give coherence to narrative. Higher level head injured patients have executive functioning or metacognitive skill impairments that make them appear unusual to others in the community. Executive functioning refers to the ability to formulate goals, develop plans, and effectively execute a plan (Lezak, 1982). Executive or metacognitive skills include self-awareness in goal-setting, planning, self-directing/initiating, self-

Table 13–1. Selected Instruments Available to Measure Cognitive Processes: Attention/ Orientation, Perception/Discrimination, Memory, Organization and Reasoning; Personality and Behavior; Over-all Outcome; Social Adjustment and Severity of Injury.

SKILLS MEASURED	TESTS
I. Attention/Orientation	Digit Span (WAIS-R) (Wechsler, 1981)
	Trail Making Test, A&B (Reitan & Davison, 1958, 1974)
	Symbol Digit Modalities Test: Written & Oral (Smith, 1968, 1973)
	Paced Auditory Serial Addition (PASA) (Levin, 1983)
	Wisconsin Card Sorting Test (WCST) (Nelson, 1976)
	Galveston Orientation and Amnesia Test (GOAT) (Levin et al. 1975)
	Glasgow Coma Scale (GCS) (Jennett & Teasdale, 1981)
II. Perception/Discrimination	Facial Recognition Test
	Color Form Sorting Test (Goldstein & Scheerer, 1945)
	Developmental Test of Visual Perception (Frostig, 1963)
	G-F-W Test of Auditory Discumination and Sound Symbol Tests (Goldman, 1974)
	Southern California Figure-Ground Visual Perception Test (Ayres, 1966)
III. Memory	Wechsler Memory Scale (WMS) (Wechsler & Stone, 1945)
	Revised Benton Visual Retention Test (RBVRT) (Benton, 1974)
	Randt Memory Test (RMT) (Randt, Brown, & Osborne, 1980)
	Denman Neuropsychology Memory Scale (DNMS) (Denman, 1984)
	Rey-Osterrieth Complex Figure (Osterrieth, 1944)
	Paced Auditory Serial Addition Task (PASAT) (Gronwall, 1977)
	Rivermead Behavioral Memory Test (Wilson, Cockburn & Baddeley, 1985)
	Controlled Word Association Test (Benton Hamsher, 1976)
	Visual Retention Test (Benton, 1974, 1992)
	G-F-W Auditory Memory Test (Goldman, Fristoe, Woodcock, 1974)
	Word Fluency Test (Borkowski, Benton & Spreen 1967)
	Auditory—Verbal Learning Task (Rey, 1964)
	Symbol Digit Modalities Test (Smith, 1973)
	Tactual Performance Test (Halstead, 1947)
	Facial Recognition Test (Benton, Deshamsher, Varney & Spreen, 1983)
	Benton Visual Retention Test (Benton, 1974)
	Post Traumatic Amnesia (PTA) (Teasdale & Jennett, 1974)

Skills Measured	Tests
IV. Organization & Reasoning	Wisconsin Card Sorting Test (WCST) (Nelson, 1976)
	Auditory Verbal Learning (Rey, 1964)
	Category Test (Halstead, 1947)
	Controlled Oral Word Association Test (COWAT) (Malec et al. 1993)
	Raven's Progressive Matrices (Raven, 1960)
	Ross Test of Higher Cognitive Processes (Ross & Ross, 1976)
	Detroit Tests of Learning Aptitude (Baker & Leland, 1935)
	Hooper Visual Organization Test (Hooper, 1958)
	Hooper Test of Visual Organization (Hooper, 1966)
	Rey-Osterrieth Complex Figure Test (Osterrieth, 1944)
V. Test Batteries Designed to Measure Several Cognitive Processes	Wechsler Adult Intelligence Scale (WAISR) (Wechsler, 1981)
	Orientation Group Monitoring System (OGMS) (Jackson, Mysin & Corrigan, 1989)
	Scales of Cognitive Ability for Traumatic Brain Injury (SCATBI) (Adamovich & Henderson, 1992)
	Neurobehavioral Rating Scale (NRS) (Levin, 1987)
	Detroit Test of Learning Aptitude (Baker & Leland, 1935)
	Ross Test of Higher Cognitive Processes (Ross & Ross, 1976)
VI. Personality and Behavior	Minnesota Multiphasic Personality Inventory (MMPI, 1992)
	Brief Psychiatric Rating Scale (BPRS) (Overall & Gorham, 1962)
VII. Independence	Glasgow Outcome Scale (GOS) (Jennett & Bond, 1975)
	Glasgow Assessment Schedule (GAS) (Livingston & Livingston, 1985)
	Disability Rating Scale (DRS) (Rappaport et al., 1982)
	Functional Independence Measure (FIM) (State University of New York at Buffalo, 1993)
VIII. Social Adjustment	The Katz Adjustment Scale (Katz & Lyerly, 1963)
	The Katz Adjustment Scale—Relatives Form (KAS-R) (Katz & Lyerly, 1963)
	Social Adjustment Scale—Self Report (SAS-SR) (Weissman, 1975)
IX. Severity of Injury	Glasgow Coma Scale (GCS) (Teasdale & Jennett, 1974)
	Post-Traumatic Amnesia (PTA) (Russell, 1932)
	Rancho Los Amigos Scale of Cognitive Function (Hagen, 1982)

inhibiting, self-monitoring, self-evaluating, and flexible problem solving (Ylvisaker, 1989). A person who lacks these skills appears to be egocentric, rude, impulsive, disinhibited, stubborn, denying, or incoherent.

Social disabilities can also occur following TBI due to personality, emotional, and behavioral impairments, which can range from mild mood and personality changes to severe psychosis. The most severe impairments tend to be secondary to frontal lobe injury. Depending on the severity of injury, frontal lobe injuries can cause a range of disorders including impulsivity, irrational behavior, and apathy (Freedman, Kaplan, & Saddock, 1976; Auerback, 1986). Wood (1987) suggested that disinhibition is the most common outcome of frontal lobe injury, which results in coarse behavior, over-familiarity, inappropriate sexual behavior, gross errors of judgment, tactlessness, a marked indifference to the effects of one's actions on others (empathy), and a lack of concern for future consequences of behavior.

Lezak (1978) emphasized that various personality impairments after TBI cause social disabilities. The severity and type of problems are related to the nature of the injury and were categorized as: (1) impaired capacity for social perceptiveness, resulting in self-centered behavior in which both empathy and self-reflective attitudes are greatly diminished; (2) impaired capacity for self-regulation, leading to impulsivity and impatience; (3) social dependency, resulting in difficulties in planning and organizing; and (4) emotional lability and depression. Prigatano (1987) also classified changes associated with interpersonal problems and reductions in social skills. He listed the following broad areas as interfering with social relations: (1) anxiety or "catastrophic" reaction; (2) denial of illness or anosognosia; (3) paranoia and psychomotor agitation; and (4) depression, social withdrawal, and lack of motivation. Cognitive, behavioral, and emotional impairments can result in social interaction and social adjustment disabilities. Ylkvisaker et al. (1987) attributed reduced social skills to: (1) poor awareness and perception of social and communication events; (2) inadequate retrieval of rules of social interactions; (3) reduced ability to take alternative perspectives; (4) disorganization at the level of introducing, maintaining, and terminating topics of conversation; (5) disinhibition and weak self-monitoring of verbal and nonverbal behavior, which may result in the patient repeating information, making inappropriate and offensive remarks, and demonstrating poor comprehension for spoken utterances.

Functional rehabilitation programs focus on disabilities that affect an individual's ability to perform functional day-to-day activities in the home, community, school, and/or workplace. These programs are generally post-acute rehabilitation programs that are integrated community networks of care that include day treatment, transitional living, and supervised living in the community and home. The programs focus on behavior management, activities of daily living (ADL), self-management, substance abuse; social, academic, and vocational skills training; counseling; and family education. Clinical and psychological treatment occurs in a "real world" environment resulting in increased patient motivation and acceptance of treatment and improved generalization of treatment strategies (Cope et al., 1991). Fryer and Fralish (1989) and Ben-Yishay and Prigatano (1990) stressed a cognitive rehabilitation approach that focused on the elimination of impairments and the removal of barriers, which would improve functional disabilities that would reduce competence in everyday life. Treatment focuses on relating impairments to functional, community reentry activities in naturalistic settings. Treatment programs are usually individualized programs based on an individual's functioning in his or her own community during which clinicians provide knowledge, training, opportunities, resources, and encouragement to facilitate patients and families to become empowered to regain control, make decisions regarding treatment goals, and be as independent as possible.

In addition to individual treatment focused on an individual's cognitive impairments as they relate to functional activities, group therapy is frequently used to focus on the interaction of cognitive functioning and psychosocial behavior. Group treatment sessions will be of greater focus in the future. Group treatment sessions are less expensive and are effective for working on metacognitive/executive functioning skills. Groups can be designed to focus on interpersonal interaction, social skills, empathic abilities, and social awareness. Group sessions provide an opportunity for peer support, peer review, and the practice of compensatory techniques that were established in individual therapy sessions in a more natural setting (Adamovich, 1991). They also provide an opportunity to work on programmatic skills such as behavior appropriate to a situation, eye contact, turn-taking, use of gestures, affect, social distance, rate, and intonation, all of which are necessary skills for effective community reentry.

Handicaps

Handicaps following TBI that prevent the fulfillment of a normal life role involve physical independence, vocational status or return to work, return to school, return to family roles, and establishment of a support network. The ability to return to work or school is often used as an index of outcome following TBI since survivors are often young adults of work or school age with an average life span. Webb et al. (1995) studied 116 TBI subjects two years after injury. Their findings suggested that employment was the strongest contributor of improved quality of life.

Vocational/educational outcome after injury is crucial because it helps to reduce financial and emotional stress to brain-injured individuals and their families, as well as costs to society. A significant proportion of the costs of TBI can be directly linked to discouraging rates of postinjury employment (Wehman, 1990). Less than 30% of persons with TBI will enter or reenter the competitive work force (Brooks, McKinlay, Symington, Beattie & Campsie, 1987). As a result of their research, Wehman, Kreutzer, et al. (1989) found that TBI individuals who return to work often take less demanding or menial positions in a sheltered environment or do volunteer work. Many activities that were previously handled automatically and easily prior to the head injury will require a great deal of concentration and effort, with some tasks beyond current capabilities after the head injury.

Wehman, Kreutzer and colleagues (1989) developed the use of supported employment as a method of vocational rehabilitation. Supported employment emphasizes placement into actual competitive employment sites with necessary support to succeed. The support includes a job coach who works with the individual and the employer to educate coworkers and to make accommodations on the job (Willer & Corrigan, 1993). Sowers and Powers (1989) and Wehman (1990 & 1995) reported that supported employment is an effective treatment approach to return persons with TBI to work.

Wehman et al. (1989) suggested that key barriers to employability relate to cognitive issues such as new learning and memory, impaired self-awareness, preexisting and postinjury dysfunctional behavior including substance abuse, and other psychological problems. People lose jobs due to poor social or interpersonal skills, not due to deficient task performance. Getting along with coworkers, accepting criticisms and supervision, following instructions, completing tasks, and being consistent in attendance and attitude are qualities desired by most employers (Wilms, 1984). Haffey and Lewis (1989) listed barriers to job placement and retention following TBI, including cognitive-communicative disorders; emotional and social behavior control problems, psychomotor and cognitive processing slowness, and inadequate interpersonal/social skills.

Adolescents and young adults experience a disproportionately high incidence of head injury compared to other age groups. Residual cognitive and behavioral deficits, even if subtle, can interfere with successful return to school. Head-injured students who return to high school, adult education, trade schools, community colleges, or 4-year colleges and universities have unique needs. For example, they often need assistance getting to classes, organizing their notebook, planning their assignments, and recognizing problems when they arise; they may require cognitive remediation classes, socialization groups, transportation tutors, adaptive equipment and note-taking, counseling, and job placement. The key to success in educational endeavors often depends on the awareness of the institution of the unique learning needs following TBI and the willingness of the institution to accommodate resources to meet these needs (Ip, Dornan & Schentag, 1995). Return to work programs and work hardening programs, which have been developed for injured workers who have not experienced brain injury, can be adapted quite effectively for patients with TBI. They need to include vocational testing to determine specific job potentials, work hardening to train job-specific skills, job coaching, and on the job training and evaluation. Special considerations include determination of a program to meet each individual's needs, education of each individual regarding specific limitations, training of necessary skills including job application and interviewing and job-related strengths and weaknesses, and supervised work trials provided through job simulation, sheltered workshops, and community work sites.

Clinical Research

Impairment

The prediction of outcomes is complicated by the uniqueness of every injury. One person with a serious injury may appear to make excellent recovery while another person with a mild injury may show long-lasting deficits. Outcomes measurement is further complicated by the heterogeneity of the head-injured population with differing severities of neuropsychological and emotional deficits and differing premorbid factors such as age, educational level, family support, financial status, educational skills, and so forth. Recovery rates vary depending on variables such as age, severity of injury, site or location of injury, preinjury intellectual abilities, physical and mental status, time since injury, and postinjury social and medical support systems (Stratton & Gregory, 1994).

Cognitive rehabilitation refers to a systematic approach to (1) remediate specific cognitive impairments including perception, memory and reasoning (Gianutsos & Gianutsos, 1979) and (2) apply specific cuing systems to improve performance on specific functional tasks (Kreutzer, et al. 1989). Zangwill (1947) distinguished between direct retraining and substitutive retraining. Benedict (1989) referred to a similar dichotomy in his classification of restorative versus compensatory approaches to cognitive rehabilitation. This distinction is analogous to treating an impairment or a disturbance in the structure of an organism due to underlying pathology versus treating a disability or a difficulty in carrying out a functional act in a given situation (Diller, 1987). Restorative approaches designed to treat impairments have been highly criticized particularly with regard to their impact on functional outcomes. Substitutive or compensatory approaches are more accepted than restorative approaches because they are generally used to improve functioning in real life, daily activities.

To date, there is a lack of empirical evidence supporting the efficacy of cognitive remediation on the restoration of overall cognitive impairments, as well as the efficacy of direct cognitive retraining of specific impairments such as memory (Miller, 1990; Schacter & Glisky, 1986; Newcombe, 1985). Several investigators have found that basic skill training or treatment of general cognitive processes or cognitive impairments has resulted in an improvement in functional skills or a reduction in functional disabilities and handicaps (Ben-Yishay et al., 1978; Diller et al., 1974; Levin, 1991). Other investigators advocate for direct skill training of functional tasks following TBI (Wilson, 1984). Gordon and Hibbard (1991) suggested that a combined treatment approach with the treatment of cognitive impairments and treatment focused on specific skill training would result in the most efficacious approach to treatment following TBI. Combined treatment would include training of cognitive processes in conjunction with the learning of actual functional skills during simulated and community-based activities. Because it is impossible to train every skill that a person will encounter following TBI, the cognitive processes provide a basic foundation that cross over many skills and behaviors and are necessary if generalization is to occur.

Bond and Brooks (1976) administered the Wechsler Adult Intelligence Scale (WAIS) to 40 patients following TBI at 3-month intervals up to 2 years postinjury. They reported that most of the recovery on the cognitive impairments assessed by the WAIS occurred during the first 6 months post-TBI. Klonoff, Low and Clark (1977) reported that 76.3% of brain-injured children and adolescents made statistically significant improvements in the recovery of cognitive functions over 5 years. Thomsen (1981) evaluated a 44-year old male two years post-TBI and reported marked cognitive impairments. Twelve years later, he was found to have only mild cognitive impairments, suggesting continuous and gradual improvement in cognitive functioning for 14 years postinjury. Sbordone et al. (1995) and Terayama et al. (1991) studied 20 patients and 42 patients, respectively, following TBI and reported that the majority of subjects showed cognitive improvements for as long as 10 years postinjury.

Studies designed to measure the effectiveness of cognitive retraining reported statistically significant improvements in scores on a number of tests of cognitive impairments that were the targets of the remedial training. However, some investigators found that the cognitive improvements did not generalize and did not result in large, clinically meaningful changes in the patients' overall capacity in the functional domains studied (Prigatano, 1986; Scherzer, 1986; Ben-Yishay, et al. 1980; Ben-Yishay et al. 1982; Ezrachi, et al. 1983; Ben-Yishay and Piasetsky, 1985; Ben-Yishay and Piasetsky, 1986; Prigatano et al. 1984). These investigators concluded that cognitive remediation is meaningful only if it is embedded in and systematically coordinated with other rehabilitation interventions and if cognitive remedial exercises are done in such a way as to improve overall problem-solving abilities in a more holistic approach.

Kaplan and Corrigan (1994) conducted a study to determine if measures of impairment reflected disturbances in functional outcome after head injury. Ratings on the Orientation Group Monitoring System (OGMS) were compared to ratings on the FIM. The OGMS is a scale developed to prospectively measure cognitive impairment after coma to the end of PTA. The FIM is a measure of disability. Significant positive relationships were found between measures of cognition (OGMS) and measures of functional status (FIM). The authors suggested that cognition contributes to and can be used as a predictor of functional abilities.

Attention and memory impairments. Ponsford et al. (1995) reported the existence of memory problems, reduced speed of thinking, concentration difficulties, problems with planning and organization, impulsiveness, and decreased initiative in the majority of 175 TBI patients studied 2 years after injury. Memory remediation studies have been problematic because (1) the specific nature of the memory impairments have not been adequately isolated and (2) there is little agreement about how to define a memory deficit (Gordon & Hibbard, 1991). Ryan and Ruff (1988) found that attention/memory training was effective for mildly/moderately impaired persons with TBI, but not for a severely impaired group. This suggests that individual differences can be an implied variable in treatment effectiveness.

Glasgow et al. (1977) utilized the Preview, Question, Read, State and Test (PQRST) approach with a 22-year-old female with high-level memory deficits following a CHI 3.5 years earlier to improve the recall of written material. These investigators reported a consistent improvement in memory over a 10-day period with the generalization of the strategy to everyday life activities. Wilson (1987) also provided experimental evidence that the PQRST approach improved retention of written material. Other techniques found to improve attention and recall include reality orientation group therapy (Wilson, 1984), attention training (Sohlberg & Mateer, 1987), subvocal rehearsal of information (Parenté & DiCesare, 1991), and prospective memory training (Sohlberg et al., 1992).

Jones (1974) studied the effects of visual imagery in patients with right, left, and bilateral temporal lobe lesions compared to a normal control group. Recall was measured immediately and two hours later. Three lists were presented containing either no imagery potential, imagery potential with instructions and visual stimuli to prompt imagery, and the free generation of mnemonics with high imagery items. This investigator suggested that all groups evidenced increased recall with imagery with the exception of patients with bilateral temporal lobe lesions. Other investigators have reported good outcomes utilizing visual imagery to improve memory impairments [Wilson (1987); Patten (1972); Crovitz (1979); Kovner, Mathis and Pass (1983); Moffat (1984); Parenté and DiCesare (1991)].

Lorayne and Lucus (1974) studied the benefits of imagery on the recall of 19 brain-injured subjects and 22 non-brain-injured subjects. Paired associate learning tasks to associate names and faces were used to train visual imagery. Recall was tested at 30 minutes and one week. A three-stage visual training technique was used: image of single words, image linking the word pairs, and image linking the name with the face. The results suggested that memory improved with visual imagery for both groups at 30 minutes, but not at 1 week. Lewinsohn, Danaher, and Kikel (1977) found that the effects of imagery-facilitated recall did not last beyond a 30-minute retention interval.

Patten (1972) studied the benefit of associations for patients with dominant hemisphere lesions. A peg system was used in which 10 peg words were learned and 10 random words were associated to constant images. This investigator suggested that the Peg System technique resulted in improved memory for patients with TBI. Wilson and Moffat (1984) suggested that mild head-injured patients benefit from this technique; however, they suggested that patients with pronounced unilateral damage in either hemisphere may not benefit because they may fail to recall the words or the peg words due to difficulty forming verbal or visual associations.

Disability

Defining and measuring functional outcomes is difficult because goals and interventions that focus on community reentry and the reduction of functional disabilities are individualized. Cognitive remediation is a relatively new field and there is little research regarding the effectiveness of cognitive rehabilitation on the improvement of functional activities. Even though several studies have documented the efficacy of cognitive remediation, the lack of generalization, the slow pace of learning, and/or the finding of improved test scores, rather than improved functional behavioral outcomes (Gordon and Hibbard, 1991; Gloag, 1985; Hart & Hayden, 1986) are often criticized. Functional gains that improve the level of independence in day-to-day activities are used to judge the benefit of rehabilitation. However, many existing functional assessment tools lack reliability and validity. Adamovich (1992) conducted a study to compare the functional communication ratings of registered nurses and SLPs on the FIM. Fourteen patients with left-hemisphere brain damage and 14 patients with right-hemisphere brain damage served as subjects. The nurses assigned significantly higher FIM scores than SLPs when rating the communication of left hemisphere-damaged patients. However, the average ranking of patients from least to most impaired were the same for nurses and SLPs, who were measuring different skills. Follow-up analysis revealed potential reasons for the discrepancies including the fact that the nurses and SLPs were measuring different skills.

Adamovich (1994) conducted a retrospective review of admission and discharge scores on on the FIM scores for 479 patients representing seven diagnostic groups: left cerebrovascular accident (CVA), right CVA, TBI, other neurological disorders, and spinal cord injury. The TBI group improved significantly beyond the levels of the RCVA, LCVA, and other neurological disorders groups. The greatest improvements for the TBI group were found in the following categories: upper body dressing, memory, problem solving, social interaction, comprehension, and expression.

The most efficacious approach to the retraining of complex behavior is one that includes retraining of both cognitive impairments and specific functional disabilities. Training of cognitive processes provides the necessary foundation for the more complex task of learning new skills and behaviors. Adamovich (1996) conducted an investigation to compare communicative effectiveness in a traditional therapeutic clinical setting versus a functional community-based setting using a standardized scoring system (Nicholas & Brookshire, 1993) to quantify the informativeness and efficiency of connected speech. Thirteen brain injured subjects comprised three groups: LCVA (N = 5), RCVA (N = 4), and TBI (N = 4). A younger normal group (N = 4) and an older normal group (N = 5) served as controls. All groups, non-brain-injured and brain-injured, evidenced better performance during the functional community-based activity condition compared to the picture description task based on an increase in the number and percentage of correct information units (CIUs).

Schacter and Glisky (1986) successfully utilized domain-specific training to improve skills of head-injured individuals in functional tasks. This technique requires the matching of task demands to those in the real world by simulating what the person will encounter in the real world. An A–B: A^1–B^1 paradigm was used that predicts maximum positive transfer using training materials similar to the evaluation world. The investigators reported the successful training of functions at task after the tasks were simulated and trained. Schacter and Glisky (1986) and Parenté & DiCesare (1991) used an A–B: C–B intervention model such that the therapy and real-world materials differed. This training approach was found to improve reading. Persons with head injury were taught to scan the iconic store in brief glimpses that are too fast to rely on eye muscle control to scan the letters. This training improved performance on tests of reading comprehension and word recognition.

Several investigators (Wilson 1987; Patten, 1972; Jones, 1974) successfully trained persons with head injury to use memory strategies to improve functional memory abilities using an A–B: C–B transfer model, with phase B representing a particular memory strategy. Phase A involves specific items practiced in therapy and the response set B, which should work as effectively with phase C items encountered in activities of daily living as it did with the phase A items. Other investigators suggest that memory techniques such as imagery do not meet the maintenance and generalization criteria necessary for positive functional outcomes (Schacter & Crovitz, 1977, Schacter & Glisky, 1986, Lewinsohn, Danaher, & Kikel, 1977, and Glasgow, Zeiss, Barrera, & Lewinsohn, 1977).

External compensation techniques are an important intervention in the treatment of functional disabilities following TBI. Internal compensation techniques pertain to specific cognitive deficits. External techniques include environmental modifications or restructuring consisting of modifying any aspect of a person's environment to facilitate effective functioning. A variety of prosthetic memory aides have been successfully used by head injury persons as memory cues for daily activities including checklists, electronic signaling devices, telememo devices, and personal directories (Kreutzer, Wehman, Morton & Stonnington, 1988; Wilson, 1987, Parenté & DiCesare 1991; and Fowler, Hart, & Sheahan, 1972). Other investigators report that the successful use of external memory aids is limited because the head injured person forgets the aide or does not fully utilize it (Harris 1978; Moffat, 1984). Metacognitive skills or "knowing about knowing" (Flavell, 1979) are necessary to appropriately utilize compensatory strategies for impaired executive functions.

Several investigators reported functional improvements in social skills as a result of group treatment that addressed interpersonal interactions (giving compliments, asking questions) and verbal and nonverbal communication and pragmatic skills (Alexy, Foster, & Baker, 1983; Helffenstein & Wechsler, 1982; Brotherton, Thomas, Wisotzek & Milan, 1988; Gajar, Schloss, Schloss & Thompson, 1984; Schloss, Thompson, Gajar & Schloss, 1985; Giles, Fussey & Burgess, 1988; Hartley & Griffith, 1989; Sohlberg & Mateer 1990). Ben-Yishay et al. (1982) studied the prediction ability of a cognitive retraining program consisting of a small-group therapy approach designed to improve interpersonal communication skills, self-awareness, and acceptance of one's disability with regard to the post-rehabilitation vocational attainments of 20 brain-injured subjects. The results revealed that the group assimilation was the most potent predictor of post- rehabilitation vocational attainments.

Ponsford, Olver and Curran (1994) stressed the need for ongoing community-based support and assistance in dealing with practical difficulties and psychological problems that individuals experience after return to the community. These investigators studied 175 TBI patients who had undergone intensive rehabilitation 2 years after injury. Two-thirds of these individuals reported cognitive, behavioral, and emotional deterioration even though the majority of the individuals were physically independent and competent in personal and domestic activities of daily living. A third of the group still relied on assistance with community skills and transport. More than half of those who previously had a job were not working 2 years postinjury. Cope, Cole, Hall and Barkan (1991) measured the outcomes of 192 brain-injured subjects post-discharge from a community-based rehabilitation program that focused on ADL in as close to a real-world environment as possible. The results of this investigation comparing admission to postprogram discharge status revealed a significant increase in residence at home, competitive employment, productive activities, and overall independence.

Johnston and Lewis (1991) conducted an outcome study of 82 head-injured subjects one year after discharge from a residential community reentry program. Results revealed an improvement in independent living activities such as self-care, mobility, and communication, with a decrease in emotional distress and maladaptive social behaviors.

Handicap

Dawson and Chipman (1995) surveyed 454 individuals withTBI who were 13 years, on average, postinjury. The study was designed to investigate the determinants of three handicaps: physical independence, work, and social integration. The prevalence of long-term handicap was high with 66% of the sample reporting the need for ongoing assistance with some ADLs, 75% not working, and 90% reporting some limitations or dissatisfaction with their social integration. The determinants of the handicaps included age, gender, level of education (primary school or less), living alone, physical environmental barriers, and specific motor and personal care disabilities. Limited data were collected on behavioral dysfunction or cognitive impairment in this study. The only behavioral dysfunction included was learning disability and the only cognitive impairment included was memory difficulty.

Ip, Dornan and Schentag (1995) studied factors predicting return to work or school following TBI. They studied 45 subjects retrospectively with regard to sociodemographics, chronicity, indices of severity, physical impairment, and cognitive functioning. The generalizability of the predictive model was then tested on a sample of 20 subjects. The performance IQ score of the *Wechsler Adult Intelligence Scale—Revised* was found to be the most significant predictor of return to work or school. Other variables causing brain-injured individuals to be most at risk for not returning to work or school were age, a high percentage of reported alcohol abuse, and lower levels of performance on perceptual-motor tasks in psychometric testing. Brain injury severity as measured by the GCS and coma length, time postinjury, and physical impairment were not significantly related to return to work or school. Ponsford et al. (1995) studied 254 TBI patients 2 years postinjury. Their results revealed that the Disability Rating Scale score, GCS score and age correlated significantly with employment status two years after TBI.

Crépeau and Scherzer (1993) conducted a review of the literature and used a meta-analysis to combine and compare the results of available independent studies. Of 140 studies identified, 41 met inclusion criteria of studies limited exclusively to individuals with TBI, at least one quantitative predictor or severity indicator measure, and one measure of return to work. Among the pretrauma predictors, age was only related to work status in studies that included subjects over the age of 60 years, while gender and number of years of education had a minimal relationship to employment outcome. Global cognitive functioning measures, language and visual-spatial abilities, flexibility, emotional and behavioral indicators, aggressiveness, depression, global ratings of dependency, and driving status moderately correlated with employment outcome. Executive functioning and flexibility were highly correlated to employment outcome. Memory correlations with return to work were divergent among the 10 studies in the analysis. Pretrauma and early recovery predictors such as coma duration and PTA were only marginally associated with vocational outcome. Better predictors were postcoma activity level, posttrauma neurological and motor sequelae, and duration of hospitalization.

Ben-Yishay and Prigatano (1990) and Prigatano et al. (1986) suggested a model for a post-acute brain injury rehabilitation program that focused on return to work or school. The program focused on insight into disabilities and on emotional and behavioral problems that provide significant barriers to the rehabilitation of cognitive and physical disabilities. Their assumption was that a major cause of the inability to return to work was the lack of understanding and awareness of their higher cerebral deficits. Prigatano et al. (1984) reported that 50% of 18 graduates were in age-appropriate activities (work, homemaking, or school) at follow-up 8 to 33 months after program completion. Ben-Yishay et al. (1987) reported that 56% of 94 graduates were competitively employed and an additional 21% were in sheltered or supported work 12 months following program completion.

Malec, Smigielski, DePompolo and Thompson (1991) evaluated the outcomes of 29 individuals with brain injuries following a group-oriented treatment program. A comprehensive integrated postacute outpatient rehabilitation program similar to those described by Ben-Yishay and Prigatano (1990) was followed with these exceptions: participants were admitted continuously, not as a group; there was no set length of treatment; and work trials were provided in actual community placements rather than clinical work activities. From admission to program completion, those living with no supervision increased from 59 to 93%, those in transitional or competitive work placements increased from 7% to 59%, and unemployment decreased from 76 to 31%. At 1 year follow-up, independent living and employment gains were maintained. Individuals entering treatment less than 1 year after injury showed greater gains than those individuals injured more than 1 year prior to admission. However, both the early and late intervention groups made significant changes on the outcome measures. Other neuropsychological measures on admission did not significantly predict outcome. More extensive disabilities had a negative impact on outcome. Cope et al. (1991) and Johnson and Lewis (1991) also found outcome was related to severity of disability.

Fraser and Wehman (1995) suggested that the TBI vocational rehabilitation literature revealed variable outcomes due to methodological differences such as a lack of uniformity in severity of TBI, neuropsychological test batteries, operational definitions of successful employment outcome, pre- and postinjury, emotional and behavioral functioning, varying periods of follow-up, and vocational interventions. These authors suggested the need for a standardized protocol for assessing functional vocational outcomes.

Outcomes Measurement Needs

Future research should include controlled, well-designed clinical studies with regard to the efficacy or effectiveness of specific treatment techniques intended to improve functional outcomes. Controls should include consideration of age, educational skills, severity of injury, site or location of injury, preinjury intellectual abilities, emotional deficits, time postinjury, and postinjury social support. The measurement of functional outcomes will require the use of functional assessment tools that are reliable and valid. Future research should focus on a comparison of gains and cost-effectiveness in traditional versus nontraditional community-based programs. Programs that focus on return to school and work should be emphasized.

All practitioners will need to be knowledgeable of efficacy and outcomes research and will need to advocate for coverage of services with third party payers. University training programs will need to educate students regarding the interdisciplinary treatment approach, functional assessments, goal-setting, outcomes measurement, and group treatment.

Because TBI survivors tend to be young adults, educational and vocational programs are essential for successful community reentry. Education and vocational programs that result in the best functional outcomes should be developed. Work reentry programs should include work hardening designed to train job-specific skills and job coaching.

SECTION 2 : RIGHT-HEMISPHERE BRAIN DAMAGE

Connie A. Tompkins and
Margaret T. Lehman

RBD has the same etiologies as left-hemisphere damage. Cerebrovascular accidents are the leading cause of RBD, but relatively focal symptoms can be associated with tumors and some types of head trauma as well. Cerebrovascular disease is distributed fairly equally between the right and left hemispheres of the brain. Though we know little about the epidemiology of RBD per se, perhaps we can extrapolate from the existing data about stroke in general. The term "stroke" refers to a number of related disorders characterized by sudden onset of prominent and often persistent neurologic deficit due to impaired circulation in the brain. Mlcoch and Metter (1994) summarize much of the relevant epidemiologic data. They note an annual incidence of stroke in North America of approximately 1–2 per 1,000 people; each year in the United States, stroke leaves more than 250,000 people with permanent disability. At any one time, approximately 6 of every 1,000 people are living with the consequences of stroke. For a population of 265 million, this translates to more than 1.5 million people at any given time. It has been estimated that, in today's dollars, stroke care costs run at least $5 to 10 billion per year. Also important, as our population ages, is the fact that the incidence of stroke increases dramatically with age. Thus, minor increases in the mean age of the population result in large increases in stroke incidence.

Outcome Measures

Various aspects of cognitive and communicative behavior may be affected by RBD, though RBD does not inevitably lead to disorders in these areas. Indeed, the RBD population is a heterogenous one: only approximately one-half of patients with RBD will have communication disorders, and in those who do, the manifestations of cognitive-communicative impairments, disabilities, and handicaps will be quite varied (see Tompkins, 1995). That said, the most common *impairments* include, broadly speaking, those noted in Table 13–2 (Tompkins, 1995 provides a detailed discussion of these and other areas of impairment).

As Frattali notes (Chapter 3), there is no one-to-one correspondence between the concepts of impairment, disability, and handicap. Personal circumstances (e.g., social support, financial situation), attitudes (e.g., coping styles, religiosity), and affective responses (e.g., depression, anxiety) can play major roles in determining how disabling or handicapping any individual's impairments might be (cf., Schulz & Williamson, 1993). While few studies exist that attempt to predict functional outcomes from typical impairments after RBD, unilateral neglect[1] frequently has been linked to poor recovery of everyday life functions (cf., Chen Sea, Henderson & Cermak, 1993; Kinsella, Olver, Ng, Packer & Stark, 1993). In general, the major categories of impairment for the RBD population could possibly be associated with *disabilities* in the manner described in Table 13–2.

It is also possible that any of the impairments or disabilities in Table 13–2 could be linked with a variety of *handicaps* for patients and their families and friends. Adults with RBD may be stigmatized as bizarre, inappropriate, uncaring, humorless, lewd, or otherwise uncomfortable to be around. These kinds of judgments may take as much of a toll on family and significant others, perhaps to the greatest extent when patients are unaware of their own problems and of others' reactions. Affected persons, whether patients or families, may experience financial insecurity and social isolation due to loss of job and income, loss of friends, and loss of intimacy. Specific disabilities, such as limitations on independent mobility or on activities associated with safety concerns, can create burdens for families and friends who must assume additional responsibilities and oversight for the patients under their care. Such limitations may foster unwarranted dependency and passivity in the patients, as well as depression and other negative psychological responses in patients and their caregivers. Further, patients who are aware of their difficulties may harbor a variety of negative self-evaluations associated with, for example, loss of control, problems fitting in with others, and inhibitions related to fear of looking different. In addition, any affected individuals may confront spiritual crises at any time after the etiologic episode.

Tables 13–3 and 13–4 summarize the few available cognitive-communicative outcome measures for adults with RBD. Unfortunately, for the most part, the development and standardization of these measures are inadequate. Theoretical foundations for these measures are often underdeveloped and out-of-date. Standardization samples are typically small and poorly characterized, thus weakening assertions of reliabil-

---

[1] unilateral neglect, also called hemispatial neglect, visuospatial neglect, visual neglect, hemineglect, hemi-inattention, and other variants, is a constellation of disorders of spatial exploration/representation and selective attention. It has often been associated with communication difficulties after RBD (see Tompkins, 1995, for further detail).

Table 13–2. Examples of Potential Links between Impairment
and Disability for Adults with RBD

IMPAIRMENT	DISABILITY
Pragmatics; Social comprehension/ communication/ judgment	Difficulty participating in social interactions of all kinds (e.g., miss indirect "hints," emotional and nonverbal nuances, etc.; lose or alienate listeners through disinhibition & other unusual behavior; create embarrassment for family)
Discourse and conversation	Difficulty participating in social interactions (e.g., being misunderstood or misunderstanding others due to problems with cohesion, coherence, determination and designation of relevant information, turn-taking and topic control, etc.)
Reading and writing	Difficulty reading/writing for daily activities and interests (newspapers, recipes, instructions, phone books, schedules, messages/letters, checks, appointments, diary entries, lists, etc.)
Cognitive/perceptual, such as anosognosia, visuoperceptual and visuospatial problems, executive function deficits, neglect and other facets of attention, impulsivity	Difficulty participating in social interactions; loss of independence in daily activities due to families' concerns about awareness, planning, safety, etc. (e.g., driving or other independent ambulation, cooking, handling money, shopping, keeping records, keeping track of belongings); diminished participation in hobbies involving visual perception or construction (e.g., woodworking; painting) or musical ability; diminished concentration for various social, recreational, and vocational activities.

ity and validity. Reliability and validity data also are diluted by questionable evidence and methods for deriving them. Most of the measures in the tables are reviewed in some detail by Tompkins (1995). Tompkins (1995) also describes some nonstandardized tasks and approaches for assessing specific areas of impairment and disability in adults with RBD, and a variety of tools that could be adapted for the RBD population with appropriate cautions. Some examples include pragmatic measures originally devised for aphasic adults, such as the CETI (Lomas et al., 1989), CADL (Holland, 1980 and under revision); and Assessment Protocol of Pragmatic Linguistic Skills (Gerber & Gurland, 1989). (See Frattali, Chapter 3, for more information on CADL and CETI.) Several other potentially relevant connected speech measures include Nicholas and Brookshire's Main Concepts (1993a) and Correct Information Unit (1993b) analyses. Finally, some of the general disability measures described by Frattali (Chapter 3) also are routinely used with RBD adults (e.g., RICFAS), though for the most part it is not clear the extent to which their communication components were designed and validated for this population.

Some of the most common measures of health-related quality of life are reviewed in Chapter 3. Though there are currently no measures of communicative handicap that have been tailored for people with RBD, there are some encouraging signs that SLPs are beginning to consider the relationships between communication treatment and quality of life issues. For instance, O'Keefe (1995) highlighted the clinician's role in helping

Table 13–3. Measures of Impairment for Adults with RBD

INSTRUMENT	INSTRUMENT TYPE	ASPECTS OF COMMUNICATION/ RELATED AREAS ADDRESSED	ASSESSMENT METHOD	APPLICABLE POPULATION	STANDARDIZATION/RELIABILITY/ VALIDITY
Right Hemisphere Language Battery (RHLB; Bryan, 1989)	Overall measure cognitive/ communicative abilities	Metaphor comprehension, appreciation of humor and other inferred meanings, lexical/ semantic recognition, emphatic stress production, discourse production	0–1 scale for subtests, with notes regarding error types (not specified); rating 11 discourse parameters on 5-point scales	RBD	40 RBD patients; few details regarding sample characteristics. Reliability and validity data mostly lacking. Partial, though question-able, evidence of content validity; interjudge reliability for discourse subtest, and test-retest reliability.
Mini Inventory of Right Brain Damage (MIRBI; Pimental & Kingsbury, 1989)	Screening tool, cognitive/ communicative abilities	Visual scanning; gnosis; body image/body schema; visuoverbal & visuosymbolic processing; praxis; affective language; higher level language skills (humor and conversation; incongruities, absurdities, figurative language, similarities); emotion and affect processing; general behavior and psychic integrity (impulsivity, distractibility, eye contact)	0–1 to 0–3 point scales for subtests; examiner observation for neglect, emotion/affect, general behavior	RBD	Standardized on 30 ill-described RBD subjects. Content, construct, and concurrent validity are claimed but questionable. Good internal consistency. Interrater reliability, standard error of measurement (for total scores only) are reported but questionable.
Rehabilitation Institute of Chi-cago Evaluation of Communication Problems in Right Hemisphere Dysfunction— Revised (RICE-R; Halper, Cherney, Burns & Mogil, in press)	Screening tool for cognitive/ communicative abilities	General behavioral patterns, visual scanning/tracking, assessment & analysis of writing errors, pragmat-ic communication violations, metaphorical language	0–2 to 0–4 point scales for subtests; severity ratings for narrative discourse based upon information units	RBD, non-brain damaged adults	Standardized on 40 RBD patients. Interrater reliability high for trained investigators. Subtest cutoff scores accurately classify over 70% of RBD patients. Correlations of subtest items to subtest totals adequate for most tasks. No test-retest reliability information available.

Test	Purpose	Scoring	Population	Comments
New York University normative data (Gordon, et al., 1984)	Compendium of norms for standardized and experimental tests and evaluation procedures	Visual scanning/inattention; basic ADLs including address copying, oral word reading and scanning, and reading comprehension; sensory-motor integration; visual perceptual integration; higher cognitive and perceptual functions; language and cognitive flexibility (conceptual analogies, word fluency, Token Test, immediate story retelling); evaluation of affect state	Varies with each test/measure	RBD	Authors do not evaluate or describe psychometric adequacy of original measures. Do describe measures, special administration and scoring instructions, and normative data for large samples of RBD patients (total N = 385), stratified for age, extent of visual field deficit, and education when appropriate. Some test-retest reliability data provided.
Barrow Neurological Institute Screen for Higher Cerebral Functions (Prigatano, Amin & Rosenstein, 1991)	Screening tool for higher level cognitive functions	Speech & language abilities, orientation, attention/concentration, memory; visuospatial skills, affect and awareness	0–1 to 0–4 point scales	RBD, LBD, TBI	Assessment of performance by 14 RBD and 14 LBD patients; groups evidenced differential scores on language versus visuospatial subtests. Test-retest reliability poor for orientation & awareness, fair to good for other subtests. High interrater reliability for experienced testers.
Revised Token Test (RTT; McNeil & Prescott, 1978)	Auditory processing of de-contextualized stimuli	Auditory processing abilities; patterns of impairment such as problems with tuning in or noise build-up	15-point multidimensional scoring system to capture qualitative aspects of responding	RBD, aphasia, non-brain-damaged elderly	Standardized on 30 RBD males. Reliability and validity data are generally strong, though test-retest data are based on a small subset of subjects, and predictive validity is not addressed.

Table 13–4. Measures of disability for adults with RBD

INSTRUMENT	INSTRUMENT TYPE	ASPECTS OF COMMUNICATION/ RELATED AREAS ADDRESSED	ASSESSMENT METHOD	APPLICABLE POPULATION	STANDARDIZATION/RELIABILITY/ VALIDITY
Pragmatic Protocol (Prutting & Kirchner, 1987)	general index of pragmatic abilities in conversation	30 parameters representing 3 aspects of communication: verbal (speech acts, topic skills, turn taking, lexical selection/use, stylistic variations); paralinguistic (intelligibility and prosodies); and nonverbal (kinesics, proxemics)	rate parameters as appropriate, inappropriate, or no opportunity to observe, based on 15-minute, unstructured conversation	RBD, LBD, non-brain-damaged elderly	Interscorer agreement high for raters who received 8–10 hours of training and reached a 90% criterion during training.
Discourse Comprehension Test (DCT; Brookshire & Nicholas, 1993)	auditory or silent reading comprehension/ retention of narrative discourse	Stated and implied main ideas and details in narratives	patient answers yes/no questions	RBD, aphasia, TBI	20 adults with RBD in standardization sample. Extensive evidence/ arguments regarding validity and reliability, though test-retest and standard error data based on overall scores only, for extremely small samples.
Behavioural Inattention Test (BIT; Wilson, Cockburn & Halligan, 1987)	measure of hemi-inattention/ neglect; impairment and disability	Conventional & functional assessments of neglect. Conventional measures: paper/ pencil line bisection, cancellation, and drawing tasks. Functional tasks: reading menus & newspaper articles, dialing a telephone, navigating by map	score number of omissions for conventional & functional scanning, reading & writing tasks; 0–1 rating for copying/drawing tasks	RBD, LBD, non-brain-damaged adults	Standardized on 54 subjects with RBD due to CVAs; good interrater and test-retest reliability. High correlation between behavioral and conventional subtests; moderate correlation between behavioral subtest scores and general questionnaire completed by patients' therapists.

Test		Measures	Scoring	Population	Standardization/Reliability/Validity
Test of Everyday Attention (TEA; Robertson, Ward, Ridgeway & Nimmo-Smith, 1994)	measure of everyday attentional abilities	Sustained, selective, divided attention and attentional switching, using functional tasks such as map and phone book search, and counting floor indicators on elevator	Score number correct for each task, calculate dual task decrement for divided attention tasks. Some timed subtests	RBD, LBD, TBI, non-brain-damaged adults	80 unilateral CVA patients in standardization sample. Adequate parallel forms reliability on most tasks for which it was claculated, but poor for dual task decrement. Most subtests correlate with at least one of 3 scales rating ADLs or attentional behavior.
Rivermead Behavioural Memory Test (RBMT; Wilson, Cockburn & Smith, 1991)	measure of "everyday memory abilities"	Some pertinent aspects of everyday memory function: recalling a route, remembering a name, remembering to do something in the future (prospective memory), orientation, story recall, face recognition	0–1 or 0–2 scale for most subtests; number of items/ideas for recall tasks	undefined TBI & CVA adults, non-brain-damaged adults	200 brain-damaged subjects; normative data for 90. Perfect interrater reliability(N=19); moderate to good parallel form reliability (four forms available). Validity: low to good correlations with Wechsler memory scales; good correlation with behavioral observations of memory lapses.

Note: RBD = right brain damage; LBD = left brain damage; TBI = traumatic brain injury; CVA = cerebrovascular accident; ADLs = activities of daily living clients to achieve communicative skills necessary to, for example, achieve a feeling of wellness and health, enjoy work and leisure, take on life roles, appreciate culture, feel safe, be productive, and enjoy good relationships. In another example, Lyon and Cariski (1994) described a Communication Readiness and Use Index (CRUI) and a Psychosocial Well-Being Index (PWI) that they use in community reintegration efforts for adults with aphasia. The CRUI asks respondents how comfortably, confidently, independently, and effectively they approach communication with family members, friends, and strangers. The PWI focuses on more general questions about satisfaction with activities, self-esteem, and basic contentment. Though nonstandardized, tools like these could provide models for instruments aimed at RBD adults.

Clinical Research

Ten years ago it was rare for SLPs to assess or treat patients with RBD. Since then, there has been an explosion of such patients in clinical caseloads, and with good reason, considering the kinds of disabilities and handicaps that these patients may face as a result of their cognitive-communicative impairments. Unfortunately, though there has been an acceleration of research designed to understand the problems of RBD patients, treatment efficacy and outcomes research is woefully sparse. To date, published efforts have focused almost exclusively on treatments for unilateral neglect. Table 13–5 provides a brief description of available studies, most of which are summarized and evaluated in more detail by Robertson, Halligan and Marshall (1993) and Tompkins (1995).

This literature must be interpreted with caution due to a variety of limitations. First, the bulk of these studies represents a "one-size-fits-all" approach to treatment, providing specified numbers of sessions rather than crafting optimal treatment plans that unfold according to performance criteria (though, sadly, the former approach is becoming more common in these days of cost-conscious health care coverage). In addition, most of this work does not separate patients with and without visual field cuts, so it is not clear whether changes that are reported have had their impact on compensating for neglect or for visual field deficits. Further, many of the reports suffer from weak designs (e.g., case studies; simple pretest-posttest; AB baseline-treatment designs), a failure to demonstrate stability of performance before beginning treatment (particularly for patients in the acute post-onset phase), and/or lack of documentation of test-retest reliability for their outcome measures. Finally, few of these reports assess even short-term maintenance of gains or generalization to functional tasks and contexts, while none deals with social validation or other consumer satisfaction issues.

Occasional case reports of more generalized consequences of RBD are also available. For example, Klonoff, Sheperd, O'Brien, Chiapello and Hodak (1990) describe vocational, behavioral, and social outcomes of three well-educated RBD adults of working age, each of whom reportedly had significant deficits in awareness (anosognosia) and other cognitive-communicative areas. These patients were enrolled in an intensive, interdisciplinary rehabilitation program that incorporated individual and group sessions addressing physical, emotional, speech, and language function; volunteer work trials; and family education and support. Each patient demonstrated great strides in independent living and transportation skills; two of the three were able to resume living alone. Each returned to work, though in greatly reduced capacities. Their acknowledgment of deficits was improved, but their actions exposed a persisting dis-

Table 13–5. Chronological Summary of Efficacy and Outcomes Research on Treatment for Hemispatial Neglect in Patients with RBD

AUTHORS	TREATMENT FOCUS	DESIGN/SAMPLE	REPORTED EFFECTS
Lawson (1962)	Cuing for full spatial exploration; exploiting meaning in reading	Case reports of 2 subjects	Gains on reading material similar to that trained; poor generalization to other materials and tasks
Weinberg et al. (1977)	Automaticity and systematicity of visual scanning	Group pretest-posttest ($N = 57$)	Experimental group: gains on simple academic-type tasks & paper/pencil measures
Weinberg et al. (1979)	Visual scanning as in 1977 report; plus sensory awareness/ spatial organization	Same as above ($N = 53$)	Same as above
Horner (1980)	Visuospatial scanning and active task exploration/ participation	Case report of 1 subject	Clinically significant gains on simple naming, reading, and drawing/copying tasks
Stanton et al. (1981)	Self-instruction to cue attention to the left	Case reports of 2 subjects	Gains in oral paragraph reading; maintainance over 8 months in 1 case; anecdotal information re: generalization
Young et al. (1983)	Visual scanning and cancellation training; block design training for some	Group pretest-posttest ($N = 27$)	Gains on scanning, oral reading, copying; moreso when block design training added to scanning training
Webster et al. (1984)	Modified Weinberg visual scanning to emphasize wheelchair navigation/mobility	Multiple baseline across 3 subjects; 1-year follow-up	All decreased direct hits with left-side obstacles in obstacle course (though not sideswipes). Above baseline at follow-up.
Gouvier et al. (1984)	Visual scanning: stationary, mobile, and with verbal mediation or distance estimation	Case reports of 2 subjects; 6 week follow-up	Wheelchair navigation task: decreased frontal collisions with obstacles, especially after mobile scanning and distance estimation.
Gordon et al. (1985)	Same as Weinberg et al. (1979) plus visual perceptual training for visual exploration and examination	Same as Weinberg; and follow up 4 months post discharge ($N = 77$).	Similar to Weinberg at immediate evaluation; at follow up, groups equivalent.
Gouvier et al. (1987)	Visual scanning and search	Case studies of 5 subjects [baseline plus treatment(s)]; probes between phases	Gains on assessment tasks similar to training tasks. Erratic generalization to tasks of reading, writing, wheelchair navigation.

Table 13–5 *(Continued)*

Authors	Treatment Focus	Design/Sample	Reported Effects
Robertson et al. (1988)	Visuospatial search, scanning, and reasoning	Multiple baseline for 2 patients with RBD	Gains on paper/pencil tasks, telephone dialing, prose reading; little concurrent change on control tasks
Robertson at al. (1990)	Same as above	Group pretest-posttest; follow up 6 months later ($N = 36$)	No improvement for experimental or control subjects (after very little training)
Lennon (1991)	Clinician- & self-directed verbal mediation on wheel-chair transfer task	Modified ABACA design (alternating baseline/treatment phases) for 1 patient	Improvement on transfer with both treatments, anecdotal report that progress enabled home visits
Robertson et al. (1992)	Activation of and perceptual anchoring with left (hemiparetic) arm in left hemispace	AB design (baseline-treatment) with repeated probes, for 3 patients	Gains on cancellation tasks for all; in family-rated mobility for 2; telephone dialing/reading for 1
Pizzamiglio et al. (1992)	Visual-spatial scanning; covert and overt cues	Pretest-posttest ($N = 13$)	Gains on paper/pencil tests and functional observation measure (e.g., serving tea, using objects for grooming, etc); anecdote re: maintenance 5 months later for 50% of patients
Lennon (1994)	Visual cuing for obstacle course performance; tactile cuing for spatial awareness	ABAB withdrawal design implemented for 1 of 5 tasks, for 1 patient; 3 month follow-up	Task-specific treatment effects on obstacle course, maintained at follow-up. No effects of tactile cuing. Spontaneously improved baselines for other tasks.
Ladavas et al. (1994)	Visual attentional orienting, covert and overt conditions	Pretest-posttest (2 experimental and 1 control groups; $N = 12$)	Experimental group: gains on paper/pencil measures. Undocumented claims of generalization to reading/writing.
Antonucci et al. (1995)	Visual scanning, reading/copying, picture description	Pretest-posttest; a delayed treatment group first received general cognitive stimulation ($N = 20$)	Gains on paper/pencil tasks, sentence reading, functional evaluation scale for immediate group, and for delayed group after specific treatment
Robertson et al. (1995)	Self-alerting vigilance tasks	Multiple baseline by function/patient for 8 subjects	Gains on "baking tray task" (analog to arranging biscuits on a tray for baking)

Note. $N =$ total sample size, for all groups/conditions

connection between their intellectual awareness and the application of beneficial strategies. Significantly, all reported social isolation, family conflict, extended depressive reactions, and suicidal ideation.

The observations of Klonoff and colleagues (1990) suggest that neuropsychological and language/communication measures may not predict functional living skills, relationships to family, or return to work for such patients. They catalogued a variety of deficits, similar to the list of pragmatic and cognitive problems in Table 13–2, that were either not readily measurable on tests, or for which the rehabilitation specialists had underestimated the impact on daily function. Though this report is limited by its lack of design and its results cannot be generalized to a wide range of patients, it offers testimony to the pervasive disabilities and handicaps potentially affecting this population.

Outcomes Measurement Needs

From the discussion above, it is evident that there are major gaps in the area of outcomes measurement for adults with RBD and cognitive-communicative disorders. Basic research, treatment studies, and instrument development are all sorely needed. One of the most obvious gaps at present is the lack of well-controlled efficacy research to evaluate treatments provided to adults with RBD. Such research should incorporate a range of measures at each level of outcome; evaluate evidence of maintenance and generalization to functional tasks and contexts; and include social validation assessments for patients and family members.

It is also strikingly apparent that we need solid information about the potentially handicapping outcomes for RBD adults and the relationship of perceived handicaps to impairments, disabilities, and psychosocial attributes of patients and their families. Clinical experience and anecdotal evidence suggest that forays into this area should include family conflict and other psychosocial and vocational consequences of the patients' cognitive-communicative difficulties. It will be crucial to obtain the perspective of family members and significant others in addition to that of the patients, particularly because many persons with RBD may not recognize their deficits and/or may be poor judges of the consequences of their behavior. In addition, investigation and measurement of handicap should be done longitudinally, because potential problems may not become evident until patient and/or family have begun to experience them, perhaps some time well after discharge. Anosognosia will present special difficulties for gathering patient input about handicap. In evaluating the contribution of anosognosia to handicapping conditions for patients and families, we must keep in mind that unawareness is notoriously difficult to measure. As another challenge, anosognosia may recover only partially or in phases (e.g., Barco, Crosson, Bolesta, Werts & Stout, 1991). That is, patients may express awareness at some basic level (e.g., intellectual acknowledgement of discrete deficits) without corollary changes in behavior.

Another conspicuous problem at present is the lack of social validation and consumer satisfaction information, at all levels of measurement. Ideally, fundamental research on the nature of disability and handicap will help point the way for instrument development. In addition, clinicians should work with patients and families to the extent possible to identify their needs and wishes for the outcomes of treatment. We should also evaluate whether different patient/family units have different priorities for evaluating treatment outcomes. It is possible, for example, that some people will be less concerned than others with achieving independence in communicative activities and more welcoming of assistance from others that helps them to establish and optimize vocational and recreational communication opportunities. Again, these preferences may evolve over time, as patients and families confront new challenges. As we ascertain relationships among these levels of concern and measurement and explore priorities expressed by affected individuals and their families, we should resist the urge to impose a single, standard model of outcome planning and assessment on everyone.

To promote flexibility in tracking the functional and quality-of-life ramifications of treatment, we should work toward developing general tools that could be fine-tuned according to individually relevant functional contexts and consumer valuations. As an example, such a general tool might provide blank lines in which clinicians entered individually designated compensatory strategies and documented their acquisition, generalization, and maintenance in individually valued contexts. As noted above, we should begin by selecting treatment targets and approaches in consultation with the patient and family and in recognition of social and vocational needs, wishes, and responsibilities. Tailoring both treatments and target measures for specific patients would be ideal for documenting relevant outcomes. Of course, such an approach has drawbacks, as individuation eliminates the uniformity that is necessary to make comparisons among patients and to ensure measurement reliability and validity. Thus, we need to remember that different kinds of tools (e.g., individualized vs. general measures) will serve different purposes, each of which may be important for gaining a complete picture of treatment efficacy and outcome.

Two final cautionary notes will complete this section. First, there is little doubt that nonstandardized measures will proliferate as clinicians grapple with unmet needs for assessment tools. Indeed, nonstandard measurement is dictated by an individualized approach such as that advocated above. We need to be vigilant in recognizing the limitations of using and interpeting such tools and in maximizing their reliability and validity when we resort to them (see Tompkins, 1995, for suggestions). Second, we must exercise caution in analyzing and interpreting the ordinal data that derive from most of the existing functional outcome and quality-of-life measures. Because the magnitude of difference between ordinal scale points is unknown and potentially unequal for different pairs of scale comparisons and different patients, total scores or change scores generated from ordinal data may be meaningless (cf., Merbitz, Morris & Grip, 1989). There is great controversy over the analysis and interpretation of ordinal data (see Frattali, Thompson, Holland, Wohl & Ferketic, 1995, for further discussion). Some recommend statistical procedures such as Rasch analysis to compensate for the troublesome properties of ordinal data (cf., Wright & Linacre, 1989; McArthur, Cohen & Schandler, 1991), while others suggest that ordinal scores can be treated as equal interval data with little consequence (e.g., Labovitz, 1967). However, we concur with those who maintain that interval scale development will be essential to advance both the process and the products of outcomes measurement (Hamilton & Granger, 1989; Merbitz et al., 1989).

SECTION 3 : DEMENTIA

Michelle Bourgeois

The WHO (1989) defines dementia as a cognitive decline from a previously higher level of functioning and manifested by impairment of memory and two or more other cognitive domains. These domains include orientation, attention, language, visuospatial functions, executive functions, motor control, and praxis. The deficits should be severe enough to interfere at least to some extent with ADL, but not be due to the physical effects of stroke alone. Approximately 2 to 4 million Americans are estimated to suffer from dementia (Cross & Gurland, 1985), with the prevalence of one type, Alzheimer's disease (AD), ranging from 10.3% overall to 47.2% for those over age 85 years (Evans et al., 1989). Cummings (1987) has identified 11 principal dementia syndromes or subtypes, and the incidence of reversible dementias is estimated to be 11% (Clarfield, 1988). Of the irreversible dementias, AD and multi-infarct dementia are the most common and the acquired immunodeficiency syndrome (AIDS) dementia complex is the most recent syndrome associated with progressive cognitive impairment (Navia, Jordan, & Price, 1986). The challenges of differential diagnosis led to the development of a work group [the National Institute of Neurological and Communicative Disorders and Stroke (NINCDS) and the Alzheimer's Disease and Related Disorders Association (ADRDA)] that was charged with proposing uniform clinical criteria for AD. Their criteria for probable, possible, and definite Alzheimer's disease have been particularly important in the design and interpretation of treatment studies with this population (McKhann et al., 1984). (For a review of clinical definitions, diagnostic criteria, and symptomatology of dementia, see Molloy and Lubinski, 1991.)

From the perspective of the SLP, the diagnostic potential of this population has sparked considerable interest in the past 15 years, particularly with respect to the breadth of cognitive-communication impairments represented in the various syndrome subtypes. A sizable amount of literature has evolved in the pursuit of describing, documenting, and understanding the relationships among pathophysiologic changes in the brain and behavioral deficits of patients with dementia (cf. Bayles & Kaszniak, 1987). These efforts have resulted in a fair number of measures of impairment and disability designed specifically for use by speech-language clinicians. Overwhelmingly, however, the measures developed to date have served a descriptive/diagnostic purpose, and very few have been used as outcome measures for interventions. Either by design, or by default, many of the published measures are not intended to gauge the often subtle changes in behavior that result from treatment. As a result, outcome measurement is typically specific to the behaviors modified by the intervention. Nonetheless, interest in intervention has lagged behind the interest in diagnosis because of the inevitable and irreversible worsening of symptoms for which there is no known pharmacologic antidote. Recently, however, SLPs have been admonished to overcome the attitude of "therapeutic nihilism" regarding the intervention potential of patients with the progressive and irreversible condition of dementia; there is clearly a financial and humanistic need to shift our treatment paradigm from the traditional medical model based on assessing pathology and restoring/remediating dysfunction to a holistic and humanistic model based on maintaining function and preventing excess disability (Clark, 1995, p. 48). ASHA's Committee on Communication Problems of the Aging has called for increasing involvement in the evaluation and management of patients with AD, including the development of treatment programs designed to facilitate or maintain functional communication for as long as possible and of services designed to improve the quality of life/quality of care (ASHA, 1988 a, b). However, in stark contrast to this encouragement from within our profession, more recent fiscal and political initiatives are threatening to halt our burgeoning efforts with this population; an article broadcast by the Associated Press (Duston, 1996) used "speech therapy with Alzheimer's patients" as an example of Medicare fraud. This potential (funding) crisis necessitates a critical analysis of our abilities to design and implement robust and efficacious interventions that will make a significant difference in the lives of patients with dementia and their families. The first step of this self-analysis is to review our ability to document, or measure, change or outcome as a result of treatment.

Outcome Measures

Impairments

On the surface there appear to be ample measures of impairment for the specific cognitive-communicative deficits typical of dementia. The most pervasive symptom of dementia, memory impairment, has been measured extensively from various theoretical viewpoints. Deficits in explicit and implicit memory, episodic and semantic memory, and remote memory, as well as relatively "preserved" procedural memory skills, have been documented through a variety of performance-based tasks, such as lexical, semantic and verbal priming, category fluency, stem-completion, and motor-skill learning tasks, usually developed by researchers for a specific investigation (for an excellent review, see Salmon, Heindel, & Butters, 1991). Traditionally, memory functioning has been assessed with the Wechsler Memory Scale (WMS) (Wechsler, 1945) and the Revised Wechsler Memory Scale (WMS-R) (Russell, 1975). While there are data supporting the differentiation of normal and demented persons using the WMS-R (Haaland, Linn, Hunt, & Goodwin, 1983), Bayles and Kaszniak (1987) raise concerns about the limitations of the norms due to educational differences of the sample. Bayles and Kaszniak (1987) also provide an excellent review of several other instruments that have been used to document the memory deficits of patients with dementia, including the Benton Revised Visual Retention Test (BVRT-R) (Benton, 1974), the Guild Memory Test (GMT) (Crook, Gilbert, & Ferris, 1980), the Misplaced Objects Test (Crook, Ferris, & McCarthy, 1979), the Fuld Object Memory Evaluation (Fuld, 1981), and the New York University Memory Test (Osborne, Brown, & Randt, 1982). It is important to note that, while these instruments may be popular in diagnostic settings, their use as outcome measures has not been reported. The increasing interest in memory, both from a theoretical and an applied perspective, has led to the recent publication of measures of episodic or semantic memory (e.g., Pyramids and Palm Trees Test; Howard & Patterson, 1992), recognition memory (Recognition Span Test; Moss, Alberts, Butters, & Payne, 1986), retrograde amnesia (The Autobiographical Memory Interview (AMI); Kopelman, Wilson, & Baddeley, 1990), long-term memory (Doors and People; Baddeley, Emslie, & Nimmo-Smith, 1994), and everyday memory functioning (Rivermead Behavioral Memory Test (RBMT); Wilson, Cockburn, & Baddeley, 1991), to name a few. Similarly, these measures have not functioned as outcome measures to date.

Memory assessment is also one domain of many comprehensive measures of cognition (see below). Most cognitive measures include several brief memory subtests; for example, the Severe Impairment Battery (Saxton, McGonigle-Gibson, Swihart, Miller, & Boller, 1990) includes sentence, shape and color recall, and immediate and delayed recall of examiner name and objects.

Many measures of cognition, of which two domains must be impaired for a diagnosis of dementia, have also been developed. (For a recent review of assessments of cognitive function in the elderly, see Albert, 1994.) Brief standardized measures of cognition, or mental status, are most useful as a baseline measure against which other testing can be compared; therefore, these measures are often considered screening measures. Performance based cognitive measures include the Mini-mental Status Exam (MMSE) (Folstein, Folstein & McHugh, 1975), the Blessed Dementia Scale (BDS) (Blessed, Tomlinson, & Roth, 1968), the Short Portable Mental Status Questionnaire (SPMSQ) (Zilmer et al., 1990), Cambridge Cognitive Examination (CAMCOG) (Blessed, Block, Butter, & Kay, 1991), the Severe Impairment Battery (SIB) (Saxton et al., 1990), and the Test for Severe Impairment (TSI) (Albert & Cohen, 1992). These measures all cover a broad range of cognitive abilities, including memory, language (naming, repetition, auditory comprehension, writing), spatial ability/praxis, set-shifting/calculation, orientation, personal knowledge, abstract thinking, construction, perception, concentration, and attention. Although these measures are useful for quantifying cognitive performance in a standardized and reliable manner, the constraints of these global measures limit their usefulness as outcome measures for a number of reasons. First, age, educational level, and racial background of the patient being assessed are known to influence patient performance and accuracy of identification of cognitive dysfunction (Gurland et al., 1992; Mungas, Marshall, Weldon, Haan, & Reed, 1996). Second, some individuals, particularly those in chronic care facilities, cannot complete some test items because of physical disability (e.g., vision-impaired) or focal cognitive deficits (e.g., aphasia) (Teresi, Lawton, Ory, & Holmes, in press). Finally, because these measures are designed to be brief, most cognitive domains are assessed with a single item, severely limiting the potential to measure change due to an intervention.

Mental status rating scales, such as the Clinical Dementia Rating Scale (CDR) (Hughes, Berg, Danziger, Coben, & Martin, 1982), the Brief Cognitive Rating Scale (BCRS) (Reisberg, 1983), the Mattis Dementia Rating Scale (Mattis, 1976), and the Global Deterioration Scale for Age Related Cognitive Decline and Alzheimer's Disease (GDS) (Reisberg, Ferris, deLeon, & Crook, 1982), involve a comprehensive evaluation of patients' cognitive skills (e.g., memory, orientation, judgment, problem solving, community affairs, home and hobbies, personal care, psychiatric symptoms, and performance on psychometric tests) by a skilled clinician who may also query family and other caregivers about behavioral functioning. Rating scales translate cognitive impairment into stages of disability, which can be useful for classifying patients and predicting relative treatment outcomes. Again, however, these global measures may not be sensitive enough to detect subtle changes in patient performance.

The need to demonstrate the clinical outcomes of pharmacologic treatments for cognitive impairment has led to the development of several comprehensive assessments of cognitive and behavioral functioning. The Alzheimer's Disease Assessment Scale (ADAS) (Rosen, Mohs, & Davis, 1984) evaluates cognitive (memory, language, and praxis) and noncognitive (mood and behavior) functioning. A comprehensive, neuropsychological battery particularly sensitive to early stage dementia was developed and validated by the Consortium to Establish a Registry for Alzheimer's Disease (CERAD) (Morris et al., 1989; Welsh et al., 1994). CERAD includes subtests of fluency, naming, praxis, memory (free-recall and delayed recall), word recognition, and the MMSE. Another recent development has been the sponsorship by the National Institute on Aging (NIA) of a 30-site clinical trials consortium, the Alzheimer's Disease Cooperative Study (ADCS), whose major objective is the development of improved outcome measures for AD clinical trials (Ferris et al., 1996). Specifically, the study will determine the utility, sensitivity, reliability, and validity of newly developed or improved assessment instruments in six domains: clinical global improvement, cognitive function, behavioral symptoms, ADLs, the SIB, and Spanish versions of the measures. This timely study is especially needed for the validation of several subjective measures currently in use. The Clinical Global Impression of Change (CGIC) (Guy, 1976) is a subjective scale of clinician or caregiver impression of a patient's clinical change relative to screening, based on a brief interview with the patient. Other subjective measures of outcome include the Clinician Interview-Based Impression (CIBI) and the Final Comprehensive Consensus Assessment (FCCA), two rating scales used by Knapp et al. (1994) in an efficacy study of the drug tacrine. Unfortunately neither the psychometric properties nor the reliability of these measures has been reported to date.

The language and communication impairments of patients with dementia have been documented with a variety of comprehensive measures, most of which were designed for patients with language impairments due to focal brain damage [e.g., Boston Diagnostic Aphasia Examination (Goodglass & Kaplan, 1983), Western Aphasia Battery (Kertesz, 1982), Porch Index of Communicative Ability (Porch, 1967)]. The Arizona Battery for Communication Disorders of Dementia (ABCD) (Bayles & Kaszniak, 1987) is the only comprehensive assessment tool designed specifically to measure the receptive and expressive oral and written language deficits of patients with dementia and is therefore used extensively in diagnostic settings. Overall, comprehensive assessment tools are important in the differential diagnosis of language impairments due brain damage because they sample a wide range of behaviors efficiently (although the administration of an entire comprehensive measure in one sitting may not be possible due to the attentional limitations of patients with dementia). However, for the same reasons, they may be less useful as outcome measures. While it may not be realistic to use an entire comprehensive measure for documenting outcomes, researchers have used specific subtests of these measures as treatment outcomes with some success, as will be discussed below. To document impairments in specific language domains, such as pragmatics, discourse, semantics, syntax, and phonology, a wide variety of measures have been "borrowed" from the aphasia assessment toolbox and administered to patients with dementia. As a result, while some normative data may have been generated for patients with dementia, the limited sample sizes of these studies warrant cautious interpretation of test results. For an analysis of dementia patient performance on standardized language measures, such as the Peabody Picture Vocabulary Test (Dunn & Dunn, 1981), the Boston Naming Test (Kaplan, Goodglass, & Weintraub, 1983), the FAS Word Fluency Measure (Borkowski, Benton, & Spreen, 1967), the Auditory Comprehension Test of Sentences (Shewan, 1979), and the Token Test (DeRenzi & Faglioni, 1978), see Bayles and Kaszniak (1987). It is precisely because of the many limitations on the use of these measures with patients with dementia that Bayles and colleagues developed their comprehensive assessment battery (the ABCD) and standardized it with an extensive population of patients across the cognitive continuum. For other useful reviews of language and communication impairment measures, see Lubinski (1991) and Ripich (1991).

Disabilities

The assessment of the functional, everyday status of patients with dementia has been of paramount importance to clinicians and third-party payment sources alike due to the recognized limitations of the medical community to reverse or halt the degenerative course of dementia. Disability in this population can be documented for a variety of functional behaviors such as language, daily living skills, and problem behaviors, and in a variety of settings (e.g., hospital, work, home, and nursing home). While speech-language clinicians may be most concerned with measures specific to language functioning from the SLP's perspective, it is important to be familiar with measures of functional status from other disciplines, as there is considerable overlap in assessed domains, particularly language domains.

In the language arena, functional disability of patients with dementia has been assessed with measures specifically designed for this population, such as the Functional Linguistic Communication Inventory (FLCI) (Bayles & Tomoeda, 1994), those developed for patients with aphasia, the CADL (Holland, 1980), or one currently under development for adults with cognitive impairments due to a variety of etiologies, ASHA-FACS (Frattali et al., 1995). While the first two measures are performance-based, the ASHA-FACS and other measures of social language and discourse are observation-based rating scales [e.g., Communication Observation Scale for Cognitively Impaired (COS) and Communication Assessment Scale for the Cognitively Impaired (CAS) (Friedman & Tappen, 1991) and the Communication Effectiveness Index (Loman et al., 1989), and Discourse Abilities Profile (Terrell & Ripich, 1989)]. To date, the only published study using these language disability measures has been Friedman and Tappen (1991).

The need to assess the rehabilitation potential of chronically ill older people and the potential of institutionalized people to regain functioning led to the development of measures of ADL, including dressing, bathing, toileting, transfer, feeding, and mobility (for a review of measures, see Kane & Kane, 1981) and IADL, such as using the telephone, managing money, meal preparation, housework, and shopping (for a review of measures and critical analysis of disability assessment, see Kovar & Lawton, 1994). Because IADL items often include behaviors that necessitate communication skills (using the telephone) and higher order cognitive skills (money management, shopping), subtests of certain IADL measures may be relevant outcome measures for communication treatments. As visual and graphic cuing strategies are more widely used in rehabilitation programming, ADL measures will be appropriate measures of skill generalization. Some relevant ADL and IADL measures to become familiar with include the FIM (State University of New York at Buffalo, 1993), the Older Americans Resources and Services (OARS) (Duke University, 1978), and the Lawton & Brody IADL Scale (Lawton & Brody, 1969). More recent performance-based IADL measures include the Direct Assessment of Functional Status (DAFS) (Lowenstein et al., 1989) and the Structured Assessment of Independent Living Skills (SAILS) (Mahurin et al., 1991); the latter has subtests for expressive and receptive language, as well as social interaction skills.

The behavioral disturbances of patients with dementia, which could be considered as impairments, also impact on their everyday functional status. Teri and Logsdon (1994) review 28 different measures of behavioral disturbance; some of the more popular rating scales include the Behavioral Pathology in Alzheimer's Disease Rating Scale (BEHAVE-AD) (Reisberg et al., 1987), the Cohen-Mansfield Agitation Inventory (Cohen-Mansfield, 1986), the Nursing Home Behavior Problem Scale (Ray, Taylor, Lichtenstein, & Meador, 1992), and the Multidimensional Observation Scale for Elderly Subjects (MOSES) (Helmes, Csapo, & Short, 1987), which also measures cognitive and psychosocial functioning. Many of these measures are currently being used in studies of behaviorally based interventions and will provide important outcome data in the future.

Handicaps

The degree to which the impairments and disabilities of patients with dementia impact on their quality of life (QL), and the quality of the lives of persons in their environment, is one gauge of the handicapping effects of the illness. It is often assumed by clinicians that intervention efforts, even regardless of outcome, will be valued by the patient and their family, the consumers, and will positively impact the life of all involved. Interventions, by design, are planned to either eradicate, ameliorate, or lessen the impact of impairments and disabilities; therefore, it can be difficult to comprehend when the consumer is less than satisfied with the outcome or finds some side effect of the treatment more salient than the clinician-measured effects (Bourgeois, 1990). It is increasingly important that consumer satisfaction, as well as other measures of QL and social impact, are directly measured alongside of the intended behavioral changes of the treatment.

QL is a broad concept that Lawton (1991) has proposed include measures of objective environment, self-perceived QL, psychological well-being, and behavioral competence (health, functional health, cognition, time use, and social behavior). In their review of QL measures used in anti-dementia drug trials for AD, Howard and Rockwood (1995) found that only one, the Progressive Deterioration Scale (PDS) (DeJong, Osterlund & Roy, 1989), had been used as an outcome measure, and its content validity is questionable. The remaining measures reviewed (4 QL measures in 36 studies read) were not adequately validated with the population, suggesting the need for both conceptual and practical development in the assessment of QL in dementia. When QL is assessed, either self-report questionnaire or observational techniques are used, raising the question of the ability of patients with dementia, who may have memory and communication constraints, to reliably report their feelings. Many researchers circumvent the reliability of self-report data with observational measures and caregiver-completed rating scales of behaviors believed to approximate QL indicators, such as affect, mood, depressive symptomatology, and pleasant events.

Schulz, O'Brien, and Tompkins (1994) reviewed tools for measuring the emotions, moods, and feeling states of the elderly; while most were self-report measures, the Philadelphia Geriatric Center Affect Rating Scale (Lawton, Van Haitsma, & Klapper, 1996) is completed by a clinician after a 10-minute observation period, during which the duration of affective states (pleasure, anger, anxiety/fear, sadness, interest, and contentment) are rated on a 5-point scale. Similarly, ratings of depressive symptomatology are obtained from interviews with both patients and staff members for the Cornell Scale for Depression in Dementia (Alexopoulos, Abrams, Young, & Shamoian, 1988). The Dementia Mood Assessment Scale (Sunderland et al., 1988) is a clinician-completed rating scale that combines direct observations of the patient in different settings and a semistructured interview. An instrument that measures behaviors that have the potential to contribute to pleasant experiences of patients with dementia is the Pleasant Events Schedule-AD (PES-AD) (Teri & Logsdon, 1991). This caregiver-completed inventory of pleasant experiences rates each of 54 items on their frequency, availability, and enjoyability during the past month and has the potential to document change in patients' positive experiences.

The impact of a dementing illness on the patient's caregivers cannot be minimized when evaluating the contributions of social and environmental factors to QL indicators. There is significant literature regarding the caregivers' role in maintaining the patient in quality surroundings and the impact caregiving has on the care provider (for reviews of the impact of dementia on caregivers, see Bourgeois, 1994; see Deimling, 1994 for a review of caregiving assessment tools). Multidimensional, comprehensive assessments of caregiving functioning relate caregiving variables such as age, gender, relationship to patient, competing responsibilities, and living arrangements to self-reported effects of caregiving, such as physical and mental health, burden or strain, and caregiving satisfaction. Although caregiving for any disabled individual is burdensome, the range, frequency, and severity of cognitive deficits and problem behaviors associated with dementia can produce stresses that are physically demanding and unremitting (George & Gwyther, 1986). As level of patient dysfunction increases, caregiver outcomes such as perceived burden and depression have been found to increase (Schulz & Williamson, 1991). As a result, a plethora of caregiving interventions have appeared in the literature (for reviews, see Bourgeois, Schulz, & Burgio, 1996; Knight, Lutszky, & Macofsky-Urban, 1993; and Zarit & Teri, 1992), whose outcomes measurement issues have sparked considerable debate and collaboration among research programs (Ory & Schulz, 1996). While it is too early for strong causal relationships to be seen, a working hypothesis of caregiver interventionists is that a happier, or less burdened, caregiver will make for a happy, or more contented, patient and an overall improvement in the QL of all members of the patient's environment.

Unfortunately, caregivers' QL may turn out to be resistant to changes of a magnitude that are measurable or clinically significant. In spite of efforts to ameliorate the burdens of caregiving, until the caregiver is fully relinquished from the caregiving role (i.e, by the death of the patient), it may be unrealistic to expect to change much, if anything, with intervention efforts. Therefore, researchers and clinicians are beginning to look at measures of consumer satisfaction as a way to gauge intervention success. Questionnaires, rating scales, and exit interviews are providing some social validity data from which outcome effects can be evaluated (Bourgeois, Schulz, & Burgio, 1995; McMahon & Forehand, 1983; Wolf, 1978). In contrast, intervention studies in nursing homes have shown positive effects on caregivers due to delivering the intervention; nurses' aides reported increased job satisfaction when delivering reality orientation and reminiscence therapy to residents with dementia (Baines, Saxby, & Ehlert, 1987; Powell-Proctor & Miller, 1982).

Clinical Research

Given that SLPs have only seriously considered the diagnostic potential of the population with dementia within the past decade, it is not surprising that therapeutic efforts have lagged behind. Nevertheless, patients with dementia have participated in a wide variety of therapeutic regimens in many treatment settings; reviews of literature dating from the 1960s and 1970s revealed interventions delivered by nurses, social workers, psychologists, recreation and occupational therapists, and families that suggested changes, and sometimes improvements, in patients' speech and language behaviors (Bourgeois, 1991; Clark, 1995; Clark & Witte, 1991; Miller & Morris, 1993). As Clark and Witte (1991) outlined, the range of treatments include reality orientation, psychotherapy, resocialization, remotivation, pet therapy, reminiscence and validation therapy, operant/behavioral techniques, memory retraining and cognitive stimulation, external memory aids, sensory training, and music, dance, and art therapies, with reported effects on environmental awareness, emotional security, cognitive functioning, communication skills, appropriate behavior, physical functioning, and social skills. Unfortunately, this literature is plagued by methodological and design flaws that seriously limit the validity of techniques for which there has not been much systematic development and programmatic evaluation, with the exception of reality orientation (Greene, 1984) and reminiscence therapy (see Berghorn & Schafer (1987) and Taft & Nehrke (1990) for a review of 90 group-designed studies). Studies have either used group designs to evaluate poorly described and implemented procedures with mixed-etiology populations or small-N designs, and even case studies, with questionable generalizability. This diversity of therapeutic efforts, while suggestive of potential benefits to patients, requires considerable attention to the development of theoretically driven, programmatic and systematic evaluations of well-described and implemented interventions for progress to be made in identifying treatments with robust outcomes. Several researchers are currently working on interventions in a programmatic fashion and their efforts will be described below.

The focus of this book on impairment, disability, and handicap as it relates to outcomes and intervention efficacy requires some understanding on the part of the reader that the state of the current literature precludes a cleanly categorized analysis; there simply is too much overlap in impairment/disability and disability/handicap outcomes in published studies. In fact, some studies, in an effort to report any significant findings, use a multiple outcomes assessment strategy to cover all the bases, rendering uneven results difficult to interpret. Nevertheless, recent intervention studies will be described below relative to the major predicted, or desired, treatment outcomes.

Impairments

Interventions designed specifically to reduce the impairment of dementia have taken either a pharmacologic or behavioral approach to treatment. In spite of the fact that effective therapeutic interventions based on emergent genetic and environmental risk factors are not yet available, pharmacologic interventions designed to modify pathophysiologic processes are beginning to demonstrate some progress in ameliorating the cognitive impairments associated with dementia (Mohs, 1995). Several recent multicenter clinical trials of the cholinesterase inhibitor tacrine have demonstrated reductions, albeit small, in the severity of cognitive symptoms in AD patients and related functional improvements (Davis et al., 1992; Farlow et al., 1992). Their major dependent measures have typically been performance-based cognitive instruments (e.g., MMSE, ADAS, and CERAD) that globally assess changes in memory, language, praxis, and orientation. However, the clinical significance of small changes on these tests are not always obvious, necessitating a "dual outcome" strategy. In addition to cognitive measures, several measures of the global severity or change in the patient as determined through office-interactions with a trained clinician are commonly used

(CGIC, CBI, and FCCA). Reliability problems with this approach are undeniable and are being addressed.

Other efforts to remediate memory impairments, as measured by improved scores on standardized cognitive measures, have shown initially promising results and then disappointing long-term regression. For example, Quayhagen and Quayhagen (1989), in their first study of a home-based program of cognitive stimulation, found that experimental subjects maintained their levels of cognitive and behavioral functioning during the 8-month study relative to comparison group patients who deteriorated on measures of cognition [Dementia Rating Scale (DRS; Coblentz et al., 1973) and Wechsler Memory Scale, Form II (Stone et al., 1946)] and behavioral functioning [the Memory and Behavior Problems Checklist (MBPC; Zarit et al., 1980)]. In a subsequent study, Quayhagen and colleagues (1995) evaluated the long-term effects of a 12-week cognitive remediation intervention using the DRS, WMS-R, FAS, and the MBPC. Experimental subjects improved in cognitive and behavioral functioning immediately postintervention when compared to the control and placebo groups, but subjects returned to their former level of functioning by the ninth month postintervention. Similarly, Scherder, Bouma, and Steen (1995) demonstrated significant improvements in visual short-term, visual long-term, and verbal long-term memory, and fluency in 16 AD patients who received 30 minutes per day for 6 weeks of tactile stimulation by massage (on the patient's back between Th1 and Th12) when compared to a placebo control group who received false electro stimulation in the same area. However, after 6 weeks without stimulation no noticeable effects remained. Findings of cognitive improvements resulting from cognitively based treatments are reported by Camp, Foss, O'Hanlon, and Stevens (1995), who have programmatically evaluated a spaced-retrieval method of learning and retraining information by recalling that information over increasingly longer periods of time. Believed to engage a relatively intact memory process, implicit memory, spaced-retrieval procedures have been used to train tasks such as face-name association (Foss & Camp, 1994), object-location associations (Camp & Stevens, 1990), and calendar use (Camp, Foss, Stevens, & O'Hanlon, 1995).

In an effort to ameliorate the comprehension impairments of patients with AD, Obler, Obermann, Samuels, and Albert (1985) investigated the use of written input with nine early-middle- to middle-staged patients. Eight of the nine patients demonstrated improved comprehension of the comprehension sections of the *Boston Diagnostic Aphasia Examination* (Goodglass & Kaplan, 1972) when they were administered as written stimuli alone or in combination with auditory input. This demonstration of improvement in an impaired language function through appropriate cuing certainly has potential functional, disability-reducing applications (i.e., ADL). In contrast, the demonstration of improved recall of numbers in a list by subjects who received a multicomponent cognitive skills training intervention (Beck et al., 1988) stretches the imagination for functional applications and should raise cost/benefit concerns.

Disabilities

Efforts to reduce the disabilities resulting from dementia have spawned a larger pool of treatment studies comprised of either communication-enhancing or disruptive behavior-reducing interventions. The memory and language impairment effects of dementia render the individual communication-disabled, particularly with respect to conversational behavior. When the disabling effects of dementia are the focus of intervention, measurement of outcomes is largely behavior-based; that is, the performance of targeted or trained behaviors is observed and monitored for change and not performance on a global measure of cognition or language. Stimulus-cuing interventions predominate, although caregiver-training approaches are also popular. Bourgeois (1990, 1992, 1993) and Bourgeois and Mason (1996) have demonstrated that memory aids (collections of picture and sentence stimuli in a book or wallet format) are used by patients to prompt significantly more statements of fact (including novel statements) and fewer ambiguous utterances during conversations. Continued use of the memory aids in a variety of settings, including adult day care centers, nursing homes, and other social situations, was thought to contribute to long-term maintenance effects; in the Bourgeois (1992) study several subjects were reassessed on conversational and cognitive measures 24- or 30-months postintervention and demonstrated rates of conversational behaviors virtually identical to their earlier rates, but significant decline in cognitive functioning as measured by the MMSE. Pragmatic behaviors of conversational interactions were the focus of the Bourgeois (1993) study in which patient dyads were evaluated during conversational interactions with and without their personalized memory aid. Turn-taking, topic maintenance, topic redirection, and partner prompting behaviors were significantly more frequent during sessions with memory aids. Bourgeois has systematically evaluated a variety of intervention features in this series of studies, including training, cognitive severity, setting, intervention agent, and stimulus dimension variables in an effort to develop an efficacious and robust treatment strategy. Generalized application of this treatment approach to other communicative disabilities produced the Bourgeois et al. (1997) study of the reduction of disruptive vocalization (i.e., repetitive questions and demands) using written stimulus cues in the form of index cards, memo boards, and memory book pages. An extension of this work is the recently funded, group-design study of the effects on the quality and quantity of communicative interactions between patients with dementia and nursing aides using written stimulus cues in a variety of formats (Bourgeois, 1996). In addition to disability outcome measures (i.e., frequency of positive and negative conversational behaviors), this study incorporates several "handicap" (i.e., QL) measures such as the Philadelphia Geriatric Center Affect Rating Scale (Lawton et al., 1996) and the Nursing Home Satisfaction Scale (Kane, Reigler, Bell, Potter, & Koshland, 1982), and measures documenting the effects of the intervention on caregivers (attitude, morale, satisfaction).

In another study of treatment for communicative disability, Santo Pietro and Boczko (1994) developed a "Breakfast Club" intervention for nursing home residents with dementia, which was compared with a traditional group conversational intervention. Subjects in the experimental group demonstrated increases in cross-conversation, questioning, use of each other's name, eye contact, and topic maintenance relative to the traditional group. In addition, increases in some subscales of the ABCD were found as a function of participation in the Breakfast Club, suggesting the possible generalized effect of structured interactions on the maintenance of cognitive skills. Subjects appeared to benefit from controlled stimulation by maintaining cognitive and communicative functioning in a nursing intervention designed to evaluate the effects of "planned walking" on nursing home residents. Friedman and Tappen (1991) conducted a group-designed evaluation of two communication interventions; one group of subjects participated in daily conversational interactions with staff while walking around the facility and the other group conversed with staff while seated at a table in a quiet room. Using staff-completed rating scales, COS and CAS, the results indicated that residents in the experimental walking group were perceived to be significantly more alert, more communicative, and functioning at a higher level than the sedentary group. However, the absence of reliability measures and environmental measures limits the interpretability of this study.

Other disability indicators, such as disruptive vocalization, finger-to-mouth self-stimulation, and agitation have been addressed in a variety of music-based interventions. Casby & Holm (1994) successfully reduced the disruptive vocalizations of nursing home residents with individualized musical selections delivered via headphones. Norberg et al (1986) decreased the frequency of finger-to-mouth self-stimulation with a music intervention; and Goddaer and Abraham (1994) reduced residents' level of agitation (as measured by the Cohen-Mansfield Agitation Inventory) during meals by playing music in the dining room.

Handicaps

Interventions designed to address the handicaps associated with dementia have been far fewer. Treatments directly addressing the QL of patients with dementia include the Teri and Uomoto (1991) study to reduce patient depression by training caregivers to engage the patient in pleasant activities and the Lund, Hill, Caserta, and Wright (1995) study of the effects on patients of watching "Video Respite" tapes. Teri and Uomoto (1991) demonstrated significant decreases in depressive symptomatology as measured by the Beck Depression Scale (Beck et al., 1961) and the Hamilton Depression Scale (Hamilton, 1960) due to measured increases in the frequency and duration of pleasant activities of patients (which included the viewing of Lund's Video Respite tapes). Preliminary results of an evaluation of Video Respite tapes on patients with dementia revealed that 84% of patients remained seated during the tape, were paying attention, and were verbally responding (Lund et al., 1995). Caregivers' anecdotal reports of agitated patients being calmed within minutes of listening to the tape, of viewers smiling, laughing, and making comments like "Thank-you," support the claims of improved QL in these patients. Lord and Garner (1993) conducted an evaluative study of the relative effects on mood and social interaction of three different interventions: Big Band music, puzzles, and drawing/painting during recreation periods. Results showed that subjects in the music group were judged to be more alert and happier than subjects in the other two groups, and these effects persisted after the sessions were over. In contrast, while it might be assumed that patients whose caregivers received training in functional communication strategies that improved their attitude toward the patient and their knowledge of AD, and increased their use of appropriate communication strategies would benefit from a more competent caregiver (Ripich, 1994), one can never be sure without measuring directly the effects of the intervention on the patient.

Outcomes Measurement Needs

It should be obvious from the above review of outcome measures and intervention studies in dementia that additional, quality work is needed across the board. However, pockets of strength exist. The most developed measurement area is the impairment domain, reflecting the skills and training of SLPs. As diagnosticians, we have more fully developed tools for describing and differentiating neurologically based language impairments, and we adopt as our own a range of measures from our colleagues in neuropsychology. As outcome measures, however, these assessment tools fall short in their ability to measure small and/or subtle changes as a result of intervention; too many of them are global assessments, limiting subjects to one performance exemplar in some cases. Others sample skills that may have little to no functional importance; unless there is a strong theoretical or functional rationale, measurement of some behaviors borders on frivolous. At the very least, unless these sorts of measurement issues are taken seriously, interventions are doomed to failure, or mediocre effects at best. An example of the struggle to develop sensitive measures is the memory-enhancing drug studies that have resorted to a multiple outcomes strategy, using standardized cognitive measures and more subjective, clinician-impression measures in order to show some effects with some patients. In some respects, the intervention technology is advancing at a faster rate than improvements in measurement.

In the disability and handicap measurement domains, a wide variety of tools exist to measure an even wider range of behaviors; however, many of them lack adequate psychometric validation or have not been used enough to provide interpretable data. More handicap measures are particularly needed; there is the potential to demonstrate significant outcomes due to intervention with low functioning individuals if affective variables, such as smiling, laughing, and calm demeanor, can be documented reliably. However, SLPs will be at a significant disadvantage if they limit themselves to specific language and communication measures for measuring intervention outcomes. Increasingly funding agents are demanding more robust and significant treatment effects, effects that generalize to a range of related behaviors, and effects that impact on skills of importance to consumers. It will be futile to present data documenting the increased frequency of conversational behaviors in a therapy setting unless there is supplemental data documenting improved conversational behavior in the dining room or hallways, and with family and staff on all shifts, and further evidence of reduced agitation or disruptive behavior. This necessitates an active exploration of all available measures, across disciplines, even if the result is the decision to develop a new measure (eg., the ASHA-FACS). While many of the measures of disability and handicap utilize rating scales, it will be increasingly important to develop performance-based and observational-based assessments. This is particularly relevant to outcomes assessment of specific treatments. As many of the treatment studies demonstrated, the most likely indicator of change as a result of treatment is the direct measurement of changes in the targeted behaviors. Including relatively indirect measures of treatment outcome may be beneficial in some instances, such as Bourgeois' documentation of maintenance of specific conversational behaviors (eg., statements of fact) in spite of concomitant decline in MMSE scores overtime.

While there is a great need for quality intervention studies from a variety of theoretical perspectives, it is important to take inventory of the many existing studies and build on them in a systematic way. Attention to design, methodology, and implementation issues is of paramount importance; many anecdotal findings could yield robust outcomes under the optimum experimental conditions. However, novel treatments should not be rushed into group design evaluations without first conducting carefully controlled efficacy studies with well-defined subjects and treatment procedures under microanalytic scrutiny. Single-subject methodology is ideally suited to developmental efforts of this sort.

CONCLUSION

Outcome measurements of cognitive-communication disorders following TBI, RBD, and dementia were reviewed pertaining to resulting impairments, disabilities, and handicaps as defined by the WHO. The need for additional research was identified, particularly with regard to the development of treatment techniques designed to improve functional outcomes and reduce disabilities and handicaps. Research is also needed to enable the early identification of persons most likely to return to home, work, and/or school, and the cost effectiveness of treatment programs.

Determining outcome predictors should improve the rehabilitation process, resulting in improved quality of life for persons with neurogenic disorders. However, caution must be exercised to avoid oversimplifying the complex variations that occur in people with neurologic deficits. It is possible that reimbursement for rehabilitation services will be based on outcome predictors. If care is not taken to account for the diverse nature of the disorders, individuals may be unjustly denied necessary services.

REFERENCES

Adamovich, B.L.B. (1991). Cognition, Language, Attention, and Information Processing Following Closed Head Injury. In P. Wehman & S. Kreutzer (Eds.), *Cognitive Rehabilitation for persons with traumatic brain injury.* Baltimore: Paul Brookes Publishing Company, 1991.

Adamovich, B.L.B. (1992). Pitfalls in Functional Assessment: A Comparison of FIM Ratings by Speech-Language Pathologists and Nurses. NeuroRehabilitation, Reading, MA: Andover Medical Publishers, Inc., November, 1992, 2(4):42–51.

Adamovich, B.L.B. (1992). The Role of the Speech-Language Pathologist in the Evaluation and Treatment of Adolescents and Adults with Traumatic Brain Injury. In B.B. Adamovich, (Ed.), American Speech-Language-Hearing Association, Special Interest Division: *Neurophysiology and Neurogenic Speech and Language Disorders,* 2,1:1–6, July, 1992.

Adamovich, B.L.B., & Henderson, J. (1992). Scales of Cognitive Ability for Traumatic Brain Injury, (SCATBI), Chicago: The Riverside Publishing Company.

Adamovich, B.L.B. (1994). *"Functional Outcomes: Assessment and Intervention Considerations"* (unpublished).

Adamovich, B.L.B. (1996). *Comparisons of connected speech effectiveness using traditional therapeutic methods and functional community based activities with neurologically impaired adults.* Article presented at the Clinical Aphasiology Conference, Newport, RI.

Albert, M., & Cohen, C. (1992). The test for severe impairment: An instrument for the assessment of patients with severe cognitive dysfunction. *Journal of the American Geriatrics Society, 40,* 449–453.

Albert, M. S. (1994). Brief assessments of cognitive function in the elderly. In M. P. Lawton & J. A. Teresi (Eds.), *Annual Review of Gerontology and Geriatrics Focus on Assessment Techniques 4,* (pp. 93–106). New York: Springer.

Alexy, W.D., Foster, M., and Baker, A. (1983). Audio-visual feedback: An exercise in self-awareness for the head injured patient. *Cognitive Rehabilitation, 1*(6), 8–10.

Alexopoulos, G. S., Abrams, R. C., Young, R. C., & Shamoian, C. A. (1988). Cornell scale for depression in dementia. *Biological Psychiatry, 23,* 271–284.

American Speech-Language-Hearing Association, Task Force on Cognitive-Communicative Impairments. (1987). *Working draft of the role of speech-language pathologists in the habilitation and rehabilitation of cognitively impaired individuals. Unpublished manuscript.*

ASHA Committee on Communication Problems of the Aging. (1988a). The roles of speech-language pathologists and audiologists in working with older persons. *Asha, 30,* 80–84.

ASHA Committee on Communication Problems of the Aging. (1988b, March). Provision of audiology and speech-language pathology services to older persons in the nursing home. *Asha,* 72–74.

Antonucci, G., Guariglia, C., Judica, A., Magnotti, L., Paolucci, S., Pizzamiglio, L. & Zoccolotti, P. (1995). Effectiveness of neglect rehabilitation in a randomized group study. *Journal of Clinical and Experimental Neuropsychology, 17,* 383–389.

Auerback, S.H. (1986). Neuroanatomical correlates of attention and memory disorders in traumatic brain injury: an application of neurobehavioral subtypes. *Journal of Head Trauma Rehabilitation, 3:* 1–12.

Ayres, A.J. (1966). *Southern California Figure-Ground Visual Perception Test.* Los Angeles: Western Psychological Services.

Baddeley, A., Emslie, H., & Nimmo-Smith, I. (1994). *Doors and People.* Bury St. Edmunds, Suffolk, England: Thames Valley Test Company.

Baines, S., Saxby, P., & Ehlert, K. (1987). Reality orientation and reminiscence therapy. *British Journal of Psychiatry, 151,* 222–231.

Baker, H., & Leland, B. (1967). *Detroit Test of Learning Abilities.* Indianapolis: Bobbs-Merrill Company.

Barco, P. P., Crosson, B., Bolesta, M. M., Werts, D., & Stout, R. (1991). Training awareness and compensation in postacute head injury rehabilitation. In J. S. Kreutzer & P. H. Wehman (Eds.), *Cognitive rehabilitation for persons with traumatic brain injury: A functional approach.* Baltimore: Paul H. Brookes, (pp. 129–146).

Bayles, K. A., & Kaszniak, A. W. (1987). *Communication and cognition in normal aging and dementia.* Boston, MA: College-Hill Press.

Bayles, K. A., & Tomoeda, C. (1994). *Functional Linguistic Communication Inventory.* Tucson, AR: Canyonlands Publishing.

Beck, C., Heacock, P., Mercer, S., Thatcher, R., & Sparkman, C. (1988). The impact of cognitive skills remediation training on persons with Alzheimer's disease or mixed dementia. *Journal of Geriatric Psychiatry, 21,* 73–88.

Beck, A. T., Ward, C. H., Mendelson, M., Mock, J., & Erbaugh, J. (1961). An inventory for measuring depression. *Archives of General Psychiatry, 4,* 561–571.

Benedict R.R. (1989). The effectiveness of cognitive remediation strategies for victims of traumatic head injury: a review of the literature. *Clinical Psychological Review, 9:*608–626.

Benton, A.L. (1974). *Revised visual retention test: Clinical and experimental application,* (4th ed.). New York: The Psychological Corporation.

Benton, A.L., and Hamsher, K, Eds. (1976). *Multilingual Aphasia Examination.* Iowa City: University of Iowa.

Ben-Yishay, Y., et al. (1978). Digest of a two year comprehensive clinical rehabilitation research program for out-patient head injured Israeli veterans. In NYU Rehabilitation Monograph, No. 59, 1. New York University Medical Center, Dept. of Behavioral Sciences. (Studies for Grant 12P-55623).

Ben-Yishay, Y., et al. (1980). Relationships between aspects of anterograde amnesia and vocational aptitude in traumatically brain damaged patients: Preliminary findings. In Ben-Yishay, Y. (ed): NYU Rehabilitation Monograph, No. 61, 55.

Ben-Yishay, Y. & Diller, L., (1981). Rehabilitation of cognitive and perceptual defects in people with traumatic brain damage. *International Journal of Rehabilitation Research, 4*(3), 20.

Ben-Yishay, Y., & Piasetsky, E. (1985). Rehabilitation of cognitive and perceptual deficits in persons with chronic brain damage. A comparative study. In L. Diller, et al. (Eds): Annual Progress Report. R.T. Center, NIHR Grant No. G008300039, 4.

Ben-Yishay, Y., & Piasetsky, E. (1986). Rehabilitation of cognitive and perceptual deficits in persons with chronic brain damage. A comparative study. In L. Diller, et al. (Eds): Annual Progress Report. R.T. Center, NIHR Grant No. G008300039, 4.

Ben-Yishay, Y. Silver, S., Piasetsky, E., & Rattok, J. (1987). Relationship between employability and vocational outcome after intensive holistic cognitive rehabilitation. *Journal of Head Trauma Rehabilitation, 2,* 35–49.

Ben-Yishay, Y. & Prigatano, G.P. (1990). Cognitive Remediation. In Rosenthal, M., Griffith E.R., Bond, M.R., Miller J.D., Eds. *Rehabilitation of the adult and child with traumatic brain injury.* 2nd ed. Philadelphia: Davis. 393–400.

Berghorn, F., & Schafer, D. (1987). Reminiscence intervention in nursing homes: What and who changes? *International Journal of Aging and Human Development, 24,* 113–127.

Bigler, E.D. (Ed.). (1990). "Neuropathology of Traumatic Brain Injury," Traumatic Brain Injury, Mechanisms of Damage, Assessment, Intervention, and Outcome, 13

Blessed, G., Tomlinson, B. E., & Roth, M. (1968). The association between quantitative measures of dementia and of senile changes in the cerebral grey matter of elderly subjects. *Journal of Psychiatry, 114,* 797–811.

Blessed, G., Black, S., Butler, T., & Kay, D. (1991). The diagnosis of dementia in the elderly: A comparison of CAMCOG (the Cognitive Section of the CAMDEX), the AGE-CAT Program, DSM-II, the Mini-Mental State examination and some short rating scales. *British Journal of Psychiatry, 159,* 193–198.

Bond, M.R., & Brooks, D.N. (1976). Understanding the process of recovery as a basis for the investigation of rehabilitation for the brain injured. *Scandinavian Journal of Rehabilitation Medicine, 8,* 127–133.

Bond, M.R. (1990). Standardized methods of assessing and predicting outcome. In M. Rosenthal, E. R. Griffith, M. R. Bond, & J. D. Miller (Eds.), *Rehabilitation of the adult and child with traumatic brain injury.* (2nd ed.; pp. 59–74). Philadelphia: Davis.

Borkowski, J. G., Benton, A. L., & Spreen, O. (1967). Word fluency and brain damage. *Neuropsychologia, 5,* 135–140.

Bourgeois, M. (1990). Enhancing conversation skills in Alzheimer's Disease using a prosthetic memory aid. *Journal of Applied Behavior Analysis, 23,* 29–42.

Bourgeois, M. (1991). Communication treatment for adults with dementia. *Journal of Speech and Hearing Research, 34,* 831–844.

Bourgeois, M. (1992). Evaluating memory wallets in conversations with patients with dementia. *Journal of Speech and Hearing Research, 35,* 1344–1357.

Bourgeois, M. (1993). Effects of memory aids on the dyadic conversations of individuals with dementia. *Journal of Applied Behavior Analysis, 26,* 77–87.

Bourgeois, M. (Ed.) (1994). Caregiving in Alzheimer's Disease I: Caregiver Characteristics. *Seminars in Speech and Language, 15,* 185–346.

Bourgeois, M., Burgio, L., Schulz, R ., Beach, S., & Palmer, B. (1997). Modifying repetitive verbalization of community dwelling patients with AD. *The Gerontologist, 37,* 30–39.

Bourgeois, M., & Mason, L. A. (1996). Memory wallet intervention in an adult day care setting. *Behavioral Interventions, 11,* 3–18.

Bourgeois, M. (1996). Increasing effective communication in nursing homes. [Grant No. 1R01Ag13008–01A1, funded by the National Institute on Aging].

Bourgeois, M., Schulz, R., & Burgio, L. (1995, November.). Improving outcomes by monitoring the intervention process. In L. Boise (Chair), *Measuring outcomes of caregiver interventions*. Symposium paper presented at the Gerontological Society of America Conference, Los Angeles, CA.

Bourgeois, M. S., Schulz, R., & Burgio, L. (1996). Interventions for caregivers of patients with Alzheimer's disease: A review and analysis of content, process, and outcomes. *The Journal of Aging and Human Development, 43*, 35–92.

Brooks, N., McKinlay, W., Symington, D., Beattie A., & Campsie L. (1987). Return to work within the first seven years of severe head injury. *Brain Injury; 1*, 5–19.

Brookshire, R. H., & Nicholas, L. E. (1993). *Discourse Comprehension Test*. Tucson, AZ: Communication Skill Builders.

Brotherton, F.A., Thomas, L.L., Wisotzek, I.E., & Milan, M.A. (1988). Social skills training in the rehabilitation of patients with traumatic closed head injury. *Archives of Physical Medicine and Rehabilitation, 69*, 827–832.

Bruner, J.S. (1966). Toward a theory of instruction. Cambridge: Belknap.

Bryan, K. L. (1989). *The Right Hemisphere Language Battery*. Kibworth, England: Far Communications.

Camp, C., Foss, J. W., O'Hanlon, A. M., & Stevens, A. B. (1996). Memory interventions for persons with dementia. *Applied Cognitive Psychology, 9*, 193–210.

Camp, C., Foss, J., Stevens, A. B., & O'Hanlon, A. M. (1995). Improving prospective memory task performance in persons with Alzheimer's disease. In M. McDaniel and G. Einstein (Eds.), *Prospective memory: Theory and applications*. Hillsdale, NJ: Lawrence Erlbaum.

Camp, C. J., & Stevens, A. B. (1990). Spaced-retrieval: A memory intervention for dementia of the Alzheimer's type (DAT). *Clinical Gerontologist, 10*, 658–661.

Casby, J. A., & Holm, M. B. (1994). The effect of music on repetitive disruptive vocalizations of persons with dementia. *American Journal of Occupational Therapy, 48*, 883–889.

Chen Sea, M.-J., Henderson, A., & Cermak, S. A. (1993). Patterns of visual spatial inattention and their functional significance in stroke patients. *Archives of Physical Medicine and Rehabilitation, 74*, 355–360.

Clarfield, A. M. (1988). The reversible dementias: Do they reverse? *Annals of Internal Medicine, 104*, 476–486.

Clark, L. W. (1995). Interventions for persons with Alzheimer's disease: Strategies for maintaining and enhancing communicative success. *Topics in Language Disorders, 15*(2), 47–65.

Clark, L. W., & Witte, K. (1991). Nature and efficacy of communication management in Alzheimer's disease. In R. Lubinski (Ed.), *Dementia and Communication* (pp. 238–256). Philadelphia, PA: B. C. Decker, Inc.

Coblentz, J. M., Mattis, S., Zingesser, H., Kasoff, S. S., Wisniewski, H. M., & Katzman, R. (1973). Presenile dementia: Clinical aspects and evaluation of cerebro-spinal fluid dynamics. *Archives of Neurology, 29*, 299–308.

Cohen-Mansfield, J., & Billig, N. (1986). Agitated behavior in the elderly. 1. A conceptual review. *Journal of the American Geriatrics Society, 34*, 711–721.

Collins A., Brown, J.S., & Newman, S.E. (1989). Cognitive apprenticeship: teaching the crafts of reading, writing and mathematics. In: L.B. Resnick, Ed. Knowing, learning, and instruction: essays in honor of Robert Glaser. Hillsdale, NJ: Erlbaum.

Cope, D.N., Cole, J.R., Hall, K.M., & Barkan, H. (1991). Brain-injury: analysis of outcome in a post-acute rehabilitation system. Part 1: General analysis. *Brain Injury, 5*, 111–126.

Crepeau F., & Scherzer, P. (1993). Predictors and indicators of work status after traumatic brain injury: A meta-analysis. *Neuropsychological Rehabilitation, 3*, 5–35.

Crook, T., Ferris, S., & McCarthy, M. (1979). The misplaced-objects task: A brief test for memory dysfunction in the aged. *Journal of the American Geriatrics Society, 27*, 284–287.

Crook, T., Gilbert, J. G., & Ferris, S. (1980). Operationalizing memory impairment for elderly persons: The Guild Memory Test. *Psychological Reports, 47*, 1315–1318.

Cross, P.S., & Gurland, B. J. (1985). The epidemiology of dementing disorders: A report on work performed by and submitted to the U.S. Congress, Office of Technology Assessment. New York: Columbia University Center for Geriatrics,

Crovitz, L.S. (1979). Memory retraining in brain-damaged patients: The airplane list. *Cortex, 15,* 131–134.

Cummings, J. L. (1987). Dementia syndromes: Neurobehavioral and neuropsychiatric features. *Journal of Clinical Psychiatry, 48,* 3–8.

Davis, K. L., Thal, L. J., Gamzu, E. R., Davis, C. S., Woolson, R., Gracón, S. I., Drachmán, D. L., Schneider, L. S., Whitehouse, P. J., Hoover, T. M., Morris, J. C., Kawas, C. H., Knopman, D., Earl, N. L., Kumar, V., & Doody, R. S. (1992). A double-blind, placebo-controlled multicenter study of tacrine for Alzheimer's disease. *New England Journal of Medicine, 327,* 1253–1259.

Dawson, D.R., & Chipman, M. (1995). The disablement experienced by traumatically brain-injured adults living in the community. *Brain Injury, 9,* (4), 339–353.

Deimling, G. T. (1994). Caregiver Functioning. In M. P. Lawton & J. A. Teresi (Eds.), *Annual Review of Gerontology and Geriatrics: Focus on Assessment Techniques* Vol. 4, (pp. 257–280). New York: Springer.

DeJong, R., Osterlund, O. W., & Roy, G. W. (1989). Measurement of quality of life changes in patients with Alzheimer's disease. *Clinical Therapy, 11,* 545–553.

Denman, S. (1984). Denman Neuropsychology Memory Scale Manual, Sidney Denman, Charleston, SC.

DeRenzi, E., & Faglioni, P. (1978) Normative data and screening power of a shortened version of the token test. *Cortex, 14,* 41–49.

Diller, L. et al. (1974). *Studies in cognition and rehabilitation in hemiplegia* (Rehabilitation Monograph No. 50). New York: New York University, Institute for Rehabilitation Medicine.

Diller, L. (1987). Neuropsychological rehabilitation. In: M.J. Meier, A.L. Benton, L. Diller, Eds. *Neuropsychological rehabilitation. London: Churchill-Livingstone, 1–17.*

Duke University Center for the Study of Aging. (1978). Multidimensional functional assessment: The OARS methodology (2nd. ed.). Durham, NC: Duke University.

Dunn, L. M., & Dunn, L. M. (1981). *Peabody picture vocabulary test-revised.* Circle Pines, MN: American Guidance Service.

Duston, D. (1996, May). Crackdown recovers $43.2 million in Medicare and Medicaid fraud. Article broadcast and published nationwide by the Associated Press, Washington, DC.

Evans, D. A., Fundenstein, H. H., Albert, M. S., Scherr, P. A., Cook, N. R., Chown, M J., Herbert, L. E., Hennekens, C. H., & Taylor, J. (1989). Prevalence of Alzheimer's disease in a community population of older persons: Higher than previously reported. *Journal of the American Medical Association, 262,* 2551–2556.

Ezrachi, O. et al. (1983). Rehabilitation of cognitive and perceptual defects in people with traumatic brain damage: A five year clinical research study: Results of the second phase. In Ben-Yisha, Y. (ed). NYU Rehabilitation Monograph, No. 66 53.

Farlow, M., Gracon, S. I., Hershey, L. A., Lewis, K. W., Sadowsky, C. H., & Dolan-Ureno, J. (1992). A controlled trial of tacrine in Alzheimer's disease. *Journal of the American Medical Association, 268,* 2523–2529.

Ferris, S., Mackell, J., Schneider, L., Sano, M., Whitehouse, P., Schmidtt, F., Mohs, R., Ernesto, C., & Thal, L. (1996). Multi-domain assessment measures across the spectrum of Alzheimer's Disease. Submitted for publication.

Flavell, J. (1979). Metacognition and cognitive monitoring. *American Psychology, 34,* pp. 6–11.

Folstein, N. F., Folstein, S. E., & McHugh, P. R. (1975). Mini-Mental State: A practical method for grading the cognitive state of patients for the clinician. *Journal of Psychiatric Research, 12,* 189–198.

Foss, J. W., & Camp, C. J. (1994, April). "Effortless" learning in Alzheimer's disease: Evidence that spaced-retrieval training engages implicit memory. Poster presented at the Fifth Biennial Cognitive Aging Conference, Atlanta, Georgia.

Fowler, R., Hart, J., & Sheahan, M. (1972). A prosthetic: An application of the prosthetic environment concept. *Rehabilitation Counseling Bulletin, 15,* 80–85.

Fraser, R. T., & Wehman, P. (1995). Traumatic brain injury rehabilitation: Issues in vocational outcome. *NeuroRehabilitation, 5,* 39–48.

Frattali, C. M., Thompson, C. K., Holland, A. L., Wohl, C.B., & Ferketic, M. M. (1995). *Functional assessment of communication skills for adults (ASHA FACS).* Rockville, MD: American Speech-Language-Hearing Association.

Freedman, A. M., Kaplan, H.I., & Saddock, B.J. (1976). *Modern Synopsis of Comprehensive Textbook of Psychiatry, II,* 2nd Ed. Baltimore, MD: Williams and Wilkins.

Friedman, R., & Tappen, R. (1991). The effect of planned walking on communication in Alzheimer's disease. *Journal of the American Geriatrics Society, 39,* 650–654.

Frostig, M. (1963). *Developmental Test of Visual Perception.* Chicago, Follett.

Fryer, J., & Fralish, K. (1989). Cognitive rehabilitation. In P.M. Deutsch & K.B. Fralish (Eds.). *Innovations in head injury rehabilitation.* Albany, NY: Matthew Bender.

Fuld, P. A. (1981). *The Fuld object memory evaluation.* Chicago, IL: Stoelting Instrument Company.

Gajar, A., Schloss, P.J., Schloss, C.N., & Thompson, C.K. (1984). Effects of feedback and self-monitoring on head trauma youths' conversation skills. *Journal of Applied Behavior Analysis, 17,* 353–358.

Gazzaniga, M.S. (1978) Is seeing believing? Notes on clinical recovery. In S. Finger, (Ed.), *Recovery From Brain Damage.* New York: Plenum Press.

George, L. K., & Gwyther, L. P. (1986). Caregiver well-being. A multidimensional examination of family caregivers of demented adults. *The Gerontologist, 26,* 253–259.

Gerber, S., & Gurland, G. (1989). Applied pragmatics in the assessment of aphasia. *Seminars in Speech and Language: Aphasia and Pragmatics, 10,* 263–281.

Gianutsos, R., & Gianutsos, J. (1979). Rehabilitating the Verbal Recall of Brain Injured Patients by Mnemonic Training: an Experimental Demonstration Using Single Case Methodology. *Journal of Clinical Neuropsychology, 1,* 1:117.

Giles, G.M., Fussey, I., & Burgess, P. (1988). The behavioural treatment of verbal interaction skills following severe head injury: A single case study. *Brain Injury, 2,* 75–79.

Glasgow, R.E., Zeiss, R.A., Barrera, M.D, & Lewinsohn P. (1977). Case studies on remediating memory deficits in brain damaged individuals. *Journal Clinical Psychology, 33,* 1049–1054.

Gloag, D. (1985). Rehabilitation after head injury: Cognitive problems. *British Medical Journal, 290,* 834–837.

Goddaer, J., & Abraham, I. L. (1994). Effects of relaxing music on agitation during meals among nursing home residents with severe impairment. *Archives of Psychiatric Nursing, 8,* 150–158.

Goldman, R., Fristoe, M., & Woodcock, R.W. (1970). *G-F-W Test of Auditory Discrimination.* Circle Pines, MN: American Guidance Service.

Goldman, R., Fristoe, M., & Woodcock, R.W. (1974). *G-F-W Auditory Memory Test.* Circle Pines, MN: American Guidance Service.

Goldman, R., Fristoe, M., & Woodcock, R.W. (1974). *G-F-W Sound Symbol Tests.* Circle Pines, MN: American Guidance Service.

Goldstein, K., & Scheerer, M. (1945). *Goldstein-Scheerer Stick Test.* New York: Psychological Corporation.

Goodglass H., & Kaplan, E. (1983). The Boston diagnostic aphasia examination. In: Goodglass H. Kaplan E. (Eds.), *The assessment of aphasia and related disorders.* Revised Edition. Philadelphia: Lea & Febiger.

Gordon, W. A., Hibbard, M. R., Egelko, S., Diller, L., Simmens, S., Langer, K., Sano, M., Orazem, J., & Weinberg, J. (1984). *Evaluation of the deficits associated with right brain damage: Nor-*

mative data on the Institute of Rehabilitation Test Battery. New York: New York University Medical Center.

Gordon, W. A., Hibbard, M. R., Egelko, S., Diller, L., Shaver, M. S., Lieberman, A., & Ragnarsson, K. (1985). Perceptual remediation in patients with right brain damage: A comprehensive program. *Archives of Physical Medicine and Rehabilitation, 66,* 353–359.

Gordon, W.A., & Hibbard, M. (1991). The theory and practice of cognitive rehabilitation. In P.E Wehman & J. Kreutzer, (Eds.), *Cognitive rehabilitation for persons with traumatic brain injury.* Baltimore: Brookes.

Gouvier, A. D., Bua, B. G., Blanton, P. D., & Urey, J. R. (1987). Behavioral changes following visual scanning training: Observations of five cases. *International Journal of Clinical Neuropsychology, 9,* 74–80.

Gouvier, W. D., Cottam, G., Webster, J. S., Beissel, G. F., & Wofford, J. D. (1984). Behavioral interventions with stroke patients for improving wheelchair navigation. *The International Journal of Clinical Neuropsychology, 6,* 186–190.

Greene, J. G. (1984). The evaluation of reality orientation. In I. Hanley and J. Hodge (Eds.), *Psychological approaches to the care of the elderly.* London: Croom Helm.

Griffith, E. R., & Miller, J. D. (Eds.), *Rehabilitation of the adult and child with traumatic brain injury* (2nd Ed., pp. 21–49). Philadelphia: F.A. Davis.

Gronwall, D. (1977). Paced auditory serial addition task: A measure of recovery from concussion. *Perception and Motor Skills, 44,* 367.

Gurland, B., Wilder, D., Cross, P., Teresi, J., & Barrett, V. (1992). Screening scales for dementia: Toward reconciliation of conflicting cross-cultural findings. *International Journal of Geriatric Psychiatry,* 105–113.

Guy, W. (Ed.) (1976). *ECDEU Assessment Manual for Psychopharmacology* (pp. 218–222). Rockville, MD: US Dept. Of Health Education and Welfare, National Institute of Mental Health.

Haaland, K. Y., Linn, R. T., Hunt, W. C., & Goodwin, J. S. (1983). A normative study of Russell's variant of the Wechsler Memory Scale in healthy elderly population. *Journal of Consulting and Clinical Psychology, 51,* 878–881.

Haffey, W. J., & Lewis, F. D. (1989). Programming for occupational outcome following traumatic brain injury. *Rehabilitation Psychology, 34* (2), 147–159.

Halper, A. S., Cherney, L. R., Burns, M. S. & Mogil, S. I. (1996). *RIC Evaluation of Communication Problems in Right Hemisphere Dysfunction-Revised RICE-R).* Rockville, MD: Aspen.

Halstead, W.C. (1947). *Brain and intelligence.* Chicago: University of Chicago Press.

Hamilton, B. B. & Granger, C. V. (1989). Totaled functional score can be valid. *Archives of Physical Medicine and Rehabilitation, 70,* 861–862.

Hamilton, M. (1960). A rating scale for depression. *Journal of Neurology, Neurosurgery, and Psychiatry, 23,* 56–62.

Harris, J. (1978). External memory aids. In M. Gruneberg, P. Morris, & R. Sykes (Eds.), *Practical aspects of memory.* London: Academic Press, (pp. 172–179).

Hart, T., & Hayden, M.D. (1986). The ecological validity of neuropsychological assessment and remediation. In B.P. Uzzell & Y. Gross (Eds.), *Clinical neuropsychology of intervention.* Boston: Martinus Nijhoff, (pp.21–50).

Hartley, L.L., & Griffith, A. (1989). A functional approach to the cognitive-communicative deficits of closed head injured clients. *Texas Journal of Audiology and Speech Pathology, 14* (2), 37–42.

Helffenstein, D.A., & Wechsler, F.S. (1982). The use of Interpersonal Process Recall (IPR) in the remediation of interpersonal and communication skill deficits in the newly brain-injured. *Clinical Neuropsychology, 4,* 139–143.

Helmes, E., Csapo, K. G., & Short, J. A. (1987). Standardization and validation of the Multidimensional Observation Scale for Elderly Subjects (MOSES). *Journal of Gerontology, 42*, 395–405.

Holland, A. L. (1980). *Communicative Abilities in Daily Living (CADL).* Baltimore: University Park Press.

Hooper, H.D. (1966). *The Visual Organization Test.* Los Angeles, CA: Western Psychological Services.

Horner, J. (1980). Visual agnosic misnaming: Treatment of a right CVA patient one year post onset. In R. H. Brookshire (Ed.), *Clinical aphasiology: Conference proceedings* (pp. 316–330). Minneapolis: BRK Publishers.

Howard, D., & Patterson, K. (1992). *Pyramids and Palm Trees.* Bury St. Edmonds, Suffolk, England: Thames Valley Test Company.

Howard, K., & Rockwood, K. (1995). Quality of life in Alzheimer's disease. *Dementia, 6*, 113–116.

Hughes, C. P., Berg, L., Danziger, W. L., Cohen, L. A., & Martin, R. L. (1982). A new clinical scale for the staging of dementia. *British Journal of Psychiatry, 140*, 566–572.

Ip, R.Y., Dornan J., & Schentag, C. (1995). Traumatic brain injury: Factors predicting return to work or school. *Brain Injury,. 9* (5), 517–532.

Jackson, R.D., Mysiw, W.J., & Corrigan, J.D. (1989). Orientation Group Monitoring System: an indicator for reversible impairments in cognition during post-traumatic amnesia. *Archives of Physical Medicine and Rehabilitation; 70*, 33–36.

Jennett, B., & Bond, M.R. (1975). Assessment of outcome after severe brain damage. *Lancet 1*, 480.

Jennett, B., Snoek, J., Bond, M. R., & Brooks, N. (1981). Disability after severe head injury: Observations on the use of the Glasgow Outcome Scale. *Journal of Neurology, Neurosurgery, and Psychiatry, 44*, 285.

Johnston, M.V., & Lewis, F.D. (1991). Outcomes of Community Re-Entry Programmes for Brain Injury Survivors. Part 1: Independent Living and Productive Activities. *Brain Injury, 5*, 141–154.

Johnston, M.V. (1991) Outcomes of Community Re-Entry Programmes for Brain Injury Survivors. Part 2: Further investigations. *Brain Injury, 5*: 155–168.

Jones, M.K., (1974). Imagery as a mnemonic aid after left temporal lobectomy: Contrast between material specific and generalized memory disorders. *Neuropsychologia, 12*, 21–30.

Kane, R. A., & Kane, R. L. (1981). *Assessing the Elderly: A practical guide to measurement.* Lexington, MA: Lexington Books.

Kane, R., Riegler, S., Bell, R., Potter, R., & Koshland, G. (1982). *Predicting the course of nursing home patients: A progress report.* Santa Monica, CA.: Rand.

Kaplan, C.P., & Corrigan, J.D. (1994). The relationship between cognition and functional independence in adults with traumatic brain injury. *Archives of Physical Medicine and Rehabilitation, 75*(6), 643–647.

Kaplan, E., Goodglass, H., & Weintraub, S. (1983). *Boston Naming Test.* Philadelphia: Lea & Febiger.

Kertesz A. (1982). *Western aphasia battery.* New York: Grune and Stratton.

Kinsella, G., Olver, J., Ng, K., Packer, S., & Stark, R. (1993). Analysis of the syndrome of unilateral neglect. *Cortex, 29*, 135–140.

Klonoff, H., Low, M.D., & Clark, C. (1977). Head injuries in children: a perspective five year follow up. *Journal of Neurology, Neurosurgery and Psychiatry, 40*, 1211–1219.

Klonoff, P. S., Sheperd, J. C., O'Brien, K. P., Chiapello, D. A., & Hodak, J. A. (1990). Rehabilitation and outcome of right-hemisphere stroke patients: Challenges to traditional diagnostic and treatment methods. *Neuropsychology, 4*, 147–163.

Knapp, M. J., Knopman, D.S., Solomon, P. R., Pendlebury, W. W., Davis, C. S., Gracon, S. I.

(1994). A 30-week randomized controlled trial of high-dose tacrine in patients with Alzheimer's disease. *Journal of the American Medical Association, 271,* 985–991.

Knight, B. G., Lutzky, S. M., & Macofsky-Urban, F. (1993). A meta-analytic review of interventions for caregiver distress: Recommendations for future research. *The Gerontologist, 33,* 240–248.

Kopelman, M., Wilson, B., & Baddeley, A. (1990). *The Autobiographical Memory Interview.* Bury St. Edmunds, Suffolk, England: Thames Valley Test Company.

Kovar, M. G., & Lawton, M. P. (1994). Functional Disability: Activities and instrumental activities of daily living. In M. P. Lawton, & J. A. Teresi (Eds.) *Annual Review of Gerontology and Geriatrics Focus on Assessment Techniques, 4,* (pp. 57–75). New York: Springer.

Kovner, R., Mattis, S., & Pass, K. (1983). *Some amnestic patients can freely recall large amounts of information in new contexts.* Article presented at the meeting of the International Neuropsychological Society, Mexico City.

Kreutzer, J. S., Wehman, P., Morton, M. V., & Stonnington, H. H. (1988). Supported employment and compensatory strategies for enhancing vocational outcome following traumatic brain injury. Brain Injury, 3, 205–223.

Kreutzer, J. S., Gordon, W. A., & Wehman P. (1989). Cognitive Remediation Following Traumatic Brain Injury. *Rehabitation Psychology, 34,* pp 117–123.

Ladavas, E., Menghini, G., & Umilta, C. (1994). A rehabilitation study of hemispatial neglect. *Cognitive Neuropsychology, 11,* 75–95.

Lawson, I. R. (1962). Visual-spatial neglect in lesions of the right cerebral hemisphere. *Neurology, 12,* 23–33.

Lawton, M.P. (1991). A multidimensional view of quality of life in frail elderly. In J. E. Birren, J. E. Lubben, J. C. Rowe, & D. E. Deutchman (Eds.), *The concept and measurement of quality of life in the frail elderly* (pp. 3–27). San Diego: Academic Press.

Lawton, M. P., Van Haitsma, K., & Klapper, J. (1996). Observed affect in nursing home residents with Alzheimer's disease. *Journal of Gerontology: Psychological Sciences, 51B,* P3–P14.

Lawton, M. P., & Brody, E. M. (1969). Assessment of older people: Self-maintaining and instrumental activities of daily living. *Gerontologist, 9,* 176–186.

Lennon, S. (1991). Wheelchair transfer training in a stroke patient with neglect: A single case study design. *Physiotherapy Theory and Practice, 7,* 551–555.

Lennon, S. (1994). Task specific effects in the rehabilitation of unilateral neglect. In M. J. Riddoch & G. W. Humphreys (Eds.), *Cognitive neuropsychology and cognitive rehabilitation* (pp. 187–203). Hillsdale, NJ: Lawrence Erlbaum.

Levin, H. S. (1990). Cognitive rehabilitation, unproven but promising. Archives Neurology, 47, 223–224.

Levin, H. S., O'Donnell, V. M. & Grossman, R. G. (1975). The Galveston orientation and amnesia test: a practical scale to assess cognition after head injury. Journal of Nervous and Mental Disease, 167–675.

Levin, H. S. (1983). *The Paced Auditory Serial Addition Task-Revised.* Unpublished test, University of Texas at Galveston.

Levin, H. S., High, W. M., Goethe, K. E., Sisson, R. A., Overall, J. E., Rhoad, H. M., Eisenberg, H. M. (1987). The neurobehavioural rating scale: assessment of the behavioural sequelae of head injury by the clinician. *Journal of Neurology, Neurosurgery, and Psychiatry, 50,* 183.

Levin, H. S., Eisenberg, H. M., & Benton, A. L. (Eds). (1991). Frontal lobe function and dysfunction. New York: Oxford University Press.

Lewinsohn, P. M., Danaher, B. G., and Kikel, S. (1977). Visual imagery as a mnemonic aid for brain-injured persons. *Journal of Consulting and Clinical Psychology,* 45, 717–723.

Lezak, M. D. (1982). The problem of assessing executive functions. *International Journal of Psychology, 17,* 281–297.

Lezak, M. D. (1978). Living with the characterologically altered brain injured patient. *Journal of Clinical Psychiatry, 39,* 592–598.

Livingston, M. G. & Livingston, H. M. (1985). The Glasgow Assessment Schedule: Clinical and research assessment of head injury outcome. *International Rehabilitation Medicine, 7,* 145.

Lomas, J., Pickard, L., Bester, S., Elbard, H., Finlayson, A., & Zoghaib, C. (1989). The Communicative Effectiveness Index: Development and psychometric evaluation of a functional communication measure for adult aphasia. *Journal of Speech and Hearing Disorders, 54,* 113–124.

Lorayne, H., & Lucas, J. (1974). *The memory book.* New York: Ballantine Books.

Lord, T. R., & Garner, J. E. (1993). Effects of music on Alzheimer's patients. *Perceptual and Motor Skills, 76,* 451–455.

Lowenstein, D. A., Amigo, E., Duara, R., Guterman, A., Hurwitz, D., Berkowitz, N., Wilkie, F., Weinberg, G., Black, B., Gittelman, B., & Eisdorfer, C. (1989). A new scale for the assessment of functional status in Alzheimer's disease and related disorders. *Journal of Gerontology: Psychological Sciences, 44,* P114–121.

Lubinski, R. (Ed). (1991). *Dementia and Communication.* Philadelphia, PA: B.C. Decker, Inc.

Lund, D. A., Hill, R. D., Caserta, M. S., & Wright, S. D. (1995). Video Respite: An innovative resource for family, professional caregivers, and persons with dementia. *Gerontologist, 35,* 683–687.

Lyon, J. G., & Cariski, D. (1994). Communication partners: Integrating adults with aphasia back into society. Miniseminar presented at annual convention of the American Speech-Language-Hearing Association, New Orleans.

Mahurin, R. K., DeBettignies, B. H., & Pirozzolo, F. J. (1991). Structured assessment of independent living skills: Preliminary functional abilities in dementia. *Journal of Gerontology: Psychological Sciences, 46,* P58-P66.

Malec, J.F., Smigielski, J.S., & DePompolo, R. W. (1991). Goal attainment scaling and outcome measurement in postacute brain injury rehabilitation. *Archives of Physical Medicine and Rehabilitation, 72,*138–143.

Malec, J.F., Smigielski, J.S., DePompolo, R., & Thompson, J.M. (1993). Outcome Evaluation and Prediction in a comprehensive-integrated Post-Acute Outpatient Brain Injury Rehabilitation Programme. *Brain Injury, 7,* (1), 15–29.

Mattis, S. (1976). Mental status examination for organic mental syndrome in the elderly patient. In R. Bellack & B. Karasu, (Eds.), *Geriatric Psychiatry* (p. 77). New York: Grune & Stratton.

McArthur, D. L., Cohen, M. J., & Schandler, S. L. (1991). Rasch analysis of functional assessment scales: An example using pain behaviors. *Archives of Physical Medicine and Rehabilitation, 72,* 296–304.

McKhann, G., Drachman, D., Folstein, M., Katzman, R., Price, D., Stadlan, E. M. (1984). Clinical diagnosis of Alzheimer's disease: Report of the NINCDS-ADRDA Work Group under the auspices of the Department of Health and Human Services Task Force on Alzheimer's disease. *Neurology, 34,* 939–944.

Mcoch, A. G., & Metter, E. J. (1994). Medical aspects of stroke rehabilitation. In R. Chapey (Ed.), *Language intervention strategies in adult aphasia* (3rd ed., pp. 27–46). Baltimore: Williams & Wilkins.

McMahon, R. J., & Forehand, R. L. (1983). Consumer satisfaction in behavioral treatment of children: Types, issues, and recommendations. *Behavior Therapy, 14,* 209–225.

McNeil, M. R., & Prescott, T. E. (1978). *Revised Token Test.* Austin, TX: Pro-Ed.

Merbitz, C., Morris, J., & Grip, J. C. (1989). Ordinal scales and foundations of misinference. *Archives of Physical Medicine and Rehabilitation, 70,* 308–312.

Miller, J. D., Pentland, B., & Berrol, S. (1990). Early evaluation and management. In M. Rosenthal, E. R. Griffith, M. R. Bond, & J. D. Miller (Eds.). *Rehabilitation of the adult and child with Traumatic Brain Injury* (2nd ed., pp. 21–51). Philadelphia : Davis.

Miller, E., & Morris, R. (1993). *The Psychology of Dementia.* New York: John Wiley & Sons.

Moffat, N. (1984). Strategies of memory therapy. In B.A. Wilson & N. Moffat (Eds.), Clinical management of memory problems (pp. 63–88). Rockville, MD: Aspen.

Mohs, R. C. (1995). Assessment of cognition in clinical trials of drugs for the treatment of dementia (pp. 347–357). In M. Bergener, & S. J. Finkel (Eds.), *Treating Alzheimer's and other dementias.* New York: Springer.

Molloy, D. W., & Lubinski, R. (1991). Dementia: Impact and clinical perspectives. In R. Lubinski (Ed.), *Dementia and communication* (pp. 2–21). Philadelphia, PA: B. C. Decker, Inc.

Morris, J. C., Heyman, A., Mohs, R. C., Hughes, J., van Belle, G., Fillenbaum, G., Mellits, E. D., Clark, C., & the CERAD investigators (1989). The Consortium to Establish a Registry for Alzheimer's Disease (CERAD). Part I. Clinical and neuropsychological assessment of Alzheimer's disease. *Neurology, 39,* 1159–1165.

Moss, M. B., Albert, M. S., Butters, N., & Payne, M. (1986). Differential patterns of memory loss among patients with Alzheimer's disease, Huntington's disease, and alcoholic Korsakoff's syndrome. *Archives of Neurology, 43,* 239–246.

Mungas, D., Marshall, S. C., Welson, M., Haan, M., & Reed, B. R. (1996). Age and education correction of Mini-mental State Examination for English- and Spanish-speaking elderly. *Neurology, 46,* 700–706.

Navia, B. A., Jordan, B. D., & Price, R. W. (1986). The AIDS dementia complex: I. Clinical features. *Annals of Neurology, 19,* 517–524.

Nelson, H.E. (1976). A modified card sorting test sensitive to frontal lobe defects. *Cortex, 12,* 313–324.

Newcombe, F. (1985). Rehabilitation in clinical neurology: neuropsychological aspects. In Parenté, R., and DiCesare, A., (1991). *Cognitive Rehabilitation, 12,* 155.

Nicholas, L.E., & Brookshire, R.H. (1993). A system for scoring main concepts in the discourse of non-brain-damaged and aphasic speakers. *Clinical Aphasiology, 21,* 87–99.

Nicholas, L. E., & Brookshire, R. H. (1993b). A system for quantifying the informativeness and efficiency of the connected speech of adults with aphasia. *Journal of Speech and Hearing Research, 36,* 338–350.

Norberg, A., Melin, E., & Asplund, K. (1986). Reactions to music, touch, and object presentation in the final stage of dementia. An exploratory study. *International Journal of Nursing Studies, 23,* 315–323.

Obler, L. K., Obermann, L., Samuels, I., & Albert, M. L. (1985, November). Written input to enhance comprehension in Alzheimer's dementia. Article presented to the American Speech-Language-Hearing Association, Washington, DC

O'Keefe, B. M. (1995). Quality of life for people with speech and language disabilities. Article presented at annual convention of the American Speech-Language-Hearing Association, Orlando.

Ory, M., & Schulz, R. (1996, November). Resources for Enhancing Alzheimer Caregivers' Health (REACH): Innovative approaches to AD Caregiving Interventions. Symposium presented at the annual meeting of the Gerontological Association of America, Washington, DC.

Osborne, D. P., Brown, E. R., & Randt, C. T. (1982). Qualitative changes in memory function: Aging and dementia. In S. Corkin, K. L. Davis, J. H. Growdon, E. Usdin, & R. L. Wurtman (Eds.), Aging: Vol. 19. *Alzheimers disease: A report of progress.* (pp. 165–169). New York: Raven Press.

Osterrieth, P. (1944). Le test de copie d'une figure complexe, *Archives de Psychologie, 30,* 206.

Overall, J.E. & Gorham, D.R. (1962). The brief psychiatric rating scale. *Psychological Reports, 10,* 799.

Parenté R., & DiCesare A. (1991). Retraining memory: theory, evaluation and application. In J.S. Kreutzer & P.E. Wehman (Eds.), Cognitive rehabilitation for persons with traumatic brain injury: a functional approach. Baltimore: Brookes.

Patten, B.M. (1972). The ancient art of memory: Usefulness in treatment. *Archives of Neurology,* 26, 28–31.

Pimental, P. A., & Kingsbury, N. A. (1989). *Mini Inventory of Right Brain Injury.* Austin, TX: Pro-Ed.

Pizzamiglio, L., Antonucci, G., Judica, G., Montenero, P., Razzano, C., & Zoccolotti, P. (1992). Cognitive rehabilitation of the hemineglect disorder in chronic patients with unilateral right brain damage. *Journal of Clinical and Experimental Neuropsychology, 14,* 901–923.

Ponsford, J.L., & Olver, J.H. (1995). A profile of outcome: 2 years after traumatic brain injury. *Brain Injury, 9,* (1), 1–10.

Ponsford, J. L., Olver, J. H., Curran C., & Ng, K. (1994). Prediction of employment status 2 years after traumatic brain injury. *Brain Injury, 9,* (1), 11–20.

Porch, B. E. (1967). *Porch index of communicative abilities.* Palo Alto, CA: Consulting Psychologists Press.

Powell-Proctor, L., & Miller, E. (1982). Reality orientation: A critical appraisal. *British Journal of Psychiatry, 140,* 457–463.

Prigatano, G. P., Fordyce, D. J. Zeiner, H. K. Rouche, J. R., Pepping, M., & Wood, B. C. (1984) Neuropsychological Rehabilitation after closed head injury in young adults. *Journal of Neurology, Neurosurgery and Psychiatry, 47,* 505–513.

Prigatano, G. P. & Fordyce, D. J. (1986). *Neuropsychological rehabilitation after brain injury.* Baltimore: Johns Hopkins University Press.

Prigatano, G. P., Klonoff, P.S., & Bailey, I. (1987). Psychosocial adjustment associated with traumatic brain injury: Statistics BNI neuro-rehabilitation must beat. *BNI Quarterly, 3,* 10–17.

Prigatano, G. P., Amin, K., & Rosenstein, L. (1991). *Manual for the BNI Screen for higher cerebral functions.* Unpublished manual.

Prutting, C. A., & Kirchner, D. M. (1987). A clinical appraisal of the pragmatic aspects of language. *Journal of Speech and Hearing Disorders, 52,* 105–119.

Quayhagen, M. P., & Quayhagen, M. (1989). Differential effects of family-based strategies on Alzheimer's disease. *The Gerontologist, 29,* 150–155.

Quayhagen, M. P., Quayhagen, M., Corbeil, R. R., Roth, P. A., & Rodgers, J. A. (1995). A dyadic remediation program for care recipients with dementia. *Nursing Research, 44,* 153–159.

Rappaport, et al. (1982). Disability Rating Scale for severe head trauma: Coma to community *Archives of Physical Medicine and Rehabilitation, 63,* 118–123.

Ray, W. A., Taylor, J. A., Lichtenstein, M. J., & Meador, K. G. (1992). The Nursing Home Behavior Problem Scale. *Journals of Gerontology: Medical Sciences, 47,* M9-M16.

Reisberg, B. (1983). *Alzheimer's disease: The standard reference.* New York: Free Press.

Reisberg, B., Borenstein, J., Salob, S. P., Ferris, S. H., Franssen, E., & Georgotas, A. (1987). Behavioral symptoms in Alzheimer's disease: Phenomenology and treatment. *Journal of Clinical Psychiatry, 48,* (Suppl.), 9–15.

Reisberg, B., Ferris, S. H., DeLeon, M. J., & Crook, T. (1982). The global deterioration scale of assessment of primary degenerative dementia. *American Journal of Psychiatry, 139* 1136–1139.

Rey, A. (1964). *L'examen clinique en psychologie* [The clinical examination in psychology]. Paris: Presses Universitaires de France.

Ripich, D. (1991). Language and communication in dementia. In D. Ripich (Ed.), *Geriatric Communication Disorders* (pp. 255–292). Austin, TX: Pro-Ed.

Ripich, D. (1994). Functional communication with AD patients: A caregiver training program. *Alzheimer Disease and Associated Disorders, 8,* 95–109.

Robertson, I. H., Gray, J. M., & McKenzie, S. (1988). Microcomputer-based cognitive rehabilitation of visual neglect: Three multiple baseline single-case studies. *Brain Injury, 2,* 151–163.

Robertson, I. H., Gray, J. M., Pentland, B., & Waite, L. J. (1990). Microcomputer-based rehabilitation for unilateral left visual neglect: A randomized controlled trial. *Archives of Physical Medicine and Rehabilitation, 71,* 663–668.

Robertson, I. H., Halligan, P. W., & Marshall, J. C. (1993). Prospects for the rehabilitation of unilateral neglect. In I. H. Robertson & J. C. Marshall (Eds.), *Unilateral neglect: Clinical and experimental studies* (pp. 279–292). Hillsdale, NJ: Lawrence Erlbaum.

Robertson, I. H., North, N. T., & Geggie, C. (1992). Spatiomotor cueing in unilateral left neglect: Three case studies of its therapeutic effects. *Journal of Neurology, Neurosurgery and Psychiatry, 55,* 799–805.

Robertson, I. H., Tegner, R., Tham, K., Lo, A., & Nimmo-Smith, I. (1995). Sustained attention training for unilateral neglect: Theoretical and rehabilitation implications. *Journal of Clinical and Experimental Neuropsychology, 17,* 416–430.

Robertson, I. H., Ward, T., Ridgeway, V., & Nimmo-Smith, I. (1994). *The Test of Everyday Attention.* Bury St. Edmunds, Suffolk, England: Thames Valley Test Company.

Rosen, W. G., Mohs, R. C., & Davis, K. L. (1984). A new rating scale for Alzheimer's disease. *American Journal of Psychiatry, 141,* 1356–1364.

Ross, J.D., & Ross, C.M. (1976). *Ross Test of Higher Cognitive Processes.* Navato: Academic Therapy Publications.

Russell, E. W. (1975). A multiple scoring method for the assessment of complex memory functions. *Journal of Consulting & Clinical Psychology, 43,* 800–809.

Ryan T.V., & Ruff, R.M. (1988). The efficacy of structured memory retraining in a group comparison of head injured patient. *Archives of Clinical Neuropsychology, 3,* 165–179.

Salmon, D. P., Heindel, W. C., & Butters, N. (1991). Patterns of cognitive impairment in Alzheimer's disease and other dementing disorders. In R. Lubinski, (Ed.), *Dementia and Communication* (pp. 37–46). Philadelphia: B. C. Decker, Inc.

Santo Pietro, M. J., & Boczko, R. (1994, November). Preliminary examination of the Breakfast Club: A multi-modal group communication intervention for mid-stage Alzheimer's patients. Presented at the annual convention of the American Speech-Language-Hearing Association, New Orleans, LA.

Saxton, J., McGonigle-Gibson, K., Swihart, A., Miller, V., & Boller, F. (1990). Assessment of the severely impaired patient: Description and validation of a new neuropsychological test battery. *Psychological Assessment, 12,* 298–303.

Sbordone, R.J. (1984). A rehabilitation neuropsychological approach for severe traumatic brain injured patients within a private practice setting. *Professional Psychology, 15,* 165–175.

Schacter, D.L., & Crovitz, H.F. (1977). Memory function after closed head injury: A review of quantitative research. *Cortex, 13,* 150–176.

Schacter, D.L. & Glisky, E.L. (1986). Memory Remediation: Restoration, Alleviation and Acquisition of Domain Specific Knowledge. In Y. Gross & B. P. Uzzell (Eds). *Clinical Neuropsychology of Intervention* (pp. 257–282). Boston: Martinys Nijhoff.

Scherder, E., Bouma, A., & Steen, L. (1995). The effects of peripheral tactile stimulation of memory in patients with probable Alzheimer's disease. *American Journal of Alzheimer's Disease, 10,* 15–21.

Scherzer, B.P. (1986). Rehabilitation following severe head trauma: Results of a three year program. *Archives of Physical Medicine and Rehabilitation, 67,* 366.

Schloss, P.J., Thompson, C.K., Gajar, A.H., & Schloss, C.N. (1985). Influence of self-monitoring on heterosexual conversational behaviours of head trauma youth. *Applied Research in Mental Retardation, 6,* 269–282.

Schulz, R., & Williamson, G. M. (1991). A 2-year longitudinal study of depression among Alzheimer's caregivers. *Psychology and Aging, 6,* 569–578.

Schulz, R., & Williamson, G. (1993). Psychosocial and behavioral dimensions of physical frailty. *Journal of Gerontology, 48* (special issue), 39–43.

Schulz, R., O'Brien, A. T., & Tompkins, C. (1994). The measurement of affect in the elderly. In M. P. Lawton & J. A. Teresi (Eds.), *Annual Review of Gerontology and Geriatrics: Focus on Assessment Techniques* (pp. 210–233). New York: Springer.

Shewan, C. M. (1979). *Auditory comprehension test for sentences.* Chicago: Biolinguistics Clinical Institutes.

Smith (1968). The Symbol Digit Modalities Test: A neuropsychologic test for screening of learning and other cerebral disorders. *Learning Disorders, 3,* 83–91.

Smith (1973). *Symbol Digit Modalities Test manual.* Los Angeles: Western Psychological Services.

Sohlberg, M. M., & Mateer, C. A. (1987). Effectiveness of an attention training program. *Journal of Clinical and Experimental Neuropsychology,* 117–130.

Sohlberg, M. M., White, O., Evans, E., & Mateer, C. (1992). Background and initial case studies into the effects of prospective memory training. *Brain Injury, 6,* 129–138.

Sowers, J. & Powers, L. (1989). Job design strategies for persons with physical and multiple disabilities. In J. Sowers & L. Powers (Eds.), *Vocational Preparation and Employment of Students with Physical and Multiple Disabilities.* Portland: Oregon Research Institute.

Stanton, K., Yorkston, K. M., Kenyon, V. T., & Beukelman, D. R. (1981). Language utilization in teaching reading to left neglect patients. In R. H. Brookshire (Ed.), *Clinical aphasiology: Conference proceedings* (pp. 262–271). Minneapolis: BRK Publishers.

State University of New York at Buffalo, Research Foundation (1993). *Guide for Use of the Uniform Data Set for Medical Rehabilitation: Functional Independence Measure.* Buffalo: Research Foundation.

Stone, C. P., Girdner, J., & Albrecht, R. (1946). An alternate form of the Wechsler Memory Scale. *The Journal of Psychology, 22,* 199–206.

Stratton M.D., & Gregory, R.J. (1994). Review of subject after traumatic brain injury: A discussion of consequences. *Brain Injury, 8,* (7), 631–645.

Sunderland, T., Alterman, I. S., Yount, D., Hill, J. L., Tariot, P.N., Newhouse, P. A., Mueller, E. A., Mellow, A. M., & Cohen, R. M. (1988). A new scale for the assessment of depressed mood in demented patients. *American Journal of Psychiatry, 145,* 955–959.

Taft, L., & Nehrke, M. (1990). Reminiscence, life review, and ego integrity in nursing home residents. *International Journal of Aging and Human Development, 30,* 189–196.

Teasdale, G., & Jennett, B. (1974). Assessment of coma and impaired consciousness. *Lancet, 2,* 81.

Terayama, Y., Meyer, J.S. and Kawamura, J. (1991). Cognitive recovery with long-term increases of cerebral perfusion after head injury. *Surgical Neurology, 36,* 335–342.

Teresi, J., Lawton, P., Ory, M., & Holmes, D. (in press). Measurement issues in chronic care populations: Dementia special care. *Alzheimer's Disease and Associated Disorders.*

Teri, L., & Logsdon, R. G. (1991). Identifying pleasant activities for Alzheimer's disease patients: The Pleasant Events Schedule-AD. *The Gerontologist, 31,* 124–127.

Teri, L., & Logsdon, R. G. (1994). Assessment of behavioral disturbance in older adults. In M. P. Lawton & J. A. Teresi (Eds.), *Annual Review of Gerontology and Geriatrics: Focus on Assessment Techniques* (pp. 107–124). New York: Springer.

Teri, L., & Uomoto, J. M. (1991). Reducing excess disability in dementia patients: Training caregivers to manage patient depression. *Clinical Gerontologist, 10,* 49–63.

Terrell, B., & Ripich, D. (1989). Discourse competence as a variable in intervention. *Seminars in Speech and Language Disorders, 24,* 77–92.

Thissen, D., Steinberg, L., & Mooney, J.A. (1989). "Trace line for testlets: A use of multiple-categorical-response models," *Journal of Educational Measurement, 26.*

Thomsen, I.V. (1981). Neuropsychological treatment and long-term follow-up in an aphasic patient with very severe head trauma. *Journal of Clinical Neuropsychology, 3,* 43–51.

Tompkins, C. A. (1995). *Right hemisphere communication disorders: Theory and management.* San Diego: Singular.

Vinken, P., Bruyn, G.W., & Klawans, H.H. (Eds.). (1985). Handbook of Clinical Neurology. Amsterdam: Elsevier Science Publishers, p. 609.

Webb, C.R., Wrigley, M., Yoels, W., & Fine, P. (1995). Explaining quality of life for persons with traumatic brain injuries 2 years after injury. *Archives of Physical Medicine and Rehabilitation, 76.*

Webster, J. S., Cottam, G., Gouvier, W. D., Blanton, P., Beissel, G. F., & Wofford, J. (1988). Wheelchair obstacle course performance in right cerebral vascular accident victims. *Journal of Clinical and Experimental Neuropsychology, 11*, 295–310.

Webster, J. S., Jones, S., Blanton, P., Gross, R., Beissel, G. F. & Wofford, J. (1984). Visual scanning training with stroke patients. *Behavior Therapy, 15*, 129–143.

Wechsler, D., & Stone, C. (1945). A standardized memory scale for clinical use. *Journal of Psychology, 19*, 87.

Wechsler, D. (1981). *Wechsler Adult Intelligence Scale-Revised* (Manual). New York: Psychological Corporation.

Wehman, P., West, M., Kregel, J., Sherron, P., & Kreutzer, J. S. (1995). Return to work for persons with severe traumatic brain injury: A data-based approach to program development. *Journal of Head Trauma Rehabilitation, 10*(1); 27–39.

Wehman, P., Kreutzer, J., West. M., Sherron, P., Diambre, J., Fry, R., Groah, C., Sale, P., & Killams, S. (1989). Employment outcomes of persons following traumatic brain injury: pre-injury, post-injury and supported employment. *Brain Injury, 3*, 397–412.

Wehman, P. (1990). Supported employment: model implementation and evaluation. In J.S. Kreutzer & P. Wehman (Eds.), *Community Integration Following Traumatic Brain Injury* Baltimore: Paul H. Brooks, pp. 185–204.

Wehman, P.H. (1991). Cognitive rehabilitation in the workplace. *Cognitive rehabilitation for persons with traumatic brain injury, a functional approach, 20*, 269–288.

Weinberg, J., Diller, L., Gordon, W. A., Gerstman, L. J., Lieberman, A., Lakin, P., Hodges, G., & Ezrachi, O. (1977). Visual scanning training effect on reading-related tasks in acquired right brain damage. *Archives of Physical Medicine and Rehabilitation, 58*, 479–486.

Weinberg, J., Diller, L., Gordon, W. A., Gerstman, L. J., Lieberman, A., Lakin, P., Hodges, G., & Ezrachi, O. (1979). Training sensory awareness and spatial organization in people with right brain damage. *Archives of Physical Medicine and Rehabilitation, 60*, 491–496.

Welsh, K. A., Butters, N., Mohs, R. C., Beekly, D., Edland, S., Fillenbaum, G., & Heyman, A. (1994). The Consortium to Establish a Registry for Alzheimer's Disease (CERAD). Part V. A normative study of the neuropsychological battery. *Neurology, 44*, 609–614.

Willer, B., & Corrigan, J.D. (1993). New concepts Whatever It Takes: a model for community-based services. *Brain Injury, 8*, (7), 647–659.

Wilms, W. (1984). Vocational education and job success: the employer's view. *Phi Delta Kappa, 65*, 347–350.

Wilson, B. (1984). Memory therapy in practice. In B. Wilson and N. Moffatt (Eds.), *Clinical management of memory problems.* London: Croom Helm, pp. 89–112.

Wilson, B.A., and Moffat, N. (Eds). (1984). Clinical management of memory problems. Rockville, MD: Aspen Systems Corporation.

Wilson, B., Cockburn, T., & Baddeley, A.D.B. (1985). *The Rivermead Behavioural Memory Test Manual.* Thames Valley Test Company, 34 The Square, Titchfield, Hants, PO14 4 AF.

Wilson, B.A. (1987). *Rehabilitation of memory.* New York: Guilford Press.

Wilson, B. A., Cockburn, J., & Halligan, P. (1987). *Behavioural Inattention Test.* Bury St. Edmunds, Suffolk, England: Thames Valley Test Company.

Wolf, M. M. (1978). Social validity: The case for subjective measurement or how applied behavior analysis is finding its heart. *Journal of Applied Behavior Analysis, 11*, 203–214.

Wood, R.L., (1987). *Brain Injury Rehabilitation: A Neurobehavioural Approach.* London: Croom Helm.

World Health Organization (1980). *The international classification of diseases 10th revision (ICD-10).* Chapter V: Mental, behavioral and developmental disorders (pp. 25–31). Geneva: WHO typescript document MNH/MEP/87.1.

Wright, B. D. & Linacre, J. M. (1989). Observations are always ordinal; measurements, however, must be interval. *Archives of Physical Medicine and Rehabilitation, 70*, 857–860.

Ylkvisaker, M., Szekeres, Henry, K., et al. (1987). Topics in cognitive rehabilitation therapy. In M.

Ylvisaker and E. Gobble (Eds.), *Community Re-entry for Head Injured Adults* (pp. 174–175). Boston, MA: Little, Brown & Co.

Ylvisaker, M. (1989). Cognitive and psychosocial outcome following head injury in children. In J.T. Hoff, T.E. Anderson, & T.M. Cole, (Eds.), *Mild to moderate head injury.* London: Blackwell Scientific Publications, Inc.

Young, G. C., Collins, D. & Hren, M. (1983). Effect of pairing scanning training with block design training in the remediation of perceptual problems in left hemiplegics. *Journal of Clinical Neuropsychology, 5,* 201–212.

Zangwill, O.L. (1947). Psychological aspects of rehabilitation in cases of brain injury. *British Journal of Psychology, 37,* 60–69.

Zarit, S., & Teri, L. (1992). Interventions and services for family caregivers. In K. W. Schaie & M. Powell Lawton (Eds.), *Annual Review of Gerontology and Geriatrics, 11,* 287–310. New York: Springer.

Zarit, S., Reever, K. E., & Bach-Peterson, J. (1980). Relatives of the impaired elderly: Correlates of feelings of burden. *The Gerontologist, 20,* 649–655.

Zilmer, E., Fowler, P., Gutnick, H., & Becker, E. (1990). Comparison of two cognitive bed-side screening instruments in nursing home residents: A factor analytic study. *Journals of Gerontology: Psychological Science, 45,* P69-P74.

CHAPTER 14

Efficacy, Outcomes, and Cost Effectiveness in Dysphagia

JERI A. LOGEMANN

INTRODUCTION

"Can't you do something to assist my patient who has had a supraglottic laryngectomy to swallow safely enough that he can go home?" "Isn't there something you could do to help Tom Jones in 374, who's had a brainstem stroke, to eat enough by mouth so he can go home?" These were the kinds of questions asked of speech-language pathologists (SLPs) in acute care hospitals by physicians and surgeons in the late 1960s and early 1970s when a number of SLPs were becoming involved in the evaluation and treatment of patients with swallowing disorders resulting from sudden onset neurologic disorders (e.g. stroke, head injury, spinal cord injury) or from treatment for head and neck cancer. We had already been evaluating and treating these patients for their speech disorders, but the physicians' greatest concern was getting the patient back to oral feeding and out of the hospital. Thus, dysphagia assessment and treatment began with and continues to have a focus on outcomes—that is, returning the patient to full oral intake and discharging them from the hospital, rehab center, or other facility as quickly as possible, thus reducing the duration and cost of hospitalization and nonoral feedings while preventing any expensive medical complications, such as aspiration, pneumonia, or dehydration. Although these outcomes were clearly stated from the beginning of the SLP's involvement with dysphagia and continue to be the focus of each patient's care, the urgency to measure and document the exact impact of our dysphagia management on homogeneous groups of dysphagic patients was not paramount and gave way to needed studies on normal swallow physiology, and quantification of normal and abnormal swallow, swallow disorders typical of particular diagnoses, and new swallow therapy procedures. My purposes here are to define the types of efficacy and outcome

studies that are feasible in the area of dysphagia and to highlight the particular constraints and advantages in the conduct of such research in the area of evaluation and treatment of swallowing disorders.

HISTORICAL PERSPECTIVE

In the past 10 years, there has been increasing recognition that normal swallowing is not a single behavior but a set of 30+ behaviors, which vary systematically with the characteristics of the food being swallowed (e.g., bolus volume and viscosity) and the voluntary control exerted over the swallow (Cook, Dodds, Dantas, Kern, Massey, Shaker, & Hogan, 1989; Jacob, Kahrilas, Logemann, Shahn & Ita, 1989; Kahrilas, Lin, Logemann, Ergun, & Facchini, 1993; Kahrilas, Logemann, Lin & Ergun, 1992; Lazarus, Logemann, Rademaker, Kahrilas, Pajak, Lazar, & Halper, 1993; Logemann, 1989; 1993). For example, a swallow of saliva (approximately 1–2 ml) involves an oral stage followed by a pharyngeal and then an esophageal stage. In contrast, a swallow of 18–20 ml of liquid (the usual volume taken from a cup of coffee) involves simultaneous oral and pharyngeal stages. In addition, changes in swallow occur with normal aging (Robbins, Hamilton, Lof, & Kempster, 1992; Tracy, Logemann, Kahrilas, Jacob, Kobara, & Krugler, 1989). Knowledge of these predictable variations is critical to understanding the dysphagic patient's complaints of swallowing difficulties on various foods and/or volumes and in assuring an accurate assessment of the patient's dysphagia. More importantly, in terms of outcome assessment and treatment efficacy studies, the types of variables selected for measurement may need to be quite different for two groups of patients whose difficulties occur on different types of swallows. The more we understand the predictable variations in normal swallow physiology, the more accurately we will understand each patient's dysphagia and the effects of our treatment(s) on their function. Thus, research on normal swallowing physiology has and will continue to have an impact on the design and implementation of our efficacy and outcome studies in dysphagia.

Early in the development of research in the area of assessment and treatment of swallowing disorders, a variety of subjects of different ages and different diagnoses were typically presented as examples of the kinds of disruptions in oropharyngeal swallowing that could occur. Then, investigators narrowed their focus to examine single populations of dysphagic patients such as those with Parkinson's disease, stroke, amyotrophic lateral sclerosis, and so on (Barer, 1989; Gordon, Hewer, & Wade, 1987; Lazarus, 1989; Logemann, 1983; Veis & Logemann, 1985). Typically, these manuscripts described the types of swallowing disorders the patients exhibited without any measurement of the effects of the disorder on the patient's oral intake. Patterns of recovery or degeneration in the various patient groups were generally not elucidated. In fact, in any single manuscript there were often patients representing different stages of disease progression or recovery. Because the systematic changes in normal swallow physiology resulting from changes in bolus characteristics such as volume and viscosity were not yet defined, the food/bolus types used in these studies were often uncontrolled.

In the past 10 years, attempts have been made to better define dysphagic patient populations with the same etiology according to their stage of recovery or degeneration and to measure the temporal and/or biomechanical (movement over time) characteristics of the swallows of these homogeneous dysphagic subjects and to control the bolus types presented (Gisel & Alphonce, 1995; Logemann, 1987; Rademaker, Pauloski,

Logemann & Shanahan, 1994; Robbins & Levine, 1988; Wade & Hewer, 1987). These studies have largely examined the movement patterns of pharyngeal structures during the course of the swallow in order to understand the physiologic causes for inefficient or unsafe swallowing (Alberts, Horner, Gray, & Brazer, 1992; Horner, Massey, Riski, Lathrop, & Chase, 1990; Kuhlemeier, Rieve, Kirby & Siebens, 1989). In the last 5 years, these measures have also begun to be applied to studies of treatment effects (Bisch, Logemann, Rademaker, Lazarus, & Kahrilas, 1991; Lazarus, Logemann, Rademaker, Kahrilas, Pajak, Lazar, & Halper, 1993; Lazzara, Lazarus, & Logemann, 1986; Logemann, Pauloski, Colangelo, Lazarus, Fujiu, & Kahrilas, 1995; Logemann & Kahrilas, 1990; Rosenbek, Robbins, Fishback, & Levine, 1991). Data on length of treatment until the dysphagic patient with recovery potential returned to full oral intake according to diagnosis were not collected for most patient groups. For the patient with dysphagia resulting from progressive disease, the clear goal is to maintain safe and efficient oral intake for as long as possible. However, data on length of swallowing treatment in relation to length of time oral feeding is maintained as compared to untreated patients have not been collected.

There are several studies of time to return to oral intake with swallowing therapy in patients who have undergone partial laryngectomy (Logemann, Rademaker, Pauloski, Kahrilas, Bacon, Bowman, & McCracken, 1994; Logemann, Pauloski, Rademaker, Cook, Graner, Milianti, Beery, Stein, Bowman, Lazarus, Heiser, & Baker, 1992; Rademaker, Logemann, Pauloski, Bowman, Lazarus, Sisson, Milianti, Graner, Cook, Collins, Stein, Beery, Johnson, & Baker, 1993). Rademaker, Logemann, Pauloski, Bowman, Lazarus, Sisson, Milianti, Graner, Cook, Collins, Stein, Beery, Johnson, & Baker (1993) defined the average length of time until recovery of oral intake in subgroups of patients who had received postoperative swallowing therapy after partial laryngectomy. The data revealed that the duration of recovery to oral intake was significantly prolonged for patients with larger resections and that patients who underwent supraglottic laryngectomy (i.e., removal of part or all of the hyoid bone, epiglottis, false vocal folds, and aryepiglottic folds) took significantly longer to recover oral intake than patients who had undergone a hemilaryngectomy (removal of one vertical half of the larynx excluding the epiglottis). The difficulty with this study is the lack of control for spontaneous recovery. There was no control group of patients studied who did not receive swallowing therapy so the investigators could not attribute the improvements over time solely to the swallowing therapy. This problem has been true of several other investigations of treatment outcomes in dysphagic patients and is true of many studies of the outcomes of speech treatment as well.

NEGATIVE AND POSITIVE OUTCOMES

Outcomes from intervention or lack of intervention in the area of dysphagia may be negative or positive (Scheld & Mandell, 1991; Terry & Fuller, 1989). If the patient is denied intervention or if intervention is inappropriately provided or assessment is done inadequately leading to ineffective treatment, a patient may develop negative outcomes, including bronchitis, pneumonia or other pulmonary problems, malnutrition, dehydration, and death (Langmore, 1991, 1995). Currently, several studies have looked at negative outcomes from intervention according to whether or not pneumonia rates changed or patients died during the intervention (Croghan, Burke, Caplan & Denman, 1994; DePippo, Holas, Reding, Mandel, & Lesser, 1994; Kasprisin, Clumeck, & Nino-

Murcia, 1989; Martin, Corlew, Wood, Olson, Golopol, Wingo, & Kirmani, 1994; Schmidt, Holas, Halvorson, & Reding, 1994). These studies have generally not differentiated spontaneous recovery from treatment effects or have inadequately defined their treatment strategies. One of these studies will be described in more detail later.

In general, most studies of outcomes from dysphagia assessment and treatment have looked at positive outcomes (e.g., the time until return to oral intake, until return to full normal diet). In a study of partial laryngectomized patients who were assessed and managed by bedside intervention without any imaging studies versus a second group of similar patients who received dysphagia management based upon results of their videofluorographic (VFG) study, timing of nasogastric tube removal and rate of return to full oral intake for the two groups was examined (Logemann, Pauloski, Rademaker, Cook, Graner, Milianti, Beery, Stein, Bowman, Lazarus, Heiser, & Baker, 1992). Rate of return to normal swallow physiology was also an outcome measure. All patients in both groups (N = 21 in the bedside arm and 82 in the VFG arm) received a VFG study at 3 months posthealing. Interestingly, those patients whose swallowing management was based on the bedside exam had removal of the nasogastric tube and return to oral intake earlier than patients who received videofluorographic studies. This is not surprising because at bedside it is difficult if not impossible to identify the presence of aspiration or other pharyngeal swallowing problems. Patients may "look" as if they are doing well but in fact may be having significant difficulty with swallowing as observed on videofluoroscopy. If these patients had been managed with videofluoroscopy they would have been withheld from oral intake. Since videofluoroscopy reveals the patient's physiologic problems with oropharyngeal swallow, it is not surprising that patients who had their swallowing therapy based upon videofluoroscopy had significantly better swallow physiology than those who had a bedside-based approach, though their removal of the nasogastric tube and return to oral intake was delayed. Surprisingly, the rate of aspiration pneumonia was not significantly different for the two groups, highlighting the fact that we know little about the patient characteristics and degree of aspiration leading to aspiration pneumonia.

A study of long-term nonoral feeders as a result of stroke, conducted by the Speech-Language Pathology Service at the Hines V. A. Hospital in Illinois, also documents positive outcomes (Klor & Milianti, 1995). These professionals were able to restore the majority of patients to oral intake. Each patient's swallow was assessed with VFG. Treatment strategies were examined as a part of the radiographic study. Patients were then followed daily for therapy for 7 weeks. This investigation, which was reported at the 1995 ASHA Convention (Klor & Milianti, 1995), also calculated the cost savings of safe transfer to oral intake. The investigators estimated that the cost of the VFG study, therapy, and follow-up was approximately 50% less than the cost of non-oral feedings for a similar time period. These savings far outweighed the monetary investment in assessment and treatment of the dysphagia.

TYPES OF EFFICACY AND OUTCOME STUDIES USED IN DYSPHAGIA

A number of different types of research designs have been used to examine the efficacy of the SLP's assessment and treatment of oropharyngeal dysphagia, including case studies, treatment studies at the time of the diagnostic assessment, randomized studies, and quality-of-life studies (Langmore & Miller, 1994).

Single Case Studies

Several investigators have used the single case study design to describe and measure the efficacy of therapy for oropharyngeal dysphagia and the rate of return to oral intake in particular patients. Most of these studies use videofluorography to define the nature of the patient's oropharyngeal swallow physiology, followed by the introduction of one or more treatment procedures designed to eliminate symptoms such as aspiration, and /or to improve the abnormal aspects of the physiology such as reduced laryngeal elevation, poor tongue base retraction, and so on. (Lazarus, Logemann, Kahrilas, & Mittal, 1994; Robbins & Levine, 1993; Logemann & Kahrilas, 1990). These case studies have focused on brainstem stroke patients who typically exhibit more severe dysphagia poststroke than other patients with infarcts higher in the central nervous system (Logemann & Kahrilas, 1990; Robbins & Levine, 1993). Patients with brainstem strokes typically exhibit a severe delay in triggering the pharyngeal swallow (especially in the first week or two poststroke), reduced laryngeal elevation resulting in reduced cricopharyngeal opening, and a unilateral pharyngeal wall paresis or paralysis, which further contributes to poor cricopharyngeal opening. Some of these patients also exhibit a unilateral vocal fold paralysis. Some of the case studies describing swallow recovery as a result of dysphagia assessment and treatment have looked at the patients long after their stroke when one might assume there is no longer any potential for spontaneous recovery (Lazarus, Logemann, Kahrilas, & Mittal, 1994; Logemann & Kahrilas, 1990; Rosenbek, Robbins, Fishback, & Levine, 1991). Other studies have examined patients early in the poststroke period or some time after other injuries or head and neck surgery when it is difficult to separate the effects of recovery from the effects of the patient's therapy program (Logemann, Rademaker, Pauloski, Kahrilas, Bacon, Bowman, & McCracken, 1994).

Several of these case studies have shown return to oral intake in these patients long after their stroke (Logemann & Kahrilas, 1990). The case study model has also been utilized in the head and neck cancer population, with studies of individual patients again examining the effectiveness of the therapy program in returning the patient to more normal swallowing physiology and to oral intake long after spontaneous recovery has been completed. In most instances, these case studies like those in the stroke population, tend to focus on measurable effects of the treatment program over time as well as the length of time it takes to return the patient to full or partial oral intake.

Studies of Intervention Completed at the Time of Videofluorographic Assessment

One of the unique aspects of evaluation and treatment of dysphagia is that the assessment procedure, particularly videofluoroscopy, can enable the clinician to evaluate the immediate effectiveness of intervention strategies such as postural techniques, heightening sensory input, changes in bolus volume and viscosity, as well as selected therapy strategies such as swallowing maneuvers (Logemann, 1989; 1993; Logemann, Rademaker, Pauloski & Kahrilas, 1994). During the radiographic study, one can study the patient's swallowing physiology and identify disordered elements. Also, one can identify the relationship between the swallowing disorders and the symptoms of aspiration and penetration and residual food or inefficient swallowing. Then, one can ask the patient to use selected intervention strategies to eliminate the symptoms of the dysphagia and to improve the oropharyngeal swallowing physiology in some cases. In general, postural procedures are introduced first because they are relatively easy for the patient to use immediately and do not require increased muscular effort on the part of the patient.

Several studies have looked at the immediate effectiveness of postural strategies on the patient's ability to swallow thin liquids of various volumes safely (without aspiration) (Rasley, Logemann, Kahrilas, Rademaker, Pauloski, & Dodds, 1993; Logemann, Rademaker, Pauloski, & Kahrilas, 1994). In these studies, patients were presented with 1 ml of thin liquid and their swallow performance assessed videofluoroscopically. If these liquid swallows were safe and efficient, patients were then given several swallows of 3 ml volumes of thin liquid. The volumes were progressively increased to 10 ml and then to cup drinking as long as the patient was producing safe and efficient swallows. However, if the patient aspirated, a postural procedure appropriate to the cause of the aspiration was introduced and the patient was then reexamined using the postural technique while swallowing the same volume of thin liquid on which he/she had previously aspirated. If the postural technique eliminated the aspiration, several more swallows of that liquid volume were presented and the volume was then increased to examine the continued effectiveness of the postural procedure. Results of both studies indicated that the introduction of postural procedures was effective in eliminating aspiration of thin liquids on at least one bolus volume over 70% of both patient groups. Further, 25% of the patients who aspirated on thin liquids were able to swallow all volumes of thin liquid, including cup drinking using a postural change.

Following these studies, patients exhibited no pulmonary problems from the potential increase in number of swallows on which they aspirated during the radiographic study if the postural procedure(s) failed to eliminate aspiration. Despite the apparent success of some of these therapy procedures, as defined videofluoroscopically, data on the final outcome of these patients' eating status and speed of return to full or partial oral intake have not been described in the literature. It is important for the patient's physician and others in the health care system to understand the potential immediate impact of these studies of intervention effects on the patient's swallow safety and efficiency during the diagnostic procedure. This model of treatment efficacy and outcome research in fact may also be the most cost-effective type of intervention as it can enable patients to return quickly to partial or full oral intake.

Randomized Studies of Treatment Efficacy

There are only two randomized studies of swallowing treatments that are available at this time (DePippo, Holas, Reding, Mandel, & Lesser, 1994; Jacobs, Logemann, Pajak, Pauloski, Collins, Casiano, & Schuller, in preparation). The first is not a study of treatment as much as it is a study of several models for patient follow-up (i.e., reminding patients to utilize the treatment strategies identified as optimum for them during videofluorographic studies). *Dysphagia Therapy Following Stroke: A Controlled Trial,* as it is titled (DePippo, Holas, Reding, Mandel, & Lesser, 1994), provided radiographic studies to each of 90 patients after stroke and identified the optimum posture and diet for each patient. This intervention by videofluoroscopy was conducted by an SLP. Then, patients were randomized into one of three groups for follow-up: Group 1 received information on optimum diet and postural procedures but received no reminders from family or clinician (i.e., they were "self-monitoring"); Group 2 received regular reminders by family as to the correct posture and diet to be used for eating; Group 3 received a regular weekly therapy session in which the SLP provided reminders regarding the posture and diet to be used. Outcome measures were rates of pneumonia, other chest infections, dehydration, and death over a 6-month period. The three groups of patients were not significantly different on any of these measures. This is not surprising because swallowing therapy, as defined by most clinicians, was not given to any of the three groups. Rather, follow-up consisted of reminders for the patient regarding the optimum postures and diet identified by the SLP. Therefore, the study was actually comparing 3 different follow-up/reminder strategies, that is, (1) follow-up by a caregiver; (2) self-monitoring by the patient themselves; and (3) reminder by the SLP who did not provide any change in therapy but rather simply reminded the patient about the postural procedures and diets to be used. Unfortunately, while the study is interesting and would indicate that follow-up by an aide or caregiver can be effective once the appropriate diet and postures are identified by an SLP, it is not a study of therapy since active exercise programs were not initiated and evaluated by an SLP. In fact, every group of patients in this study received a careful assessment with compensatory treatments (diet modification and posture) designed by an SLP. The intervention process was identical except for follow-up.

A second randomized study, which has been completed but has not yet been published, is a study of cricopharyngeal myotomy attached to the surgical treatment for posterior oral cavity cancer and for laryngeal cancer requiring a partial laryngectomy (Jacobs, Logemann, Pajak, Pauloski, Collins, Casiano, & Schuller, in preparation). In this randomized study, patients with base of tongue or supraglottic malignant tumors were randomized to either receive or not receive a myotomy as a part of their definitive surgical treatment. Most head and neck surgeons perform a cricopharyngeal myotomy as a part of their definitive tumor surgery for these two types of tumors in order to "improve swallowing." Yet, no studies have determined whether cricopharyngeal myotomy does improve the patient's postoperative swallow. In fact, there are several nonrandomized studies that indicate highly variable results as a result of this procedure which vertically cuts across the fibers of the cricopharyngeal muscle by way of an external neck incision and dissection down to the cricopharyngeal muscle fibers (Buchholz, 1995; Chodosh, 1975; Sessions, Zill, & Schwartz, 1979). There is no control of healing in this surgical procedure. In this study, 67 patients were randomized to myotomy versus no myotomy arms, and videofluorographic studies were collected preoperatively and at 1 and 3 months postoperatively. The outcome measure for the trial was oropharyngeal swallow efficiency, which is a summary swallow measure that is calculated by dividing oropharyngeal transit time into the percentage of bolus swallowed. The percentage of bolus swallowed into the esophagus does not include any material that is aspirated or left in the mouth or pharynx. The videofluoroscopic studies were sent to a single reference laboratory that was blinded to the arm of the study to which each patient was randomized. The swallow laboratory then analyzed the patient swallow measures on 1 ml boluses of liquid and pudding and sent these data to the statistical center for analysis.

Results of the study indicate that there were no significant differences in oropharyngeal swallow efficiency for patients who did or did not receive the cricopharyngeal myotomy or any of the bolus types (liquid, paste, or cookie). These results do not support the use of cricopharyngeal myotomy as a part of the definitive surgery for tumor treatment in these tumor types. This study also has cost implications, since myotomy adds operating room time to the basic surgical procedure to resect the tumor and reconstruct the area.

It is clear that additional randomized studies of treatment efficacy and outcomes of treatment on oropharyngeal dysphagia are necessary. Several are underway, including a study of swallowing therapy for treated head and neck cancer patients with significant dysphagia 12 months or more after their initial tumor treatment (Pauloski, Logemann, Rademaker, McConnel, Stein, Beery, Johnson, Heiser, Cardinale, Shedd, Graner, Cook, Milianti, Collins, & Baker, 1994). The delay in accessing patients until 12 months or more posttreatment should eliminate the issue of spontaneous recovery effect(s) versus treatment effect(s). Patients with a specific level of swallow dysfunction will be randomized to an immediate treatment versus delayed treatment group. Those receiving dysphagia treatment by an SLP will have a prescribed therapy program for 16 weeks. Patients in both the treated and untreated arms will receive assessment at the beginning of the study and at the end of 16 weeks of therapy. At that time the patients who received swallowing treatment will serve as a control group and the patients who were randomized to delayed treatment will receive the 16-week treatment program. Both groups will again be reassessed after the second group completes treatment to define immediate treatment effects as well as the more lasting effects of treatment. A total of 150 patients will be treated in this study.

Quality-of-Life Instruments

In the last 10 years, there has been an increasing emphasis and understanding of the importance of the patient's perceived quality-of-life after a neurologic insult, head and neck cancer treatment, and other clinical conditions and interventions. As a result, there have been a number of quality-of-life instruments, as well as assessments of disability developed, such as the *Performance Status Scale for Head and Neck Cancer Patients* (PSS-HNC) (Browman, Levine, Hodson, et al., 1993; Cella, Tulsky, & Gray, 1993; List, Ritter-Sterr, & Lansky, 1990), which ask an independent observer to define the patient's level of function in a variety of areas including eating and diet. The ultimate goal of a swallowing rehabilitation program is to return the patient to the most normal diet possible. Quality-of-life instruments tend to be self-administered paper-and-pencil questionnaires or are to be completed in a relaxed, face-to-face discussion between the patient and the SLP. Questions regarding the patient's typical ability to eat a variety of foods in a variety of locations are usually included. An alternative to the quality-of-life assessments in the area of dysphagia are the nutritional diet calendars or notebooks, which request patients to note their oral intake according to type and amount of food on a meal-by-meal, day-by-day basis. This can then provide the basis for analysis of adequacy of oral intake, hydration, and nutrition. Though these types of instruments have been applied in several studies of head and neck surgical patients, there are still no typical patient outcome profiles on return to oral intake available for patients who have received particular types of treatment for head and neck cancer according to their original site and stage of disease.

LIMITATIONS ON TREATMENT EFFICACY AND OUTCOME STUDY DESIGNS SPECIFIC TO DYSPHAGIA

Because the intervention or lack thereof for oropharyngeal dysphagia can cause serious and costly health complications, the types of research designs that can be utilized in this population is somewhat more limited than in other disorder types. For example, randomizing patients to a treatment/no treatment paradigm if they are known to aspirate can cause a serious health problem for patients in the no-treatment group.

Another limitation in dysphagia research studies is the number of repetitions of both the number of swallows studied within each assessment and the physiologic assessment procedure itself. The use of videofluoroscopy as the major assessment tool for measurement of efficacy and outcome is a major limiting factor because of radiation exposure. The number of swallows that can be studied in a single session and the number of repeated radiographic studies that can be done, especially in young adults and children, is limited. Therefore, the clinician or clinical investigator must be careful to select those procedures for assessment and treatment that are most likely to improve the patient's status. This decision, in itself, is a limitation in that the clinician cannot deliver three or four different treatments in a randomized paradigm to the patient. The clinician must attempt to select the treatment procedures that he or she believes are most likely to be effective in the particular patient in order to reduce the risk of aspiration and pulmonary consequences.

Establishing a control group for treatment efficacy studies in dysphagia is difficult because of the potential risk of medical complications such as pneumonia, malnutrition, or dehydration, that may result from withholding swallowing therapy. Also, patients with swallowing disorders are often desperate to eat and are not willing to delay their rehabilitation as part of a study. If they agree to participate in a randomized study of immediate versus delayed swallowing therapy so that therapy versus recovery can be assessed, and they are randomized to the delayed treatment group, patients often drop out of the study and seek swallowing therapy elsewhere.

As in other areas of clinical research, separation of the patient's natural recovery process from the effects of treatment is a challenge (Cooper, 1990; Ingham, 1990; Judson, 1980; Medawan, 1979; Rimm, Hartz, Kalbfleisch, Anderson, & Hoffman, 1980). However, the model of introduction and assessment of treatment procedures during a single radiographic study does eliminate the recovery factor. Unfortunately, several of the studies in which postural procedures have been introduced in x-ray did not necessarily follow the patient to the point of return to oral intake. Neither did these studies follow the patients long enough to ensure that pneumonia did not occur because of noncompliance. Patients may have been instructed in effective treatment procedures but may not have continued to use these techniques because they erroneously think that they have recovered and don't need to use the posture change any longer during their meal times.

CONCLUSION

Many more studies on the efficacy, outcomes, and cost-effectiveness of treatment for oropharyngeal dysphagia are needed in well specified populations. In addition, investigations of the "carry over" effect(s) of treatment for swallowing on speech understandability are also needed. Since both speech and swallowing exist in the same mechanism, it is important for us to understand the effect(s) of a single therapy on both of these functions. In this way, research on treatment efficacy, outcomes and cost may result in multiple benefits, including expansion of our knowledge on sensorimotor control of the mechanism and identification of treatments which result in the best functional outcomes for our dysphagic patients.

REFERENCES

Alberts, M. J., Horner, J., Gray, L., & Brazer, S. R. (1992). Aspiration after stroke: Lesion analysis by brain MRI. *Dysphagia, 7,* 170–173.

Barer, D. (1989). The natural history and functional consequences of dysphagia after hemispheric stroke. *Journal of Neurology, Neurosurgery and Psychiatry, 52,* 236–241.

Bisch, E. M., Logemann, J. A., Rademaker, A. W., Lazarus, C., & Kahrilas, P. J. (1991, November). *Pharyngeal Effects of Bolus Temperature.* Paper presented at American Speech-Language-Hearing Association (ASHA) annual convention.

Browman, G. P., Levine, M. N., Hodson, D. I., et al. (1993). The head and neck radiotherapy questionnaire: A morbidity/quality-of-life instrument for clinical trials of radiation therapy in locally advanced head and neck cancer. *Journal of Clinical Oncology, 11,* 863–872.

Buchholz, D. W. (1995). Cricopharyngeal myotomy may be effective treatment for selected patients with neurogenic oropharyngeal dysphagia. *Dysphagia, 10,* 255–258.

Cella, D. F., Tulsky, D. S., Gray, G., et al. (1993). The functional assessment of cancer therapy scale: Development and validation of the general measure. *Journal of Clinical Oncology, 11,* 570–579.

Chodosh, P. (1975). Cricopharyngeal myotomy in the treatment of dysphagia. *Laryngoscope, 85,* 1862–1873.

Cook, I. J., Dodds, W. J., Dantas, R. O., Kern, M. K., Massey, B. T., Shaker, R., & Hogan, W. J. (1989). Timing of videofluoroscopic, manometric events and bolus transit during the oral and pharyngeal phases of swallowing. *Dysphagia, 4,* 8–15.

Cooper, J. A. (1990). Treatment studies and research design: An NIH perspective. In L. B. Olswang, C. K. Thompson, S. F. Warren, & N. J. Minghetti (Eds.), *Treatment Efficacy Research in Communication Disorders.* Rockville, MD: ASHA Foundation.

Croghan, J. E., Burke, E. M., Caplan, S., & Denman, S. (1994). Pilot study of 12-month outcomes of nursing home patients with aspiration on videofluoroscopy. *Dysphagia, 9,* 141–146.

DePippo, K. L., Holas, M. A., Reding, M. J., Mandel, F. S., & Lesser, M. L. (1994). Dysphagia therapy following stroke: A controlled trial. *Neurology, 44,* 1655–1660.

Gisel, E. G., & Alphonce, E. (1995). Classification of eating impairments based on eating efficiency in children with cerebral palsy. *Dysphagia, 10,* 268–274.

Goldstein, H. (1990). Assessing clinical significance. In L. B. Olswang, C. K. Thompson, S. F. Warren, & N. J. Minghetti (Eds.), *Treatment Efficacy Research in Communication Disorders.* Rockville, MD: ASHA Foundation.

Gordon, C., Hewer, R., & Wade, D. (1987). Dysphagia in acute stroke. *British Medical Journal, 295,* 411–414.

Horner, J., Massey, E. W., Riski, J. E., Lathrop, D. L., & Chase, K. N. (1990). Aspiration following stroke: Clinical correlates and outcome. *Neurology, 38,* 1359–1362.

Ingham, J. C. (1990). Issues of treatment efficacy: Design and experimental control. In L. B. Olswang, C. K. Thompson, S. F. Warren, & N. J. Minghetti (Eds.), *Treatment efficacy research in communication disorders* (pp. 51–61). Rockville, MD: ASHA Foundation.

Jacob, P., Kahrilas, P. J., Logemann, J. A., Shah, V., & Ha, T. (1989). Upper esophageal sphincter opening and modulation during swallowing. *Gastroenterology, 97*, 1469–1478.

Jacobs, J., Logemann, J., Pajak, T., Pauloski, B., Collins, S., Casiano, R., & Schwiller, D. (in preparation). Failure of cricopharyngeal myotomy to improve dysphagia: Results of a randomized clinical trial.

Judson, H. F. (1980). *The search for solutions* (p. 171). New York: Holt, Rinehart and Winston.

Kahrilas, P. J., Lin, S., Logemann, J. A., Ergun, G. A., & Facchini, F. (1993). Deglutitive tongue action: Volume accommodation and bolus propulsion. *Gastroenterology, 104,* 152–162.

Kahrilas, P. J., Logemann, J. A., Lin, S., & Ergun, G. A. (1992). Pharyngeal clearance during swallow: A combined manometric and videofluoroscopic study. *Gastroenterology, 103,* 128–136.

Kasprisin, A. T., Clumeck, H., & Nino-Murcia, M. (1989). The efficacy of rehabilitative management of dysphagia. *Dysphagia, 4,* 48–52.

Klor, B., Milianti, F. (1995) Rehabilitation of dysphagia in patients with G-tubes. Presented at the 1995 ASHA convention in Orlando, FL.

Kuhlemeier, K., Rieve, J., Kirby, N., & Siebens, A. (1989). Clinical correlates of dysphagia in stroke patients. *Archives of Physical Medicine and Rehabilitation, 70* (special annual meeting issue, A–56).

Langmore, S. E. (1995). Efficacy of behavioral treatment for oropharyngeal dysphagia. *Dysphagia, 10,* 259–262.

Langmore, S. E. (1991). Managing the complications of aspiration in dysphagic adults. *Seminars in Speech and Language, 12,* 199–207.

Langmore, S. E., & Miller, R. M. (1994). Behavioral treatment for adults with oropharyngeal dysphagia. *Archives of Physical Medicine and Rehabilitation, 75,* 1154–1160.

Lazarus, C. L. (1989). Swallowing disorders after traumatic brain injury. *Journal of Head Trauma Rehabilitation, 4*(4), 34–43.

Lazarus, C. L., Logemann, J. A., Rademaker, A. W., Kahrilas, P. J., Pajak, T., Lazar, R., & Halper, A. (1993). Effects of bolus volume, viscosity and repeated swallows in non-stroke subjects and stroke patients. *Archives of Physical Medicine and Rehabilitation, 74,* 1066–1070.

Lazarus, C. L., Logemann, J. A., Kahrilas, P. J., & Mittal, B. B. (1994). Swallow recovery in an oral cancer patient following surgery, radiotherapy, and hyperthermia. *Head & Neck, 16*(3), 259–265.

Lazzara, G., Lazarus, C., & Logemann, J. A. (1986). Impact of thermal stimulation on the triggering of the swallowing reflex. *Dysphagia, 1,* 73–77.

Lindgren, S. & Ekberg, O. (1990). Cricopharyngeal myotomy in the treatment of dysphagia. *Clinical Otolaryngology, 15,* 221–227.

List, M. A., Ritter-Sterr, C. & Lansky, S. B. (1990). A performance status scale for head and neck cancer treatment. *Cancer, 66,* 564–569.

Logemann, J. A. (1987). Criteria for studies of treatment for oral-pharyngeal dysphagia. *Dysphagia, 1,* 193–199.

Logemann, J. A. (1983). *Evaluation and treatment of swallowing disorders.* Austin, TX: Pro-Ed.

Logemann, J. A. (1993). *A manual for videofluoroscopic evaluation of swallowing* (2nd ed.). Austin, TX: Pro-Ed.

Logemann, J. A. (1989). Evaluation and treatment planning for the head-injured patient with oral intake disorders. *Journal of Head Trauma Rehabilitation, 4*(4), 24–33.

Logemann, J. A. (Ed.) (1993). Dysphagia: Evaluation and treatment. *Clinics in Communication Disorders, 3*(4).

Logemann, J. A., Pauloski, B. R., Rademaker, A., Cook, B., Graner, D., Milianti, F., Beery, Q., Stein, D., Bowman, J., Lazarus, C., Heiser, M. A., & Baker, T. (1992). Impact of the diagnostic procedure on outcome measures of swallowing rehabilitation in head and neck cancer patients. *Dysphagia, 7,* 179–86.

Logemann, J.A., Rademaker, A.W., Pauloski, B.R., Kahrilas, P.J., Bacon, M., Bowman, J., & McCracken, E. (1994). Mechanisms of recovery of swallow after supraglottic laryngectomy. *Journal of Speech and Hearing Research, 37,* 965–974.

Logemann, J. A., Pauloski, B. R., Colangelo, L., Lazarus, C., Fujiu, M., & Kahrilas, P. J. (1995). Effects of a sour bolus on oropharyngeal swallowing measures in patients with neurogenic dysphagia. *Journal of Speech Hearing Research, 38*(3), 556–563.

Logemann, J. A., Rademaker, A. W., Pauloski, B. R., & Kahrilas, P. J. (1994). Effects of postural change on aspiration in head and neck surgical patients. *Otolaryngology-Head and Neck Surgery, 110,* 222–227.

Logemann, J. A., & Kahrilas, P. J. (1990). Relearning to swallow post CVA: Application of maneuvers and indirect biofeedback: A case study. *Neurology, 40,* 1136–1138.

Martin, B. J. W., Corlew, M. M., Wood, H., Olson, D., Golopol, L. A., Wingo, M., & Kirmani, N. (1994). The association of swallowing dysfunction and aspiration pneumonia. *Dysphagia, 9,* 1–6.

Medawar, P. B. (1979). *Advice to a young scientist* (p. 50). London: Basic Books.

Miller, R., M., & Langmore, S. E. (1994). Treatment efficacy for adults with oropharyngeal dysphagia. *Archives of Physical Medicine and Rehabilitation, 75,* 1256–1262.

Pauloski, B. R., Logemann, J. A., Rademaker, A. W., McConnel, F. M. S., Stein, D., Beery, Q., Johnson, J., Heiser, M. A., Cardinale, S., Shedd, D., Graner, D., Cook, B., Milianti, F., Collins, S., & Baker, T. (1994). Speech and swallowing function after oral and oropharyngeal resections: One-year follow-up. *Head & Neck, 16,* 313–322.

Rademaker, A. W., Pauloski, B. R., Logemann, J. A., & Shanahan, T. K. (1994). Oropharyngeal swallow efficiency as a representative measure of swallowing function. *Journal of Speech and Hearing Research, 37,* 314–325.

Rademaker, A. W., Logemann, J. A., Pauloski, B. R., Bowman, J., Lazarus, C., Sisson, G., Milianti, F., Graner, D., Cook, B., Collins, S., Stein, D., Beery, Q., Johnson, J., & Baker, T. (1993). Recovery of postoperative swallowing in patients undergoing partial laryngectomy. *Head & Neck, 15,* 325–334.

Rasley, A., Logemann, J. A., Kahrilas, P. J., Rademaker, A. W., Pauloski, B. R., & Dodds, W. J. (1993). Prevention of barium aspiration during videofluoroscopic swallowing studies: Value of change in posture. *American Journal of Roentgenology, 160,* 1005–9.

Rimm, A., Hartz, A., Kalbfleisch, J., Anderson, A., & Hoffmann, R. (1980). Basic biostatistics in medicine and epidemiology (pp. 296–299). London: Appleton-Century-Crofts.

Robbins, J., & Levine, R. (1988). Swallowing after unilateral stroke of the cerebral cortex: Preliminary experience. *Dysphagia, 3,* 11–17.

Robbins, J., Hamilton, J. W., Lof, G. L. & Kempster, G. B. (1992). Oropharyngeal swallowing in adults of different ages. *Gastroenterology, 103,* 823–829.

Robbins, J. & Levine, R. (1993). Swallowing after lateral medullary syndrome plus. *Clinics in Communication Disorders, 3*(4), 45–55.

Rosenbek, J. C., Robbins, J., Fishback, B., & Levine, R. L. (1991). The effects of thermal application on dysphagia after stroke. *Journal of Speech and Hearing Research, 34,* 1257–1268.

Scheld, W. M., & Mandell, G. L. (1991). Nosocomial pneumonia: Pathogenesis and recent advances in diagnosis and therapy. *Review of Infectious Disease, 13* (Suppl 9), 743–751.

Schmidt, J., Holas, M., Halvorson, K., & Reding, M. (1994). Videofluoroscopic evidence of aspiration predicts pneumonia and death but not dehydration following stroke. *Dysphagia, 9,* 7–11.

Sessions, D., Zill, R., & Schwartz, S. (1979). Deglutition after conservation surgery for cancer of the larynx and hypopharynx. *Otolaryngology-Head and Neck Surgery, 87,* 779–796.

Spilker, B. (Ed.). (1990). *Quality of life assessments in clinical trials.* New York: Raven.

Terry, P., & Fuller, S. (1989). Pulmonary consequences of aspiration. *Dysphagia, 3,* 179–183.

Tracy, J., Logemann, J., Kahrilas, P., Jacob, P., Kobara, M., & Krugler, C. (1989). Preliminary observations on the effects of age on oropharyngeal deglutition. *Dysphagia, 4,* 90–94.

Veis, S., & Logemann, J. (1985). The nature of swallowing disorders in CVA patients. *Archives of Physical Medicine and Rehabilitation, 66,* 372–375.

Wade, D., & Hewer, L. (1987). Motor loss and swallowing difficulty after stroke: Frequency, recovery and prognosis. *Acta Neurologica Scandinavia, 76,* 50–54.

Wilson, E. O. (1994). *Naturalist.* Washington, DC: Island Press/Shearwater Books.

CHAPTER 15

Outcomes Measurement in Motor Speech Disorders

DAVID R. BEUKELMAN, PAMELA MATHY,
AND KATHRYN YORKSTON

INTRODUCTION

The communication disorders that result from neurologic impairments are diverse in their nature and severity. Individuals with a variety of etiologies may experience communication disorders as a result of neuromotor, neurolinguistic, or neurocognitive impairments. This chapter focuses on outcomes measurement of a range of motor speech disorders, including disorders in the planning (apraxia of speech) and execution (the dysarthrias) of the movements of speech production. Apraxia of speech is a motor speech disorder caused by a disturbance in motor programming of sequential movement for volitional speech production. In apraxia, the speech musculature itself is not impaired; however, the apraxic speaker will have difficulty completing sequences of speech movements. In contrast, dysarthria is a motor speech disorder caused by disturbances in neuromuscular control of the components of the speech mechanism. Weakness, paralysis, or incoordination of the muscles due to damage to the central or peripheral nervous systems cause difficulty in execution of movements during speech.

When reviewing the outcomes research associated with motor speech disorders, a number of factors must be considered, including etiology, natural course of the pathology, pharmacological intervention, and possible associated cognitive deficits. These factors must be understood if the potential impact of motor speech interventions are to be evaluated. For example, individuals with amyotrophic lateral sclerosis, Parkinson's disease, and Huntington's disease experience communication disorders that become more severe as the disease progresses. For those with motor speech disorders associated with stroke, the communication disorder remains essentially stable for extended periods of time. Persons with traumatic brain injury may recover functional speech within months of their injury, others recover speech very gradually, and still others experience an essentially stable communication disorder. Thus, changes associated with speech intervention must be assessed in relation to the predicted natural course of the disease.

At times interventions are not targeted to improve speech production. For many individuals with the most severe communication disorders, communication strategies other than natural speech are required for them to meet their daily communication needs on a temporary or permanent basis. This collection of strategies and options is referred to as augmentative or alternative communication (AAC). Outcome assessment for these individuals must focus on the adequacy of communication with AAC systems rather than on natural speech.

In this chapter, we will review strategies that have been applied to outcomes measurement in motor speech disorders. It is beyond the scope of this chapter to complete an exhaustive examination of the evidence for the benefit of speech treatment for individuals with dysarthria or apraxia of speech. Rather, we will discuss the rationale and goals of outcome measures in motor speech disorders. Most clinicians and clinical researchers would agree that we do not know enough about the outcomes of our treatment. For the most part, definitive studies of treatment efficacy are lacking. Our field is not alone. Duffy (1995) suggests that well-controlled treatment efficacy studies are available for only approximately 15% of medical intervention. Despite that fact that there is much work yet to be done, it is useful to establish a framework for our questions about treatment efficacy and to use that framework to continue exploration of intervention outcomes.

CHRONIC DISABILITY MODEL

The chronic disability model conceptualized by Nagi (1991) is a particularly useful framework for considering the intervention outcomes associated with motor speech disorders. For individuals with motor speech disorders, all levels of the model—pathology, impairment, functional limitation, and disability—may be considered targets for intervention and also for outcome assessment. For example, pharmacologic interventions are focused either on the *pathology level* of the disease, such as dopamine for persons with Parkinson's disease, or the secondary pathologies, such as muscle relaxants for persons with spasticity. Outcome measures at the pathology (cellular or tissue) level usually involve chemical tests (therapeutic levels of a drug), physiological tests of tremor, strength, rate of movement, and so on.

At the *impairment level*, interventions target specific speech mechanism subsystems. For example, prosthodontic intervention, such as a palatal lift for the velopharyngeal subsystem, is not intended to effect the underlying pathology. Speech intervention may focus on the impairment level by targeting the phonatory, respiratory, velopharyngeal, or articulatory subsystems. Outcome measures at the impairment level usually involve the measurement of performance for a particular subsystem. For example, measures of respiratory performance typically include estimates of subglottal air pressure, lung volume patterns during speech, or respiratory shape during speech (Hixon, 1984). The status of the velopharyngeal subsystem is evaluated using estimates of velopharyngeal resistance, nasal emission, or nasality. Articulatory accuracy and precision are routine outcome measures used to evaluate the articulatory subsystem. Details of the physiologic assessment of motor speech disorders can be found elsewhere (Duffy, 1995; Rosenbek & LaPointe, 1985; and Yorkston, Beukelman, & Bell, 1988).

Intervention directed toward overall speech performance influence the *functional limitation level* of the disorder. For example, teaching a speaker to reduce overall speaking rate may be considered an organism level rather than a subsystem level intervention. Some dysarthric speakers are so disordered that they are unable to meet their daily communication needs on a temporary or a long-term basis. Typically, these individuals are provided with AAC options to supplement or substitute for their natural speech. AAC aids and techniques are designed to increase overall communicative function and, therefore, would be considered interventions at the functional limitation level. Outcomes at the functional limitation level have included speech intelligibility, speaking rate, and speech naturalness (Yorkston, Beukelman, & Bell, 1988).

Finally, speech interventions that focus on listener's attitudes and/or interactions between dysarthric speakers and their listeners in a variety of contexts, including school, work, and social, would be considered a *disability level* intervention. The typical goal of these interventions is not to change or improve the dysarthric speech, but to instruct or support the listener to interact more effectively with disordered speakers. Communication is made more adequate by improving interactional skills and by reducing the listener bias and prejudice. Two types of outcome measures are used to assess the disability of dysarthric speakers—message comprehensibility and ratings of communication effectiveness and comfort in various contexts (Sullivan, Brune, & Beukelman, 1995; Antonius, Beukelman, & Reid, 1996; Yorkston & Bombardier, 1992; Yorkston, Bombardier, & Hammen, 1994; Yorkston, Strand, & Kennedy, 1996).

In the previous paragraphs, specific interventions and outcome measure strategies have been associated with discrete levels of the chronic disorders model. In reality, however, the outcomes of interventions are not restricted to a single disorder level. In other words, an intervention at the pathology level may impact performance at one or more of the other levels. For example, inappropriate pharmacological intervention may negatively impact speech subsystems, overall speech performance, and social interaction with listeners. On the other hand, effective pharmacological intervention may have positive impact on all of the disorder levels. An intervention at the subsystem level (impairment) may also have far reaching outcomes. For example, a successful palatal lift fitting will not only impact velopharyngeally related outcomes (nasal emission and nasality), but usually also impact respiratory function, articulatory performance, and overall speech intelligibility. The benefits derived from successful palatal lift fittings may also improve speech intelligibility in natural communication contexts.

The relationship among the various disorder levels is difficult to predict except at the extremes. Obviously, if an intervention is so successful that speech is normalized, one would expect improvement to be observed at all levels of the disorder. However, such dramatic improvement is quite uncommon among motor speech disorders. Usually, improvements at one level may or may not be accompanied by improvements at other levels. Therefore, in outcomes research, it is necessary to assess all levels of disorder in order to document the outcomes from an intervention.

PROGRESSIVE MOTOR SPEECH DISORDERS

In the following sections, the discussion of intervention effectiveness will be organized by natural course of the motor speech disorders, that is, progressive, and recovering-stable. In each of these categories, the approach to measurement of outcome will vary as will the reasons for outcome measures. For example, it may not be appropriate to measure the outcomes of intervention for progressive diseases in the same way as those with a stable or recovering course. We will review four progressive neurological diseases (amyotrophic lateral sclerosis, multiple sclerosis, Parkinson's disease, and Huntington's disease). Although all are progressive disorders, they vary considerably in rates of degeneration, physiologic characteristics, and concomitant problems such as cognitive decline.

The Diseases

Amyotrophic Lateral Sclerosis (ALS)

Amyotrophic lateral sclerosis (ALS) is a rapidly progressive degenerative disease resulting in severe functional communication limitations due to a mixed flaccid-spastic dysarthria. The pathology of ALS is destruction of the motor neurons of the brain and spinal cord. In its classical form, the impairment is restricted to motor function, leaving sensation and cognition unimpaired. Incidence figures range from 0.4 to 1.8 per 100,000 populations with prevalence rates between 4 and 6 per 100,000 (Tandan & Bradley, 1985).

Dysarthria is a common symptom of ALS. According to Saunders, Walsh, and Smith (1981), 75% of persons with ALS are unable to speak at the time of their deaths. An even larger number experience such severe functional communication difficulties that they are unable to meet all of their daily communication needs using natural speech. Due to the prevalence of severe motor speech disorders in this population, AAC strategies are routine.

The progression of the motor speech disorder experienced in ALS is dependent upon the pattern of neurological pathology. Those individuals who have primarily bulbar ALS symptoms experience such severe communication disorders early in their disease progression that they require AAC systems at a time when they may still be able to walk and drive. Approximately one-fourth of patients experience initial symptoms classified primarily as bulbar ALS. Persons with primarily spinal involvement may be able to communicate quite effectively using their natural speech for several years, even as their ability to walk, drive, and feed themselves is deteriorating.

Multiple Sclerosis (MS)

Multiple Sclerosis (MS) is a progressive disease with pathology of the white matter of the central nervous system. The incidence is estimated at about 8000 cases per year with the mean onset age of 27 years and a ratio of females to males of 1.5:1. In the northern part of the United States the prevalence of MS is about one in 1000 of population; it is one-third to one-half that in the southern states (Arnason, 1982).

The clinical course of the pathology has been divided into five classes: benign (20%), combined relapsing/remitting with nearly full remission (15 to 20%) with incomplete remissions evolving into chronic progressive (30 to 40%), chronic progressive with insidious onset (20 to 30%), and malignant with severe, rapid progression and death within weeks to months (5% or less) (Yorkston, Miller, & Beukelman, 1995). Speech symptoms depend upon the location of the lesions. Therefore, the nature of the communication disorder is not consistent from person to person. Thirty-two to 41% of persons with MS exhibit dysarthria of speech (Darley, Brown, & Goldstein, 1972).

Approximately 4% of persons with MS report that they are unable to speak so that strangers can understand them (Beukelman, Kraft, & Freal, 1985). Of this group, 28% reported that they used AAC strategies.

Parkinson's Disease

Parkinson's disease is a syndrome with primary symptoms that include resting tremor, rigidity, paucity of movements, and impaired postural reflexes. The pathology of Parkinson's disease is a loss of dopaminergic neurons in the basal ganglia (especially the substantia nigra) and brain stem. Age-adjusted prevalence ratios range from 30 to 180 per 100,000. There are approximately 40,000 new cases per year (McDowell & Cederbaum, 1987). Rates of occurrence are similar across nationality groups and countries.

Dysarthria is typically not one of the early symptoms of Parkinson's disease; however, its prevalence increases with the course of the disorder. Logemann, Fisher, Boshes, and Blonsky (1978) reported that 89% of their sample exhibited impairment of the vocal subsystem and 45% exhibited impairment of the articulary subsystem. In 1956, Buck and Cooper studied the functional limitations of 67 individuals with Parkinson's disease and reported that 29% of their sample had severe dysarthria, 22% had moderate dysarthria, and 37% exhibited normal speech or were mildly involved.

Probably the most complete overview of the impairment of parkinsonian speech characteristics comes from the work of Darley, Aronson, and Brown (1969a and 1969b, 1975). They studied 32 individuals with Parkinson's disease and observed reduced variability in pitch and loudness, reduced loudness level overall, and decreased use of all vocal parameters for achieving stress and emphasis, markedly reduced articulatory precision, short bursts of speech, inappropriate silences, and harsh voice quality that was sometimes breathy.

Huntington's Disease

Huntington's disease is an inherited autosomal dominant degenerative disease. Symptoms of this progressive disease typically appear in the fourth decade with death occurring 15 to 20 years after onset. Huntington's disease often progresses more rapidly in juvenile than adult patients. The pathology of Huntington's disease is atrophy of the striate bodies associated with the loss of small neurons. Cortical neurons may also degenerate. Huntington's disease involves a deficiency of the neural transmitter in the basal ganglia (gamma-amino butyric acid-GABA). The reduction in GABA inhibitions may result in overactivity of the dopaminergic system. Chorea is the primary motor disorder feature of the disorder. However, rigidity and dystonia may be present in addition to chorea. Huntington's disease may also be associated with personality changes and progress to cognitive changes and memory losses. The movement and cognitive disorders associated with Huntington's disease result in a number of functional limitations, such as dysarthria, dysphagia, weight loss, feeding and swallowing problems, and abnormal gait. Dysarthria (of the hyperkinetic type) reflects the underlying choreatic movement disorder of Huntington's disease. These involuntary contractions of the muscle may affect any aspect of the speech mechanism (respiration, phonation, or articulation). The speech impairment associated with Huntington's disease may vary considerably from person to person. For some, the choreatic movements may be restricted primarily to the lower extremities without obvious speech disorder. For others, speech is so impaired that AAC strategies are required. A review of the literature reveals limited successful use of high-technology AAC systems for persons with Huntington's disease. In the authors' experience, this occurs because of the nature of the motor and cognitive impairments and the fact that intervention is typically not initiated early in the course of the disease when learning new skills is practical.

Intervention Effectiveness Analysis

Because there is no reason to assume an improvement in the neuromotor pathology for individuals with degenerative disease, *improvement* in speech performance at any level of disorder, in response to an intervention protocol, can be viewed as effective. In the face of a progressive condition such as Parkinson's disease, one would not expect spontaneous improvement in the underlying pathology, unless there was a change in response to pharmacological or surgical intervention. One might make the argument that treatment resulting in stabilization of speech performance could be judged as effective if there was a documented increase in pathology or impairment.

Some diseases, such as multiple sclerosis, are associated with an unstable neuromotor impairment. Although the overall course of the disease can be progressive, the week-to-week, month-to-month course of the disease can be quite variable with numerous periods of exacerbation and remission. In this case, improvement in speech symptoms may not be associated with intervention effectiveness but simply be a reflection of the natural course of the underlying pathology.

Why Measure Speech Outcomes?

In the following section, we will review selected studies in order to highlight different purposes or goals of outcome assessment and how outcome measures may be used to enlighten our clinical practice.

Documenting the Efficacy of Impairment-level Intervention

Although all of the disorders discussed in this section are characterized by a degenerative course, numerous positive approaches to intervention have recently been developed. These include drug intervention for ALS (Bensimon, Lacomblez, & Meininger, 1994) and MS (Goodkin, 1994; Jacobs & Johnson, 1994; Van Oosten, Truyen, Barkhof & Polman, 1995) and surgical management for individuals with Parkinson's disease (Iacono, Lonser, Oh, & Yamada, 1995; Laitinen, 1995). All of these interventions focus on reducing the pathophysiology of the disorder. Outcome measures including those that reflect speech function are necessary in order to confirm that changes at the physiologic level bring about concomitant changes at other levels of the disorder. For example, does interferon reduce the severity of respiratory, phonatory, or articulatory symptoms in dysarthric speakers with MS? Further, do changes in the speech impairment also translate into improvements in the areas of functional limitation and disability? Because of both the costs and potential risk to patients, we must confirm efficacy of impairment-level intervention across a number of levels of the disorder.

Staging of Treatment

Each of the progressive neurological disorders discussed in this section has a different rate and pattern of progression. For example, ALS is considered a rapidly progressive disease, while Parkinson's disease is considered slowly progressive. Further, there are individual differences among patients with a particular disease. In other words, not all speakers with ALS progress at a similar rate. Because of these group and individual differences, there is no overall "calendar" by which intervention should be implemented. Therefore, outcome measures that take into account the level of impairment, functional limitation, and disability are essential for appropriate staging or timing of treatment. Scales are available for ALS, Parkinson's disease, MS, and Huntington's disease (see Table 15–1) in order to rate speech function (Yorkston, Miller, & Strand, 1995). Sequencing of management insures that current problems are addressed and future problems are anticipated. Staging of treatment should be based on knowledge of disease progression and provision of that information to the patient and their families in a timely fashion.

Table 15–2 contains a summary of possible intervention for mild, moderate, and severe dysarthria associated with the degenerative diseases discussed in this chapter.

Table 15–1. Summary of Speech Severity Scales for Amytrophic Lateral Sclerosis (ALS) and Parkinson's Disease (PD)

SCALE SCORE	ALS	PD
10	Normal speech	Normal speech
9	Nominal speech abnormality	Speech entirely adequate; minor voice disturbances present
8	Perceived speech changes	Speech easily understood, but voice or speech rhythm may be disturbed
7	Obvious speech abnormalities	Communication accomplished with ease, although speech impairment detracts from content
6	Repeats messages on occasion	Speech can always be understood if listener pays close attention; both articulation and voice may be defective
5	Frequent repetition required	Speech always employed for communication, but articulation is very poor; usually uses complete sentences
4	Speech plus augmentative communication	Uses speech for most communication, but articulation is highly unintelligible; may have occasional difficulty in initiating speech; usually speaks in single words or short phrases
3	Limits speech to one-word response	Attempts to use speech for communication, but has difficulty initiating vocalization; may stop speaking in middle of phrase and be unable to continue
2	Vocalizes for emotional expression	Vocalizes to call attention to self
1	Nonvocal	Vocalizes, but rarely for communicative purposes
0		Does not vocalize at all

Adapted from Yorkston, Miller, & Strand, 1995.

Table 15–2. Summary of the Staging of Speech Intervention for Degenerative Motor Speech Disorders

SEVERITY OF DYSARTHRIA

	MILD	MODERATE	SEVERE
Amyotrophic Lateral Sclerosis			
Presenting Features	Changes noted by unfamiliar partners	Imprecise consonant production and reduced speech intelligibility	Speech no longer functional
Intervention	Avoid environmental adversities, established context, maximize hearing of partners	Energy conservation techniques, break-down resolution strategies	AAC systems including alerting system, alphabet boards, writing systems
Parkinson's Disease			
Presenting Features	Reduced loudness, monotony, & breathiness	Reduced loudness, monotony, breathiness, reduced intelligibility	Difficulty initiating voice, poor intelligibility
Intervention	Techniques to increase vocal fold adduction	Rate control, techniques to improve vocal fold adduction	Alphabet supplementation, AAC devices
Multiple Sclerosis			
Presenting Features	Voice tremor, harsh voice, symptoms worsen with fatigue	Harsh voice, reduced speaking rate, decreased speech naturalness	Natural speech is no longer functional
Intervention	Energy & loudness regulation techniques	Speaking rate control, respiratory patterning techniques, alphabet board supplementation	Compensation for visual and motor problems; vocabulary selection
Huntington's Disease			
Presenting Features	Choreic movements superimposed on speech	Choreic movements interfere with intelligibility	Natural speech is no longer functional
Intervention	Prosody drill, techniques to reduce phonatory stenosis	Techniques to resolve communication breakdowns	Supported communication, alphabet board, choice-making, conversational starters

Adapted from Yorkston, Miller, & Strand, 1995.

Note that the symptoms of mild and moderate dysarthria vary among the diseases as do the commonly employed treatment techniques. Also note that treatment approaches vary markedly as a function of the severity of the dysarthria. Techniques whose goals are to improve speech production are useful for individuals with mild dysarthria, while for those with severe dysarthria augmentative communication techniques are appropriate.

Planning the appropriate "next" steps that would be appropriate if impairment worsens is critical in the management of degenerative disease. There is an unfortunate tendency to wait until the individual is experiencing decreases in intelligibility before investigating AAC options. Typically, this strategy results in an intervention that is delayed. By the time an assessment is completed and AAC options are determined, the individuals are usually so severely communicatively impaired that they must attempt to use the "new AAC system" to meet their communication needs while they are no longer able to speak functionally in the majority of communicative situations. Clinical research has suggested that marked changes in the intelligibility of dysarthric speakers with ALS are often preceded by reduction in their speaking rate (Yorkston, Miller, & Strand, 1995). In other words, speakers will experience a phase of the disorder where their speech is intelligible but slow before speech intelligibility scores decline markedly. There is a "rule of thumb" for ALS patients that has gained increasing acceptance in the AAC community. According to this rule, the consideration of an AAC system should be implemented when the rate of natural speech is 50% of the habitual rate. In this way, speakers with ALS and proceeding their families can make informed decisions about assistive technology, rather than proceeding only after crises have occurred.

Documenting the Efficacy of Speech Treatment

Being diagnosed with a degenerative disease should not be equated with a loss of hope. Especially with slowly progressive disease such as Parkinson's disease, speakers with mild or moderate dysarthria may choose to invest considerable time and effort in maintaining adequate speech. A long history of behavioral intervention for parkinsonian dysarthria can be found in the literature. This history is reviewed in detail elsewhere (Yorkston, in press). In the late 1960s and early 1970s, general speech treatment programs were felt to bring about positive changes during the treatment sessions, but these changes were not felt to be maintained outside the therapy room (Allan, Turner, & Gadea-Ciria, 1970; Sarno, Buonaguro, & Levita, 1986). Perhaps because of the lack of carryover in the earlier studies, case studies followed which document the effectiveness of devices such as pacing boards (Helm, 1979) and delayed auditory feedback devices (Downie, Low, & Lindsay, 1981). These cases were useful because they not only suggested the effectiveness of these devices, but also provided guidelines suggesting who might be the best candidates for this type of intervention. In the 1980s and early 1990s, prospective studies of speech treatment reported both immediate improvement and some maintenance of progress (Scott & Caird, 1981; LeDorze, Dioone, Ryalls, Julien, & Ouellet, 1992).

Most recently in a series of studies, Ramig and colleagues (1995) have reported positive findings following a voice intervention program for dysarthric speakers due to Parkinson's disease. Specifically, Ramig, Countryman, Thompson, and Horii (1995) have reported the effect of two forms of intensive speech intervention: (1) respiratory only, and (2) respiratory and voice on the speech performance of hypokinetic speakers due to idiopathic Parkinson's disease. The authors conclude that intensive respiration and voice intervention was more effective than respiration intervention alone for improving vocal intensity and decreasing the impact of Parkinson's disease on communication. Ramig's work is particularly notable in that it is an example of a treatment outcome study where multiple levels of the disease are measured. Although the treatment focuses on a single aspect of the impairment, that is, respiratory/phonatory function, the effectiveness of this intervention is measured at a number of levels including at the level of the impairment, functional limitation, and disability. The Ramig work also represents an advancement over earlier treatment studies in that it goes beyond the simple question: Does treatment work?; and asks a more sophisticated question: Does one form of treatment work better than another?

Studies are also becoming available that document the long-term impact of these speech intervention strategies on speakers with Parkinson's disease. Sullivan, Brune, and Beukelman (1995) found that five of six participants improved their speech performance and maintained the improvements for up to 10 months (the point when follow-up was terminated) following intervention. Thus recent intervention studies are not only documenting the immediate effectiveness of intervention but also its long-term benefit, even in the face of gradual progression of the underlying pathophysiology.

Documenting the Patterns of Using Augmentative Communication Systems

AAC intervention may be applicable when natural speech is no longer functional. Studies of use patterns are needed in order to develop better devices that are well-suited to the needs of the speaker. For example, Mathy and Brune (1993) studied use patterns of 11 individuals with ALS who were unable to speak. They were questioned about their daily use of AAC strategies across typical communicative activities/needs. Results are illustrated in Figure 15–1. The activities included: communicating immediate needs, face-to-face conversation, communicating needs in detail, communicating detailed information, interacting on the telephone, and written communication. All of the individuals were experienced users of multimodal AAC systems, which included no technology (e.g., answering yes/no questions), low-tech strategies (e.g., alphabet boards), and multipurpose high-tech devices, which provided speech output and written communication. When asked which of their AAC strategies/devices they used most frequently based on communicative activity, all subjects indicated that they relied primarily on their no-tech and low-tech strategies for conversation and to communicate immediate needs. High-tech strategies were used primarily for indicating needs in detail, providing detailed information, for the telephone and for written communication activities.

NONPROGRESSIVE MOTOR SPEECH DISORDERS

Many individuals with motor speech disorders are diagnosed with nonprogressive diseases. These disease may have either a stable or an improving course. For example, an individual with dysarthria associated with traumatic brain injury may initially experience a period of recovery followed by later stabilization. We will review three nonprogressive neurological diseases (stroke, traumatic brain injury, and cerebral palsy).

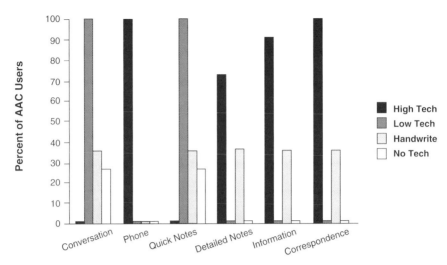

Figure 15–1. AAC use patterns in 11 persons with amyotrophic lateral sclerosis.

The Diseases

Stroke

A stroke or cerebrovascular accident is caused by a disruption of the blood flow to the brain. Ischemic strokes may result from several conditions including a sudden blockage of a major blood vessel, a blood or air embolus that lodges in a vessel, or a microinfarct (lacune), which results from the effect of chronic hypertension. Hemorrhagic infarcts may be caused by subarachnoid hemorrhages due to a congenital defect or hypertension, intracerebral hemorrhage, or arteriovenous malformations. The incidence of stroke increases with age. Although aphasia is commonly associated with cortical stroke, motor speech disorders, including apraxia of speech and dysarthria, are also a frequent sequelae of stroke. The prevalence of motor speech disorders following stroke is not well documented. Duffy (1995) reports that the primary diagnosis of apraxia of speech accounted for 9% of the motor speech disorders seen at the Mayo Clinic. Apraxia of speech is more frequently a secondary diagnosis, often occurring concomitantly with aphasia and dysarthria. The perceptual characteristics of apraxia of speech include disturbances in articulation, rate, prosody, and rhythm of spoken utterance (Wertz, LaPointe, & Rosenbek, 1984). Severity varies extensively from speakers who are unable to imitate vowels to mild disruptions of speech naturalness.

Several types of dysarthria are associated with stroke, depending on the site and extent of the lesion. Unilateral upper motor neuron lesions result in a mild and often temporary dysarthria characterized by imprecise consonant production, slow speech, and oral movement rates (Duffy, 1995). Bilateral cortical lesions may result in a pseudobulbar dysarthria characterized by a strained-strangled voice quality, velopharyngeal dysfunction, as well as articulatory impairment. Brainstem lesions are characterized by two major muscular abnormalities, weakness and hypotonia, and may lead to flaccid dysarthria. The distinguishing features of this type of dysarthria include marked hypernasality, breathy voice, and audible inspiration, as well as articulatory imprecision (Darley, Aronson, & Brown, 1975).

Traumatic Brain Injury (TBI)

The incidence of TBI that results in moderate to severe physical or behavioral impairment is 20 per 100,000 or 44,000 new cases per year (Kraus et al., 1984). The TBI population is bimodal with peak incidence in young adulthood and old age. Because of the diffuse and variable neuropathology associated with TBI, a number of communication problems are common. Language is frequently disrupted as part of a complex constellation of memory and cognitive deficits. Dysarthria is also common in TBI. Approximately one-third of persons with TBI exhibit dysarthria (Rusk, Block, & Lowman, 1969; Sarno, Buonaguro, & Levita, 1986). Other reports suggest that the prevalence of dysarthria following TBI ranges from over 60% in acute rehabilitation to approximately 10% long-term (Yorkston, Honsinger, Mitsuda, & Hammen, 1989).

Cerebral Palsy

Cerebral palsy is a nonprogressive motor disorder resulting from pathology to the central nervous system during the prenatal or paranatal period. The prevalence is between 2 and 2.5 per 1,000 (Erenberg (1984). The reports of dysarthria prevalence vary greatly from 31 to 39% (Wolfe, 1950) to 88% (Achilles, 1955). Approximately 75% of the children studied by Murphy and colleagues had at least one of the following disorders: mental retardation, epilepsy, visual impairment, and hearing impairment (Murphy, Yeargin-Allsopp, Decoufl'e, & Drews, 1993). The severity and pattern of dysarthria in cerebral palsy is dependent upon the underlying pathophysiology. Spastic dysarthria is the most common and is characterized by low pitch hypernasality, pitch breaks, breathy voice, and excess and equal stress. Speech in athetoid cerebral palsy is characterized by irregular articulatory breakdowns, inappropriate silences, prolonged interval and speech sounds, excessive loudness variation, and voice stoppage (Workinger & Kent, 1991).

Intervention Effectiveness Analysis

Stable Pathologies

For conditions with stable pathologies, outcome analysis is more straightforward than it is with degenerative pathologies. Interventions that are associated with improved performance at any of the levels of disorder might be considered effective. Obviously, improvements in functional limitations and disability are usually most valued, as they are generally associated with increased functional communication for dysarthric speakers.

Improving Pathologies

Outcome analysis of individuals with improving disorders has its unique considerations. Obviously, if the disorder is improving gradually, one would assume that speech performance might improve concomitantly. In order for an intervention to be effective in this situation, it will be necessary to show that the improvement occurs at a rate that is more rapid than would be expected given the natural improvement in the disorder.

Why Measure Speech Outcomes?

Documenting the Extent and Pattern of Recovery

Outcome assessment at just one level or at one static point in time misses some important aspects of outcome (Hammel, 1996). Serial measures of functional outcome are useful for tracking the clinical course of individuals with nonprogressive motor speech disorders. They allow clinicians to answer a variety of questions. Is this patient with a severe brainstem stroke continuing to improve in speech function? If the answer is "no," then aggressive pursuit of an AAC system might be warranted. Is this patient with TBI worsening in speech function despite the fact that an improving or stable course is expected? If the answer is "yes," then aggressive attempts should be made to identify the underlying causes for the decline.

Studies have been reported that follow the long-term course of individuals with severe dysarthria. These studies are useful in that they provide clinicians with some general guidelines for the timing and focus of management. Culp and Ladtkow (1992) have provided a rather complete description of the 16 patients with locked-in-syndrome (LIS) whom they followed for at least 1 year. Fifteen of these patients presented with LIS following stroke. All remain nonambulatory and half of them have experienced visual difficulties sufficient to interfere with AAC interventions. Only three remained dependent on gastric tubes and two remained ventilator dependent. The communication needs of these 16 people were met in a variety of ways. Eight of them developed adequate vision and motor skills for direct selection access to AAC systems. This means they were able to directly select their message of choice from the display on their AAC system. Eight other patients had to rely on a scanning interface for the AAC system. This required them to have their message options scanned and they made their choices by activating a switch. Thirteen of the 16 patients chose to pursue high technology options; three of the 16 did not.

In 1992 Ladtkow and Culp followed 138 persons with traumatic brain injury over an 18-month period. Twenty-one percent of these individuals were classified as "nonspeaking" at some time during their recovery. Of this nonspeaking group, 55% became functional speakers during the middle stage of recover (Rancho Levels IV & V) and 45% did not. Dongilli, Hakel, and Beukelman (1991) followed 27 persons with traumatic brain injury who were unable to speak functionally when they were admitted to active rehabilitation. Fifty-nine percent of these individuals became functional speakers during inpatient rehabilitation, all during Rancho levels V & VI. Of the 41% who failed to regain functional speech during inpatient rehabilitation, one experienced a severe language impairment and the others experienced severe motor speech impairments.

Documenting the Effectiveness of Specific Interventions

Group studies focusing on intervention effectiveness are uncommon in the field of motor speech disorders, perhaps because patterns of communication deficits vary extensively from person to person. Wertz (1984) examined the response to treatment in groups of individuals with apraxia of speech and aphasia as part of the Veterans Administration Cooperative

Study of Aphasia. Although some trends were suggestive of treatment effectiveness, a number of issues made interpretation of the results difficult. First, a proportion of subjects changed diagnostic categories during the course of the 44-week investigation. Subjects in this study also varied considerably in the relative severity of aphasia versus apraxia of speech. Finally, the drop-out rates reduced the numbers of speech subjects in the treatment groups to the point where meaningful statistical analyses were not always possible.

A variety of case reports are available which document the impact of specific intervention on individuals with motor speech disorders. These studies provide the clinician with insights into which speakers are candidates for specific interventions. The literature contains several detailed descriptions of the AAC intervention with persons with severe communication disorders following brainstem stroke. Beukelman and Yorkston (1977) describe a man with brainstem stroke whose speech intelligibility was 16% as measured by a sentence intelligibility task developed for this study. He was taught to use a supplemented speech approach during which he pointed to the first letter of each word on an alphabet board. Using this approach, his comprehensibility was 65%, which was adequate for most conversations with familiar listeners. Beukelman, Yorkston, and Dowden (1985) describe the outcomes of two women with brainstem stroke who were unable to speak or produce voluntary vocalization. Each of the women progressed through a series of low-tech AAC systems, eventually using electronic AAC systems for most of their communication needs.

Because the patterns of dysarthria vary extensively from person to person with TBI, it is unlikely that a single type of intervention would be appropriate with all individuals who experience dysarthria secondary to TBI. A variety of different intervention approaches have been reported to be effective with some dysarthria speakers: physiological approaches (Aten, 1988; Crow & Enderby, 1989; Harris & Murry, 1984; Hartman, Day, Pecora, 1979; Olswang, 1990; Simpson, Till, & Goff, 1988; Workinger & Netsell, 1992), feedback of acoustic information (Caligiuri & Murry, 1983; Simmons, 1983), and rate control and breath patterning (Bellaire, Yorkston, & Beukelman, 1986; Berry & Goshorn, 1983; Yorkston & Beukelman, 1981). Several clinical researchers have documented that important changes in speech performance can be obtained many years post injury (Aten, 1988; Enderby & Crow, 1990; Harris & Murry, 1984; Keenen & Barnhart, 1993; Workinger & Netsell, 1992). Palatal lifts have also been shown to be effective for persons with TBI (Aten, McDonald, Simpson, & Gutierrez, 1984; Bedwinek & O'Brian, 1985; Brand, Matsko, & Avart, 1988; Gonzalez & Aronson, 1970; Simpson, Till, & Goff, 1988; Yorkston, Honsinger, Beukelman, & Taylor, 1989).

Outcomes of these intervention studies are measured in a variety of ways, including improvement in muscle strength and control (Harris & Murry, 1984; Nemec & Cohen, 1984), reduction in selected deviant features (Brand, Matsko, & Avart, 1988; Kuehn & Wachtel, 1994; Netsell & Daniel, 1979; Yorkston & Beukelman, 1981a; Yorkston, Honsinger, Beukelman, & Taylor, 1989), and changes in overall features such as speech intelligibility (Aten, 1988; Berry & Goshorn, 1983), and speaking rate (Yorkston & Beukelman, 1981b).

Moving Toward More Well Designed AAC Systems

The field of AAC has changed extensively in the last decade in its ability to enhance the communication of individuals with severe motor speech disorders. Research in this area has focused on the features of the AAC system (particularly in identifying those features that are most beneficial), and on training of nonspeaking individuals and their communication partners in system use (Yorkston, in press).

In 1987, DeRuyter and Fontaine reported on 66 nonspeaking clients with cerebral palsy, 57.5 percent used low-tech strategies while the remainder used electronic AAC systems. Treatment studies focused on learning to use AAC systems have recently received considerable attention in the literature. Learning of AAC systems has been documented in groups of individuals with cerebral palsy (Udwin & Yule, 1991a, 1991b) using single-subject research designs (Dattilo & Camarata, 1991; Gies-Zaborowski & Silverman, 1986), and case reports (Ferrier, 1991; Goossens, 1989; Spiegel, Benjamin, & Siegel, 1993). Outcomes have been documented using a variety of parameters including increased conversational participation (Dattilo & Camarata, 1991), increased spontaneously initiated requests (Glennen, & Calculator, 1985; Spiegel, Benjamin, & Siegel, 1993), and percentage of hours in the day that systems were used (Culp, Ambrosi, Berninger, & Mitchell, 1986). Light and Lindsay (1992) studied message encoding strategies and found that letter encoding resulted in more accurate learning than iconic techniques.

CONCLUSION

Intervention Effectiveness Value

It is clear from this review and from other discussions (Hammel, 1996) that most of our focus in measurement has been at the level of the pathology and the impairment. Although one should measure outcomes for communication disorders at the various levels of disorder in order to document the overall impact of an intervention, one should not assume that change at all levels of intervention are of equal value to all stakeholders. Stakeholders include the patient, his or her family, medical personnel, rehabilitation personnel, the payer, the community, and so forth. The authors have worked in medical centers for many years and have watched conflict among the various stakeholders regarding the value of an intervention. For instance, Yorkston, Beukelman, and Bell (1988) describe an episode in which a man with Parkinson's disease was hospitalized so the neurological staff could adjust his medication regime. After a couple of weeks, the medical staff reported improved blood chemistry values, and the physical therapists reported less tremor and increased movement ranges, while the SLPs also noted less tremor but no changes in speech intelligibility. The man's family, however, reported no changes in his mobility, communication, or self care that they considered important enough to justify the hospitalization! The "take home" message from this example is that patient and family stakeholders may not choose to spend time and money on rehabilitation unless they can achieve functional gains. This underscores the need to develop and use outcome measures in the motor speech disorders area at the functional limitation and disability levels, as well as the impairment and pathology levels, of the chronic disease model.

ACKNOWLEDGMENT

The preparation of this chapter was funded in part by grant number MCJ-319152 awarded to the Meyer Rehabilitation Institute by the Bureau of Maternal and Child Health Services and by the Barkley Trust.

REFERENCES

Achilles, R. (1955). Communication anomalies of individuals with cerebral palsy: I. Analysis of communication processes in 151 cases of cerebral palsy. *Cerebral Palsy Review, 16,* 15–24.

Allan, C., Turner, J., & Gadea-Ciria, M. (1970). Investigations into speech disturbances following stereotaxic surgery for Parkinsonism. *British Journal of Communication Disorders, 1,* 55–59.

Antonius, K., Beukelman, D., & Reid, R. (1996). The communication disability of Parkinson's disease. In D. Robin, K. Yorkston, & D. Beukelman (Eds.), *Motor speech disorders* (pp. 275–286). Baltimore: Paul H. Brookes Publishers.

Arnason, B. (1982). Multiple sclerosis: Current concepts and management. *Hospital Practice, 17*(2), 81–89.

Aten, J. (1988). Spastic dysarthria: Revising understanding of the disorder and speech treatment procedures. *Journal of Head Trauma Rehabilitation, 3,* 63–73.

Aten, J., McDonald, A., Simpson, M., & Gutierrez, R. (1984). Efficacy of modified palatal lifts for improved resonance. In M. McNeil, J. Rosenbek, & A. Aronson (Eds.), *The Dysarthrias: Physiology, Acoustics, Perception, Management* (pp. 231–242). Boston: College-Hill Press.

Bedwinek, A. P., & O'Brian, R. L. (1985). A patient selection profile for the use of speech prosthesis in adult disorders. *Journal of Communication Disorders, 18*(3).

Bellaire, K., Yorkston, K., & Beukelman, D. (1986). Modification of breath patterning to increase naturalness of a mildly dysarthric speaker. *Journal of Communication Disorders, 19,* 271–280.

Bensimon, G., Lacomblez, L., & Meininger, V. (1994). A controlled trial of riluzole in amyotrophic lateral sclerosis. *New England Journal of Medicine, 330*(9), 585–591.

Berry, W., & Goshron, E. (1983). Immediate visual feedback in the treatment of ataxic dysarthria: A case study. In W. Berry (Ed.), *Clinical Dysarthria* (pp. 253–266). Boston: College-Hill Press.

Beukelman, D., Kraft, G., & Freal, J. (1985). Expressive communication disorders in persons with multiple sclerosis: A survey. *Archives of Physical and Rehabilitation Medicine, 66,* 675–677.

Beukelman, D., & Yorkston, K. (1977). A communication system for the severely dysarthric speaker with an intact language system. *Journal of Speech and Hearing Disorders, 42,* 265–270.

Beukelman, D., Yorkston, K., & Dowden, P. (1985). *Communication augmentation: A casebook of clinical management.* Austin, TX: Pro-ed.

Brand, H., Matsko, T., & Avart, H. (1988). Speech prosthesis retention problems in dysarthria: Case report. *Archives of Physical Medicine and Rehabilitation,* 213–214.

Buck, J., & Cooper, I. (1956). Speech problems in parkinsonian patients undergoing anterior choroidal artery occlusion or chemopallidectomy. *Journal of the American Geriatric Society, 4,* 1285–1290.

Caligiuri, M. P., & Murry, T. (1983). The use of visual feedback to enhance prosodic control in dysarthria. In W. Berry (Ed.), *Clinical Dysarthria.* Austin, TX: Pro-ed.

Crow, E., & Enderby, P. (1989). The effects of an alphabet chart on the speaking rate and intelligibility of speakers with dysarthria. In K. M. Yorkston & D. R. Beukelman (Eds.), *Recent Advances in Clinical Dysarthria.* Austin, TX: Pro-ed.

Culp, D., Ambrosi, D., Berninger, T., & Mitchell, J. (1986). Augmentative communication aid use: A follow-up study. *Augmentative and Alternative Communication, 2,* 19–24.

Culp, D., & Ladtkow. M (1992). Locked in syndrome and augmentative communication. In K. Yorkston (Ed.), *Augmentative Communication in the Medical Setting* (pp. 59–138). San Antonio, TX: Psychological Corporation.

Darley, F., Aronson, A., & Brown, J. (1969a). Differential diagnostic patterns of dysarthria. *Journal of Speech & Hearing Research, 12,* 246–269.

Darley, F., Aronson, A., & Brown. J. (1969b). Clusters of deviant speech dimensions in the dysarthrias. *Journal of Speech & Hearing Research, 12,* 462–496.

Darley, F., Aronson, A., & Brown. J. (1975). *Motor speech disorders.* Philadelphia: Saunders.

Darley, F., Brown, J., & Goldstein, N. (1972). Dysarthria in multiple sclerosis. *Journal of Speech and Hearing Research, 15,* 229–245.

Dattilo, J., & Camarata, S. (1991). Facilitating conversation through self-initiated augmentative communication treatment. *Journal of Applied Behavior Analysis, 24,* 369–378.

DeRuyter, F., & Fontaine, L. (1987). The nonspeaking brain-injured: A clinical and demographic database report. *Augmentative and Alternative Communication, 3,* 18–35.

Dongilli, Jr., P., Hakel, M., & Beukelman, D. (1992). Recovery of functional speech following traumatic brain injury. *Journal of Head Trauma Rehabilitation, 7,* 91–101.

Downie, A., Low, J., & Lindsay. D. (1981). Speech disorders in parkinsonism: Usefulness of delayed auditory feedback. *American Journal of Medical Science, 251,* 600–616.

Duffy, J. (1995). *Motor speech disorders: Substrates, differential diagnosis, and management.* St. Louis: Mosby.

Enderby, P., & Crow, E. (1990). Long-term recovery patterns of severe dysarthria following head injury. *British Journal of Disorders of Communication, 25*(3), 341–354.

Erenberg, G. (1984). Cerebral Palsy. *Postgraduate Medicine, 75,* 87–93.

Ferrier, L. (1991). Clinical study of a dysarthric adult using a Touch Talker with words strategy. *Augmentative and Alternative Communication, 7,* 266–274.

Gies-Zaborowski, J., & Silverman, F. (1986). Documenting the impact of a mild dysarthria on peer perception. *Speech & Hearing Services in Schools, 17*(2), 143.

Glennen, S., & Calculator, S. (1985). Training functional communication board use: A pragmatic approach. *Augmentative and Alternative Communication, 1,* 131–141.

Gonzalez, J., & Aronson, A. (1970). Palatal lift prosthesis for treatment of anatomic and neurologic palatopharyngeal insufficiency. *Cleft Palate Journal, 7,* 91–104.

Goodkin, D. E. (1994). Role of steroid and immunosuppression and effects of interferon beta-1b in multiple sclerosis. *Western Journal of Medicine, 161,* 292–298.

Goossens', C. (1989). Aided communication intervention before assessment: A case study of a child with cerebral palsy. *Augmentative and Alternative Communication, 5,* 14–26.

Hammel, J. (1996). What's the outcome? Multiple variables complicate the measurement of assistive technology outcomes. *Rehabilitation Management, February/March,* 97–99.

Harris, B., & Murry, T. (1984). Dysarthria an aphasia: A case study of neuromuscular treatment. *Archives of Physical and Medical Rehabilitation, 65,* 408–411.

Hartman, D., Day, M., & Pecora, R. (1979). Treatment of dysarthria: A case report. *Journal of Communication Disorders, 12,* 167–173.

Helm, N. (1979). Management of palilalia with a pacing board. *Journal of Speech and Hearing Disorders, 44,* 350–353.

Hixon, T. (1984). Parameter-based evaluation of speech breathing functions in dysarthria. Presentation at the annual convention of The American Speech-Language-Hearing Convention, San Francisco, CA.

Iacono, R. P., Lonser, R. R., Oh, A., & Yamada, S. (1995). New pathophysiology of Parkinson's disease revealed by posteroventral pallidotomy. *Neurological Research, 17*(3), 178–180.

Jacobs, L., & Johnson, K. P. (1994). A brief history of the use of interferons as treatment of multiple sclerosis. *Archives of Neurology, 51,* 1245–1252.

Keenan, J. E., & Barnhart, K. S. (1993). Development of yes/no systems in individuals with severe traumatic brain injuries. *Augmentative and Alternative Communication, 9,* 184–190.

Kraus, J. F., Black, M. S., Hessel, N., et al. (1984). The incidence of acute brain injury and serious impairment in a defined population. *American Journal of Epidemiology, 119,* 186–201.

Kuehn, D. P., & Wachtel, J. M. (1994). CPAP therapy for treating hypernasality following closed head injury. In J. A. Till, K. M. Yorkston, & D. R. Beukelman (Eds.), *Motor speech disorders: Advances in assessment and treatment* (pp. 207–212). Baltimore: Paul H. Brookes Publishing.

Ladtkow, M. & Culp (1992). Augmentative communication with traumatic brain injury. In K.

Yorkston (Ed.), *Augmentative Communication in the Medical Setting*. San Antonio, TX: Psychological Corporation.

Laitinen, L. V. (1995). Pallidotomy for Parkinson's disease. *Neurosurgery Clinics of North America, 6*, 105–112.

LeDorze, L., Dioone, L., Ryalls, J., Julien, M., & Ouellet, L. (1992). The effects of speech pathology language therapy for a case of dysarthria associated with Parkinson's disease. *European Journal of Disorders of Communication, 27*, 313–324.

Light, J., & Lindsay, P. (1992). Message-encoding techniques for augmentative communication system: The recall performance of adults with severe speech impairments. *Journal of Speech and Hearing Research, 35*, 853–864.

Logemann, J., Fisher, H., Boshes, B., & Blonsky, E. (1978). Frequency and concurrence of vocal tract dysfunctions in the speech of a large sample of parkinsonian patients. *Journal of Speech & Hearing Disorders, 42*, 47–57.

Mathy P., & Brune, P. (1993). Using personal computers as AAC devices. Presented at the RESNA 1993 Annual Conference, Las Vegas, NV.

McDowell, F., & Cederbaum, J. (1987). The extrapyramidal system and disorders of movement. In A.B. Baker & R. Joynt (Eds.), *Clinical Neurology*. Philadelphia: J. B. Lippincott.

Murphy, C. C., Yeargin-Allsopp, M., Decoufl'e, P., & Drews, C. D. (1993). Prevalence of cerebral palsy among ten-year-old children in metropolitan Atlanta, 1985 through 1987. *Journal of Pediatrics, 123*, S13–20.

Nagi, S. (1991). Disability concepts revisited: Implications for prevention. In A. Pope & A. Tarlov (Eds.), *Disability in America: Toward a national agenda for prevention* (pp. 309–327). Washington, DC: National Academy Press.

Nemec, R. E., & Cohen, K. (1984). EMG biofeedback in the modification of hypertonia in spastic dysarthria: Case report. *Archives of Physical Medicine & Rehabilitation, 65*, 103–104.

Netsell, R., & Daniel, B. (1979). Dysarthria in adults: Physiologic approach to rehabilitation. *Archives of Physical Medicine and Rehabilitation, 60*, 502–508.

Olswang, L. B. (1990). Treatment efficacy: The breadth of research. In L. B. Olswang, C. K. Thompson, S. F. Warren, & N. J. Minghetti (Eds.), *Treatment efficacy research in communication disorders*. Rockville, MD: American Speech-Language-Hearing Foundation.

Poser, C. (Ed.). (1984). *The diagnosis of multiple sclerosis*. New York Theme-Stratton.

Ramig, L., Countryman, S., Thompson, L., & Horii, Y. (1995) Comparison of two forms of intensive speech treatment for Parkinson's disease. *Journal of Speech and Hearing Research, 38*, 1232–1251.

Rosenbek, J., & LaPointe, L. (1985). The dysarthrias: Description diagnosis and treatment. In D. F. Johns (Ed.), *Clinical management of neurogenic communication disorders*. Boston: Little, Brown.

Rusk, H., Block, J., & Lowmann, E. (1969). Rehabilitation of the brain injured patient: A report of 157 cases with long term follow-up of 118. In E. Walker, W. Caveness, & M. Critchley (Eds.), *The late effect of head injury*. Springfield: Charles C. Thomas.

Sarno, M. T., Buonaguro, A., & Levita, E. (1986). Characteristics of verbal impairment in closed head injured patients. *Archives of Physical Medicine & Rehabilitation, 67*, 400–405.

Saunders, C., Walsh, T., & Smith, M. (1981). Hospice care in the motor neuron disease. In C. Saunders & J. Teller, (Eds.), *Hospice: The living idea*. London: Edward Arnold Publishers.

Scott, S., & Caird, F. (1981). Speech therapy for patients with Parkinson's disease. *British Journal of Communication Disorders, 2*, 1088.

Simmons, N. (1983). Acoustic analysis of ataxic dysarthria: An approach to monitoring treatment. In W. Berry (Ed.), *Clinical dysarthria* (pp. 283–294). Austin, TX: Pro-ed.

Simpson, M. B., Till, J. A., & Goff, A. M. (1988). Long-term treatment of severe dysarthria: A case study. *Journal of Speech & Hearing Disorders, 53*, 433–440.

Spiegel, B. B., Benjamin, B. J., & Siegel, S. A. (1993). One method to increase spontaneous use of an assistive communication device: Case Study. *Augmentative and Alternative Communication, 9,* 111–118.

Sullivan, M., Brune, P., & Beukelman, D. (1995). Maintenance of speech changes following group treatment for hyokinetic dysarthria of Parkinson's disease. In D. Robin, K. Yorkston, & D. Beukelman (Eds.), *Disorders of Motor Speech: Assessment, Treatment, & Clinical Characterization* (pp. 287–307). Baltimore: Paul H. Brookes Publishing Company.

Tandan, R., & Bradley, W. G. (1985). Amyotrophic lateral sclerosis: Part 1. Clinical features, pathology, and ethical issues in management. *Annals of Neurology, 18,* 271–280.

Udwin, O., & Yule, W. (1991a). Augmentative communication systems taught to cerebral-palsied children—a longitudinal study. II. Pragmatic features of sign and symbol use. *British Journal of Disorders of Communication, 26,* 137–148.

Udwin, O., & Yule, W. (1991b). Augmentative communication systems taught to cerebral-palsied children—a longitudinal study. III. Teaching practices and exposure to sign and symbol use in schools and homes. *British Journal of Disorders of Communication, 26,* 149–162.

Van Oosten, B. W., Truyen, L., Barkhof, F., & Polman, C. H. (1995). Multiple sclerosis therapy. A practical guide. *Drugs, 49*(2), 200–212.

Wertz, R. T. (1984). Response to treatment in patients with apraxia of speech. In J. Rosenbek, M. McNeil, & A.E. Aronson (Eds.), *Apraxia of speech: Physiology, acoustics, linguistics, management* (pp. 257–276). San Diego: College-Hill Press.

Wertz, R., LaPointe, L., & Rosenbek, J. (1984). *Apraxia of speech in adults: The Disorder and its management.* Orlando, FL: Grune and Stratton.

Wolfe, W. (1950). A comprehensive evaluation of fifty cases of cerebral palsy. *Journal of Speech and Hearing Disorders, 15,* 234–251.

Workinger, M. S., & Kent, R. D. (1991). Perceptual analysis of the dysarthria in children with athetoid and spastic cerebral palsy. In C. A. Moore, K. M. Yorkston, & D. R. Beukelman (Eds.), *Dysarthria and apraxia of speech: Perspectives on management* (pp. 109–126). Baltimore, MD: ProEd.

Workinger, M. S., & Netsell, R. (1992). Restoration of intelligible speech 13 years post-head injury. *Brain Injury, 6,* 183–187.

Yorkston, K. M. (in press). Treatment efficacy in dysarthria. *Journal of Speech & Hearing Research.*

Yorkston, K., & Beukelman, D. (1981). Ataxic dysarthria: Treatment sequences based on intelligibility and prosodic considerations. *Journal of Speech and Hearing Disorders, 46,* 398–404.

Yorkston, K., & Beukelman, D. (1981a). Communication efficiency of dysarthric speakers as measured by sentence intelligibility and speaking. *Journal of Speech and Hearing Disorders, 46,* 296–301.

Yorkston, K. M., & Beukelman, D. R. (1981b). Ataxic dysarthria: Treatment sequences based on intelligibility and prosodic consideration. *Journal of Speech and Hearing Disorders, 46,* 398–404.

Yorkston, K. M., Beukelman, D. R., & Bell, K. (1988). *Clinical management of dysarthric speakers.* Austin, TX: Pro-ed.

Yorkston, K., & Bombardier, C. (1992). *The communication profile for speakers with motor speech disorders.* Unpublished questionnaire. Seattle: University of Washington.

Yorkston, K., Bombardier, C., & Hammen, V. (1994). Dysarthria from the viewpoint of individuals with dysarthria. In J. Till, K. Yorkston, & D. Beukelman (Eds.), *Motor speech disorders: Advances in assessment and treatment* (pp. 19–36). Baltimore: Paul H. Brookes Publishing Company.

Yorkston, K. M., Honsinger, M. J., Mitsuda, P. M., & Hammen, V. (1989). The relationship between speech and swallowing disorders in head-injured patients. *Journal of Head Trauma Rehabilitation, 4,* 1–16.

Yorkston, K. M., Honsinger, M. J., Mitsuda, P. M., & Taylor, T. (1989). The effects of palatal lift fitting on the perceived articulatory adequacy of dysarthric speakers. In K. M. Yorkston & D. R. Beukelman (Eds.), *Recent Advances in Clinical Dysarthria* (pp. 85–98). Austin, TX: Pro-ed.

Yorkston, K. M., Beukelman, D., & Taylor, T. (1989). The effects of palatal lift fitting on the perceived articulatory adequacy of dysarthric speakers. In K. M. Yorkston & D. R. Beukelman (Eds.), *Recent Advances in Clinical Dysarthria* (pp. 85–98). Boston: College-Hill Press.

Yorkston, K., Miller, R., & Strand, E. (1995). *Management of speech and swallowing disorders in degenerative disease.* San Antonio, TX: Psychological Corporation.

Yorkston, K. M., Strand, E. A., & Kennedy, M. R. T. (1996). Comprehensibility of dysarthric speech: Implications for assessment and treatment planning. *American Journal of Speech-Language Pathology, 5,* 55–66.

CHAPTER 16

Outcomes Measurement in Voice Disorders

KATHERINE VERDOLINI, LORRAINE RAMIG,
AND BARBARA JACOBSON

INTRODUCTION

The history of clinical research in voice disorders is fundamentally similar to the history of clinical research in communication disorders in general. Echoing Leija McReynolds' apt comments, the research is "sparse and short. Very little treatment research has been conducted" (1990, p. 5). However, as McReynolds also noted, "There is a new breeze blowing" (p. 5). In voice disorders, the number and quality of outcomes studies have steadily increased over the past five decades.

Tables 16–1 and 16–2 reveal the developmental story. The few treatment outcome studies that were published in the 1940s were nonexperimental, and were largely characterized by "expert opinions." Since then, a transition has taken place, with the appearance of quasi-experimental and experimental study designs. Further, there has been the appearance of: (1) operationalized measures of therapy results; (2) detailed, operationalized descriptions of therapy itself; (3) information about the results of therapy at extended follow-up intervals; (4) large N studies; (5) consideration of instrumental as well as intermediate and ultimate outcomes; (6) the use of clinical data bases; (7) functional outcome measures, including job performance and patient satisfaction with treatment; (8) cohesive, theoretically motivated therapy models; and (9) investigational series, which examine therapy issues at multiple levels across several experiments.

In sum, although the number of published reports regarding the results of voice therapy remains decisively modest, trends show clear quantitative and qualitative increments. We appear to be on the brink of a new era in voice therapy research. This chapter's purpose is twofold: (1) to inform about specific design features and findings in voice therapy research, and (2) to provide direction for future research.

This review is organized by decade, showing how early "expert opinions" have been folded into later, more formal research. Far from decrying expert opinions, it is our impression that these opinions motivate the experimental infrastructures that are increasingly used to assess them.

As a framework for the present discussion, we first addressed the ideal characteristics of a voice therapy study. Efficacy studies address cause-effect relations. They are experimental and prospective, involving matched or randomized assignment to treatment or control groups or phases. Double-blind, placebo-controlled studies remain the gold standard. Effectiveness studies assess trends and relationships in typical clinical settings. They are non- or quasi-experimental, often data-based. Beyond these distinguishing factors, ideal treatment studies of any type have similar characteristics. Large N, cross-clinic observations should be used to assess treatment effects across settings, clinicians, and diverse clinical populations. Therapies should be well described and theoretically based where possible. Measures should be reliable, valid, and standardized. Outcome measures should be reported and reflect not only perceptual, acoustic, and physiologic information pertinent to voice, but also functional status and well-being at long-term follow-up.

We have elected to provide details about the studies' designs and results. We have adopted this approach for several reasons. First, we would like the chapter to serve as a resource of specific information for clinical, research, and reimbursement purposes. Second, we view the reader as a collaborator who independently evaluates the extent to which the studies' findings are accepted or rejected. To that end, details about subject numbers, study methodologies, and specific results are required. Third, the detail should highlight specific strengths and weaknesses in voice therapy research, enhancing our ability to conduct voice research in the future.

In this chapter, we have elected to review only the findings for laryngeal speech. Laryngectomy rehabilitation is a critical topic with sufficiently distinct issues and problems, which requires a separate review.

1940s

Introductory Comments

Consistent with early medical research, voice therapy studies in the 1940s were exclusively characterized by expert opinions. The studies were few in number, and all were nonexperimental (Table 16–1). Most lacked operational descriptions of treatment and outcomes. However, some important elements did appear. One was the assertion that voice therapy works. Another was the call for service delivery by certified clinicians (Peacher & Holinger, 1947). Finally, in one study series (Peacher, 1947; Peacher & Holinger, 1947), systematic observation emerged through the use of retrospective case data. The reporting of actual numbers of subjects obtaining and not obtaining a benefit from voice therapy, and the use of a control group, were noted.

Review of Studies

Among the few studies published, Wyatt (1941) discussed the results of combined voice therapy and psychoanalytic therapy, versus voice therapy alone, in the treatment of functional voice disorders. Seven adult subjects with functional voice disorders were described retrospectively. Wyatt's clinical observations indicated that five patients who received combined voice therapy and psychoanalytic therapy obtained normal voice as the result of treatment. In contrast, two patients who received voice therapy alone did

Table 16–1. Number of Nonexperimental, Quasi-experimental, and Experimental Studies in Voice Therapy Research, by Decade

DECADE	NONEXPERIMENTAL STUDIES	QUASI-EXPERIMENTAL STUDIES	EXPERIMENTAL STUDIES	TOTAL
1940s	4	0	0	4
1950s	7	0	0	7
1960s	15	0	0	15
1970s	12	0	0	12
1980s	26	2	5	33
1990s to 1996	13	1	15	29
Total	77	3	20	100

Note: The number of studies in the table are limited by those that were included in the literature review for this chapter.

not improve. Therapy was vaguely described, and specifically defined outcome measures were not provided. Consistent with other studies from this decade, there was no concern for the problem of potentially biased observations by clinicians who both treated patients and reported on their outcomes.

Another characteristic study from the 1940s addressed the treatment of hyperfunctional voice disorders (Froeschels, 1943). Retrospective case studies were used to describe the effect of the "chewing" method in treatment. Outcomes involved the author's impressions that voice improved to being, for example, "sufficiently loud" or "normal and pleasing" in five of five treated patients. The distinguishing factor in this report was the relatively detailed discussion of the actual therapy provided. Specifically, chewing was described as the evolutionary basis for phonation, with the argument that the use of chewing in therapy should promote nonhyperfunctional voicing patterns.

A departure from the tone of the early studies was found in work by Peacher and colleagues (Peacher & Holinger, 1947; Peacher, 1947). Peacher, using a retrospective case study design, examined the effect of voice therapy on laryngeal contact ulcers and granulomas. However, in contrast to other studies of her era, and indeed, from studies for the next 40 years, a control group was included. Sixteen patients with contact ulcers were examined. Six received voice therapy (experimental group), and 10 did not (control group). Regrettably by today's standards, group assignment was determined by transportation availability rather than randomly. Arguably, factors associated with transportation issues partly could have mediated the results. Peacher observed that six of six patients who received therapy (and transportation) obtained normal or near-normal larynx and symptom status subsequent to voice therapy. In contrast, six of 10 no-therapy (no-transportation) patients experienced a recurrence of lesion and of symptoms. These findings strengthened the argument that therapy has value in the treatment of voice disorders. The therapy itself was broadly described as ". . . instruction in the correct use of the speaking voice" (Peacher & Holinger, 1947, p. 617), ". . . [including] . . . relaxation, ear training, control of breathing, easy initiation of tone, optimum pitch, easy vocal production, melody pattern, rate, volume, and purity of tone" (Peacher, 1947, p. 179). Outcome measures were not operationalized. In addition to discussing the putative value of voice therapy, Peacher argued the need for service delivery by qualified personnel with "advanced rating in the American Speech Correction Association" (Peacher & Holinger, 1947, p. 617).

1950s

Introductory Comments

As in the 1940s, voice therapy studies in the 1950s were exclusively characterized by reports of expert opinion. However, the scope of investigated voice disorders increased in this decade. Studied disorders included contact ulcers (Baker, 1954), nodules (Brodnitz & Froeschels, 1954), benign laryngeal lesions in general (Brodnitz, 1958); polypoid laryngitis (Lowenthal, 1958); soft palate and laryngeal paralyses (Froeschels, Kastein, & Weiss, 1955); Parkinson disease (Froeschels et al., 1955); and hyperfunctional voice disorders, mutational falsetto, and voice problems in hearing-impaired persons (Froeschels, 1952). Also, learning variables in therapy were addressed (Froeschels, 1952).

Review of Studies

Several studies demonstrate the persistence of retrospective case studies. Baker (1954) retrospectively described the result of "vocal reeducation" in the treatment of contact ulcers with and without surgery. "Most" of the 12 patients who received voice rest alone, without vocal reeducation, "did well," but were frustrated by a long clinical process. In contrast, 7/7 patients who received therapy "did well."

Brodnitz and Froeschels (1954) reported that five of six patients with nodules obtained complete clinical resolution with the "chewing method" of therapy. Again, details of therapy were sparse, and outcome "measures" were not operationally defined.

Finally, Lowenthal (1958) reported that "recurrences [were] uncommon" in 20 patients with polypoid laryngitis, following a combination of surgery, voice rest, and "voice correction therapy, if indicated."

Froeschels et al. (1955) departed from the tone of other reports in the 1950s, describing "pushing therapy" in the treatment of voice disorders associated with palatal paralysis, laryngeal paralysis, laryngeal ablation, Parkinson disease, and neurologically based swallowing disorders. Contained in this study was a thorough description of the "pushing" therapy, the training hierarchy, and the number of repetitions to be performed daily (about 600). Case discussion of 7 patients and comments about an additional 40 led to the conclusion that some patients improved with this treatment.

Froeschels (1952) further introduced an important theme of learning variables and cognitive simplification in voice therapy. Froeschels criticized traditional treatment which calls attention to individual parts of the speech and voice mechanism ("Drop the jaw;" flatten the tongue;" "take a deep breath;" "direct the tone up to the hard palate . . ."). He considered these approaches fragmented and mechanical, and implied that they may be ineffectual as well. In contrast, he proposed that a single gesture be used in voice training and rehabilitation: easy, voiced chewing, to ". . . [bring] forth a hygienic voice . . . [with a single stroke]." (p. 430). He reported success with the chewing method in many cases of voice disorders, based on 17 years of clinical experience (see also Tarneaud, 1958, for contrasting opinion).

<u>1960s</u>

Introductory Comments

As in the preceding decades, nonexperimental studies of voice therapy were conducted in the 1960s. However, large N, quasi-experimental designs appeared in voice disorder incidence studies (Baynes, 1966; Senturia & Wilson, 1968), and a true experimental design was further used in a voice categorization study (Aronson, Peterson, & Litin, 1964). Operationalized perceptual measures of voice were developed, and statistical data management was used, in another voice categorization study (Aronson, Brown, Litin, & Pearson, 1968). Thus, the overall rigor of therapy studies increased in the 1960s. Several prospective research designs appeared (e.g., Aronson, Peterson, & Litin, 1964). Although measurement operationalization remained limited in many studies (e.g., Barton, 1960; Cooper & Nahum 1967), distinctly operationalized measures did appear in at least one treatment study (Arnold, 1962a). Some large N therapy studies were reported (Holinger & Johnston, 1960; Peacher, 1961; Pahn, 1966). Therapy details were increasingly provided (e.g., Aronson, 1969; Arnold, 1962b; Boone, 1965; Cooper & Nahum, 1967; Wilson, 1962; Wolski & Wiley, 1965). In some cases, patients were examined at extended posttherapy intervals (Aronson et al, 1964; Boone, 1965; Peacher, 1961). Finally, the principle of converging evidence appeared across treatment studies (Boone, 1965; Aronson, 1969).

Review of Studies

Quasi-experimental designs. At least two large incidence studies were conducted in the 1960s, assessing the frequency of dysphonia in children (Baynes, 1966, N = 1012; Senturia & Wilson, 1968, N = 32,500). These studies are important for two reasons. First, both indicated an approximately 6 to 7% rate of hoarseness noted in children, thus signaling the need for public attention to a prevalent public health issue. Second, the studies introduced large N, epidemiological methods to the study of voice disorders.

Operationalized measures, and statistical data management. In 1968, Aronson et al. published a study introducing two important elements in voice disorders research: operationalized perceptual measures of voice, and statistical data management. Specifically, an attempt was made to statistically differentiate operationalized, multidimensional perceptual characteristics of "spastic dysphonia," essential tremor, and other neurogenic and psychogenic dysphonias. The reliability of perceptual measures was also addressed, perhaps for the first time.

In 1962, Arnold utilized operationalized ratio[1] measures reflecting acoustic and physiologic performance to describe therapy effects in patients with paralytic dysphonia (Arnold, 1962a). Treatment involved medical therapy, physical therapy (heat treat-

---

[1]Ratio measures arise from ratio scales, which are equal-interval scales with an absolute zero value, which represents the absence of the measured phenomenon. The value of ratio measures in research is that they permit the use of high-powered parametric statistical analyses, which maximize the likelihood of detecting effects if they are present.

ments, electrical stimulation, vibration, and massage), laryngeal manipulation with lateral compression, and pushing exercises. All 18 patients improved in maximum phonation time, with many achieving normal performance at the end of therapy, according to today's standards (norms were not provided in the article). Most of the patients also improved in pitch range with treatment. Regrettably, the lack of a control group precluded the possibility of addressing the extent to which the results were due to treatment versus maturational or learning factors.

Prospective experimental design. One study from the 1960s used a prospective, experimental study design (Aronson et al., 1964). One of its purposes was to assess the ability of voice therapy and hypnotherapy to eliminate symptoms of hysterical aphonia, with long-term follow-up, in 20 adult patients. The order of voice therapy and hypnotherapy was counterbalanced across subjects, with the alternative therapy offered in the event of therapy failure. Long-term results were assessed with a questionnaire approximately 6 months after therapy termination.

Unfortunately, the results of therapy were not provided in this published report. Instead, the report focused on operationalized perceptual findings, with the conclusion that hysterical aphonia is characterized by a range of voice characteristics in addition to mutism and whisper.

Larger N therapy studies. Several studies in the 1960s were based on considerably larger subject pools than previously. Holinger and Johnston (1960), addressed the etiology, pathology, and treatment of contact ulcers, retrospectively describing 92 cases presenting clinically over a 10-year period. The features of voice therapy and treatment outcomes were not described. The authors simply stated that previous findings of a benefit from voice therapy (Peacher & Holinger, 1947) were confirmed in the present series.

A similar study was reported by Peacher (1961), who provided follow-up information to her earlier reports on patients with contact ulcers 16 years earlier (Peacher, 1947; Peacher & Holinger, 1947). Using a retrospective case study design, Peacher (1961) described 70 patients who had been followed over a 12-year period. All had received voice therapy. Outcome measures were more systematically defined than in her earlier reports: voice quality, the ability to generate and sustain loud voice, patient-reported voice fatigue, overall symptom occurrence, and laryngeal appearance were described. The results indicated that 65 of the 70 patients had no lesion recurrence. The implication was that therapy was beneficial, because the literature usually indicated that ulcer recurrence was generally common. Peacher's study was valuable particularly because of the relatively large N and the long-term follow-up interval. However, little information was provided about the actual effect of voice therapy, because of the almost complete lack of experimental controls, including a control group.

Another ambitious, large N study was reported by Pahn (1966). This German phoniatrician described an observational study of approximately 1500 children in their development of voice skills. While observational methods were not provided, based on his findings he described a voice training model, including attention to shoulder and back posturing, phonation and ear training, and chewing exercises. Applied results also were not available, but the study is important because it addresses therapy issues in a large patient population.

Studies yielding converging evidence. The principle of cross-clinic, converging evidence was demonstrated by one set of therapy studies in the 1960s, which used retrospective, nonoperationalized case study approaches. Specifically, Boone (1965) and Aronson (1969) described the results of therapy for five cases of functional (psychogenic) aphonia. In both reports, the use of vegetative functions including coughing and inhalation phonation successfully elicited voice. Voicing was then stabilized within a few days or less, using a standard hierarchy from simple to complex speech tasks. Voice symptoms did not recur over a 1- to 2-year follow-up period (Boone, 1965), nor did conversion symptoms occur in other physical systems (Aronson, 1969). Aronson further reported similar levels of success in 39 of 40 cases. (See also Wolski & Wiley, 1965, for a description of a longer therapy period for a psychiatrically involved boy.)

These reports are important because they describe similar therapy techniques, yielding qualitatively similar results, across clinicians and settings. Although experimental controls were lacking, the converging evidence across the studies constitutes a type of reliability. The main problems in the studies was the failure to consider maturational effects and treatment specificity.

1970s

Introductory Comments

Voice therapy research in the 1970s reflected a clear change in the overall investigational level compared to previous decades. On the surface, there appeared to be a fascination with instrumentation. For the first time, there was also a distinct appeal to basic science to address clinical questions. Some instrumental ratio measures were used to indicate therapy results (e.g., Fisher & Logemann, 1970; Smith & Thyme, 1976). Instrument-driven biofeedback was introduced (Holbrook, Rolnick, & Bailey, 1974; Prosek, Montgomery, Walden, & Schwartz, 1978). In tandem, programmatic therapy approaches used in biofeedback studies emerged in other work, reflecting the influence of behaviorism (e.g., Deal, McClain, & Sudderth, 1976).

Although not emphasized, concerns about learning variables in treatment were also mentioned in the 1970s (Shearer, 1972; Drudge & Philips, 1976). Instrumental outcomes, and their relation to ultimate outcomes, were formally addressed perhaps for the first time (Drudge & Philips, 1976; Fisher & Logemann, 1970; Prosek et al., 1978). Prospective study designs were occasionally used (e.g., Fisher & Logemann, 1970; Smith & Thyme, 1976; Prosek et al., 1976). Occasionally, therapies were differentially assessed, albeit without random assignment (Toohill, 1975). Finally, some therapy studies utilized relatively larger subject pools than most studies in the preceding decades (Deal et al., 1976; Smith & Thyme, 1976).

Based on these observations, there is reason for encouragement in the development of voice therapy studies in the 1970s. But, despite technological advances, virtually all the studies reviewed from this decade remained fully nonexperimental: Control groups were entirely lacking, as were principled single-subject designs. Numerous, unoperationalized retrospective case studies were also reported (e.g., Brewer & McCall, 1974; Shearer, 1972; Strandberg, Griffith, & Hallowell, 1971; Zwitman, 1979; Zwitman & Calcaterra, 1973).

The review that follows focuses on the studies illustrating the advances made in voice therapy research in the 1970s.

Review of Studies

Operationalized ratio measures rooted in basic voice science. Therapy studies in the 1970s were ushered in with a report by Fisher and Logemann (1970) using highly operationalized, instrumentally derived measures of voice function. In the cited study, an adult female with nodules received "optimal pitch" therapy over an 18-month period. At 6-month intervals, her larynx was filmed at her modal pitch (190 Hz) and at what was considered her optimal pitch (250 Hz) (Fairbanks, 1949; Fisher, 1966). In each measurement session, the open quotient (OQ), the speed quotient (SQ), and cycle-to-cycle changes in successive glottal periods were extracted from filmed laryngeal images (Lieberman, 1961; Luchsinger & Pfister, 1959; Moore & Thompson, 1965; Sonesson, 1960; Timcke, von Leden, & Moore, 1958; von Leden, Moore, & Timcke, 1960). The experimental hypothesis was that optimal pitch should decrease laryngeal adductor and/or internal tension, resulting in increased OQ (decreased adduction) and decreased SQ (decreasing vocal fold closing speed). As laryngeal appearance and dysphonia improved, there should further be a reduction in cycle-to-cycle variability in the vibratory period.

The results were consistent with expectations. OQs for the optimal pitch were consistently greater than for the modal pitch, and OQs tended to increase over therapy time, at both pitches. SQs were consistently smaller for the optimal pitch than for the modal pitch, with SQs for the two pitches converging over therapy time. Cycle-to-cycle variations in the vocal fold period also decreased over time, at the optimal pitch. Subsequently, the patient resumed her acting career, and "encountered no difficulty in vocal projection or expressiveness" (p. 284). A laryngeal examination revealed a reduction in her nodules.

This study represents a significant step forward in the history of voice therapy studies. The study was conducted with thoughtful experimental hypotheses, and operationalized physiological outcome measures. Yet, despite rigorous attention to the objective measurement of intermediate and instrumental outcomes,[2] conspicuously limited

---

[2]Intermediate, instrumental, and ultimate outcomes are globally defined by Frattali in Chapter 1 (see also Olswang chapter; Olswang, 1990; Rosen & Proctor, 1981). A review of their definitions, with specific reference to voice therapy, may be useful here. Intermediate outcomes indicate the patient's session-to-session progress. Intermediate outcomes discussed by Fisher and Logemann (1970) were OQs, SQs, and periodicity, for several sessions during therapy. Instrumental outcomes are those which activate learning, and which trigger the final outcome. Although straightforward as a definition, the identification of instrumental outcomes in voice therapy is somewhat complex. In voice therapy, instrumental outcomes are divided into two types: cognitive and physiological. Instrumental cognitive outcomes involve learning processes in acquiring a new perceptual-motor voicing pattern, including attentional, perceptual, pattern recognition, and habituation processes. Instrumental physiological outcomes involve the actual production of the new voicing pattern, which will in turn influence the patient's final organic and functional status. It is this latter type of instrumental outcome that Fisher and Logemann (1970) describe, by reporting a change in OQ, SQ, and periodicity at the end of therapy. Finally, ultimate outcomes reflect the final goals of therapy. In voice therapy, such goals include perceptual, organic, and social and ecological outcomes. Fisher and Logemann (1970) refer to ultimate outcomes by describing improvements in voice quality, in nodules, and in the patient's apparent ability to resume her performing career.

information was provided about ultimate therapy outcomes ("voice improved," "nodules reduced," "career resumed"). Similarly, relatively little information was provided about the actual therapy. Finally, there were no controls for maturational or placebo effects.

Another study incorporating highly operationalized outcome measures was reported by Smith and Thyme (1976), who investigated the Accent Method of voice therapy. The Accent Method is a training approach based on accentuated speech patterns in conjunction with physiological abdominal breathing gestures. Developed over a 40-year period prior to the cited report, the method is used for both voice and fluency disorders. In the present study, a short version of this standardized therapy was applied to 220 students in a Danish teachers' college. All were evaluated before and after training, and data from 30 students were randomly selected as the basis for analysis. The findings indicated a significant increase in the intensities of spectral frequencies both above and below 1000 Hz, in reading, following Accent Method training. Thus, overall voice output was enhanced in "normal" subjects (see also Froekjaer-Jensen & Lauritzen, 1970; Smith, 1961). There was no control group.

While the foregoing studies contributed to the development of voice therapy research in important ways (e.g., use of operationalized outcome measures), both failed to provide information about the specificity of observed treatment effects, due to the lack of control groups.

The use of biofeedback. The fascination with instrumentation in the 1970s was also reflected by the introduction of biofeedback studies. For example, Holbrook, Rolnick, and Bailey (1974) assessed the use of a "vocal intensity controller (VIC)" in the treatment of patients with trauma-based laryngeal conditions, including nodules, prepolypoid formations, and vocal fold thickenings.[3] The VIC is an intensity monitor, which presents a tone through an earphone when "excessively loud speech occurs." Thirty-two subjects were fitted with the device. Four "typical" cases were reported. Subjects used the VIC intermittently over a 2- to 3-month period, as part of a more comprehensive therapy program that included general voice hygiene. The results indicated either nodule resolution (three or four subjects), and/or voice improvements (three of three subjects for whom voice information was provided). This study is laudable for the development of a potentially useful instrument in the treatment of voice disorders. However, a detailed description of the treatment was lacking, as were operationalized outcome measures. Experimental controls were also not used.

Another biofeedback study was conducted by Prosek, Montgomery, Walden, & Schwartz (1978), which may be a gem in the history of voice therapy research. The study assessed the utility of electromyographic (EMG) biofeedback in the treatment of hyperfunctional voice disorders in six adults. A prospective, repeated measures study design was used. Specifically, following a baseline session, subjects received 14 30-minute EMG

---

[3]The authors described the study's focus as "vocal abuse" disorders, further defined by pathological category. The first author of this chapter would like to register disagreement with the use of the term "abuse" in voice disorders, for several reasons. First, the term has connotations which can be morally discouraging to the patient, and thus undermine the therapeutic process. Second, and more conceptually important, vocal abuse is a circular concept: traumatic lesions are supposedly caused by abuse, but abuse can only be retrospectively determined by the appearance of lesions. What is "abusive" for one subject is not for another. For these combined reasons, this author prefers descriptive terms such as "disorders related to traumatic laryngeal lesions."

biofeedback sessions over a 4-week period, followed by a final, no-feedback session. During training sessions, surface electrodes were placed over the cricothyroid region bilaterally, with this placement considered to provide a global indication of laryngeal and perilaryngeal activity. Voltage indicators were set progressively lower throughout the experiment, as 80% criteria were successively met during speech production. Noise was presented when muscle activity exceeded threshold, and a tone was presented when muscle activity was less than threshold. The tone's pitch indicated whether tension was increasing or decreasing. The statistically managed results indicated that EMG biofeedback produced significant reductions in muscular activity in speech, for three to six subjects, as the result of training, with posttreatment EMG distributions approaching normal. The diagnostic conditions for these subjects were contact ulcers, traumatic laryngitis, and bilateral nodules. For two of the subjects, there was also an improvement in ordinally rated voice quality, assessed by multiple, naive judges. For the remaining three subjects (post-nodule surgery, spastic dysphonia, and post-carcinoma removal and radiation therapy), EMG activity did not improve appreciably, nor did voice quality.

Both of the preceding studies paid careful attention to important instrumental variables in treatment—and detailed descriptions of therapy itself—as well as to final outcomes.[4] Both studies, however, lacked experimental control conditions, and thus did not address treatment specificity.

Programmatic approaches. Behavioral science dominated training paradigms in the 1960s and 1970s, and speech-language pathology was no exception. In a study by Deal, McClain, and Sudderth (1976) 31 children with nodules underwent a systematic, multiparameter, voice therapy program based on behaviorism. Goals included reduction in amount and loudness of talking, increased breath flow and gentle adductions in speech, and auditory monitoring. Children were encouraged to bring same-age cohorts to therapy sessions to enhance carryover, and parental involvement was solicited. Each child's larynx was evaluated 2, 4, and 6 months following the initial examination. By the end of the experimental period, an ordinal rating system indicated that nodules had resolved in 20 of 31 children. No subjects had nodules that were the same size or larger (5 were lost to follow-up).

A strength of this study was the description of a training program, based on known learning principles, with ultimate outcome measures identified (nodule status). A weakness was the lack of a control group and the possible influence of observer bias in the results.

Learning variables. The interest in learning variables surfaced in the 1970s. A concern about carryover of learning was noted by Shearer (1972) in the treatment of schoolchildren with voice disorders. Further points were made about the need for patient self-evaluations based on sensory information (Drudge & Philips, 1976), and auditory monitoring (Deal et al., 1976), for skill stabilization. These issues would not be addressed theoretically or empirically until the 1990s (e.g., Ramig, Pawlas, & Countryman, 1995; Verdolini, in press).

---

[4]In these studies, instrumental variables are speech loudness (Holbrook et al., 1974) and EMG muscle activity (Prosek et al., 1978). Final variables are laryngeal status and voice quality. Social and ecological outcomes were not addressed.

Evaluation of instrumental and ultimate outcomes. Woven throughout the preceding sections is another research principle that became more prevalent in the 1970s—the evaluation of both instrumental and ultimate outcomes (Drudge & Philips, 1976; Fisher & Logemann 1970; Prosek et al., 1978). The study of the temporal aspects of treatment outcomes is critically important to reliable therapy models, and its formal beginning can be traced to this decade.

Differential assessment of therapies. In one study, an attempt was made to assess the differential effect of voice therapy treatments (Toohill, 1975). Seventy-seven children with nodules received either school therapy, "professional therapy," parental involvement and counseling, or no therapy. The results indicated that the degree of cure (not operationalized) was equivalent across the three treatment groups, and "[compared] favorably" to outcomes for the no-treatment group. Overall, 58.5% of the children had either complete resolution or improved nodules, although 72% still had nodules at the end of the study period.

This study has several positive qualities, including the attempt to examine treatment effects differentially. However, the specificity and generalizability of the results were limited by the lack of random subject assignment to treatment group, the lack of treatment description, the lack of operationalized outcome measures, and the lack of reliability and validity assessments.

Large N studies. Examples of therapy studies based on large samples included studies by Deal et al. (1976; 31 therapy subjects), Smith and Thyme (1976; 220 subjects trained, 30 formally assessed), and Toohill (1975; 77 therapy subjects), discussed above.

1980s

Introductory Comments

In the 1980s the number of studies increased sharply relative to previous decades (Table 16–2). So, too, did the studies' quality. Although retrospective case studies with limited operationalization were still reported (Boone, 1982a, 1982b; Bridger & Epstein, 1983; Fox, 1982a, 1982b; Freeman & Schaefer, 1982a, 1982b; Hartman & Aronson, 1981; Moore, 1982a, 1982b; Stone, 1982a, 1982b, 1983; see also Butcher & Elias, 1983; MacIntrye, 1981; Ranford, 1982), several operationalized, nonexperimental studies were conducted (Bastian, 1985, 1987; Bloch, Gould, & Hirano, 1981; Stemple, Weil, Whitehead, & Komray, 1980; see also Casper, Colton, Woo, & Brewer, 1989, 1990). Further, there was the appearance of quasi-experimental studies with control groups (Izdebski, Dedo, & Boles, 1984; Kay, 1982) and experiments that approached quasi-experimental designs, but without specific control groups, because of the nature of the questions explored (Elias, Raven, & Butcher, 1989; Lancer, Syder, Jones, & LeBoutillier, 1988; Koufman & Blalock, 1989; Moran & Pentz, 1987).

In the 1980s several treatment efficacy studies were conducted, using full experimental designs (Andrews, Warner, & Stewart, 1986; Lodge & Yarnall, 1981; Robertson & Thomson, 1984; Scott & Caird, 1983; see also Nilson & Schneider, 1983). Large N studies were sometimes conducted (Bridger & Epstein, 1983, 109 subjects; Elias et al., 1989, 244 subjects; Koufman & Blalock, 1989, 127 subjects; Moran & Pentz, 1987, 535 respon-

Table 16–2. Characteristics of Voice Therapy Research, by Decades

DECADE	CHARACTERISTICS
1940s	expert opinion claim that therapy works at all one retrospective study with control group
1950s	nonexperimental design, expert opinion some operationalized outcome measures learning variables embedded in some studies increased scope of disorders investigated
1960s	nonexperimental treatment studies quasi-experimental designs in incidence studies experimental design used in categorization study increased details of therapy increased details in outcome measures some large N studies some studies with extended follow-up occasional statistical management converging evidence across studies

1970s	fascination with machinery, measures, use of basic science; some outcome
	    measures highly operationalized with electronic equipment; machine-driven
	    biofeedback studies
	programmatic (Behavioral) therapy
	increased details of therapy
	learning, self-evaluation, and carryover addressed
	instrumental outcomes assessed in relation to ultimate outcomes
	occasional prospective studies, with experimental hypotheses
	therapies differentially compared
	relative increase in subject N
	no control groups in any study

1980s	large increase in number and type of study nonexperimental studies conducted with operational outcome measures quasi-experimental studies appear in therapy, with and without specific control groups data base studies some experimental studies functional measures and patient satisfaction mentioned
1990–1996	true experimental studies predominate double-blind placebo-controlled studies appear functional, quality-of-life issues surface more strongly client/clinician interface is addressed instrumental variables studied in relation to final variables learning and compliance become formal topic of interest cross-study investigations are conducted theory-based models of voice therapy are developed data base study is reported

dents; Nilson & Schneiderman, 1983, 155 subjects). Important ecological issues were introduced regarding the impact of voice disorders on everyday functions (Llewellyn-Thomas et al., 1984a, 1984b; Sutherland et al., 1984) and on general job functioning and patient satisfaction with voice treatment (Izdebski et al., 1984). Finally, there was a limited number of "As I do it" (expert opinion) papers that did not provide data but were conceptually important (Boone, 1988; Brodnitz, 1981).

Review of Studies

Operationalized nonexperimental studies, without control group. An operationalized study was reported by Stemple and colleagues in 1980. The effect of EMG biofeedback training was evaluated in seven adults with nodules. Electrodes were placed on the left thyroid lamina. Subjects first received a no-feedback session, followed by eight training sessions in 4 weeks, with feedback withdrawn for one those sessions. During each feedback session, subjects attempted to reduce EMG activity in silence for 10 minutes, and then to reduce it in rote speech for 10 minutes. Two weeks posttraining, EMG activity was measured during silence and speech. Results were compared to collected normative data.

The findings indicated that: (1) subjects with nodules initially displayed greater levels of laryngeal tension during silence and speech than normal controls; (2) subjects with nodules obtained a significant reduction in laryngeal tension during silence and speech from pre- to posttreatment, with posttherapy values similar to those for normal subjects; (3) EMG activity and voice quality were related, based on randomly ordered perceptual measures made by blind judges from tape recordings; however EMG and voice intensity were unrelated; (4) after treatment, vocal fold appearance had improved in five of six patients. Three of the patients obtained nodule resolution.

This study approached a true, prospective experimental design, with operationalized therapy, blind perceptual judgments of voice, comparison of data to control data, and evaluation of instrumental (EMG activity), as well as ultimate outcomes (auditory-perceptual status of voice and laryngeal status). However, the study was nonexperimental because no control group was used.

Another study was reported by Bloch, Gould, and Hirano (1981). Ordinal measures of laryngeal and voice improvement indicated that, at long-term follow-up (6 months to 7 years, depending on the patient), granulomas were completely eliminated in 9 of 17 surgical and nonsurgical patients who had undergone conventional voice therapy. Granulomas were reduced in 4 of 17 therapy patients, with no change in 1 of 17. Voice was normal in 4 of 17, with 6 of 17 having no voice changes. Three patients discontinued treatment and were not available for follow-up. The authors contended that excluding 5 patients who received 5 or less voice therapy sessions, the success rate for return to normal status was 11 of 11 or 100%.

This study incorporated some improved design characteristics compared with many of the earlier, retrospective case studies. In particular, there was an attempt to operationalize outcome measures. What was lacking was information about the measures' reliability and validity, and a control group.

Bastian (1985, 1987) reported on the use of rigid endoscopy in the acquisition of novel laryngeal postures, and on the use of rigid or flexible endoscopy in the reacquisition of true vocal fold voicing in clinical patients. In his first study, according to two judges, 9 of 9 singers acquired the ability to produce an epiglottic tilt, 8 of 9 acquired a glottal squeeze, and 7 of 9 acquired pseudobowing using rigid endoscopy biofeedback, during a maximum of 6-minute biofeedback trials. Interjudge reliability was good. In his second study, two patients without true vocal fold phonation acquired it with alternating biofeedback/no feedback trials. One patient with false vocal fold phonation secondary to intubation required seven 30-minute biofeedback sessions. This patient further achieved complete relief of symptoms, clinically. The second patient, who presented with psychogenic aphonia, acquired true vocal fold phonation within 10 minutes of biofeedback trials, and simultaneously gained insight into the psychological factors associated with her aphonia.

Although these studies were based on case reports, they have a different flavor with respect to many of the less formal, retrospective studies of earlier decades. First, the studies had at least some prospective component because of the relatively standardized sequence of training components across subjects. Second, a single-subject, "ABAB" design appeared, with alternating application and withdrawal of treatment (biofeedback). However, again, the methods' specificity was not addressed.

Quasi-experimental studies with control group, and no-control data base studies. In the 1980s, we see the first true attempts at quasi-experimental or clinical epidemiological studies assessing voice therapy. Kay (1982) examined the etiology and management of nodules in 42 children. For these children, chart data were inspected for age on presentation, sibling number, type and duration of voice symptoms, management characteristics, and clinical outcomes (e.g., "cured" or "cured of hoarseness"). Questionnaires were also administered to parents of 58 children being treated in various nonotolaryngological clinics, including medical, surgical, and ophthalmic clinics. The questionnaire inquired if the children screamed or shouted during play. Of 35 patients with nodules, case histories indicated "vocal abuse" in seven cases (20%). In contrast, parents of 27 of the 58 control cases (45%) indicated a positive history of screaming and shouting. The results imply that screaming and shouting are not necessarily risk factors for nodules.

This study contributed to the limited number of studies with a control group. However, especially one factor limited the interpretation of the results: The data collection method was inconsistent across patient and control groups. Retrospective chart examination was used to assess patients' voice use patterns, whereas parental questioning was used to assess voice patterns in the control subjects.

Another clinical epidemiological study was reported by Izdebski et al. (1984). Profiles for 200 persons with spasmodic dysphonia were described, with data also collected for 200 control subjects matched for age and sex. It was unclear whether data were obtained from chart review, questionnaire, or interview. Multiple parameters were evaluated, including medical history, voice history, job functioning, and satisfaction with care.

The results for job functioning and satisfaction with care focused on data from patients with spasmodic dysphonia, without comparison to control subjects. Those results indicated that 92.7% of males and 77.4% of females experienced job interferences because of their voice problems. A large proportion of patients had actually changed jobs because of these problems (25.9% of men and 36.7% of women). Nineteen percent of those who had received speech therapy thought that it had helped, with no instances of long-term cure.

As noted, this study was an ambitious one by its inclusion of a large, matched control group. Another contribution was the introduction of ecological and quality-of-life measures, including job-related functions and patient satisfaction with treatment. Unfortunately, as with many questionnaire studies, information about the measures' reliability and validity was lacking.

Koufman and Blalock (1989) also conducted a clinical epidemiological study. However, a control group was not included, and thus the data-based study is considered nonexperimental. Clinical records were examined for 127 consecutive patients receiving laryngeal microsurgery for the treatment of benign laryngeal lesions and cancer in situ. Information was tabulated regarding postoperative voice recommendations (i.e., complete voice rest or voice conservation in the immediate postoperative period). Other information included age, sex, smoking, diagnosis, laser versus knife surgery, pre- and/or posttherapy, patient compliance, and duration of postoperative dysphonia. Prolonged dysphonia was operationalized as postoperative dysphonia lasting 4 weeks or more. The data were managed statistically. Most relevant for voice therapy, 41% of patients with voice conservation postsurgery experienced prolonged postoperative dysphonia, in comparison with 27% of patients who observed complete voice rest ($p = .17$). Further, 16% of patients who received voice therapy preoperatively experienced prolonged dysphonia following surgery. In contrast, 54% of patients who did not receive preoperative therapy experienced prolonged dysphonia ($p < .001$). Finally, 86% of noncompliant patients who did not observe postoperative instructions experienced prolonged dysphonia ($p < .001$).

The study's contribution is valuable, indicating a potential positive effect on voice with preoperative voice therapy for the lesions noted (see also Lancer et al., 1988, for similar findings). The primary regret with the study is that the voice therapy was not described.

Other studies relevant for voice therapy, but not about voice therapy itself, were also conducted in an epidemiological vein, without control groups. These studies investigated otolaryngologists' opinions about voice therapy for children with nodules, the adequacy of SLPs' training (Moran & Pentz, 1987), and methods used by SLPs in the United Kingdom to treat psychologically based voice disorders (Elias, Raven, & Butcher, 1989).

Studies using full experimental designs. Three strong voice therapy studies were found using full experimental designs. The first investigated the reduction of abnormally loud voice volume in a mentally retarded adult female, using a behavioral therapy program (Large & Yarnall, 1981). A prospective, single-subject ABA experimental design was used. The subject first received three baseline sessions without reinforcers or cues. Then, during an intervention period, she received verbal and visual cues with social and food reinforcers, for productions of less than 65 dB (desired). A "Whisperlite" device was used as an aversive stimulus for loud productions (undesirable). Cues and reinforcers were systematically faded according to an established hierarchy. Following 12 treatment sessions, three reversal sessions were conducted without reinforcers or cues. A second intervention period followed similar to the first one. When 100% satisfaction was met for three consecutive sessions, three final reversal sessions were conducted (total of more than 30 sessions). Reliability checks were included in the design.

The results indicated improvements in performance during the first intervention period, and deterioration during the reversal period, confirming a treatment effect. Performance improved in the second intervention period, with improvements retained in the final, withdrawal testing period. In this study, therapy and hierarchy criteria were fully described prior to the experiment. Therapy was based on a theoretical learning paradigm. Reliability checks were included. However, because the control condition involved the successive introduction and withdrawal of treatment rather than the use of a control subject or group, it is not clear to what extent any therapy or clinical contact might have produced similar results.

The first experimental group study was reported by Scott and Caird (1983). These authors investigated the effect of prosodic exercises on speech prosody and intelligibility in persons with Parkinson disease. Twenty-six patients were prospectively, randomly assigned to one of two treatment groups. One group received prosodic exercises with a visual reinforcement device, the Vocalite (Group A), and the other group received prosodic exercises without Vocalite (Group B). Therapy was provided in-home, in five, 1-hour sessions weekly, for 2 weeks. Measures were made before and after 2 weeks of treatment in both groups. Group B further received another week of prosodic exercises, and measures were made again in that group following that week. Both groups underwent final testing 3 months later after a no-therapy period.

The results indicated no group differences in blind, ordinally rated prosody or intelligibility measures at baseline. Subjects in both groups made significant gains in prosody and intelligibility with treatment. Performance deteriorated when therapy was withdrawn, but not back to baseline. All family members thought that therapy was worthwhile.

This study incorporates all of the critical elements of true experimental design: Random, prospective assignment, control (or alternative therapy) group, and multiple blinded raters for (multidimensional perceptual) outcomes data. Other important experimental design features were long-term follow-up after therapy withdrawal, and the consideration of extraclinical validation of the data (relatives' comments about treatment outcome).

Given these factors, it is somewhat disappointing that group differences in treatment effects were not shown. An effect of treatment was shown by posttherapy deterioration in performance. However, the lack of differences in performance curves across the groups suggests the possibility that treatment effects were nonspecific placebo effects that might be obtained with any clinical contact.

Another group study using a quasi-experimental design also investigated the effect of speech/voice therapy for persons with Parkinson disease (Robertson & Thomson, 1984). Twenty-two subjects were randomly assigned to either treatment or control groups. Subjects in the therapy group received 3.5 to 4 hours of therapy daily during a 2-week period, while control subjects received no treatment. Therapy included group treatments, and individual treatments if needed, focusing on respiratory control, voice production control (pitch variations and loudness), articulatory range, strength, and speed, speech rate control, intonational and stress variations, and speech intelligibility. Standardized measures were made before treatment, immediately after a 2-week treatment (or control) period, and then at 3-month follow-up. Outcome measures, based on Robertson's (1982) ordinal-level Dysarthria Profiles, indicated the therapy group obtained significantly better average scores on the measured parameters than the control group. The therapy group further continued to show improvements after therapy but the control group did not.

A shortcoming in this otherwise strong experimental design was an inconsistency in data collection procedures in the two groups: (Nonblind) clinicians obtained the measures in the therapy subjects, whereas the authors obtained the measures for the control subjects. This factor could have biased the results.

A third experimental study was published by Andrews, Warner, and Stewart, in

1986. This study investigated the utility of EMG biofeedback and relaxation training for hyperfunction. Subjects included a total of 10 adult females with hyperfunctional voice disorders associated with nodules, vocal fold thickenings, edema, incomplete vocal fold approximation, and normal larynx. Pairs of subjects were matched for age and severity of dysphonia, and were assigned on an alternating basis to one of two treatment groups: EMG laryngeal relaxation, and conventional relaxation training.

Therapy in the two groups was described as identical, except for the method of laryngeal relaxation. Following introductory explanations, subjects were to receive weekly 45-minute therapy sessions. The number of sessions ranged from 4 to 15, over a total of 4 to 36 weeks. The therapy schedule was considered typical for many clinical settings. In the EMG group, continuous EMG feedback about laryngeal tension was provided from electrodes placed over the pars recta of the cricothyroid, apparently unilaterally. One-minute tension reduction trials were separated by 30-second intertrial periods, based on a pilot study. When predetermined criterion levels were obtained, reading trials were incorporated. A no-feedback trial ended each stage of therapy, as well as each session. In the relaxation group, progressive relaxation exercises were used based on Bernstein and Borkovec (1973). This relaxation method involves a condensation of the more familiar Jacobson progression (1968).

Measures were made before treatment initiation, after treatment, and at 3-month follow-up. The results were evaluated statistically. Both EMG and progressive relaxation groups showed improvements in voice quality (based on reliable ordinal ratings), vocal fold control (from a fundamental frequency trace), and subjects' self-ratings of voice. All improvements were retained at 3-month follow-up.

The study is exemplary in many ways. Initial subject matching for severity is critical in assessing treatment effects, particularly with smaller N studies such as this one. The delivery of identical therapy across groups with the exception of the specific modality of laryngeal relaxation has rarely been incorporated in voice therapy studies, and is critical if specificity is to be addressed. The use of subject diaries to indicate adherence to practice schedules is an instrumental variable which would help to interpret the final results, particularly in the event of group differences.

The perplexing aspect of this study lies not with the experimental design, but with the results. Both therapy groups appeared to improve equivalently with treatment. But to what extent were improvements the result of the specific therapies studied, as opposed to "placebo" or "generic therapy" effects?

Development of functional outcome measures. In addition to the consideration of the functional impacts of voice disorders reported by Izdebski et al. (1984), further efforts were made to develop formal, functional ability scales related to voice. Llewellyn-Thomas and colleagues (Llewellyn-Thomas et al., 1984a, 1984b) developed a series of linear analogue self-assessment (LASA) scales to assess the symptoms and functional abilities for voice in patients who were undergoing radiation treatment for laryngeal cancer. Patients placed a vertical mark on a 10-cm line, which was anchored at each end by statements such as "able to speak without any effort" and "able to speak only with great effort." Sixteen scales were presented to patients. While the aim of these studies was to gauge patients' evaluation of their states due to a medical intervention, this is probably the first instance of the development of a standardized tool for measuring self-assessment of function relative to voice. In an extension of this work, ratings of voice quality and functional ability were made by patients and physicians (Sutherland et al., 1984). There was often disagreement on the degree of impairment or disability between physicians and patients.

"As I do it" papers. Numerous expert opinion "As I do it" papers were published in the 1980s, as in previous decades. Two are highlighted here, which raised issues addressed in the subsequent decade.

The first of these papers was by Brodnitz (1981). In this work, an expert clinician's argument was made for the role of psychological factors in voice therapy. Brodnitz cited at least two levels of psychological issues: One was the role of potential resistance to carryover, and the second was the importance of appealing to individual patients' predominant preferred sensory modality in training. Although not data-based, the arguments were cogent ones. In particular the issue of sensory processing would reappear as an emerging, theoretically and empirically based issue in the 1990s (Verdolini, 1996).

A second paper was published by Boone in 1988. In it, he discussed respiratory training in voice therapy. An important point was that "too much knowledge about one's performance can confuse the patient" (p. 21). Instructions should be simplified in training. This theme will be reencountered in the work of Ramig and colleagues in the 1990s (Dromey, Ramig, & Johnson, 1995; Ramig, Pawlas, & Countryman, 1995), and will also be theoretically treated by Ramig (Ramig, Countryman, Thompson, & Horii, 1995; Ramig & Dromey, 1996) and Verdolini (in press).

1990s

Introductory Comments

True experimental studies predominate in the 1990s according to our literature review (see Table 16–1). To date this decade is characterized by the solid appearance of important study design features only dimly present in preceding decades. These include: double-blind, placebo controlled experimental studies in voice training and voice therapy studies (Stemple, Lee, D'Amico, & Pickup, 1994; Verdolini-Marston, Sandage, & Titze, 1994); other fully experimental studies (e.g., Johnson & Pring, 1990, and other described below); the development and assessment of cognitively simplified therapy procedures (Ramig, Countryman, Thompson, & Horii, 1995; Verdolini-Marston, Burke, Lessac, Glaze, & Caldwell, 1995); further studies on instrumental variables mediating ultimate outcomes in voice therapy, including learning and compliance variables (Andrews & Schmidt, 1995; Boone & McFarlane, 1993; Casper et al., 1989, 1990; Dromey, Ramig, & Johnson, 1995; Kotby, Shiromoto, & Hirano, 1993; Peterson, Verdolini-Marston, Barkmeier, & Hoffman, 1994; Ramig & Dromey, 1996; Schmidt & Andrews, 1993; Verdolini, Druker, Palmer, & Samawi, in press); the development of functional and quality-of-life scales pertinent to voice disorders and voice therapy (Jacobson & Bush, 1996; Jacobson et al., in press; Smith et al., 1996); multiple-study investigations of single therapy types anchored in theoretically based, cohesive therapy models (for Lee Silverman Voice Treatment (LSVT), Countryman & Ramig, 1993; Countryman, Ramig, & Pawlas, 1994; Dromey et al., 1995; Ramig, Countryman, Thompson, & Horii, 1995; Smith, Ramig, Dromey, Perez, & Samandari, 1995; for Resonant Voice Therapy, Peterson et al., 1994; Verdolini & Titze, 1995; Verdolini et al., in press; Verdolini-Marston et al., 1995; for Accent Method, Frokjaer-Jensen, & Lauritzen, 1970; Kotby, El-Sady, Basiouny, Abou-Rass, & Hegazi, 1991; Kotby, Shiromoto, & Hirano, 1993; Smith & Thyme, 1976); and the use of clinical data bases to formulate tentative impressions about the effects of voice therapy (Murry & Woodson, 1995).

Also, several nonexperimental studies without control groups, but with strongly operationalized measures, have been conducted in this decade. These include studies on EMG biofeedback for nodule and hyperfunction treatment (Allen, Bernstein, & Chait, 1991); some of the studies conducted on Lee Silverman Voice Treatment (LSVT) in patients with Parkinson disease (Countryman & Ramig, 1993; Countryman et al., 1994, Ramig, Bonitati, Lemke, & Horii, 1994, later compared to control data in King, Ramig, Lemke, & Horii, 1994); Accent Method for a range of voice disorders (Kotby et al., 1991); laryngeal manipulation for functional voice disorders (Roy & Leeper, 1993); and a pushing exercise program for glottal incompetence (Yamaguchi et al., 1993).

Review of Studies

Experimental studies using control and/or alternative therapy groups. Several group studies have been reported during the 1990s using experimental designs, with control or alternative therapy groups. Johnson and Pring (1990) investigated the effect of speech/voice therapy for persons with Parkinson disease. Twelve subjects with idiopathic Parkinson disease were matched for age and sex. One member of each pair was randomly assigned to either a treatment group or a control (no-treatment) group. Subjects in the treatment group received 10 sessions of speech/voice therapy over 4 weeks. Successive sessions focused on a relaxed, "diaphragmatic" breathing pattern and coordination of breathing and voice; the improvement of loudness and loudness contrasts in phrases; stress patterns in speech in sentences; pitch and intonation patterns in speech; bilabial and lingual articulatory work; maintenance of clear articulation with increased loudness in speech passages; speech rate; and carryover to extra-clinical circumstances. Measures were made at the beginning of treatment and 4 weeks later (i.e., 1 week following treatment termination). Measures were based on the *Frenchay Dysarthria Assessment* (Enderby, 1983). The data were statistically managed. The results indicated that dysarthria improved in the treatment group, and deteriorated over the same period in the no-treatment group ($p < .005$ for both groups). Treated patients further improved in maximum intensity, speech intensity, reading intensity, pitch range, and changed modal pitch in reading. In contrast, untreated subjects did not achieve these changes. Subjects in both groups improved in maximum intensity. The results indicate a definite effect of treatment in comparison with a control condition. However, treatment specificity was not addressed.

Another study investigated the effect of therapy on communication disorders in Parkinson disease, comparing the impact of two, alternative treatments (Ramig, Countryman, Thompson, & Horii, 1995). Specific treatment effects were shown in this work by a combination of experimental design and results. Forty-five subjects with idiopathic Parkinson disease received 16 sessions of either respiration treatment or LSVT over a 4-week period. Subjects were stratified for age, sex, Parkinson disease stage, performance on a motor examination, time since initial diagnosis, degree of glottal incompetence, and severity of speech deficits. Stratified subjects were then randomly assigned to a treatment group.

Both therapy types involved high-effort training, earlier described by Ramig, Pawlas, and Countryman (1995). In the respiratory group, high-effort training focused on maximum ribcage and abdominal excursion during nonspeech and speech tasks, to the conversational level. In the LSVT group, high-effort training focused on maximum loudness during speech tasks, also to the conversational level. Throughout training, instrumented feedback about performance was provided to subjects in both groups, and self-monitoring was encouraged.

Numerous measures were made within 1 week prior to treatment, and within 1 week following treatment. Measures included sound pressure level in isolated phonemes, reading, and monologue; maximum phoneme duration; fundamental frequency and semitone standard deviation during reading and monologue; functional vital capacity; and patient and family ratings of loudness, speech prosody, voice quality, intelligibility, and tendency to initiate conversation.

A comparison of pre- and posttreatment measures indicated that more measures improved with LSVT as compared with respiratory therapy. Further, only subjects who received LSVT indicated an improvement in the effect of Parkinson disease on their communication deficits (see also Smith, Ramig, Dromey, Perez, & Samadari, 1995, for a description of underlying changes in vocal fold adduction with LSVT). The study reveals *specific* treatment effects by showing a superior outcome of one treatment, in comparison with another treatment. Further studies indicated substantial retention of treatment benefits at long-term follow-up of 1 year and greater (Ramig, Countryman, O'Brien, Hoehn, & Thompson, 1996; Dromey, Ramig, & Johnson, 1995).

Other studies using experimental controls, but showing *non*specific treatment effects, have investigated hyperfunctional voice disorders. One was reported by Blood (1994). This author described the effect of a computer-assisted voice therapy protocol in the treatment of hyperfunction and nodules. The study used a variant of the repeated AB design, with two subjects. The experimental phases were: (A) Baseline; (B) Voice therapy protocol; (C) Voice therapy protocol + relaxation; and (D) Follow-up. The actual ordering of phases was: (A), (B), (B + C), (B), (B+C), and (D).

Voice therapy consisted of education about "abuse" reduction, breathing and easy onset phonation, and carryover activities. Voice therapy + relaxation was the same, with the addition of relaxation training. Breathing and easy-onset phonation exercises were assisted with a Computer-Aided Fluency Establishment Trainer (Goebel, 1988a, 1988b). Twelve sessions were provided. Repeated baseline measures were made, and posttherapy measures were repeated at 1, 2, and 3 months following therapy termination.

The results indicated that all measured parameters specifically improved with therapy, and tended to remain relatively stable across the extended follow-up intervals: perturbation decreased, the percent of error-free breathing groups increased, the percent of easy onset phonation trials increased, maximum phonation time increased, and relaxation ratings improved. Fundamental frequency also increased. Both subjects thought that their voices had improved with treatment, and had become normal by the final follow-up session. Multiple, naive listeners also thought that subjects' voices improved to almost normal by the end of treatment. Nodules were further eliminated in both patients. Relaxation training failed to provide additional benefits, relative to voice training alone. Thus, the treatment benefits shown were nonspecific.

A final study showing a nonspecific benefit from voice therapy using control or alternative therapy groups also investigated subjects with nodules (Verdolini-Marston et al., 1995). This study examined the effects of "resonant" and "confidential voice therapy" in the treatment of nodules. Eighteen adult females with nodules were enrolled in a prospective protocol, and were assigned to therapist x treatment conditions, or to a control (no-treatment) condition on an alternating basis, so that initial severity distributions would be equal across the experimental cells. Therapy subjects received 9 1-hour therapy sessions over 12 consecutive days. The therapy hierarchy was similar across the two therapy groups, with the exception of the use of resonant voice or confidential voice in training. Control subjects received no active treatment. All subjects were instructed to limit yelling and screaming, alcohol, caffeine, and smoke exposure, and were required to complete diaries indicating their adherence.

Measures were made prior to therapy, 1 day following therapy termination, and 2 weeks following therapy termination. Data from 13 of 18 subjects were complete and available for analysis. The findings indicated that a statistically significant proportion of treatment subjects improved across all of the measures reported: blind auditory-perceptual ratings of voice severity, blind ratings of laryngeal severity, and direct magnitude estimation of phonatory effort (Wright & Colton, 1972; Colton & Brown, 1972), from baseline to 2-week follow-up. The same statistical improvement was not obtained in the control group. Thus, a benefit from therapy was shown. However, the likelihood of a treatment benefit was nonspecific: It did not depend on which treatment was provided. Rather, the likelihood of a relatively longer-term treatment benefit depended on whether subjects reported that they did or did not use the trained phonation technique outside the clinic following therapy termination.

Experimental studies using double-blind, placebo-controls. Placebo effects are those due to receiving treatment in general, such as increased motivation. The first double-blind, placebo-controlled study was conducted by Verdolini-Marston et al. (1994). The effects of hydration on laryngeal nodules and polyps and voice were studied. Six adult females with nodules received both hydration and placebo treatments for 5 days each, with the order of treatments counterbalanced across subjects. The hydration treatment consisted of eight 16-ounce glasses of water (128 ounces) or more daily, 1 teaspoon of Robitussin expectorant three times daily, and daily 2-hour exposures to 90 to 100% relative humidity environments. The placebo treatment consisted of 8 sets of 20 bilateral forefinger flexions daily, 1 teaspoon of a placebo drug (cherry syrup) daily, and 2-hour daily exposures to what was described to subjects as an "airfiltered" environment daily (airfilter devices were employed, but filtering mechanisms were deactivated). All subjects were instructed to limit heavy voice use including yelling and screaming, alcohol and caffeine intake, and exposure to smoke during the experimental period. Subjects kept daily diaries to indicate their adherence to the instructions. An experimenter who was blind to the experimental hypotheses provided all instructions and was unaware that a placebo treatment was involved. Experimenters who elicited and tabulated all measures were blind to subjects' experimental condition. Multiple blind raters made perceptual measures with reliability checks. Subjects were unaware that a placebo treatment was involved in the experiment.

The results indicated significant improvements in voice and laryngeal measures with both hydration and placebo treatments. However, significantly greater improvements were obtained with the hydration treatment. Specifically, jitter improved significantly in both placebo and hydration treatments, but significantly more with hydration.

Perceived phonatory effort, laryngeal appearance, and shimmer indicated similar trends, but with statistically paradoxical results. The signal-to-noise ratio showed statistically equivalent improvements with both hydration and placebo treatments. The results were interpreted in light of earlier, physical models predicting a decrease in vocal fold tissue viscosity, and thus a decrease in phonatory subglottic pressures and effort (Titze, 1988) and in vocal fold edema (Titze, 1981) with hydration treatments.

There are three caveats regarding these data. First, the type of hydration treatment studied in this experiment was more intensive than treatments used in most clinical situations. Second, although some robust hydration effects were detected, the magnitude of those effects was relatively small, for the brief treatment period studied. A third caution is that when hydration treatments were withdrawn, there was some degree of a "wash-out" or reversal effect: Hydration treatments produced their maximum apparent benefit only so long as the treatments continued to be administered.

A second study using a double-blind placebo-controlled design pertained to voice training in normal subjects (Stemple et al., 1994). Thirty-five healthy female graduate students without any history of voice or laryngeal disorder were randomly assigned to treatment, placebo, or control groups. Treatment consisted of exercises designed to improve various aspects of laryngeal control. In the treatment group, subjects performed several vocal exercises daily, including maximally sustained /i/ on F4, pitch glides from lowest to highest note and the reverse on /o/; and successive, maximally sustained C4, D4, E4, F4, and G4 on /a/. Each exercise was repeated twice, two times daily, for 4 weeks. Three practice sessions each week were taped for clinician review, and subjects also met three times weekly with a clinician for exercise checks. In the placebo group, subjects read a short passage at a comfortable pitch, and further chanted a series of sentences at specified pitches near the habitual pitch. Practice and clinical check-up schedule was the same as for the treatment group. The control group performed no vocal exercises during the protocol period.

The results indicated "significant changes in phonation volume flow rate, maximum phonation time, and frequency range for the experimental group. No significant changes were noted in the measurements of the control and placebo groups" (p. 271). Similar results were obtained in a parallel study assessing a group of singers who underwent the vocal function exercise program, in comparison to a control group who did not (Sabol, Lee, & Stemple, 1995).

Essentially, the placebo-controlled study by Stemple and colleagues (1994) showed an improvement in specific, practiced parameters—and necessary physiological correlates—across a practice period. The design is an excellent one for experimental purposes. A question that was not addressed was whether treatment affected not only the specific functions trained, but also affected vocal abilities in conversation or singing. The study also did not address the applicability of the findings to subjects with voice disorders. Data collection in this population is currently underway (Stemple, personal communication).

Studies including learning and compliance variables. Several studies in the 1990s have investigated instrumental variables that may mediate ultimate therapy outcomes. As an overview, primary topics have included client and clinician characteristics in voice therapy (Andrews & Schmidt, 1995; Schmidt & Andrews, 1993), physiological variables underlying potential treatment effects (Boone & McFarlane, 1993; Casper et al., 1989,

1990; Kotby et al., 1993; Peterson et al., 1994; Dromey et al., 1995; Ramig & Dromey, 1996; Verdolini, Druker, Palmer, & Samawi, in press), learning variables in treatment (Verdolini, in press), and patient compliance (Verdolini-Marston et al., 1995).

New therapy models. Voice therapy is changing in several ways, including the number of variables directly manipulated in treatment. Traditionally, multiple treatment goals have been used. Although there have been exceptions such as the "chewing method" (Froeschels, 1952), simplified respiration training (Boone, 1988), and focused biofeedback procedures (e.g., Stemple et al., 1980), voice therapies have traditionally targeted multiple parameters ranging from explanations to counseling to postural, respiratory, phonatory, resonatory, and even articulatory adjustments. A new emphasis is found on cognitive simplification in treatment.

There is a trend for single or few training parameters to be targeted in therapy, with those parameters simultaneously affecting multiple levels of the voice production mechanism. An example is found in the LSVT. This treatment focuses almost exclusively on stimulating the global "loud" variable in speech, resulting in voice and also speech improvements, in persons with Parkinson disease (Dromey, Ramig, & Johnson, 1995; Ramig, Countryman, Thompson, & Horii, 1995; Ramig, Pawlas, & Countryman, 1995). Another example is Resonant Voice Therapy (Verdolini & Titze, 1995; Verdolini-Marston et al., 1995). In this therapy, the singular focus in the production of voice with anterior oral vibratory sensations, in the context of easy phonation. The approach may be relevant for a range of conditions, including hypo- and hyperadducted disorders (Verdolini & Titze, 1995). A third example is the use of vocal function exercises described earlier in this chapter in the treatment of phonasthenia and other conditions (see Sabol, Lee, & Stemple, 1995; Stemple et al., 1994). Finally, the Accent Method, which has been widely used in Europe, northern Africa, and Japan, is a cognitively simplified method used to treat a range of dysphonia conditions (Kotby et al., 1991; Smith & Thyme, 1976), and which focuses on rhythmic speech production providing a timing base for the production of efficient voice production.

There are both empirical and theoretical reasons for this shift towards cognitively simplified therapy. Empirically, there are hard data indicating benefits from this type of treatment, with such data lacking for most others. Second, current theoretical models point to the likelihood that skill acquisition is governed by an experiential system, fundamentally driven by sensory data and at least partly governed by basal ganglia (see review by Verdolini, in press); see also Salmon & Butters, 1995; Epstein, 1994). Although the processes underlying skill acquisition appear to largely lay outside of conscious awareness, attention to sensory information may be required in initial acquisition phases (e.g., Verdolini-Marston & Balota, 1994). A minimization in the number of training targets should increase the likelihood of full attention to those targets, and thus support skill acquisition. In particular, in-depth verbal explanations, which sometimes accompany multidimensional or micromanagement therapy, are particularly questionable as the basis for acquiring new perceptual-motor skills in voice therapy or otherwise (Verdolini, in press).

Another related theme that has been recently emphasized is the issue of self-monitoring or "calibration" to new sensory information as a key to carryover. This treatment key is one of the essential concepts in LSVT for Parkinson disease and is suggested as a critical element in long-term treatment success (for example, Ramig, Pawlas, & Countryman, 1995).

The development of functional and quality-of-life assessments. The development of scales assessing functional effects of voice disorders continues in the 1990s. One example is the *Voice Handicap Index* (VHI; Jacobson et al., in press). This index is a 30-item, 120-point maximum, standardized self-assessment scale which measures patients' perceptions about the impact of a voice disorder upon function, emotional, and physical aspects of daily living. The scale has good internal consistency and good test-retest reliability, and correlates well with patients' judgments of voice disorder severity. Its major application is to measure change in the perception of daily functioning with behavioral, medical, or surgical intervention. In a study by Jacobson and Bush (1996), scores on the VHI did not correlate well with judgments by clinicians about the severity of the voice disorder.

A study by Smith et al. (1996) utilized another, original assessment scale to assess the frequency and effects of voice problems on quality of life in different domains: job, social, psychological, physical, and communicative. Questionnaire data from 174 adult patients presenting to a hospital ENT clinic were compared to data from 173 nonpatients, of whom 2% described hoarseness. The questionnaire had previously been tested for reliability. Only responses indicating moderate or greater impairment were tabulated as "a problem" in data management.

Patients were more likely than controls to report adverse quality-of-life effects as the result of a voice disorder. Most patients considered that voice problems negatively affected past (53%), current (49%), and future (76%) job performance. In contrast, subjects in the comparison group indicated a 2 to 4% rate of negative effects on job functions. Seventy-five percent of patients considered that voice problems negatively affected social functioning, in comparison with only 11% in the comparison group. Patients further described depression related to voice functions more commonly than nonpatients (65% versus 4%).

The development of such scales and associated results speak to a critical issue, and that is the functional impact of voice disorders. It might be easy to consider voice problems as less serious than other medical problems which produce visible effects of disease, such as cancer, amputation, heart disease, and AIDS, to name a few. Clinicians working with voice patients know that voice disorders are sometimes literally devastating to the patient, producing debilitating psychological effects and professional incapacitation, in some cases. Studies exploring the functional effects of voice disorders make the critical point that such disorders constitute a legitimate and important topic of public interest and investigation.

Investigations on single topics and theoretically based therapy models. One investigational series already mentioned has systematically examined multiple aspects of LSVT in the treatment of communication disorders from Parkinson disease, based on theoretical considerations. As previously discussed, a specific benefit of LSVT has been shown, relative to alternative respiratory exercise therapy (Ramig, Countryman, Thompson, & Horii, 1995). The treatment's physiological basis has been investigated, with documented physiological changes, including increases in laryngeal adduction and phonatory efficiency, and a corresponding increase in voice output intensity (Dromey, Ramig, & Johnson, 1995; Ramig & Dromey, 1996; Smith, Ramig, Dromey, Perez, & Samadari, 1995). Improved articulation and speech rate also frequently occur with this treatment, as a by-product of voice manipulations (Ramig, Countryman, Thompson, &

Horii, 1995). The proposed theoretical basis for the results involves the suggestion that there may be a neurologic hierarchy, in which voice changes govern articulatory changes, but not the reverse. Yet other studies have examined the utility of LSVT in the treatment of other neurologic disorders such as Parkinson Plus Syndrome (Countryman et al., 1994) and status post-bilateral thalamotomy (Countryman & Ramig, 1993).

Another investigational series based on theoretical considerations has been conducted on "resonant voice." In this series, the physiological properties of resonant voice have been explored, the clinical effect of resonant voice therapy has been experimentally examined, and a theoretical model has been proposed for the utility of this therapy type. Specifically, Peterson et al. (1994) and Verdolini et al. (in press) found that both skilled normal subjects and skilled subjects with nodules tend to produce resonant voice with a barely abducted laryngeal configuration during vowel production. As discussed earlier, Resonant Voice Therapy appeared as effective as Confidential Voice Therapy in the treatment of nodules, and more effective than no treatment (Verdolini-Marston et al., 1995). Finally, a theoretical model was proposed indicating that the barely abducted laryngeal configuration, apparently used to produce resonant voice, should produce an optimum trade-off between voice output (maximized) and intra-vocal fold impact stress (minimized; Verdolini & Titze, 1995), or maximum vocal economy. That model was embedded in a more comprehensive one proposed by Verdolini-Marston and colleagues (1995), that posits three fundamental parameters in voice therapy: (1) Physiology ("what" should the patient do?), (2) Learning ("how" will the patient acquire that behavior?) and (3) Compliance ("if" the patient will utilize the behavior consistently outside the clinic). The physiological aspect of the model has further been operationalized into (a) Vocal economy, described above (Verdolini & Titze, 1995), (b) Vocal fold tissue viscosity, influenced by hydration (Titze, 1981, 1988; Verdolini-Marston et al., 1994); and (c) Vocal fold tissue integrity (e.g., Gray, 1991; Gray, Hirano, & Sato, 1993; Gray, Pignatari, & Harding, 1994; Gray & Titze, 1988). Learning and compliance aspects of the model have been more tentatively framed in terms of sensory processing (Verdolini, in press) and personal versus cultural influences in treatment behavior (White & Verdolini, 1995). A third investigational series is demonstrated in independent work by different author groups, who have studied the Accent Method of voice therapy. Mentioned earlier in this chapter, Smith & Thyme (1976) described changes in the spectral content of speech, with enhancements above and below 1000 Hz, following a brief program of Accent Method training in teaching students. Kotby et al. (1991) further described improvements in dysphonia and laryngeal appearance, as well as in maximum phonation time, mean flow rate, phonatory subglottic pressure, and glottal efficiency with Accent Method therapy, in a variety of clinical patients. Neither of these studies included a control group, so the treatment's specificity was not addressed. However, since then at least one physiological study was reported (Kotby et al., 1993), indicating an increase in glottal airflow with Accent Method training, in healthy subjects.

Investigational series such as these are important for the progressive and systematic exploration of therapy types, ultimately to develop and distribute information about reliable and effective treatment means and their causal mechanisms.

Use of clinical data bases. Similar to work by Koufman and Blalock in the 1980s (1989), Murry and Woodson (1995) recently provided an example of how clinical data bases can be used in contemporary science to indicate the results of voice therapy. Such studies may be particularly useful for intrainstitutional and third-party payer inquiries. Murry and Woodson described the effect of botox and voice therapy for 27 patients with adductory spasmodic dysphonia. Seventeen received botox injections plus post-injection voice therapy, and 10 received botox only. The basic therapy program involved five sessions, with work on reducing voice onset effort, pitch glides using /h/ and other fricatives, continuous airflow during voice production, anterior tongue positioning, and easy articulation. Patients were encouraged to continue home training after therapy termination, and were offered follow-up sessions as needed. Voice measures were made prior to treatment, 2 to 3 weeks later, and then again upon symptom return.

Patients returned for repeat botox injections based on their perception of when an injection was required: that is, upon self-perceived symptom return. The results indicated that 65% of patients who received therapy returned for reinjection more than 25 weeks after the earlier one. In comparison, only 30% of patients who did not receive therapy waited longer than 25 weeks for reinjection. Treated patients further demonstrated "significantly higher mean airflow rates for significantly longer periods" (p. 460).

This study is encouraging regarding the potential value of voice therapy in this patient population. An important point is made that a benefit from therapy does not necessarily require complete symptom resolution or near-resolution, in all cases, to count as a benefit. Clinicians should be aware of such cases, and of the expected type and magnitude of therapy effects.

Necessary limitations in this type of study regard the problem of why some subjects did and some subjects did not receive therapy, and the problem of patient biases in returning for repeat botox injections. In particular the former issue was addressed by the authors, who noted that this factor could have affected the results as much as therapy itself.

CONCLUSION

What Have We Learned About the Impact of Voice Therapy?

Based on this review, the following conclusions are made:

- Functional aphonias can sometimes be successfully treated with the use of facilitatory, vegetative voicing maneuvers.
- Some types of intensive therapies, including Lee Silverman Voice Treatment, may produce a benefit in communication disorders related to Parkinson disease, with benefits often most striking upon treatment termination but usually persisting to some degree.
- Conventional voice therapy may provide a protective effect against the recurrence of laryngeal lesions, in particular following surgery.
- Conventional voice therapy and resonant voice therapy may produce benefits in the treatment of nodules, beyond benefits seen for hygiene intervention alone.
- Intensive hydration treatments may be beneficial in the treatment of nodules.
- Hyperfunctional voice disorders in general may benefit from systematic EMG or behavioral relaxation training of the larynx.

- Conventional voice therapy may provide a protective effect against early symptom return in spasmodic dysphonia, following botox injection.
- Vocal efficiency may improve with a vocal function exercise program.
- Loudness reduction may be facilitated by the use of a behavioral program including positive reinforcement and aversive stimulation, at least in cognitively impaired individuals.
- Voice therapy is a useful and important topic of investigation, given reports of functional impairments and disruptions to quality of life subsequent to voice problems.

Current trends in voice therapy research are discernible and promote promise for the future. Numerous needs remain. First, the number and quality of studies must continue to increase. As this literature review reveals, controlled studies, including blind, placebo-controlled studies, are needed. Large N studies likely will arise from clinical data bases and cross-center investigations. Studies should be based in theoretical models, where possible. Perceptual, acoustic, physiologic, and functional measures should be valid and reliable. Outcome measures should include functional status and quality-of-life instruments. Intervening variables, such as patient compliance and motivation, should be examined.

Finally, the review in this chapter reveals a conspicuous absence of multicultural studies in voice therapy. We are personally and ethically mandated to develop and investigate therapy models for all sectors of the population in order to represent its rich diversity and to serve all of its constituents.

ACKNOWLEDGMENTS

The authors gratefully acknowledge Alison Holman for her critical assistance with library and references searches.

REFERENCES

Allen, K.D., Bernstein, B., & Chait, D.H. (1991). EMG biofeedback treatment of pediatric hyperfunctional dysphonia. *Journal of Behavior Therapy and Experimental Psychiatry, 22,* 97–101.

Andrews, M.L., & Schmidt, C.P. (1995). Congruence in personality between clinician and client: Relationship to ratings of voice treatment. *Journal of Voice, 9,* 261–269.

Andrews, S., Warner, J., & Stewart, R. (1986). EMG biofeedback and relaxation in the treatment of hyperfunctional dysphonia. *British Journal of Disorders of Communication, 21,* 353–369.

Arnold, G.E. (1962a). Vocal rehabilitation of paralytic dysphonia. *Archives of Otolaryngology, LXXVI,* 76–83.

Arnold, G.E. (1962b). Vocal nodules and polyps: Laryngeal tissue reaction to habitual hyperkinetic dysphonia. *Journal of Speech and Hearing Disorders, 27,* 205–217.

Aronson, A.E. (1969). Speech pathology and symptom therapy in the interdisciplinary treatment of psychogenic aphonia. *Journal of Speech and Hearing Disorders, 34,* 321–341.

Aronson, A.E., Brown, J.R., Litin, E.M., & Pearson, J.S. (1968). Spastic dysphonia. II. Comparison with essential (voice) tremor and other neurologic and psychogenic dysphonias. *Journal of Speech and Hearing Disorders, 33,* 220–231.

Aronson, A.E., Peterson, H.W., & Litin, E.M. (1964). Voice symptomatology in functional dysphonia and aphonia. *Journal of Speech and Hearing Disorders, 29,* 367–380.

Baker, D.C. (1954). Contact ulcers of the larynx. *Laryngoscope, 64,* 73–78.

Barton, R.T. (1960). The whispering syndrome of hysterical dysphonia. *Annals of Otology, Rhinology, and Laryngology, LXIX,* 156–164.

Bastian, R.W. (1985). Laryngeal image biofeedback for voice modification. In V.L. Lawrence (Ed.), *Transcripts of the Fourteenth Symposium: Care of the Professional Voice,* pp. 330–333. New York: The Voice Foundation.

Bastian, R.W. (1987). Laryngeal image biofeedback for voice disorder patients. *Journal of Voice, 1,* 279–282.

Baynes, R.A. (1966). An incidence study of chronic hoarseness among children. *Journal of Speech and Hearing Disorders, 31,* 172–176.

Bernstein, D.A., & Borkovec, T.D. (1973). *Progressive relaxation training: A manual for the helping professions.* Champaign, Illinois: Research Press.

Bloch, C.S., Gould, W.J., Hirano, M. (1981). Effect of voice therapy on contact granuloma of the vocal fold. *Annals of Otology, Rhinology, and Laryngology, 90,* 48–52.

Blood, G.W. (1994). Efficacy of a computer-assisted voice treatment protocol. *American Journal of Speech-Language Pathology, 3,* 57–66.

Boone, D.R. (1965). Treatment of functional aphonia in a child and an adult. *Journal of Speech and Hearing Disorders, 30,* 69–74.

Boone, D.R. (1982a). Symptomatic voice therapy: Theory and research. In V.L. Lawrence (Ed.), *Transcripts of the Eleventh Symposium: Care of the Professional Voice,* pp. 1–6. New York: The Voice Foundation.

Boone, D.R. (1982b). Symptomatic voice therapy: Diagnosis and therapy. In V.L. Lawrence (Ed.), *Transcripts of the Eleventh Symposium: Care of the Professional Voice,* pp. 67–72. New York: The Voice Foundation.

Boone, D.R. (1988). Respiratory training in voice therapy. *Journal of Voice, 2,* 20–25.

Boone, D.R., & McFarlane, S.C. (1993). A critical view of the yawn-sigh as a voice therapy technique. *Journal of Voice, 7,* 75–80.

Brewer, D.W., & McCall (1974). Visible laryngeal changes during voice therapy. *Annals of Otology, Rhinology, 83,* 423–427.

Bridger, M.W., & Epstein, R. (1983). Functional voice disorders. A review of 109 patients. *Journal of Laryngology and Otology, 97,* 1145–1148.

Brodnitz, F.S. (1958). Vocal rehabilitation in benign lesions of the vocal cords. *Journal of Speech and Hearing Disorders, 23,* 112–117.

Brodnitz, F.S. (1981). Psychological considerations in vocal rehabilitation. *Journal of Speech and Hearing Disorders, 46,* 21–26.

Brodnitz, F.S., & Froeschels, E. (1954). Treatment of nodules of vocal cords by chewing method. *Archives of Otolaryngology, LIX,* 560–565.

Butcher, P., & Elias, A. (1983). Cognitive-behavioural therapy with dysphonic patients: An exploratory investigation. *Bulletin of the College of Speech Therapists, 377,* 1–3.

Casper, J.K., Colton, R.H., Woo, P., & Brewer, D. (1989, 1990). *Investigation of selected voice therapy techniques.* Amalgamation of two articles presented at the 18th and 19th Symposia: Care of the Professional Voice, 1989, 1990, Philadelphia, PA.

Colton, R.H., & Brown, W.S. *Some relationships between vocal effort and intra-oral air pressure.* Paper presented at the 84th meeting of the Acoustical Society of America, Miami, FL, November, 1972.

Cooper, M., & Nahum, A.M. (1967). Vocal rehabilitation for contact ulcer of the larynx. *Annals of Otolaryngology, 85,* 41–46.

Countryman, S., & Ramig, L.O. (1993). Effects of intensive voice therapy on voice deficits associated with bilateral thalamotomy in Parkinson disease: A case study. *Journal of Medical Speech-Language Pathology, 1*, 233–250.

Countryman, S., Ramig, L.O., & Pawlas, A. (1994). Speech voice deficits in Parkinsonian plus syndromes: Can they be treated? *Journal of Medical Speech-Language Pathology, 1*(4), 227–240.

Deal, R.E., McClain, B., & Sudderth, J.F. (1976). Identification, evaluation, therapy, and follow-up for children with vocal nodules in a public school setting.

Dossey, L. (1993). *Healing words: The power of prayer and the practice of medicine.* San Francisco: Harper.

Dromey, C., Ramig, L.O., & Johnson, A.B. (1995). Phonatory and articulatory changes associated with increased vocal intensity in Parkinson disease: A case study. *Journal of Speech and Hearing Research, 38*, 751–764.

Drudge, M.K., & Philips, B.J. (1976). Shaping behavior in voice therapy. *Journal of Speech and Hearing Disorders, 49*, 398–411.

Elias, A., Raven, R., & Butcher, P. (1989). Speech therapy for psychogenic voice disorder: A survey of current practice and training. *British Journal of Disorders of Communication, 24*, 61–76.

Enderby, P. (1983). *The Frenchay Dysarthria Assessment.* San Diego: College Hill Press.

Epstein, S. (1994). Integration of the cognitive and the psychodynamic unconscious. *American Psychologist, 49*, 709–724.

Fairbanks, G. (1949). *Voice and articulation drillbook.* New York: Harper.

Fisher, H. (1966). *Improving voice and articulation.* Boston: Houghton-Mifflin.

Fisher, H.B., & Logemann, J.A. (1970). Objective evaluation of therapy for vocal nodules: A case report. *Journal of Speech and Hearing Disorders, 35*, 277–285.

Fox, D.R. (1982a). Theory and research of the Fox approach. In V.L. Lawrence (Ed.), *Transcripts of the Eleventh Symposium: Care of the Professional Voice,* pp. 7–13. New York: The Voice Foundation.

Fox, D.R. (1982b). Methods of Fox approach to voice therapy. In V.L. Lawrence (Ed.), *Transcripts of the Eleventh Symposium: Care of the Professional Voice,* pp. 73–77. New York: The Voice Foundation.

Freeman, F.J., & Schaefer, S.D. (1982a). Disorders of voice: Theory and research. In V.L. Lawrence (Ed.), *Transcripts of the Eleventh Symposium: Care of the Professional Voice,* pp. 14–24. New York: The Voice Foundation.

Freeman, F.J., & Schaefer, S.D. (1982b). Voice disorders: Diagnosis and treatment. In V.L. Lawrence (Ed.), *Transcripts of the Eleventh Symposium: Care of the Professional Voice,* pp. 78–88. New York: The Voice Foundation.

Frokjaer-Jensen, B., & Lauritzen, K. (1970). Fonetisk-akustisk analyse af recurrens-stemmer for og efter paedagogisk og operativ behandling. *NTTS, 2*, 57–72.

Froeschels, E. (1943). Hygiene of the voice. *Archives of Otolaryngology, XXXVIII*, 122–130.

Froeschels, E. (1952). Chewing method as therapy. *Archives of Otolaryngology, LVI*, 427–434.

Froeschels, E., Kastein, S., & Weiss, D.A. (1955). A method of therapy for paralytic conditions of the mechanisms of phonation respiration and glutition. *Journal of Speech and Hearing Disorders, 20*, 365–370.

Goebel, M.D. (1988a). *Computer aided fluency establishment trainer.* Annandale, VA: Annandale Fluency Clinic, Inc.

Goebel, M.D. (1988b). CAFET-A computer-aided fluency establishment trainer: A clinician's perspective. *Clinical Connection, 2*, 1–5.

Gray, S. (1991). Basement membrane zone injury in vocal nodules. In: Gauffin, J., & Hammarberg, B. (Eds.), *Vocal fold physiology conference* (pp. 21–28). San Diego: Singular Publishing Group.

Gray, S.D., Hirano, M., & Sato, K. (1993). Molecular and cellular structure of vocal fold tissue. In I.R. Titze (Ed.), *Vocal fold physiology: Frontiers in Basic Science* (pp. 1–33). San Diego: Singular Publishing Group, Inc.

Gray, S.D., Pignatari, S.N., & Harding, P. (1994). Morphologic ultrastructure of anchoring fibers in normal vocal fold basement membrane zone. *Journal of Voice, 8,* 48–52.

Gray, S., & Titze, I.R. (1988). Histologic investigation of hyperphonated canine vocal cords. *Annals of Otology, Rhinology, and Laryngology, 97,* 381–388.

Hartman, D.E., & Aronson, A.E. (1981). Clinical investigations of intermittent breathy dysphonia. *Journal of Speech and Hearing Disorders, 46,* 428–432.

Holbrook, A., Rolnick, M.I., & Bailey, C.W. (1974). Treatment of vocal abuse disorders using a vocal intensity controller. *Journal of Speech and Hearing Disorders, 39,* 298–303.

Holinger, P.H., & Johnston, K.C. (1960). Contact ulcer of the larynx. *Journal of the American Medical Association, 172,* 511–555.

Izdebski, K., Dedo, H.H., & Boles, L. (1984). Spastic dysphonia: A patient profile of 200 cases. *American Journal of Otolaryngology, 5,* 7–14.

Jacobson, E. (1968). *Progressive relaxation (2nd ed.).* Chicago: University of Chicago Press.

Jacobson, B.H., & Bush, C. (1996). *Voice Handicap Index and clinicians' perceptual judgments: A comparison.* Paper presented at the ASHA Convention, Seattle, Washington, November, 1996.

Jacobson, B.H. Johnson, A., Grywalski, C., Silbergleit, A., Jacobson, G., Benninger, M.S., & Newman, C.W. (in press). The Voice Handicap Index (VHI): Development and Validation. *American Journal of Speech-Language Pathology.*

Johnson, J.A., & Pring, T.R. (1990). Speech therapy and Parkinson's disease: A review and further data. *British Journal of Disorders of Communication, 25,* 183–194.

Kay, N.J. (1982). Vocal nodules in children-aetiology and management. *Journal of Laryngology and Otology, 96,* 731–736.

King, J.B., Ramig, L.O., Lemke, J., & Horii, Y. (1994). Parkinson's disease: Longitudinal variability in acoustic parameters of phonation. *Journal of Medical Speech-Language Pathology, 2,* 29–42.

Kotby, M.N., El-Sady, S.R., Basiouny, S.E., Abou-Rass, Y.A., & Hegazi, M.A. (1991). Efficacy of the Accent Method of voice therapy. *Journal of Voice, 5,* 316–320.

Kotby, M.N., Shiromoto, O., & Hirano, M. (1993). The Accent Method of voice therapy: Effect of accentuations on Fo, SPL, and airflow. *Journal of Voice, 7,* 319–325.

Koufman, J.A., & Blalock, P.D. (1989). Is voice rest never indicated? *Journal of Voice, 3,* 87–91.

Lancer, J.M., Syder, D., & LeBoutillier, A. (1988). The outcome of different management patterns for vocal cord nodules. *Journal of Laryngology and Otology, 102,* 423–427.

Lieberman, P. (1961). Perturbations in vocal pitch. *Journal of the Acoustical Society of America, 33,* 597–603.

Llewellyn-Thomas, H.A., Sutherland, H.J., Ciampi, A., Etezad-Amoli, J., Boyd, N.F., & Till, J.E. (1984a). The assessment of values in laryngeal cancer: Reliability of measurement methods. *Journal of Chronic Diseases, 37,* 283–291.

Llewellyn-Thomas, H.A., Sutherland, H.J., Hogg, S.A. Ciampi, A., Harwood, A.R., Keane, T.J., Till, J.E., & Boyd, N.F. (1984b). Linear analogue self-assessment of voice quality in laryngeal cancer. *Journal of Chronic Diseases, 37,* 917–924.

Lodge, J.M., & Yarnall, G.D. (1981). A case study in vocal volume reduction. *Journal of Speech and Hearing Disorders, 46,* 317–319.

Lowenthal, G. (1958). The treatment of polypoid laryngitis. *Laryngoscope, LSVIII,* 1095–1104.

Luchsinger, R., & Pfister, K. (1959). Ergebnisse von Kehlkopfaufnahmen mit einer zeitdehner Apparatur. *Bulletin Der Schweizerrischen Der Medizinischen, 15,* 164–177.

MacIntyre, J. (1981). Therapy for a straightforward case of mechanical dysphonia. *Bulletin of the College of Speech Therapists, 351,* 2–4.

McReynolds, L. (1990). Historical perspective of treatment efficacy research. In L.B. Olswang, C.K. Thompson, S.F. Warren, & N.J. Minghetti (Eds.), *Treatment efficacy research in communication disorders* (pp. 5–14). Rockville, MD: American Speech-Language-Hearing Foundation.

Moore, G.P. (1982a). Theory and research of the Moore approach. In V.L. Lawrence (Ed.), *Transcripts of the Eleventh Symposium: Care of the Professional Voice*, pp. 25–28. New York: The Voice Foundation.

Moore, G.P. (1982b). Methods of Moore approach to voice therapy. In V.L. Lawrence (Ed.), *Transcripts of the Eleventh Symposium: Care of the Professional Voice*, pp. 89–96. New York: The Voice Foundation.

Moore, G.P., & Thompson, C. (1965). Comments on the physiology of hoarseness. *Archives of Otology, Rhinology, and Laryngology, 81*, 97–102.

Moran, M.J., & Pentz, A.L. (1987). Otolaryngologists' opinions of voice therapy for vocal nodules in children. *Language, Speech, and Hearing Services in Schools, 18*, 172–178.

Murry, T., & Woodson, G.E. (1995). Combined-modality treatment of adductor spasmodic dysphonia with botulinum toxin and voice therapy. *Journal of Voice, 9*, 460–465.

Nilson, H., & Schneiderman, C.R. (1983). Classroom program for the prevention of vocal abuse and hoarseness in elementary school children. *Language, Speech, and Hearing Services in Schools, 14*, 121–127.

Olswang, L. (1990). Treatment efficacy: The breadth of research. In L.B. Olswang, C.K. Thompson, S.F. Warren, N.J. Minghetti (Eds.), *Treatment efficacy research in communication disorders* (pp. 99–103). Rockville, MD: American Speech-Language-Hearing Foundation.

Pahn, V.J. (1966). Zur Entwicklung und Behandlung funktioneller Singstimmerkrankungen. *Folia Phoniatrica, 18*, 117–130.

Peacher, G. (1947). Contact ulcer of the larynx Part IV. A clinical study of vocal re-education. *Journal of Speech and Hearing Disorders, 12*, 179–190.

Peacher, G.M. (1961). Vocal therapy for contact ulcer of the larynx. A follow-up of 70 patients. *Laryngoscope, 71*, 37–47.

Peacher, G., & Holinger, P. (1947). Contact ulcer of the Larynx II. The role of vocal reeducation. *Archives of Otolaryngology, 46*, 617–623.

Peterson, K.L., Verdolini-Marston, K., Barkmeier, J., & Hoffman, H. (1994). Comparison of aerodynamic and electroglottographic parameters in evaluating clinically relevant voicing patterns. *Annals of Otology, Rhinology, and Laryngology, 103*, 335–346.

Prosek, R.A., Montgomery, A.A., Walden, B.E., & Schwartz, D.M. (1978). EMG biofeedback in the treatment of hyperfunctional voice disorders. *Journal of Speech and Hearing Disorders, 43*, 282–294.

Ramig, L., Countryman, S., O'Brien, C., Hoehn, M., & Thompson, L. (1996). Intensive speech treatment for patients with Parkinson disease: Short and long-term comparison of two techniques. *Neurology, 47*, 1496–1504.

Ramig, L.O. Countryman, S., Thompson, L.L., & Horii, Y. (1995). Comparison of two forms of intensive speech treatment for Parkinson disease. *Journal of Speech and Hearing Research, 38*, 1232–1251.

Ramig, L.O., & Dromey, C. (1996). Aerodynamic mechanisms underlying treatment-related changes in vocal intensity in patients with Parkinson disease. *Journal of Speech and Hearing Research, 39*, 798–807.

Ramig, L.O., Pawlas, A., & Countryman, S. (1995). The Lee Silverman Voice Treatment. *A practical guide to treating the voice and speech disorders in Parkinson Disease.* Iowa City, IA: National Center for Voice and Speech, University of Iowa.

Ranford, H.J. (1982). Casebook: 'Larynx-NAD'? *Bulletin of the College of Speech Therapists, 359*, 5. (Erratum: *361, 3*).

Robertson, S.J., & Thomson, F. (1984). Speech therapy in Parkinson's disease: A study of the efficacy and long term effects of intensive treatment. *British Journal of Disorders of Communication, 19*, 213–224.

Rosen, A., & Proctor, E. (1981). Distinctions between treatment outcome and their implications for treatment evaluation. *Journal of Consulting and Clinical Psychology, 49*, 418–425.

Roy, N., & Leeper, H.A. (1993). Effects of the manual laryngeal musculoskeletal tension reduction technique as a treatment for functional voice disorders: Perceptual and acoustic measures. *Journal of Voice, 7,* 242–249.

Sabol, J.W., Lee, L., & Stemple, J.C. (1995). The value of vocal function exercises in the practice regimen of singers. *Journal of Voice, 9,* 27–36.

Salmon, D.P., & Butters, N. (1995). Neurobiology of skill and habit learning. *Current Opinion in Neurobiology, 5,* 184–190.

Schmidt, C.P., & Andrews, M.L. (1993). Consistency in clinicians' and clients' behavior in voice therapy: An exploratory study. *Journal of Voice, 7,* 354–358.

Scott, S., & Caird, F.L. (1983). Speech therapy for Parkinson's disease. *Journal of Neurology, Neurosurgery, and Psychiatry, 46,* 140–144.

Senturia, B.H., & Wilson, F.B. (1968). Otorhinologic findings in children with voice deviations. *Annals of Otology, Rhinology, and Laryngology, 77,* 1027–1042.

Shearer, W.M. (1972). Diagnosis and treatment of voice disorders in school children. *Journal of Speech and Hearing Disorders, 37,* 215–221.

Smith, S. (1961). On artificial voice production. *Proc. 4th Int. Congr. Phon.,* pp. 96–110. Helsinki.

Smith, M.E., Ramig, L.O., Dromey, C., Perez, K., & Samandari, R. (1995). Intensive voice treatment in Parkinson disease: Laryngostroboscopic findings. *Journal of Voice, 9,* 453–459.

Smith, S., & Thyme, K. (1976). Statistic research on changes in speech due to pedagogic treatment (the Accent Method). *Folia Phoniatrica, 28,* 98–103.

Smith, E., Verdolini, K., et al. (1996). Effect of voice disorders on quality of life. *Journal of Medical Speech-Language Pathology, 4,* 223–244.

Sonesson, B. (1960). On the anatomy and vibratory movements of the human vocal folds. *Acta Otolaryngologica, Supplement 156,* 1–80.

Stemple, J.C., Lee, L., D'Amico, B., & Pickup, B. (1994). Efficacy of vocal function exercises as a method of improving voice production. *Journal of Voice, 8,* 271–278.

Stemple, J.C., Weiler, E., Whitehead, W., & Komray, R. (1980). Electromyographic biofeedback training with patients exhibiting a hyperfunctional voice disorder. *Laryngoscope, 90,* 471–476.

Stone, R.E. (1982a). Bases of an intervention approach in recalcitrant functional dysphonias. In V.L. Lawrence (Ed.), *Transcripts of the Eleventh Symposium: Care of the Professional Voice,* pp. 29–39. New York: The Voice Foundation.

Stone, R.E. (1982b). Considerations in assessing functional dysphonia and demonstration of intervention procedures. In V.L. Lawrence (Ed.), *Transcripts of the Eleventh Symposium: Care of the Professional Voice,* pp. 97–100. New York: The Voice Foundation.

Stone, R.E. (1983). Application of intervention in functional dysphonia. In V.L. Lawrence (Ed.), *Transcripts of the Twelfth Symposium: Care of the Professional Voice,* pp. 175–183. New York: The Voice Foundation.

Strandberg, T.E., Griffith, J., & Hollowell, M.W. (1971). A case study of psychogenic hoarseness. *Journal of Speech and Hearing Disorders, 36,* 281–286.

Sutherland, H.J., Llewellyn-Thomas, H., Hogg, S.A., Keane, T.J., Harwood, A.R., Till, J.E., Boyd, N.F. (1984). Do patients and physicians agree on the assessment of voice quality in laryngeal cancer? *Journal of Otolaryngology, 13,* 325–330.

Tarneaud, J. (1958). The fundamental principles of vocal cultivation and therapeutics of the voice. *Logos, I,* 7–10.

Timcke, R., von Leden, H., & Moore, G.P. (1958). Laryngeal vibrations: Measurements of the glottic wave. Part I: The normal vibratory cycle. *Archives of Otology, Rhinology, and Laryngology, 68,* 1–19.

Titze, I.R. (1981). Heat generation in the vocal folds and its possible effect on vocal endurance. In V.L. Lawrence (Ed.), *Transcripts of the Tenth Symposium: Care of the Professional Voice. Part I: Instrumentation in Voice Research* (pp. 52–65). New York: The Voice Foundation.

Titze, I.R. (1988). The physics of small-amplitude oscillation of the vocal folds. *Journal of the Acoustical Society of America, 83,* 1536–1552.

Toohill, R.J. (1975). The psychosomatic aspects of children with vocal nodules. *Archives of Oto-laryngology, 101,* 591–595.

Verdolini, K. (in press). Principles of skill acquisition applied to voice training. In M. Hampton & B. Acker (Eds.), *The vocal vision.*

Verdolini, K., Druker, D.G., Palmer, P.M., & Samawi, H. (in press). Laryngeal adduction in resonant voice. *Journal of Voice.*

Verdolini, K., & Titze, I.R. (1995). The application of laboratory formulas to clinical voice management. *American Journal of Speech-Language Pathology, 4,* 62–69.

Verdolini-Marston, K., & Balota, D.A. (1994). The role of elaborative and perceptual integrative processes in perceptual-motor performance. *Journal of Experimental Psychology: Learning, Memory, and Cognition, 20,* 739–749.

Verdolini-Marston, K., Burke, M.K., Lessac, A., Glaze, L., & Caldwell, E. (1995). Preliminary study of two methods of treatment for laryngeal nodules. *Journal of Voice, 9,* 74–85.

Verdolini-Marston, K., Sandage, M., & Titze, I.R. (1994). Effect of hydration treatments on laryngeal nodules and polyps and related voice measures. *Journal of Voice, 8,* 30–47.

von Leden, H., Moore, P., & Timcke, R. (1960). Laryngeal vibrations: Measurements of the glottic wave. Part III: The pathological larynx. *Archives of Otology, Rhinology, and Laryngology, 71,* 16–35.

White, E., & Verdolini, K. (1995). *Frequency of voice problems in gospel versus non-gospel choral singers.* Paper presented at the Twenty-Fourth Annual Symposium: Care of the Professional Voice, June 5–10, 1995, Philadelphia, PA.

Wilson, D.K. (1962). Voice reeducation of adolescents with vocal nodules. *Archives of Otolaryngology, LXXVI,* 19–26.

Wolski, W., & Wiley, J. (1965). Functional aphonia in a fourteen-year-old boy: A case report. *Journal of Speech and Hearing Disorders, 30,* 71–75.

Wright, H.N., & Colton, R.H. (1972). *Some parameters of autophonic level.* Paper presented at the American Speech and Hearing Association Convention, November, 1972.

Wyatt, G.L. (1941). Voice disorders and personality conflicts. *Mental Hygiene, XXV,* 237–250.

Yamaguchi, H., Yotsukura, Y., Sata, H., Watanabe, Y., Hirose, H., Sobayashi, & Bless, D.M. (1993). Pushing exercise program to correct glottal incompetence. *Journal of Voice, 7,* 250–256.

Zwitman, D.H. (1979). Bilateral cord dysfunctions: Abductor type spastic dysphonia. *Journal of Speech and Hearing Disorders, 44,* 373–378.

Zwitman, D.H., & Calcaterra, T.C. (1973). The "silent cough" method for vocal hyperfunction. *Journal of Speech and Hearing Disorders, 38,* 119–125.

CHAPTER 17

Outcomes Measurement Issues in Fluency Disorders

GORDON W. BLOOD
AND EDWARD G. CONTURE

INTRODUCTION

The purpose of this chapter is to broadly review literature pertaining to treatment efficacy for stuttering and to describe a conceptual model to help clinicians as well as
researchers evaluate, design, and conduct treatment outcomes research that addresses
all, not merely behavioral, aspects of stuttering influenced by treatment. To begin, it
seems safe to say that every person who stutters poses an interesting challenge in planning and treatment for speech-language pathologists (SLPs). As clients become more
fluent, clinicians address the stability and longevity of the current treatment changes,
long-term planning, dismissal criterion, and optimization of environmental factors
which may affect the fluency disorder. Many variables are considered by SLPs when
determining progress following treatment. For instance, clinicians examine overt and
covert measures of changes in the frequency of instances of stuttering, avoidance, and
reaction to speaking situations, the possibility of relapse, amount and need of continued and sustained effort to maintain the changes, associated mannerisms that accompany stuttering (e.g., facial grimaces). Clinicians also examine client's adjustment to
their "new" role as a fluent speaker, listener's adjustments to the "new" speaker, the
cyclical nature of stuttering, negative attitudes and feelings as a speaker, and support
groups (Andrews, 1984; Boberg, 1981; Manning, 1991, 1996). As SLPs' planning has
become less focused on behavioral change in clinic treatment rooms and more
focused on the process of integrating the individual who stutters into the classroom,
work force, and community (Blood, 1995b; Manning, 1996; Watson, 1995), there has
developed an increased need for appropriate outcome measures. These comprehensive
treatment programs view communication as an integral part of socialization. As such,
the goals of rehabilitation include changes in speech behavior, attitudes, and feelings.
The ongoing examination of treatment planning includes four critical concepts: (1)
treatment processes, (2) outcomes, (3) efficacy, and (4) effectiveness.

387

Table 17–1. Summary of Desirable Goals in the Management of Fluency Disorders from the Guidelines for Practice in Stuttering Treatment

Management Goal 1
Reduce the frequency with which stuttering behaviors occur without increasing the use of other behaviors that are not a part of normal speech production.

Management Goal 2
Reduce the severity, duration, and abnormality of stuttering behaviors until they are or resemble normal speech discontinuities.

Management Goal 3
Reduce the use of defensive behaviors.

Management Goal 4
Remove or reduce processes serving to create, exacerbate, or maintain stuttering behaviors.

Management Goal 5
Help the person who stutters make treatment (e.g., adaptive) decisions about how to handle speech and social situations in everyday living.

Management Goal 6
Increase the frequency of social activity and speaking.

Management Goal 7
Reduce attitudes, beliefs, and thought processes that interfere with fluent speech production or that hinder the achievement of other treatment goals.

Management Goal 8
Reduce emotional reactions to specific stimuli when these have a negative impact on stuttering behavior or on attempts to modify stuttering behavior.

Management Goal 9
Where necessary, seek helpful combinations and sequences of treatments, including referral, for problems other than stuttering that may accompany the fluency disorder, such as cluttering, learning disability, language/phonological disorder, voice disorder, psychoemotional disturbance.

Management Goal 10
Provide information and guidance to clients, families, and other significant persons about the nature of stuttering, normal fluency and disfluency, and the course of treatment and prognosis for recovery.

Source: Starkweather et al., 1995.

DEFINITIONS

The purpose of this section is to set the context for the remainder of the chapter. These definitions will enhance the understanding of measurement issues relevant to stuttering.

1. *Process* research examines "what happens" during the treatment sessions (Blood, 1993). In the area of stuttering, process variables that contribute to the dynamic exchanges occurring in treatment include: (a) *client behaviors* (e.g., client motivation levels for therapy, attribution for the disorder, expectations for therapy, levels of suggestibility, locus of control, social integration, gender, intelligence, trait as well as state anxiety levels, educational status, social class, and previous experience in stuttering therapy), (b) *clinician behaviors* (e.g., clinician's age,

Table 17–2. Summary of Desirable Goals in the Transfer and Maintenance of Acquired Fluency Behaviors from the Guidelines for Practice in Stuttering Treatment

Transfer and Maintenance Goal 1
Generalization of the behavioral changes learned in the treatment setting to speech situations in the client's everyday life.

Transfer and Maintenance Goal 2
A sense of committed interest and self-reliance on the part of clients in managing their own speech behavior, balanced against an awareness of the need for occasional help (professional or otherwise) as needed.

Transfer and Maintenance Goal 3
Ability on the client's part at recognizing the earliest signs of returning emotional reactions and/or stuttering behaviors and knowledge and skill for dealing with these occurrences.

Transfer and Maintenance Goal 4
In parents, knowledge and skills needed to facilitate their child's further development of fluency.

Source: Starkweather et al., 1995.

experience, empathy, warmth, expectations, ability to convey the rationale for the therapy, gender, amount and type of self-disclosure, locus of control, level of trust, credibility, and knowledge of treatment), and (c) *client-clinician* interactions and relationships (e.g., client-clinician shared goals, expectations, preferred treatment types, locus of control, beliefs about stuttering).

2. *Outcomes* research explores the quantifiable events that occur as a result of the structure and processes of treatment. This usually includes both immediate and long-term changes. Outcome measures in stuttering examine changes during and immediately after "formal treatment," and then 3, 6, 12, or more months after formal treatment has been concluded. Increasingly, issues pertaining to relapse and maintenance are the focus of treatment outcome measurements for stuttering, with maintenance of speech behavior changes in persons who stutter continuing to be an important variable in determining successful intervention (Blood, 1995 a, b; Boberg, 1981, 1983, 1986; Boberg, Howie, & Woods, 1979; Craig & Calvert, 1991; Guitar & Bass, 1978; Ingham, 1984; Kuhr & Rustin, 1985; Silverman, 1981).

3. The concept of *efficacy* in the clinical treatment area essentially attempts to answer the question "Does treatment work?" It addresses a specific level of benefit that can be expected when the treatment is applied under *ideal* circumstances (Benjamin, 1995). In the area of stuttering, Bloodstein (1995) described a set of 12 "rules" that must be satisfied for a treatment to be efficacious. These rules include: (a) adequate sample size; (b) objective and reliable measures of speech behaviors; (c) repeated evaluations and adequate sample of speech; (d) stability of changes demonstrated through long-term follow-up; use of control groups; (e) speech naturalness and spontaneity; (f) freedom by clients from the necessity of monitoring their speech; (g) removal of fears, anticipations, and self-concepts of persons who stutter; (h) realistic assessment of the success of the program, including dropouts from the study protocol; (i) similar results in the hands of any qualified clinician; and (j) the treatment should endure the test of "newness" and "novelty." Conture and Wolk (1990) used these criteria for their discussion

on treatment efficacy and stated that "few if any presently used treatment methods for stuttering could pass all of these (Bloodstein's) tests, but once again we are discussing the ideal" (p. 202). Indeed, the concept of *ideal* is what distinguishes *efficacy* from *effectiveness*.

4. Finally the concept of *effectiveness* deals with the level of benefit that can be expected from treatment services offered under *typical* circumstances by *typical* practitioners for *typical* patients (Benjamin, 1995). Bloodstein (1995) reviewed the effectiveness of over 160 studies of children and adults who stutter and concluded that (a) stuttering is a very difficult disorder to treat, especially in adults, and (b) "at face value one would be inclined to infer that substantial improvement, as defined in these studies, typically occurs as a result of almost *any kind of therapy* in about 60 to 80% of cases" (p. 438). Recently, Blood (1995a) empirically tested a behavioral-cognitive treatment approach specifically for use with adolescents who stutter using a single-subject research design. Examining the role of relapse management with adolescents who stutter, Blood suggested that considerations for designing effective interventions with adolescents who stutter should include issues about peer pressure, parental involvement, individual autonomy and control, and perceived as well as anticipated stressors. Blood (1995b) also reported on the effectiveness of a behavioral-cognitive program for adults who stutter. The program combined a commercially available computer-assisted biofeedback program for the reduction of stuttering and a relapse management program for counseling and attitude change. Four adults participated in a multiple baseline across subjects single-subject design. Results showed that all subjects maintained their posttreatment fluency levels, as well as their positive changes in feelings and attitudes at 6- and 12-month follow-up assessments.

Other single-subject client-centered treatment studies examining behaviors, feelings, and attitudes (using multiple measures) across different time segments, with follow-up periods evaluating social validation measures at a minimum of one year after formal treatment, have also been reported recently (Dembrowski & Watson, 1991; Hillis, 1993). These studies of effectiveness represent considerable advances from early anecdotal reports in clinician-centered treatments in the earlier part of this century that simply stated that "clients had improved their speech." This brief review demonstrates that the concepts of processes, outcomes, efficacy, and effectiveness are not new in the stuttering literature. In fact, one major problem in the area of stuttering is the lack of agreement not only on the definition and etiology of stuttering, but also a strategy for organizing and selecting outcome measures.

CHALLENGES WITH OUTCOME MEASUREMENTS IN STUTTERING

Outcome measurements may be effected by numerous variables, including the researchers' or practitioners' theoretical perspectives and qualifications, the reliability of the measures selected, format of treatment, duration of the treatment, percent of clients lost at follow-up, client characteristics, and the goals of the principal treatment protocols. Part of the difficulty with outcomes measurement in stuttering is the confusion caused by the researchers and practitioners' orientation to, definitions, and beliefs about the disorder. J. C. Ingham (1993) in reviewing behavior modification and stuttering suggested that researchers and practitioners needed to develop reliable listener-derived measures of stuttering. She emphasized the need to be able to accurately identify, observe, reinforce and/or punish stuttering behavior. Unfortunately her review produced 17 studies utilizing perceptual threshold definitions of stuttering and 22 studies using different behavioral definitions of stuttering. Thus, it becomes very difficult to evaluate treatment outcomes, efficacy, and effectiveness when the basic definition of stuttering is not agreed upon. Ingham also states that an adequately comprehensive behavioral definition would be exceedingly cumbersome, if not impossible, to achieve.

A brief review of different theoretical perspectives demonstrates one of the challenges in establishing and selecting outcome measures in stuttering. According to Silverman (1996) most persons who stutter consult an SLP because they either want to reduce the severity of their stuttering or to "cure" it. Treatment outcomes for these individuals would include achieving optimal performance levels in the reduction and/or absence of stuttering behaviors. Cooper (1987, 1993) has suggested that stuttering is a clinical syndrome characterized by abnormal and persistent disfluencies in speech accompanied by fluency-related affective and cognitive responses. Stuttering syndromes can be described as one of three types: developmental, remediable, and chronic. These syndromes appear to be related to the age of the clients and the type of professional assistance required from the SLP. *Developmental stuttering* is typically experienced in preschool children. Without significant professional help, but with appropriate parental change and assistance, this type of stuttering often dissipates by the age of seven. *Remediable stuttering* describes the speech disfluencies observed in children after seven years of age. With parental support and professional assistance, these children usually learn to apply techniques for fluency control and do not typically consider themselves "as people who stutter" during adulthood. Finally, *chronic stuttering* is observed in adolescents and adults, and the demand of maintaining fluency is a lifelong challenge. With professional support, these individuals learn techniques that help them monitor their fluency and adapt their feelings and beliefs. These individuals define themselves as "people who stutter" (Cooper & Cooper, 1995). The chronicity of the disorder in persons who stutter, as defined by Cooper, would require that outcome measurements include reductions or changes in stuttering behaviors as well as coping strategies to deal with a lifelong challenge of stuttering. Bloodstein (1995) and others view stuttering at least in part as a learned behavior that is precipitated by the "anticipation and fear" of the stuttering event. Accordingly, stuttering is thought to be maintained by both the anticipation of the event and the struggle to avoid it. Outcome measurements for proponents of this orientation to stuttering would not only include reductions in the stuttering behaviors, but also attitude and cognitive changes dealing with avoidance, fear, and struggle.

Ingham (1984) reviewed the relevant research and concluded that stuttering acts like an operant behavior most of the time. Ingham and Costello (1985) developed a model to assist researchers and practitioners identify and measure treatment outcomes. Their approach included stuttering counts, speech rate and quality measures, within- and beyond-clinic measures, multiple baseline, interactive designs, and covert assessment during follow-up treatment phases. The Ingham and Costello model evaluated stuttering from a very behavioral, operant perspective. Subsequently, Ingham (1993a), when assessing why their model did not appear to be widely embraced by researchers and practitioners in fluency disorders, critiqued the Ingham and Costello model by stating "that these procedures were not shining examples of user-friendliness (p. 137)." Ingham pointed out that these outcome measures based on strict behavioral speech targets may be too difficult to apply in certain clinical settings. He further mentioned that some of the outcome models suggested "in operation, may almost preempt therapy!" The lack of agreement on a set of outcome criteria implies that researchers and practitioners will probably only adopt measures consistent with their own beliefs and orientation to stuttering. Ingham (1993) reviewed the current status of stuttering and behavior modification in "modern times" and concluded that programs incorporating prolonged speech treatment packages resulted in immediate and long-term reductions in the frequency of stuttering. She also included drop-out rates, maintenance of reduced stuttering during follow-up periods, relapse, and speech naturalness as part of her outcome measures.

Some Relationships between Outcome Measures and Orientation to Problem

Starkweather and his colleagues (1990) suggested that the demands placed on children who stutter may exceed their motoric, cognitive, and linguistic capacities, resulting in disfluent speech. Presumably, therefore, their outcome measurements would include evaluation of these multiple capacities. Webster's research (1993) suggested that stuttering was the result of disturbances in the supplementary motor area. Logan (1991) reported that stuttering results from behavioral reactions to emotional responses, both of which arise from common cortical and subcortical sites of the central nervous system. It seems safe to say, therefore, that these authors would utilize different outcome measures than "pure" behavioralists. Conture (1990) has suggested that learned helplessness and loss of control may significantly contribute to the disability of stuttering. Conture and Wolk (1990) in their discussion on treatment effectiveness in stuttering included a measurement hierarchy of speech behavior and attitudes. They concluded that although attitudes and feelings were more difficult to measure and quantify, they were an integral component of many treatment models. According to Conture and Wolk, constructs like locus of control and learned helplessness needed to be empirically examined and included as outcome measures for the long-term success of stuttering treatments. Similarly, Perkins, Kent, and Curlee (1991) defined stuttering as "a disruption of speech experienced by the speaker as loss of control" (p. 734). These authors would also include some type of attitude and locus of control measures as outcome variables. Recently, Stewart (1996) reported on the link between the acquisition and maintenance of a fluency-enhancing speech technique and personal construct psychology. This perspective suggests that disfluencies will decrease as the relevance of the role of fluent speaker increases. Building on previous work (Evesham & Fransella, 1985; Fransella, 1987), Stewart reported on two individuals who stuttered using a brief longitudinal design (2 years). It is not surprising that her outcome measurements included the following statements, "At the end of the course (of treatment) he construed himself as a positive fluent speaker with good communication skills and an ability to listen to others" (p. 40). This outcome statement is quite different from statements made by her colleagues with operant or behavioral perspectives in stuttering. The call for a battery or systematic protocol to assess effectiveness (Bloodstein, 1995; Conture & Wolk, 1990; Ingham & Costello, 1985) continues to go largely unheeded by researchers and practitioners alike. Blood (1993) recommended a systematic protocol be developed to assess treatment effectiveness in adults who stutter. He provided a detailed model based on improvement criteria, qualitative and quantitative measurements, and client, clinician, and treatment variables.

This brief review of contrasting orientations to stuttering and differing perspectives regarding the definition and etiology of stuttering is extremely relevant to the discussion of outcomes research. Is stuttering a syndrome, a learned behavior, a multifactorial problem, inherited, spasms of laryngeal muscles, deficits in auditory temporal processing or combinations of two or more of the above? In essence, we are suggesting that orientation and perspective oftentimes determine expected outcomes. Treatment for persons who stutter should be dedicated to the enhancement of communicative performance. Communicative performance may be facilitated by changes in the speaker's motor behavior, attitudes, and feelings (Blood, 1993, 1995 a, b, c).

CURRENT STATUS OF OUTCOMES RESEARCH

Numerous reviews of studies examining treatment outcomes can be found for adults and children who stutter (Blood, 1993; Bloodstein, 1995; Conture, 1990, 1996; Conture & Guitar, 1993; Conture & Wolk, 1990; Curlee, 1993; Ingham, 1984, 1985, 1993 a, b; Ingham & Costello, 1985, 1987; Perkins, 1981; Prins, 1984, 1993; Sheehan, 1984, St. Louis & Westbrook, 1987, Van Riper, 1973).

Studies have been conducted attempting to sort out the important variables that contribute to overall treatment effectiveness. For example, Andrews, Guitar, and Howie (1980) completed a meta-analysis of the effects of stuttering treatment on the data of 756 persons who stuttered. From their review of 42 studies, results revealed that prolonged speech, gentle onset, rhythm, airflow, attitude change, and desensitization were the six most common principal treatment formats. The greatest treatment effectiveness (for immediate and long-term results) was reported using prolonged speech and gentle onset techniques. This study suggested that the most effective treatment programs were those that utilized these techniques. However, Sheehan (1984) criticized these findings and the meta-analyses performed. He suggested that the strong positive results for the prolonged speech and gentle onset studies may have resulted from the evaluation measures used by the researchers because their criteria for effectiveness was strongly based on frequency and rate measures. According to Sheehan, other studies and treatment models utilize attitude changes, desensitization, and relaxation as criteria for treatment effectiveness. If these criteria had been entered into the meta-analyses employed by Andrews, Guitar, and Howie, the primary treatment strategies predicting treatment effectiveness would probably differ. For example, Silverman (1996) stated that it was possible to reduce a client's speech disfluencies by modifying his or her attitude toward stuttering, that changes in attitudes would result in a reduced severity of stuttering. He also suggested that techniques reported in the literature included: reduced avoidance of stuttering, increased acceptance and/or acknowledgment of the problem, developing better self-concept as a speaker, anticipation of fluency instead of stuttering, realistic expectations for speech and self, reduced embarrassment, guilt, and shame, and increased sense of ownership and humor. If changes in these attitudes were selected as primary outcome measures, perhaps Silverman's counseling techniques might then surface as the most effective treatment techniques according to Sheehan. Sheehan's (1984) critique highlights the necessity of carefully examining the selection of the outcome criteria. Similarly, Prins (1984), after reviewing six different program outcome studies for adults who stuttered, identified four potential sources of error in outcome measurements: outcome criteria used, sampling, measurement procedures, and experimenter bias.

Howie and Andrews (1984) suggested that the *minimal* requirements for treatment outcome measures for stuttering should include at least three measurements: (a) reliable measures of frequency, (b) measures of speech rate, and (c) measures of the extent of handicap (avoidance of speech and negative self concept). These authors suggested that a formal evaluation of a "social or psychological component" be included as an outcome measure. Indeed, review of treatment studies strongly suggest that social, cognitive, or psychological variables are seldom included in outcome measures. Instead, most practitioners and researchers focus outcome measures on the stuttering or stuttered speech motor event. Most recently, excellent studies have been conducted by Packman, Onslow, and van Doorn (1994) examining unresolved outcome issues associated with prolonged speech treatment programs.

Shift from Behavioral to Cognitive Outcome Measures

A shift in examining only the behavioral components of stuttering occurred in the 1980s. Increasingly, researchers began to focus on cognitive changes during treatment that occurred as a result of assuming personal responsibility and control. At present, a cognitive-behavioral orientation is evident in many current approaches to stuttering treatment. Fransella (1987) discussed personal construct therapy using controlled elaboration and personal change to alter the client's self-perceptions. Researchers and practitioners began to utilize specific tests that could evaluate cognitive and attitudinal constructs. For instance, Webster (1984) discussed the use of the *Perceptions of Stuttering Inventory* (Woolf, 1967) with adults who stuttered as treatment outcome measures of changes in attitudes. Locus of control refers to the individuals' perceptions and generalized expectancies concerning behavior and the reinforcements associated with it (Foon, 1987). Dhariti (1985) administered Rotter's *Internal-External Locus of Control Scale (REF)* to adults who stuttered and found a relationship between internality and therapeutic progress. McDonough and Quesal (1988) devised their own scales for speech locus of control for use with persons who stutter. Craig et al. (1984) administered a 17-item locus of control scale to evaluate the effect of locus of control on relapse following treatment for stuttering—that is, to determine a relationship between outcome (maintenance of reduced stuttering) and locus of control. Craig and Andrews (1985) reported that adults who were treated with a behavioral program and demonstrated *internal* locus of control maintained their speech improvement over long-term assessment. Madison, Budd, and Itzkowitz (1986) reported that pretreatment locus of control scores were related to changes in stuttering for a group of 7- to 16-year-old clients. DeNil and Kroll (1995) examined locus of control and speech fluency in 21 adults who stuttered. They examined the speech changes 2 years after an intensive fluency shaping program. While they reported no relationship between internality and ability to maintain speech fluency, they did report that locus of control scores were predictive of the clients' fluency self-evaluations. They suggested that locus of control contributed to the prediction of long-term outcome as perceived by the client. This study suggests that outcome measurements must consider not only the clinician's assessment, but also the client's perceptions of effective treatment. Outcome measurements should establish hierarchies of importance for both client's and clinician's perceptions. Conture and Guitar (1993) reviewed 10 treatment studies with school-age children who stuttered and suggested that a key variable in examining the efficacy of treatment was the assessment of the manner in which clinicians accurately deliver treatment programs. Other authors have suggested that measures for anxiety, assertiveness, self-efficacy, and depression be included as outcomes (Blood, 1995 a, b; Craig, 1990; Hillis, 1993).

OUTCOMES AND THE WHO MODEL

In 1991, Prins suggested that a useful conceptual framework for evaluating outcome studies in stuttering was the model of health proposed by the World Health Orgainzation (WHO). He recommended that by using the WHO model and definitions, stuttering could be conceptualized on three separate levels: *impairment* (including neurophysiological events that preceded and accompany the stuttering event); *disability* (which included the visible and audible manifestations of stuttering behavior that affect communication), and *handicap* (which would include the reactions from an individual's stuttering and their reactions to their stuttering). His recommendation was an attempt to resolve one of the major stumbling blocks in this area of clinical research for practitioners and researchers—a mutually agreed-upon model and set of definitions.

In 1993, Curlee described a method for assessing the disability of stuttering based on the WHO model. He suggested that because the common goal of current treatments was to reduce or eliminate stuttering behavior in order to communicate effectively, the evaluation of treatment efficacy should be related to measures on the disability level of the WHO model. Curlee provided an outline for assessment of the disability level of stuttering including the following basic measures: frequency of stuttering (in stuttered syllables or percentage of words stuttered), ratings of speech naturalness (Martin, Haroldson, & Triden, 1984), and the administrations of the S-24 scale (Andrews & Cutler, 1974). He also suggests a number of optional measures including: duration of the typical and longest stuttering events; length of stutter-free segments; rate of speech and administration of the standardized severity rating scale. This model was similar to the one described by Ingham and Costello (1985) and others examining and reporting on the changes in the behavioral aspects of stuttering. Curlee also recommended one measure assessing the client's perception of the disorder.

Stuttering involves several different levels of interrelated events. It should be noted, however, that the motor speech (disability) level cannot readily be separated from the general well-being and social interaction level (handicap) or the neurophysiological functioning level (impairment). One strength of the WHO model is that it focuses on individuals' functioning, overall well-being, and complex behaviors and attitudes. In particular, this model reflects a strong commitment to quality-of-life issues which tend to be overlooked or not evaluated in treatment outcome studies solely based on behavioral measures. Quality of life as defined by the WHO is "a state of complete physical, mental, and social well-being and not merely the absence of disease or infirmity." This definition deals with the individual's overall satisfaction with life, and with one's general sense of personal well-being. Quality of life is not really separate from physical functioning, psychological status, social interactions, employment, or economic status. All of these components interact. Outcome measures must be broad enough to answer questions about treatments at a number of different levels. The problem with the WHO classification model for the disorder of stuttering is that it does not clearly show or emphasize the *interactions* among the different levels of the problem (i.e., impairment, disability, handicap).

SUGGESTIONS AND MODELS FOR OUTCOMES RESEARCH IN STUTTERING

In view of the fact that definitions of stuttering may not be "formally" agreed upon because of considerable variability observed in persons who stutter, a starting point for agreement may be the *Guidelines for Practice in Stuttering Treatment* developed by the Special Interest Division in Fluency and Fluency Disorders of the American Speech-Language-Hearing Association (Starkweather, St. Louis, Blood, Peters, Westbrook, Gregory, Cooper, & Healey, 1995). The Guidelines do not take a position on stuttering theory or advocate a specific philosophy of treatment. They provide a set of 10 desirable goals in the management of fluency disorders and 4 desirable goals in the transfer and maintenance of acquired fluency behaviors and the procedures that are used to achieve them. These desirable goals are presented in Tables 17–1 and 17–2. It is suggested that outcome measurements be developed for each of these goals. For example, *Management Goal 1* is to reduce the frequency with which stuttering behaviors occur without increasing the use of other behaviors that are not a part of normal speech production. Many of the outcome measures reported by Costello and Ingham (1984), Howie and Andrews (1984), Prins (1991), and Packman, Onslow, and van Doorn (1994) could be included. These might include: frequency of stuttering in stuttered syllables or percentage of words stuttered (Curlee, 1993), ratings of speech naturalness (Martin, Haroldson, & Triden, 1984), stuttering counts, and speech rate (Costello & Ingham, 1984). *Management Goal 7* is to reduce attitudes, beliefs, and thought processes that interfere with fluent speech production or that hinder the achievement of other treatment goals. Outcome measures could include a number of scales for locus of control, assertiveness, and perceptions of stuttering such as: Shumak's (1955) *Stutterer's Self-Ratings of Reactions to Speech Situations,* Woolf's (1967) *Perceptions of Stuttering Inventory,* Spielberger, Gorsuch, and Lushen's (1970) *State-Trait Anxiety Scale,* Erickson's (1969) *S-scale,* Craig, Franklin and Andrews's (1984) *Locus of Control of Behavior,* Silverman's (1980) *Stuttering Problem Profile,* Rathus's (1973) *Assertiveness Scale,* Orstein and Manning's (1985) *Self-Efficacy Scale for Adult Stutterers,* Brutten and Dunham's (1989) *Communication Attitude Test,* and DeNil and Brutten's (1991) *Child's Attitude Test (Revised),* among others. Researchers and practitioners could examine the remaining treatment and transfer goals and recommend a series of instruments that would evaluate each of these goals.

Expansion of WHO Model through Wilson and Cleary (1995) Model

Another recommendation for outcomes measurement is to expand on the excellent preliminary work already conducted in this area. Building on Prins' (1990) and Curlee's

(1993) work that outcome assessment should be conceptually motivated, we recommend the use of a recently developed model in the health literature. Wilson and Cleary (1995) developed a conceptual model of patient outcomes expanding on the WHO model (see Chapter 1 for schematic). Their model included specific sections of the quality of life and general client perceptions. We believe that the Wilson and Cleary model provides a clearer and more comprehensive model of how different levels or domains of impairment, disability, and handicap *interact*. This model also shows the influence of individual and environmental characteristics. If treatment outcomes research in stuttering is to be continued, then a conceptual model needs to be adopted that researchers and practitioners with differing viewpoints and orientations can more easily relate to and/or use.

The Wilson and Cleary model is presented in Table 17–3 with our adaptations for stuttering treatment and research. Instead of three levels of the WHO model (impairment, disability and handicap), this model includes five domains, and addresses how the characteristics of the environment (social, economic and psychological supports) and the individual (personal values, preferences, personality, motivation) interact among these five domains. Using this model, one would evaluate outcome measures along a continuum of biological, social, and psychological functioning. In essence, we have combined the Wilson and Cleary model with the *Guidelines for Practice in Stuttering Treatment* (Starkweather, St. Louis, Blood, Peters, Westbrook, Gregory, Cooper, & Healey, 1995). The arrows in the model presented in Table 17–3 suggest possible interrelationships among the five domains posited by Wilson and Cleary. For example, biological variables (i.e., genetic markers, voice onset times, laterality preferences) may have an effect on the symptom status or overall quality of life of individuals who stutter. Similarly, functional communicative competence, which could be related to intrapersonal skills, symptom status, and general life satisfaction, could determine the effectiveness of treatment. This model suggests that despite interrelationships among the domains, researchers and clinicians may not (or cannot) evaluate all the domains during a particular treatment or study. However, we do recommend that treatment studies attempt to identify the domains under investigation, with ideal treatment involving all five domains. We have also included as a final adaptation to the Wilson and Cleary model, the management and transfer/maintenance goals from the *Guidelines*. This will allow clinicians and researchers a framework to evaluate their treatments using common goals.

A brief explanation of the expanded model is included. The first thing to notice in Table 17–3 is the three classifications from the WHO model and their relationships to Wilson and Cleary's five domains. The five domains clarify the impairment, disability, and handicap domains of the WHO classification. The first of the five domains is labeled *biological* and *physiological* variables. This first domain could include measures that range from simple tests of laterality and galvanic skin responses to electroencephalographic studies, electromyographic measurements, voice onset and voice initiation time, brainstem auditory responses, and more complex variables, including positron emission tomography testing and hormone levels (e.g., Blood et al. 1994; Ingham et al., 1996). This domain is placed at the beginning stage for the outcome model and most closely parallels the "impairment" level of the WHO model. These biological/physiological factors would play an integral part in the outcome and effectiveness studies, but other domains along the continuum could affect these factors. In the Wil-

Table 17–3. Overview of Possible Relationships among the Three Domains of World Health Organization's Model and the Five Domains of Wilson and Cleary Model, as Well as Goals from the Guidelines for Practice in Stuttering Treatment

WHO MODEL (3 DOMAINS)		
Impairment	*Disability*	*Handicap*

WILSON AND CLEARY MODEL (5 DOMAINS)				
Biological and Physiological Variables $\rightarrow$	*Symptom Status* $\leftarrow\rightarrow$ $\leftarrow\rightarrow$	*Functional Status* $\leftarrow\rightarrow$ $\leftarrow\rightarrow$	*General Perceptions* $\leftarrow\rightarrow$ $\leftarrow\rightarrow$	*Overall Quality of Life* $\leftarrow$

$\updownarrow$ These above five *domains* of the Wilson and Cleary model are affected by: $\updownarrow$

Characteristics of the Individual:	*Characteristics of the Environment:*
Symptom Amplification, Personality, Motivation, Preferences, and Values	Psychological Supports, Economic Supports, Social Supports

Which result in the following *treatment outcome* measurements:

Biological and Physiological Variables:	*Symptom Status:*	*Functional Status:*	*General Perceptions:*	*Overall Quality of Life:*
Traditional and experimental acoustic, physiological, and behavioral measurements of stuttering	Traditional measures of frequency, severity, rate, audible and visible symptoms, concomitant behaviors and attitudes	Functional communication competence measures	Intrapersonal and self-efficacy scales and inventories	Scales and questionnaires dealing with satisfaction with communicative competence, relationships between stuttering and life

Which are related to the *management* goals and the *transfer* and *maintenance* goals:

Biological and Physiological Variables:	*Symptom Status:*	*Functional Status:*	*General Perceptions:*	*Overall Quality of Life:*
Management Goal - 4	Management Goals - 1, 2 & 3	Management Goals - 5 & 6 Transfer and Maintenance Goal 1	Management Goal - 7 & 8 Transfer and Maintenance Goal 2	Management Goals - 9 & 10 Transfer and Maintenance Goal 4

son and Cleary model, this domain may interact with general health perceptions, attributions, or beliefs about stuttering on the other end of the continuum. Inspection of the arrows reveals that the physiological, biological, or predisposition of the individual to stutter influences all other domains. However, this domain by itself would provide only a partial view of the stuttering problem and only some information for outcome measurements for individuals who stutter.

The second domain (*symptom status*) included in this model could help to explain and determine immediate and long-term outcomes. The symptoms domain is defined as "the patient's perception of abnormal physical, emotional, or cognitive states" (Wilson & Cleary, 1995, p. 61). Symptoms could include physical (audible and visible) symptoms of the stuttering problem, something that has been the focus of numerous research and treatment studies. Disfluency analyses, rate of speech, and frequency counts, and severity ratings would be included. However, using this conceptual model, clinicians and researchers would also evaluate feelings and thoughts about stuttering. This might include scales mentioned earlier, including: Spielberger, Gorsuch, and Lushene (1970) *State-Trait Anxiety Scale,* Erickson's (1969) *S-scale,* Silverman's (1980) *Stuttering Problem Profile,* and Orstein and Manning's (1985) *Self-Efficacy Scale for Adult Stutterers.* These measures could help to quantify symptoms status.

The third domain (*functional status*) in this model would include how stuttering is effecting everyday communication. It is relatively easy to measure a client's stuttering behavior (number of words, prolongations, etc.), but we should also evaluate his functional (Conture & Guitar, 1993) communicative competence. Although the symptoms of stuttering may be very severe, this may not result in an inability to communicate. For instance, a client's symptoms may reveal a considerable number of speech disfluencies with highly visible facial contortions and physical concomitants, but her overall communicative functioning may be significantly influenced by such factors as her personality, her view of perceived threat or challenge, her ability to approach her communication problem, her motivation to communicate, and her social support network (membership in self-help groups). Therefore, the effectiveness of the treatment should not be *solely* evaluated in terms of measurable speech behaviors or even the attitude changes, but must include the day-to-day situations and environments which improve her overall communicative functioning. The present model provides a framework for researchers and clinicians to examine the relationships among these measures. There is a need to develop protocols and measures that can be used to determine the relationships among the different domains. For instance, it is possible that a significant contribution to successful long-term outcomes for individuals who stutter may be membership in self-help groups or a supportive social environment. The other important point about this domain is that although functioning is related to the first and second domains (physiology and symptoms) in the Wilson and Cleary model, there are also no definitive studies in stuttering that prove this relationship. There are no data that establish whether persons, for example, with a specific voice onset time, specific amounts of muscle tension, or specific types of laterality *always* stutter.

The fourth domain of this model is *general perceptions.* This domain includes subjective impressions, previous histories of treatments, previous experiences with clinicians, and general ideas about health, disorders, and treatments. This domain has been suggested by a number of authors as extremely important in treatment effectiveness. Prins (1993) in describing the work of Bandura (1969) states that to alter how clients behave, the clinician must alter how the client thinks. Although the mastery of the behavioral skill is the treatment "vehicle," the medium for change is cognitive. These ideas are similar to Williams' (1957) treatment approach. He suggested that individuals' language reflects their thoughts. By changing language, individuals influence their thoughts, which in turn influence how they behave. This refers to the general impressions and beliefs individuals bring to the treatment sessions. These cognitive influences on the changing and maintaining of behavior suggest a major shift from traditional therapy (e.g., models based on stimulus-response conceptualizations). Prins (1993) recommends that intrapersonal factors and a self-efficacy (expectations) model could help explain changes in the behavior of individuals who stutter. This domain includes some of Bandura's key contributions to treatment outcomes: individuals' motivation and *belief* in their ability to accomplish the act, and their *belief* in the outcome of the behavior. Clients' expectations of their own abilities may play a critical role in the outcome of the many, many treatment studies reviewed by Bloodstein (1995). Also included in general health perceptions are the individual's coping skills and strategies. Rosenbaum (1990) developed the concept of "learned resourcefulness" to explain a self-control model that examined what people did when stressful circumstances call for self-control. Meichenbaum (1985) developed Stress Inoculation Training, designed to nurture and develop coping skills for current and future problems. Individuals went from states of "learned helplessness" to effective use of "psychological antibodies." The training of coping skills is not new to stuttering therapy. Many proponents of this type of counseling can be found in the literature on stuttering (Blood, 1995a; Conture, 1990; Cooper, 1983; Daly, 1988; Dell, 1990; Fraser, 1990; Peters & Guitar, 1991; Sheehan, 1975; Van Riper, 1982).

The fifth domain (*overall quality of life*) of this model for stuttering outcomes research examines how happy or satisfied individuals are with their lives at the present time. The disorder of stuttering is too often evaluated in a vacuum, with such evaluation failing to recognize the importance stuttering has on the everyday lives of individuals. The "rules of thirds" could be applied to the overall quality of life and its relationship to stuttering. We can probably assume that for one-third of the individuals who stutter, the disorder has *no negative effect* on their general well-being or satisfaction. For another one-third, stuttering probably has *little to some negative effect* on general well-being or life satisfaction. And for the last one-third of the individuals who stutter, the disorder has an *appreciable negative* impact on their overall quality of life. Individuals who stutter may cross the boundaries of the "thirds" based on expectations, aspirations, social and psychological supports, or other events in their lives.

The adaptation of the Wilson and Cleary model for outcomes measurement in stuttering also examines how the characteristics of the individual and environment affect stuttering, and assesses the role of clients' preferences, clients' values, personality, and motivation. It is possible that clients and clinicians who share similar ideas and expectations about treatment may fare better on long-term outcomes. Clients' attribution for the disorder may also play an important role in their "coping" with the disorder, or reducing and eliminating the stuttering behavior. Likewise, the ability to reduce, talk about, or disclose negative emotions can also mediate the treatment processes. Similarly, one should evaluate the characteristics of the environment (e.g., listener). Psychological and social support from self-help groups may enhance speech fluency skills. Financial and economic constraints and issues may also affect treatment. All of these relationships are explored in the Wilson and Cleary model. This model suggests that one should evaluate stuttering outcome along a complex continuum across five domains. These five domains are all effected by various potential mediating factors. It would seem that researchers and practitioners would profit from considering ways to test each of these domains and their interrelationships.

CONCLUSION

Treatment outcome measurements must include a number of useful dimensions. The clarification of five specific areas of outcome (biological and physiological variables, symptom status, functional status, general perceptions, and overall quality of life) suggested by Wilson and Cleary provide an excellent framework for researchers and practitioners in the area of stuttering. One could conduct a thorough examination of the professional literature to determine which tests, measurements, questionnaires, and scales are reported most frequently and demonstrate the highest level of measurement validity and reliability. Researchers should be encouraged to develop new measures to evaluate each of these outcome domains. Blood (1993) has presented a model for evaluating outcome measurements including a *temporal* dimension (immediate outcome, session outcome and long-term outcome), *respondent* dimension (client evaluations, clinician's ratings, significant others ratings, community/employment/societal ratings), and *disorder* dimension (speaking, feeling, and thinking).

Development of a uniform protocol for measuring treatment outcomes would make it easier for practitioners to clarify what type of change had taken place during treatments. The protocol could also motivate researchers to compare studies from different sites and centers on similar dimensions. These protocols, based on conceptual models like the one presented in this chapter, should be designed to carefully evaluate these various outcome domains. We need to answer questions regarding "clinical significance and real change," specific speech and attitude targets, and direct and indirect effects of treatment. Well-defined studies involving relatively few subjects examining real-life differences need to be completed using similar outcome measurements. In this way, fluency specialists can become more accountable to clients who stutter by identifying clients at greater risk (and hence most in need of treatment) by assisting clients in selecting optimal treatment programs, and by developing a thorough understanding of the impact stuttering has on the *everyday* functioning and quality of life of people who stutter.

REFERENCES

Andrews, G. (1984). The epidemiology of stuttering. In R. Curlee & W. Perkins (Eds.), *Nature and treatment of stuttering* (pp. 1–12). San Diego, CA: College Hill.

Andrews, G., & Cutler, J. (1974). Stuttering therapy: The relation between changes in symptom levels and attitudes. *Journal of Speech and Hearing Disorders, 39,* 309–311.

Andrews, G., Guitar, B., & Howie, P. (1980). Meta-analysis of the effects of stuttering treatment. *Journal of Speech and Hearing Disorders, 45,* 287–307.

Bandura, A. (1969). *Principles of behavior modification.* New York: Holt, Rinehart, and Winston.

Benjamin, K. (1995). *What is an outcome? The role of structure, process, and outcome. The continuum of physiologic, functional, general health perceptions and quality of life outcomes.* Proceedings of the Clinical Outcomes Institute, Convened by the Association of Schools of Allied Health Professions and Towson State University, College of Allied Health Sciences and Physical Education, Towson, MD.

Blood, G. W. (1993). Treatment efficacy in adults who stutter: Review and recommendations. *Journal of Fluency Disorders, 18,* 303–318.

Blood, G. W. (1995a). POWER²: Relapse management with adolescents who stutter. *Language Speech Hearing Services in the Schools, 26,* 169–179.

Blood, G. W. (1995b). A behavioral-cognitive therapy program for adults who stutter: Computers and counseling. *Journal of Communication Disorders, 28,* 165–180.

Blood, G. W. (1995c). *The POWERᴿ game: Dealing with stuttering.* Psychological Corporation/ Communication Skills Builders.

Blood, G. W., Blood, I. M., Simpson, S. C., Bennett, S. L., & Susman, E. J. (1994). Subjective anxiety measurements and cortisol responses in adults who stutter. *Journal of Speech and Hearing Research 37,* 561–570.

Bloodstein, O. (1995). *A handbook on stuttering* (5th Ed.). San Diego: Singular Publishing Group, Inc.

Boberg, E. (Ed.). (1981). *Maintenance of fluency.* New York: Elsevier North Holland, Inc.

Boberg, E. (1983). Behavioral transfer and maintenance programs for adolescent and adult stutterers. In J. Fraser Gruss (Ed.), *Stuttering therapy: Transfer and maintenance* (Publication No. 19) (pp. 41–61). Memphis,TN: Stuttering Foundation of America.

Boberg, E. (1986). *Maintenance of fluency.* New York: Elsevier.

Boberg, E., Howie, P., & Woods, L. (1979). Maintenance of fluency: A review. *Journal of Fluency Disorders, 4,* 93–116.

Brutten, G. J., & Dunham, S. L. (1989). The communication attitude test. *Journal of Fluency Disorders, 14,* 371–377.

Brutten, G. J., & Shoemaker, D. J. (1967). *The modification of stuttering.* Englewood Cliffs, NJ: Prentice Hall.

Conture, E. G. (1990). *Stuttering* (2nd Ed.). Englewood Cliffs, NJ: Prentice Hall.

Conture, E. (1996). Treatment efficacy: Stuttering. *Journal of Speech and Hearing Research, 39,* 518–526.

Conture, E., & Guitar, B. (1993). Evaluating efficacy of treatment of stuttering: School-age children. *Journal of Fluency Disorders, 18,* 253–287.

Conture, E., & Wolk, L. (1990). Efficacy of intervention by speech-language pathologists: Stuttering. *Seminars in Speech and Language, 11,* 200–211.

Cooper, E. B. (1983). *Understanding the process.* Publication No. 18. Memphis, TN: Speech Foundation of America.

Cooper, E. B. (1987). The Cooper personalized fluency control therapy. In L. Rustin, H. Porser, & D. Rowley (Eds.), *Progress in the treatment of stuttering* (pp. 150–189). New York: Taylor and Francis.

Cooper, E. B. (1993). Second opinion: Chronic perseverative stuttering syndrome: A harmful or helpful construct. *American Journal of Speech Language Pathology, 2,* 11–15.

Cooper, E. B., & Cooper, C. S. (1995). Treating fluency disordered adolescents. *Journal of Communication Disorders, 28,* 125–142.

Costello, J. M., & Ingham, R. J. (1984). Assessment strategies for stuttering. In R. Curlee & W. H. Perkins (Eds.), *Nature and treatment of stuttering: New directions* (pp. 303–333). San Diego: College-Hill.

Craig, A. (1990). An investigation into the relationship between anxiety and stuttering. *Journal of Speech Hearing Disorders, 55,* 290–294.

Craig, A., & Andrews, G. (1985). The prediction and prevention of relapse in stuttering. *Behavior Modification, 9,* 427–442.

Craig, A., & Calvert, P. (1991). Following up on treated stutterers: Studies of perception of fluency and job status. *Journal of Speech and Hearing Research, 34,* 279–284.

Craig, A., Franklin, J., & Andrews, G. (1984). A scale to measure the locus of control of behavior. *British Journal of Medical Psychology, 57,* 173–180.

Curlee, R. (1993). Evaluating treatment efficacy for adults: Assessment of stuttering disability. *Journal of Fluency Disorders, 18,* 319–331.

Daly, D. A. (1988). *Freedom of fluency.* Tucson, AZ: LinguiSystems.

Dell, C. (1990). *Treating the school age stutterer: A guide for clinicians* (Publication No. 14). Memphis, TN: Speech Foundation of America.

Dembrowski, J., & Watson, B. C. (1991). An instrumented method for assessment and remediation of stuttering: A single-subject case study. *Journal of Fluency Disorders, 16,* 241–273.

DeNil, L., & Brutten, G. (1991). Speech associated attitudes of stuttering and nonstuttering children. *Journal of Speech Hearing Research, 34,* 60–66.

DeNil, L. F., & Kroll, R. M. (1995). The relationship between locus of control and long-term stuttering treatment outcome in adult stutterers. *Journal of Fluency Disorders, 20,* 345–364.

Dhariti, R. (1985). Response to therapy by stutterers in relation to their locus of control. *Indian Journal of Clinical Psychology, 12,* 37–40.

Erickson, R. L. (1969). Assessing communicative attitudes among stutterers. *Journal of Speech and Hearing Research, 12,* 711–724.

Evesham, M., & Fransella, F. (1985). Stuttering relapse: The effect of a combined speech and psychological reconstruction programme. *British Journal of Disorders of Communication, 20,* 237–248.

Foon, A. E. (1987). Review: Locus of control as a predictor of outcome in psychotherapy. *British Journal of Medical Psychology, 60,* 99–107.

Fransella, F. (1987). Stuttering to fluency via reconstruing. In R. A. Neimeyer & G. J. Neimeyer (Eds.), *Personal construct therapy casebook* (pp. 290–308). New York: Springer Publishing Company.

Fraser, M. (1990). *Self-therapy for the stutterer* (7th ed.). Memphis, TN: Speech Foundation of America.

Guitar, B., & Bass, C. (1978). Stuttering therapy: The relation between attitude change and long-term outcome. *Journal of Speech Hearing Disorders, 43,* 392–400.

Hillis, J. W. (1993). Ongoing assessment in the management of stuttering: A clinical perspective. *American Journal of Speech Language Pathology.*

Howie, P., & Andrews, G. (1984). Treatment of adult stutterers: Managing fluency. In R. F. Curlee & W. H. Perkins (Eds.), *Nature and treatment of stuttering: New Directions.* San Diego: College Hill Press.

Ingham, J. C. (1993). Current status of stuttering and behavior modification—I: Recent trends in the application of behavior modification in children and adults. *Journal of Fluency Disorders, 18,* 27–55.

Ingham, R. J. (1984). *Stuttering and behavior therapy: Current status and experimental foundations.* San Diego, CA: College-Hill Press.

Ingham, R. J. (1985). Stuttering treatment outcome evaluation: Closing the credibility gap. *Seminars in Speech and Language, 6,* 105–123.

Ingham, R. J. (1993a). Stuttering treatment efficacy: Paradigm dependent or independent? *Journal of Fluency Disorders, 18,* 133–149.

Ingham, R. J. (1993b). Current status of stuttering and behavior modification: II. Principal issues and practices in stuttering therapy. *Journal of Fluency Disorders, 18,* 57–79.

Ingham, R. J., & Costello, J. M. (1985). Stuttering treatment and outcome evaluation. In J. M. Costello (Ed.), *Speech disorders in adults* (pp. 189–223). San Diego, CA: College Hill Press.

Ihgham, R. J., Fox, P. T., Ingham, J. C., Zamarripa, F., Martin, C., Jerabek, P., & Cotton, J. (1996, December). Functional-lesion investigation of developmental stuttering with positron emission tomography. *Journal of Speech and Hearing Research, 39,* 1208–1227.

Kuhr, A., & Rustin, L. (1985). The maintenance of fluency after intensive in-patient therapy: Long-term follow-up. *Journal of Fluency Disorders, 10,* 229–236.

Logan, R. J. (1991). *The three dimensions of stuttering: Neurology, behavior, and emotion.* Austin, TX: Pro-Ed.

Madison, L. S., Budd, K. S., & Itzkowitz, J. S. (1986). Changes in stuttering in relation to children's locus of control. *Journal of Genetic Psychology, 147,* 233–240.

Manning, W. H. (1991). Making progress during and after treatment. In W. Perkins (Ed.), *Seminars in speech and language* (pp. 349–354). New York: Thieme Medical Publishers.

Manning, W. H. (1996). *Clinical decision making in the diagnosis and treatment of fluency disorders.* New York: Delmar Publishers.

Martin, R. R., Haroldson, S. K., & Triden, K. A. (1984). Stuttering and speech naturalness. *Journal of Speech and Hearing Disorders, 49,* 53–58.

McDonough, A., & Quesal, R. (1988). Locus of control orientation of stutterers and nonstutterers. *Journal of Fluency Disorders, 13,* 97–106.

Meichenbaum, D. (1985). *Stress inoculation training.* New York: Pergamon Press.

Orstein, A., & Manning, W. (1985). Self-efficacy scaling by adult stutterers. *Journal of Communication Disorders, 18,* 313–320.

Packman, A., Onslow, M., & van Doorn, J. (1994). Prolonged speech and modification of stuttering: Perceptual, acoustic, and electroglottographic data. *Journal of Speech and Hearing Research, 37,* 724–737.

Perkins, W. H. (1981). Measurement and maintenance of fluency. In E. Boberg (Ed.), *Maintenance of fluency.*

Perkins, W. H., Kent, R. D., & Curlee, R. F. (1991). A theory of neuropsycholinguistic function in stuttering. *Journal of Speech and Hearing Research, 34,* 734–752.

Peters, T. J., & Guitar, B. (1991). *Stuttering: An integrated approach to its nature and treatment.* Baltimore: Williams & Wilkins.

Prins, A. (1984). Treatment of adults: Managing stuttering. In R. F. Curlee & W. H. Perkins (Eds.), *Nature and treatment of stuttering* (pp. 397–424). San Diego, CA: College Hill Press.

Prins, D. (1991). Theories of stuttering as event and disorder: Implications for speech production processes. In H. Peters, W. Hulstijn, & C. W. Starkweather (Eds.), *Speech motor control and stuttering* (pp. 571–580). Amsterdam: The Netherlands: Elsevier.

Prins, D. (1993). Models for treatment efficacy studies of adult stutterers. *Journal of Fluency Disorders, 18,* 333–350.

Rathus, S. P. (1973). A 30-item scale for assessing assertive behavior. *Behavior Therapy, 4,* 398–406.

Rosenbaum, M. (1990). (Ed.). *Learned resourcefulness, on coping skills, self-control, and adaptive behavior.* New York: Springer Publishing Co.

Sheehan, J. G. (1975). Conflict theory and avoidance reduction therapy. In J. Eisenson (Ed.), *Stuttering: A second symposium* (pp. 97–198). New York: Harper and Row.

Sheehan, J. G. (1984). Problems in the evaluation of progress and outcome. In W. H. Perkins (Ed.), *Stuttering disorders* (pp. 223–239). New York: Thieme Stratton.

Shumak, I. C. (1955). A speech situation rating sheet for stutterers. In W. Johnson & R. Leutenegger (Eds.), *Stuttering in children and adults.* Minneapolis: University of Minnesota Press.

Silverman, F. H. (1980). The stuttering problem profile: A task that assists both client and clinician in defining therapy goals. *Journal of Speech Hearing Disorders, 45,* 119–123.

Silverman, F. H. (1981). Relapse following stuttering therapy. In N. J. Lass (Ed.), *Speech and language, advances in basic research and practice* (Vol. 5) (pp. 56–78). New York: Academic Press.

Silverman, F. H. (1996). *Stuttering and other fluency disorders.* Englewood Cliffs, NJ: Prentice Hall.

Spielberger, C. D., Gorsuch, R. L., & Lushene, R. E. (1970). *Manual for the state-trait anxiety inventory.* Palo Alto, CA: Consulting Psychologists Press.

Starkweather, C. W., Gottwald, S. R., & Halford, M. M. (1990). *Stuttering prevention: A clinical method.* Englewood Cliffs, NJ: Prentice Hall.

Starkweather, C. W., St. Louis, K., Blood, G. W., Peters, T., Westbrook, J., Gregory, H., Cooper, E., & Healey, C. (1995). Guidelines for practice in stuttering treatment. *ASHA, 37* (Suppl. 14), 26.

Stewart, T. (1996). Good maintainers and poor maintainers: A personal construct approach to an old problem. *Journal of Fluency Disorders, 21,* 33–48.

St. Louis, K., & Westbrook, J. (1987). The effects of treatment for stuttering. In L. Rustin, H. Purser, & D. Rowley (Eds.), *Progress in the treatment of fluency disorders* (pp. 233–257). London: Taylor & Francis.

Van Riper, C. (1973). *The treatment of stuttering.* Englewood Cliffs, NJ: Prentice-Hall.

Van Riper, C. (1982). *The nature of stuttering.* Englewood Cliffs, NJ: Prentice-Hall.

Watson, J. B. (1995). Exploring the attitudes of adults who stutter. *Journal of Communication Disorders, 28,* 143–164.

Webster, R. L. (1984). Empirical considerations regarding stuttering therapy. In H. G. Gregory (Ed.), *Controversies about stuttering therapy* (pp. 209–239). Baltimore: University Park Press.

Webster, W. G. (1993). Hurried hands and tangled tongues: Implications of current research for the management of stuttering. In E. B. Boberg (Ed.), *Neuropsychology of stuttering* (pp. 73–127). Canada: University of Alberta Press.

Williams, D. E. (1957). A point of view about stuttering. *Journal of Speech and Hearing Disorders, 22,* 390–397.

Wilson, I. B., & Cleary, P. D. (1995). Linking clinical variables with health-related quality of life. *Journal of the American Medical Association, 273,* 59–65.

Woolf, G. (1967). The assessment of stuttering as struggle, avoidance and expectancy. *British Journal of Communication Disorders, 2,* 158–171.

CHAPTER 18

Outcomes Measurement in Child Language and Phonological Disorders

HOWARD GOLDSTEIN AND JUDITH GIERUT

INTRODUCTION

Many of the approximately 11% of students in public schools who receive special education services require speech and language services. Over 5 million children between birth and 21 years receive services under the Individuals with Disabilities Education Act (IDEA) and 22% of those students are eligible because of speech or language disorders (Terman, Larner, Stevenson, & Behrman, 1996). Approximately half of these students have phonological disorders. This underestimates the number of children with speech and language impairments who are considered IDEA-eligible because of other diagnoses: learning disabilities (51%), mental retardation (11%), emotional disturbance (9%), and hearing or visual impairments, orthopedic impairments, autism, traumatic brain injury, or multiple disabilities (7%). Impairments in child language are commonly associated with a variety of etiologies, including mental retardation, hearing impairment, autism, paralysis, malformation of the vocal apparatus, emotional disturbance, and neurological conditions (such as seizure disorders or brain lesions). In addition, a diagnosis of Specific Language Impairment (SLI) differs from the majority of child language disorders, in that children exhibit a significant limitation in language ability that cannot be attributed to deficits in hearing, general intelligence, oral structure and function, or obvious brain damage. An estimated 5% of preschool children are diagnosed with specific language impairment (National Institute on Deafness and Other Communication Disorders, 1991). An estimated 10% of preschool and early school-age children are diagnosed with functional phonological impairments (National Institute on Deafness and Other Communication Disorders, 1994); for 80% of these children, the disorder is sufficiently severe to require clinical treatment. Finally, it should be noted that developmental language disorders occur three to four times more often in boys than in girls (National Institutes of Health, National Advisory Neurological Disorders and Stroke Council, 1990).

Despite the obvious fact that child language and phonological disorders affect a significant portion of the population of children, it is difficult to estimate incidence and prevalence rates. This problem relates not only to the overlap with other handicapping conditions, but also to a myriad of measurement issues. The problem is exacerbated by widespread ambiguity in definitions, the absence of standard criteria for diagnosis, and lack of stability in diagnoses (see Cole, Schwartz, Notari, Dale, & Mills, 1995). Nevertheless, there is a great need to evaluate and manage children with language and phonological disorders. This chapter focuses on measurement strategies and especially on issues that relate to the evaluation of outcomes. We discuss measurement tools and approaches within the context of a conceptual outcomes framework offered by Frattali in this volume (Chapter 1). In addition, we discuss some of the treatment efficacy research that demonstrates intermediate, instrumental, and ultimate outcomes of treatment for child language and phonological disorders.

DEFINITIONS OF CHILD LANGUAGE AND PHONOLOGICAL DISORDERS

Language Disorders

Language disorders refer to a heterogeneous group of developmental and/or acquired disorders principally characterized by deficits in comprehension, production, and/or use of language. These deficits may be manifested in the development of form (e.g., phonology, syntax, morphology), content (semantics), and/or use of language (pragmatics). The following are examples of some of these deficits:

Deficits in *syntax* could be reflected in problems comprehending or producing syntactic structures. For example, a passive structure, "Jeff was kissed by his dog" might be misinterpreted as meaning the same as "Jeff kissed his dog." Deficits in *morphology* refer to a lack of knowledge or understanding that certain sounds or groups of sounds have meaning. Such a deficit might result in the omission of morphemes. An utterance such as "He walk his dog," might be missing a tense marker, *-ing* or *-ed;* possibly an auxiliary verb, *was* or *is;* and the plural marker *-s.* An SLP is careful to assess whether such omissions reflect a morphological deficit rather than a phonological deficit or a dialectical difference.

Semantic deficits might be reflected in inappropriate use or meaning of words, especially words that differ according to the context. For example, children may be confused about the use of subject versus object pronouns, saying "him went to the park" for "he went to the park." Another example might entail confusions between *here* and *there,* as the place being indicated depends on who is speaking; this shifting of reference in relation to the speaker is an example of deixis.

Pragmatic deficits refer to inappropriate social uses of language. A variety of pragmatic problems can cause misunderstandings or even rejection by the people with whom one wishes to communicate. For example, lack of eye contact during conversation may indicate disinterest; the inability to take turns appropriately may result in monopolizing the conversation or too little participation; and not recognizing the need to maintain topics may lead to disjointed conversation.

Phonological Disorders

Phonological disorders can be defined as a breakdown in a speaker's production and/or mental representation of speech sounds of the target language (Bernthal & Bankson, 1993; Edwards & Shriberg, 1983; Ferguson, Menn, & Stoel-Gammon, 1992; Fey, 1992; Folkins & Bleile, 1990; Hoffman & Daniloff, 1990; Ingram, 1989; Leonard, 1973; Locke, 1983; Shriberg & Kwiatkowski, 1982a). Specifically, a phonological disorder may reflect an inability to articulate speech sounds, with the communication difficulty involving a motoric component. Disorders of this type have been described as *phonetic* in nature; that is, the difficulty lies in how sounds are produced (Dinnsen, 1984; Elbert, 1992; Hoffman, Schuckers & Daniloff, 1989; Stoel-Gammon, 1985). A phonological disorder may also affect the way in which speech sound information is stored and represented in the mental lexicon, or is accessed and retrieved cognitively (Bernhardt, 1992a, 1992b; Chiat, 1994; Dean, Howell, Waters, & Reid, 1995; Dinnsen, 1984; Dodd, Leahy, & Hambly, 1989; Leonard, Schwartz, Swanson, & Loeb, 1987; McGregor & Schwartz, 1992; Schwartz, 1992; Stackhouse & Wells, 1993). In this case, the communication difficulty may have a linguistic or cognitive basis. Disorders of this type may be termed *phonemic* because the difficulties can involve the way in which sounds are used to signal meaning differences among words (Dinnsen, 1984; Elbert, 1992). It must be acknowledged that phonetically and phonemically based phonological disorders are not mutually exclusive. Consequently, a phonological disorder may have a broad impact on both a child's articulation (i.e., performance) and internalized knowledge (i.e., competence) of the sound system of the target language (Gierut, 1990b; Kamhi, 1992).

In a majority of cases, phonological disorders in children are *functional,* that is, with no known cause for the communication breakdown (Shriberg, Kwiatkowski, Best, Hengst, & Terselic-Weber, 1986). Children generally present normal hearing, intelligence, social, emotional, and behavioral skills. Yet, for many children with functional phonological disorders, receptive and expressive language abilities are not age-appropriate (Hoffman, 1992). Semantic, syntactic, and pragmatic disorders of language have been observed in association with functional phonological disorders (Camarata & Schwartz, 1985; Campbell & Shriberg, 1982; Fey, Cleave, Ravida, Long, Dejmal, & Easton, 1994; Himmelwright-Gross, St. Louis, Ruscello, & Hull, 1985; Panagos & Prelock, 1982; Paul & Jennings, 1992; Paul & Shriberg, 1982; Ruscello, St. Louis, & Mason, 1991; Schwartz, Leonard, Folger, & Wilcox, 1980; Tyler, 1992; Tyler & Sandoval, 1994; Tyler & Watterson, 1991). In these cases, there may be more global involvement of the linguistic system.

Other co-occurring conditions have also been reported in conjunction with functional phonological disorders, including for example, early otitis media (Churchill, Hodson, Jones, & Novak, 1988; Paden, Matthies, & Novak, 1989; Paden, Novak, & Beiter, 1987; Roberts, Burchinal, Koch, Footo, & Henderson, 1988; Shriberg & Kwiatkowski, 1982a; Shriberg & Smith, 1983), perceptual deficits (Broen, Strange, Doyle, & Heller, 1983; Locke, 1980a, 1980b; Rvachew & Jamieson, 1989; Smit & Bernthal, 1983; Winitz, 1975), and disfluency (Conture, Louko, & Edwards, 1993; Louko, Edwards, & Conture, 1990; Throneburg, Yairi, & Paden, 1994; Wolk, Edwards, & Conture, 1993). To date, however, the causal and precedence relationships among these co-occurring conditions remain unknown and continue to be the focus of ongoing research (Johnson, Shelton, & Arndt, 1982; Lewis & Freebairn, 1993; Shriberg, 1993).

In summary, appropriate communication depends on the use of a vast array of linguistic skills made all the more complicated when they must be applied collectively and adapted to interactions with others. Different intervention approaches may target one of these domains, but their intent is usually to have a more general impact on a child's functional communication and intelligibility in social contexts. This intent is not always made obvious, because of the difficulty in evaluating specific effects across such a wide array of linguistic skills. However, it is important to keep in mind that children with speech and language impairments may have deficiencies across a variety of linguistic domains mentioned and the selection of intervention targets is largely a matter of establishing priorities.

MEASUREMENT ISSUES

Frattali (Chapter 1) presents three typological frameworks for characterizing on a continuum the consequences of an illness or disorder. The International Classification of Impairments, Disabilities, and Handicaps (ICIDH), developed by the World Health Organization (WHO) (1980), is presented here as one example of how these models may be applied specifically to children with language and phonological disorders.

The ICIDH utilizes these categories: impairment, disability, and handicap. Although an impairment usually results from a pathology, an identifiable pathology is not always apparent. A pathology is not identified in the case of functional phonological disorders and specific language impairment, for example. When speech and language disorders are associated with other diagnoses, e.g., mental retardation, there still may be no identifiable pathology. Nevertheless, impairment is present when children clearly deviate from the phonological and/or language norms of their age-matched peers and of their surrounding speech community. This may lead to a communication disability if children are unable to understand instructions, are unable to be understood, or are unable to communicate basic and social needs. If phonological and language disorders persist into the school-age years, there may be further deleterious social consequences and social stigmatization. These social sequelae are increasingly likely with increasingly severe disorders. Handicapping conditions affecting an individual across the lifespan may ultimately result, as demonstrated by recent retrospective studies of individuals with phonological disorders (Felsenfeld, Broen, & McGue, 1992, 1994; Felsenfeld, McGue, & Broen, 1995) and individuals with language disorders (Aram, Ekelman, & Nation, 1984; Aram & Nation, 1980; Bashir, Wiig, & Abrams, 1987; Bishop & Edmundson, 1987; Hall & Tomblin, 1978; King, Jones, & Lasky, 1982; Schery, 1985; Stark et al., 1984).

Classification frameworks such as this are relevant when considering special populations for at least two reasons: (1) specific measurement tools and systems may be identified for each level of classification, and (2) specific methods of treatment and their success may be associated with particular levels of classification. For children with speech and language disorders, outcomes research has begun to address the first issue. In the case of functional phonological disorders, there has been considerable development in the area of measurement, which has assisted in identifying certain trends within the population and in establishing relationships among apparent characteristics exhibited by these children. Despite the myriad of measures of child language development, surprisingly little attention has been paid to the development of formal measures beyond the impairment level of classification. Advances in the area of child language intervention may provide more insights into the measurement of disability and handicap. The issue of linking classification levels directly with particular methods and durations of intervention remains largely unexplored, however. We limit our discussion then to outcomes measurement as related to the categories of impairment, disability, and handicap.

Impairment-level Measurement

Primary outcomes measurement for the category of impairment is diagnostic in nature. Table 18–1 lists approximately 100 child language assessments identified in recent texts and reference books for speech-language pathologists (Lund & Duchan, 1993; Nicolosi, Harryman, & Kresheck, 1989; Owens, 1995). These assessments reflect a variety of theoretical frameworks for understanding language. As can be seen in Table 18–1, they sample different aspects of language; some are narrowly focused and others attempt to be more comprehensive. With few exceptions, these assessments reflect a developmental perspective. The tools used for testing typically compare a child's performance to age norms that reflect an average course of communication development. Significant deviation from expectations for one's age is used to judge an impairment either in language generally or in a particular aspect(s) of language. Standardized, norm-referenced assessment tools may be exclusively devoted to communication (e.g., *Sequenced Inventory of Communication Development,* Hedrick, Prather, & Tobin, 1984; *Test of Early Language Development,* Hresko, Reid, & Hammill, 1981; *Peabody Picture Vocabulary Test,* Dunn & Dunn, 1981), or may be a part of a comprehensive developmental assessment instrument (e.g., *Battelle Developmental Inventory,* Newborg, Stock, Wnek, Guidubaldi, & Svinicki, 1984). Despite the large number of formal tests, few have been thoroughly standardized, and rigorously tested (see McCauley & Demetras, 1990; McCauley & Swisher, 1984).

Some of the many procedures for analyzing communication samples are included in Table 18–1 as well. Speech-language pathologists (SLPs) commonly analyze a corpus of a child's utterances collected in a facilitative context to determine the range of forms, meanings, and/or functions that are present and absent when compared to those expected for age-matched peers. Global quantitative measures, such as Mean Length of Utterance (MLU), also have been used to make general judgments about whether a language impairment exists. Because contextual factors influence communicative performance, careful consideration should be paid to the contexts in which samples are collected (Bain, Olswang, & Johnson, 1992; Mirenda & Donnellan, 1986; Yoder & Davies, 1990). Factors including interaction partners (e.g., parent, teachers, clinicians), the setting (e.g., home, clinic, classroom), situation (e.g., structured, unstructured, predictable, unpredictable), and materials (e.g., familiar, unfamiliar) can influence performance. Computerized systems (e.g., *Systematic Analysis of Language Transcripts,* Miller & Chapman, 1986; *Child Language Data Exchange System,* MacWhinney, 1991) can assist in summarizing qualitative and quantitative information about a child's language development (e.g., MLU, type-token ratios, percentages of initiations versus responses, frequency of specific forms, content, and functions). Additional research efforts are needed, however, to better understand how to gather representative samples most effectively. Also, research is needed to determine the developmental and diagnostic signifi-

Table 18–1. Summary of Age Ranges and Areas Covered by Language Tests and Procedures

Language Assessments	Age Range	Phonology	Morphology	Syntax	Semantics	Pragmatics	Other	Expressive	Receptive
Adolescent Language Screening Test	11–17 yr	X	X	X	X	X		X	X
Ammons Full Range Picture Vocabulary Test	2–adult				X				X
Analysis of the Language of Learning	chn*	X		X	X			X	
Assessment of Children's Language Comprehension	3–6.5 yr				X	X			X
Bankson Language Screening Test	4–7 yr		X	X	X		X	X	X
Basic Concept Inventory	Pre–3rd				X				X
Basic Language Concepts Test	4.1–6.6 yr				X	X		X	X
Bellugi-Klima's Language Comprehension Test	chn				X				X
Berko Test of English Morphology	chn		X					X	
Berry-Talbott Language Test	chn		X					X	
Bilingual Syntax Measure	4–9 yr			X				X	
Boehm Test of Basic Concepts-R	K–2nd				X				X
Boehm Test of Basic Concepts-Preschool	3–5 yr				X				X
Carrow Elicited Language Inventory	3–7.11 yr		X	X				X	
The Children's Language Battery	chn	X		X	X			X	X
Clark-Madison Test of Oral Language	chn		X	X				X	
Clinical Evaluation of Language Fundamentals-R	K–12th	X		X	X		X	X	X
The Communication Screen—A Preschool Speech-Language Screening Tool	2.10–5.9				X		X	X	X
Communication Abilities Diagnostic Test and Screen	3–8.11 yr	X		X	X	X		X	X
Communication and Symbolic Behavior Scales	8–24 mos				X		X	X	
Compton Speech and Language Screening Evaluation	3–6 yr	X	X	X	X			X	X
Developmental Sentence Scoring	3–6.11 yr			X				X	
Environmental Language Inventory	Pre			X	X			X	
Environmental Pre-language Battery	0–3 yr	X			X	X	X	X	X
Evaluating Acquired Skills in Communication	chn w sev. dis.		X	X	X	X		X	X
Evaluating Communication Competence	9–17 yr			X	X	X		X	X
Expressive One-Word Picture Vocabulary Test	2–12 yr				X			X	
EOWPVT-Upper Extension	12–16 yr				X			X	
Fluharty Speech and Language Screening Test-R	2–6 yr	X			X	X		X	X
Fullerton Language Test for Adolescents	11–adult		X	X	X			X	X
Grammatical Analysis of Elicited Language	8–12 yr (hrg imp)			X				X	
Houston Test for Language Development	18 mo–6 yr							X	X
Illinois Children's Language Assessment Test	3–6 hr	X			X			X	X
Illinois Test of Psycholinguistic Abilities	2–10 yr		X		X			X	X
Interpersonal Language Skills and Assessment	8–14 yr			X	X	X	X	X	
Joliet 3-Minute Speech and Language Screen	K, 2nd, 5th	X	X	X	X		X	X	X
Kindergarten Language Screening Test	K				X			X	X
Language Assessment, Remediation, and Screening Procedure (LARSP)	chn		X	X				X	X
Language Processing Test	5–12 yr				X			X	
Language Proficiency Test	9–adult				X	X	X	X	X
Language Sampling, Analysis, and Training	chn		X	X				X	
Let's Talk Inventory for Children	9th +					X		X	
MacArthur Communication Development Inventory	0.8–2.6 yr				X			X	
Mean Length of Utterance in Morphemes (MLU)	chn		X				X		
Merrill Language Screening Test	K–1	X	X	X	X	X	X	X	X
Michigan Picture Inventory	3–7.11 yr				X			X	X
Miller-Yoder Comprehension Test	devel 4–8 yr		X	X					X
Multilevel Informal Language Inventory	K–6th		X	X	X			X	X

(continued)

411

Table 18–1. Summary of Age Ranges and Areas Covered by Language Tests and Procedures *(continued)*

Language Assessments	Age Range	Phonology	Morphology	Syntax	Semantics	Pragmatics	Other	Expressive	Receptive
Northwestern Syntax Screening Test	3–7.11 yr		X	X	X		X	X	X
Oral Language Sentence Imitation Screening Test	3–7 yr		X	X				X	
Oral Language Sentence Imitation Diagnostic Inventory	5–7 yr		X	X	X			X	
Parson Language Sample	chn				X			X	X
Patterned Elicitation Syntax Screening Test	3–7.6 yr		X	X				X	
Peabody Picture Vocabulary Test-R	2.6–18 yr				X				X
Performance Assessment of Syntax Elicited and Spontaneous	3–8 yr			X				X	
Porch Index of Communicative Abilities in Children	3–12th							X	X
Pragmatics Screening Test	3.6–8.6 yr					X		X	
Preschool Language Assessment Instrument	3–6 yr				X	X	X	X	X
Preschool Language Scale-R	1–7 yr							X	X
Psycholinguistic Rating Scale	K–8 yr						X	X	X
Quick Test	1.6–19 yr				X				X
Receptive-Expressive Emergent Language Scale	0–3 yr							X	X
Receptive-Expressive Observation Scale	5–12 yr							X	X
Receptive One Word Picture Vocabulary Test (ROWPVT)	2–12 yr				X				X
ROWPVT-Upper Extension	12–16 yr				X				X
Screening Kit of Language Development	2–5 yr			X	X			X	X
Screening Test of Adolescent Language	6th +			X	X		X	X	X
Screening Test for Auditory Comprehension of Language	3–6 yr		X	X	X				X
Sequenced Inventory of Communication Development	4 mo–4 yr	X	X	X	X		X	X	X
Slingerland Screening Tests for Identifying Children with Specific Language Disability	1st–6th						X	X	X
Stephens Oral Language Screening Test	4–7 yr	X		X				X	
Structured Photographic Expression Language Test II-P	3–9 yr				X			X	
Temple University Short Syntax Inventory	3–5 yr		X	X				X	
Test of Adolescent Language-2	12–18 yr		X	X	X		X	X	X
Test for Auditory Comprehension of Language-R	3–10 yr		X	X	X				X
Test of Early Language Development	3–7.11 yr			X	X			X	X
Test for Examining Expressive Morphology	3–8 yr		X					X	
Test of Language Competence	9–19 yr				X	X	X	X	X
Test of Language Competence for Children	4–9 yr			X	X			X	X
Test of Language Development-Intermediate	8.6–13 yr		X	X	X			X	X
Test of Language Development-Primary	4–8.11 yr	X	X	X	X			X	X
Test of Pragmatic Skills	3–8 yr					X	X	X	X
Test of Word Finding	6.6–22 yr				X			X	X
The Token Test for Children	3–12.5 yr			X	X				X
Toronto Tests of Receptive Vocabulary, English/Spanish	4–10 yr				X			X	
Utah Test of Language Development	2–14 yr			X	X			X	X
Vocabulary Comprehension Scale	2–6 yr			X	X				X
Woodcock Language Proficiency Battery	Sch Age						X		X
The Word Test	7–12 yr				X			X	X

*Children

412

cance of many of the measures that one might obtain from communication sample analyses (Klee, 1992a, b).

Formal language tests and analyses of communication samples are used most often to document impairment. However, to select target behaviors and monitor progress, SLPs usually turn to more specific assessments. For example, a number of nonstandardized tests sample certain skill areas more extensively. There are a number of commercially available tests devoted exclusively to communication skills that have not been standardized (e.g., *Environmental Prelanguage Battery,* Horstmeister & MacDonald, 1978; *Environmental Language Intervention Program,* MacDonald, 1978). A number of more global assessments include communication sections (e.g., *Assessment, Evaluation, & Programming System for Infants and Children,* Bricker, 1992; *Transdisciplinary Play-Based Assessment,* Linder, 1992).

Still more specific measurement may require SLPs to design their own nonstandardized probes to determine whether a child can comprehend or produce a specific communicative form, meaning, or function (Miller, 1981). Probes present repeated opportunities for a certain behavior to be demonstrated using somewhat different materials for each opportunity. For example, 10 different opportunities to request objects might be embedded into everyday activities (e.g., giving the child a puzzle with a piece missing; "forgetting" to distribute crackers to a hungry child; handing the child a desired toy that is sealed in a jar). Because probes of this sort embody modifications in the way natural environments are arranged, they are referred to as a "naturalistic" assessment approach. Such probes require evaluators to be good actors, emphasizing naturalness, but giving up some of the efficiency inherent in more traditional testing situations.

One can build upon nonstandardized probes to assess learning potential for more advanced communication skills. Dynamic assessment procedures can be used to introduce prompts or teaching episodes into the assessment to determine how a child's performance is enhanced through instruction (Olswang, Bain, & Johnson, 1992). Dynamic assessment is helpful in deriving information about (1) the child's learning potential for particular behaviors, (2) the factors that may influence the child's success or failure on particular tasks, and (3) strategies for facilitating the child's development or functioning (Minick, 1987). Olswang et al. (1992) provide an application of Feuerstein's *Learning Potential Assessment Device* (1979) to the dynamic assessment of two-word semantic relations.

Going beyond standardized tests of articulation (e.g., Bankson & Bernthal, 1990; Goldman & Fristoe, 1986) and established procedures of phonological analysis (e.g., Bernhardt & Stoel-Gammon, 1994; Dinnsen, 1984; Hodson, 1986; Ingram, 1981), there have been significant advances in the development of diagnostic and classification schemes (Shriberg & Kwiatkowski, 1982a, 1982b, 1982c). In particular, one long-standing question in the diagnosis of children with functional phonological disorders relates to the causal nature or the correlative factors associated with this communicative disorder. With advances in medical genetics, there has been a corresponding interest in establishing whether there may be a possible genetic basis for some subsets of phonological disorders. In order to pursue this, however, valid psychometric tools for identifying possible subtypes of phonological disorders were needed. Toward this end, Shriberg (1993) introduced and validated four speech measures for potential use in the identification of subtypes (perhaps even genetically based) of phonological disorders.

The *Speech Disorders Classification System* rates speech abilities using a 10-category continuum ranging from normal speech acquisition to speech delay to residual errors. It is appropriate for use with ages 2 through adulthood, thereby providing a longitudinal rating and comparison of a speaker's phonological system. The *Articulation Competence Index* rates the severity of phonological involvement by considering the percentage of target consonants that are produced accurately in a brief connected speech sample. This index also can be used across generations because it takes into account a speaker's age and the nature of persistent speech errors (either common or uncommon) when determining severity. A third measure is the *Speech Profile*, which provides a detailed and standard method of displaying speech performance data. There are individual Speech Profiles for consonant production, phonetic classes, and vowels, and for the nature of error patterns including substitutions and distortions by word position. The *Prosody-Voice Profile* rates suprasegmental and prosodic properties of production, including loudness, pitch, and quality of a speaker's voice and prosodic phrasing, rate, and stress. Together, these four measures provide a measurement schema for describing phonological systems. The measures are integrated because each can be completed using data from the same speech sample. They provide a unified picture of a given person's speech abilities because performance can be rated over time using the same measures. They also allow for systematic comparison and differentiation of potential subgroups of speakers with phonological disorders.

To demonstrate, Shriberg put these four speech and voice profiles to test in the diagnostic characterization and longitudinal monitoring of speech normalization of 178 children with phonological disorders (Shriberg, Gruber, & Kwiatkowski, 1994; Shriberg & Kwiatkowski, 1994; Shriberg, Kwiatkowski, & Gruber, 1994). *Speech normalization* refers specifically to the process by which sound production and use become target-appropriate relative to the surrounding speech community. From this research, several findings relevant to outcomes emerged:

(1) Apparent properties associated with phonological disorders in children ages 3 to 11 were identified. Briefly, about 8% of the subject population exhibited some type of phonological disorder. Of these children, 5% had residual errors with only one or two target sounds being produced incorrectly. The remaining 3% evidenced more involved errored sound productions. For this latter group, 50 to 75% also had some type of expressive and/or receptive language impairments. Difficulties in receptive language occurred less often than combined expressive plus receptive language disorders.

(2) Speech normalization took place at different rates for different children. Approximately 18% of the study population experienced short-term normalization, that is, adultlike productions within 1 year of the initial diagnosis of a phonological disorder. Short-term normalization, however, was not associated with any one specific variable. For example, the particular target sounds produced in error, nature of the error pattern, delivery of clinical treatment, hearing acuity, or general language abilities did not uniquely differentiate children who did from those who did not normalize within 1 year post-diagnosis. Thus, it was not possible to predict which children would remediate rapidly as based on the outcomes measurement tools.

(3) Long-term normalization spanned as much as a 5-year period of improvement. During this time, two growth spurts were observed for the children of this study. Dramatic gains took place between ages 4 and 6, and again between ages 7 and 8. The pattern of phonological improvements for these children strongly resembled that of nor-

mal phonological development and of short-term normalization. This suggested an element of phonological delay, rather than deviance, in this study population and its potential subgroups.

Disability-level Measurement

The relevant outcomes measurement of disability involves establishing the functional status of the child in the day-to-day environment. The existence of an impairment does not necessarily imply a functional restriction or lack of ability to perform common, everyday activities or daily communicative tasks. Children with impairments can learn or be taught to compensate in a number of ways so that their communication abilities match everyday demands. As Frattali (Chapter 1) points out, functional status can vary depending on personality, motivation, social supports, and even economic supports. Thus, individuals with similar impairment characteristics may function very differently depending on their personal circumstances. Indeed, differences in individuals' daily activities depend on one's age, family circumstances, social expectations, and cultural milieu. There may be different expectations in terms of the degree of independent functioning needed in relation to the social supports that are available. For example, telephone communication skills may come into play at earlier ages in some families than in others. Does a child need to communicate most often in child-adult dyads, child-child dyads, small groups, or large groups? Homework completion may depend on whether a teacher gives instructions orally or in written form.

It is hard to imagine attempting to measure disability without using parents and significant others in the child's life as informants. The most straightforward way of gathering information at the level of disability is by questioning the child's family. Questionnaires and interviews can be used to allow families to provide accounts of their child's communication abilities and needs as well as to describe the family's concerns and priorities. We should note that questions about communication usually are a part of a more comprehensive questionnaire or interview that addresses other developmental areas when an interdisciplinary, collaborative approach to assessment is possible. This is considered preferable to having families complete a stack of questionnaires or series of interviews given by different professionals.

Interviews and surveys of teachers and other professionals may be used to gather information about communicative functioning in different contexts. Information about previous communication intervention efforts and activities should also be gathered. Unfortunately, the literature has not focused extensively on this source of information (see Klein et al., 1981, for one example of a teacher questionnaire).

The few measures that purport to measure disability outcomes in children rely on interviews of parents concerning functional abilities and independence usually with a heavy emphasis on self-help and mobility skills. For example, the *Functional Independence Measure for Children* (WeeFIM; McCabe & Granger, 1990; Braun & Granger, 1991) asks for a single judgment of degree of independence/assistance for understanding spoken or written communication and a single judgment for clarity of vocal or nonvocal expression. The *Pediatric Evaluation of Disability Inventory* (PEDI; Haley et al., 1992) is a longer instrument that assesses an array of communication skills. Parents are asked to judge whether their child can perform 65 social function skills. Although many of the items mirror those found on formal language tests, they are organized into 13 areas. Many of the areas are meant to sample a variety of communicative contexts, including problem-resolution, play interaction with adults, peer interactions, self-information, time orientation, household chores, self-protection, and community function. The other areas are more developmentally based, e.g., play with objects, comprehension of word meanings, comprehension of sentence complexity, functional use of communication, and complexity of expressive communication. In addition, parents are asked to judge the amount of support needed to perform 20 complex functional activities, four of which relate to communication. These measures lack the specificity one would need to validate results via observations, but the PEDI, at least, provides information about communication functioning in a variety of contexts.

Most disability-level outcome measurements for children with language disorders involve observational coding. Children are observed interacting with people in particular contexts. For example, one might observe whether children request food and related items during snacktime and lunchtime at their preschool. Interactions with other children might be observed during playtime. Patterns of interaction at school or at home can be documented to judge the extent to which relationships or friendships are established. Much of the child language intervention research uses observational schemes for evaluating outcomes. Although some investigators use formal tests of language development to assess impairment, it would appear that much of this literature focuses on the disability level of analysis. Thus, a wealth of outcome measures are available for evaluating disability. What is lacking is a formal assessment designed to assess functional status observationally in a variety of highly relevant contexts. This is not too surprising, given the difficulty one would anticipate in trying to reach a consensus on what contexts to sample. Perhaps the idea is antithetical to the individualized nature of disability and the need to take into consideration communication in individuals' everyday social contexts.

Not only can observations yield representative information about the ways the child communicates with significant others, it also can illuminate how others may be facilitating or inhibiting the child's communication. Information about supports and the use of education strategies is highly relevant to disability measurement. For example, observations might reveal that a mother provides occasional models of phrases at her child's communicative level. An intervention program for the mother might focus on increasing the frequency of her models and targeting a specific communicative structure. Many coding protocols have been developed for research purposes (e.g., Mahoney & Powell, 1988; Rice, Sell, & Hadley, 1990), but can be adapted for practical use. Rating scales or checklists offer an alternative means of measuring the communicative supportiveness of a communication environment. These instruments attempt to identify strategies that are thought to facilitate communication development. The *Communication Environment Checklist* (Rainforth, York, & Macdonald, 1992) and the *Teacher-Child Communication Scale* (Bailey & Roberts, 1987) are two such instruments that focus on classroom environments specifically.

In some cases, general information about environmental supports is not sufficient for designing interventions and evaluating outcomes. Functional analyses can be used to specify antecedents that predict certain behaviors and to identify consequences that maintain specific behaviors (O'Neill, Horner, Albin, Storey, & Sprague, 1990; Reichle & Wacker, 1993). Functional analyses have proven especially useful in helping interventionists design effective interventions for challenging behavior (e.g., Carr & Durand,

1985; Donnellan, Mirenda, Mesaros, & Fassbender, 1984; Reichle & Wacker, 1993). In a functional analysis one records the events and circumstances that precede and follow specific behaviors. Analysis of this information may reveal that some behaviors are in fact functioning as unconventional forms of communication for a child. For example, a child may frequently approach other children and push them or grab their possessions. Functional analysis of these behaviors may reveal that they occurred only in play settings and appeared to be the way that the child entered into the ongoing play of the other children who in turn responded negatively by pushing the child away. As a result of this analysis, one could decide to restrict the focus of observations to opportunities to join group situations, as well as to teach the child more appropriate play entry behaviors (e.g., offering a toy to share; saying "Can I play too?"). If the other children respond positively to the child's new play entry skills then the invasive behavior should stop occurring (e.g., Gallagher & Craig, 1984).

Ecological inventories (Browder, 1991; Falvey, 1989; Rainforth, et al., 1992) offer an approach that acknowledges the need to evaluate the demands and supports for a child's everyday communicative functioning. Ecological inventories can be used to identify skills necessary for functioning in any present or future settings of interest (e.g., arrival or dismissal at school, bedtime or dinnertime at home, shopping at the mall, or taking swimming lessons at the community center). They also reveal how communication skills interface with other skills in the execution of specific tasks, activities, and routines (e.g., entering the classroom and greeting teachers and peers; listening to a story and saying "good night;" requesting food in the cafeteria). The behaviors needed to function in a particular setting can be determined by observing age-matched peers who are not disabled. Then the target child is observed in the same setting to identify discrepancies between the skills used by the target child and those of nondisabled peers. Both instructional objectives and adaptations to the environment can be proposed based on this analysis. An *Assessment of Student Participation in General Education Classes* (Macdonald & York, 1992) lists social and communication skills that assist children in functioning in many school settings.

Relevant functional measures for phonological disorders are intelligibility and severity of involvement. How well can the child be understood by parents, peers, relatives, and others? How severe is the child's problem relative to others with a similar problem? One available procedure for answering these questions is the calculation of percentage of consonants correct in a connected speech sample (PCC; Shriberg & Kwiatkowski, 1982c). The PCC is based on a clinician's judgment of a child's accurate versus inaccurate consonantal productions. Incorrect productions may include, for example, consonant deletions, substitutions, additions, or distortions, with dialectal and allophonic variation set aside. The actual computation involves summing the number of consonants a child produces accurately, dividing this by the number of accurate plus inaccurate consonants produced, and multiplying by 100 for a percentage. Based on the percentage, a qualitative descriptor of severity is assigned: severe, less than 50% accurate consonant production; moderate-severe, 50 to 65% accurate consonant production; mild-moderate, 65 to 85% accurate consonant production; and mild, 85% or greater accurate consonant production. The PCC has construct validity and reliability, but it is cautioned that the age of the child, serious involvements of suprasegmental and prosodic properties of speech, or disorders of expressive language may affect its adequacy (see the *Articulation Competence Index* discussed above). The PCC is recommended for use at entry to treatment, but also may be an indicator of treatment effectiveness as changes in severity may be observed with intervention.

Handicap-level Measurement

Measurement of the social consequences of an impairment or disability in children has not received much attention despite the earnest concerns expressed by families when their child does not talk or respond reliably to language at an early age. Interactions in the home and community can be significantly compromised if a child is unable to communicate effectively. If challenging behaviors, such as aggression and self-injury, develop in lieu of appropriate language skills, then young children are likely to be stigmatized and their social interaction patterns restricted. Young children with language impairments may have particular difficulty establishing positive relationships with their peers (Goldstein & Gallagher, 1992; Goldstein & Kazmarek, 1991). By the time children are of school age, it is clear to families that deficiencies in language development may have profound impacts on their child's ability to advance academically, to interact effectively with adults and children, and to establish meaningful friendships (Aram, Ekelman, & Nation, 1984; Aram & Nation, 1980; Bashir, Wiig, & Abrams, 1987; Bishop & Edmundson, 1987; Hall & Tomblin, 1978; King, Jones, & Lasky, 1982; Schery, 1985; Stark et al., 1984). Limited abilities to succeed in the classroom and in social circles ultimately put children with language disorders at risk for school dropout and low achievement generally.

Particular interest has been paid to measurement of children with specific language impairment. Controversies over the criteria for diagnosis and the poor stability of this diagnosis over time has hindered research on short- and long-term consequences (e.g., Cole et al., 1995; Fazio, Naremore, & Connell, 1996). Nevertheless, Records, Tomblin, and Freese (1992) were able to apply a number of quality-of-life measures to young adults with histories of specific language impairment who had received treatment. Items were derived from the *Index of General Affect* (Campbell, Converse, & Rodgers, 1976), the *Affect Balance Scale* (Bradburn, 1969), the *Satisfaction with Life Scale* (Diener, Emmons, Larsen & Griffin, 1985), and the *Internal-External Locus of Control Scale* (Rotter, 1982). They obtained subjective information about personal happiness and life satisfaction, as well as objective measures of educational, vocational, and family life status. Objective measures showed significant differences in educational attainment and income, as well as in all their language assessments; but no differences were shown in self-report measures of personal well-being and life satisfaction. Records and her colleagues suggest that a high salary or good language skills are not necessarily associated with greater satisfaction with one's life. Although long-term social consequences associated with child language disorders are readily detectable even with less severe disorders, perceptions of those consequences obviously will be judged differently by different people. Keep in mind that the individual with the impairment or disability often is not asked to make that judgment, especially in the case of children. Systems for developing a consensus on subjective judgments among family members may be a difficult task depending on the families, their social contexts, and their cultural backgrounds. In light of such difficulties, one might question whether professionals are in a position to judge social consequences.

It is especially difficult to design outcome measures that could be administered directly to young children, especially those with limited language skills. Measures of sociometric status and self-esteem would seem highly relevant to the handicap level of classification. Although adaptations for younger children have been developed for some of these measures (e.g., Asher, Singleton, Tinsley, & Hymel, 1979), validity and reliability tend to be questionable even with normally developing preschoolers, for example. Consequently, one usually turns to family members and teachers to ask them to judge whether a child's language impairment is resulting in social isolation or an inability to make and keep friends. Observational measures might be useful to judge social affect expressed by a child (e.g., eye contact, smiles, crying).

Another strategy entails evaluation of the impact that children with speech and language impairments have on their families. Research on children with chronic illness may serve as a model. Stein and Riessman (1980), for example, developed a scale for evaluating effects on families across a number of dimensions, such as financial effects and personal strain. They also evaluate social and familial effects, such as friends' and relatives' reactions to the child and the family, and the extent to which free time, activities outside of the home, and relationships may be more limited. The final dimension, mastery, evaluates whether learning to manage the child effectively improves self-esteem or brings the family closer.

Prospective measurement tools for assessing quality of life before and following treatment of a phonological disorder are not yet available. This notwithstanding, recent retrospective studies underscore the necessity for such outcome measurements. Of significance is the fact that these disorders appear to have long-term consequences that potentially affect an individual throughout the lifespan (Bebout & Arthur, 1992; Felsenfeld et al., 1992, 1994; Freeby & Madison, 1989; Lewis, 1990; Shriberg & Kwiatkowski, 1988). In childhood, 50 to 70% of those diagnosed with phonological disorders exhibit general academic difficulty through grade 12 (Aram, Ekelman, & Nation, 1984; Aram & Hall, 1989; Felsenfeld et al., 1994; King, Jones, & Lasky, 1982; Shriberg & Kwiatkowski, 1988). There is an observed relationship between early phonological disorders and subsequent reading, writing, spelling, and mathematic abilities (Bird, Bishop, & Freeman, 1995; Catts, 1993; Catts & Kamhi, 1986; Clarke-Klein & Hodson, 1995; Hoffman, 1990; Hoffman & Norris, 1989; King et al., 1982; Lewis & Freebairn, 1992; Shriberg et al., 1986; Webster & Plante, 1992).

These difficulties seem to persist because retrospective studies have shown that adults who were diagnosed and treated for phonological disorders in childhood continued to have global difficulties in the retrieval, manipulation, and comprehension of linguistic information (Felsenfeld et al., 1992; Felsenfeld et al., 1995; Lewis, Ekelman, & Aram, 1989; Lewis & Freebairn, 1992). On the surface, these adults did not have trouble producing speech sounds, but they had extreme difficulty processing information that pertained to language generally and the sound system in particular. These adults consistently made more errors and were slower to interpret language than other adults with no prior history of phonological disorders (i.e., controls).

Adults with a prior history of a phonological disorder may complete fewer years of formal education, and hold jobs that involve unskilled labor. In another retrospective study (Felsenfeld et al., 1994), 70% of adults with a prior history of a phonological disorder finished high school, but none went on to earn a college degree. This was in contrast to controls with no prior history of the disorder, who typically completed at least one year of college. Similarly, for adults who completed high school, 70% of those with a history of a phonological disorder held an unskilled job; whereas none of the controls with a terminal high school degree held an unskilled position.

The occurrence of a phonological disorder may even have consequences for future generations. An increased rate of phonological disorders has been observed for children when a first-degree relative has been similarly affected (Felsenfeld et al., 1995). If a parent had a phonological disorder, there is greater likelihood that his or her offspring will perform poorly on tests of articulation and will require phonological intervention. The same pattern was not generally observed for children of control parents who did not have phonological disorders in childhood.

Together, these reports hint that, for some individuals and families, a phonological disorder may become a seriously handicapping condition. It must be underscored, however, that those who receive some form of clinical treatment for their phonological disorder have better long-term social, academic, and communication prognoses than those who do not (King et al., 1982; Kwiatkowski & Shriberg, 1993; Shriberg, Gruber et al., 1994; Shriberg, Kwiatkowski et al., 1994). In light of this, we turn our attention to the results of treatment efficacy and outcomes research that document the success of clinical intervention for children with language and phonological disorders.

EFFICACY AND OUTCOMES RESEARCH

Current efficacy and outcomes research for child language and phonological disorders do not speak directly to the WHO classifications of impairment, disability, or handicap. Effective methods of teaching are not associated with these specific classifications; observed behavioral and functional effects of treatment do not differentiate among the classifications; and efficiency of treatment methods is not unique to one classification versus another. Although clinical research on treatment does not yet address the ICIDH categories, the experimental questions that have been raised do bear on the temporal ordering of outcomes, namely intermediate, instrumental, and ultimate outcomes of intervention.

Phonological Treatment

A comprehensive review of treatment efficacy for functional phonological disorders in children may be found in Gierut (in press), with exhaustive references therein. A brief summary is presented below.

Intermediate Outcomes

One line of efficacy research has examined whether phonological treatment is benefiting the child. This addresses intermediate outcomes of phonological treatment because it explores the treatment process itself. What is the structure of a "good" treatment session?

To illustrate, one observation about phonological treatment is that if a sound is taught in a limited set of words, accurate production will extend to other words that also contain that same target sound. A relevant question then is, how many words must be taught to effect this change? Elbert determined that it is necessary to teach a sound in only three to five different words for widespread lexical change (Elbert, Powell, & Swartzlander, 1991). This finding bears importantly on both the structure and economy of an effective clinical program.

As another example, the method of minimal pair treatment has come under experimental scrutiny (Gierut, 1989, 1990a, 1991, 1992; Gierut & Neumann, 1991). Minimal pairs are two words that differ by one sound, as in rhyming words like "sun"–"fun." In its conventional application, minimal pair treatment associates the target sound with its corresponding error substitute. That is, if a child produces [f] as the substitute for target /s/, then the two sounds [f] and [s] would be introduced together and contrasted during treatment. One question that could be asked is why does minimal pair treatment emphasize the errored substitute? Why focus a child's attention on the error pattern? Isn't this precisely what treatment is trying to eliminate? An alternate form of minimal pair treatment was thus introduced whereby a target sound was paired with a *correct* sound from the child's repertoire. This method was found to be more effective in promoting accurate production than the conventional structure of minimal pair treatment. Taking this one step further, why should minimal pair treatment appeal to correct or incorrect aspects of the child's grammar? Perhaps only new information should be introduced, without regard to known sounds in the child's repertoire or to errored substitutes. In answer to this, the pairing of two new target sounds with each other was shown to facilitate the greatest phonological learning. This line of investigation isolated the characteristic properties of minimal pairs that yield the greatest sound change. These conditions provide guidelines about how the method of minimal pair teaching should be structured to achieve the goal of improved sound production.

Instrumental Outcomes

Global and local changes in a child's sound system are two relevant pieces of evidence that demonstrate instrumental outcomes of phonological treatment. *Global change* refers to broad systemwide improvements in the productive sound system and is reflected by changes in untreated sounds and sound classes. *Local change* refers to limited improvements in the treated sound and treated sound class. Together, these two types of demonstrated change trigger the ultimate treatment outcome, namely, a productive sound system that is comparable to that of the surrounding speech community.

Local changes have been reported in efficacy studies that demonstrate: (1) treatment of a sound in one word position extends accurate production of that sound to other word positions; (2) treatment of a sound in syllables extends accuracy to words and, in turn, treatment in words extends accuracy to connected speech; and (3) treatment of one representative aspect of a sound category facilitates improvement across that category of similarly articulated sounds. The latter is known as *within-class generalization* and has been widely documented for all places, manners, and voicing of production. It has also been reflected in the error pattern a child exhibits. To illustrate, treatment of the fricatives /s θ/ enhanced change in other untreated errored fricatives /zð/ (Costello & Onstine, 1976). Similarly, treatment focusing on the error pattern of final consonant deletion facilitated improvements in a broad range of final consonants disrupted by the same pattern (Weiner, 1981).

Global change is associated with *across-class generalization* where improvements extend to categories other than the treated. For phonological systems in particular, across-class generalization has been associated with implicational laws of language. That is, if a language has property X (i.e., marked), it will also have property Y (i.e., unmarked) but not vice versa. This prediction has been shown to hold during treatment for children with phonological disorders in the acquisition of a wide range of known implicational relationships: (1) voiced as opposed to voiceless obstruents (i.e., stops, fricatives, and affricates), (2) voicing of stops in word-final as opposed to word-initial position, (3) fricatives as opposed to stops, (4) clusters as opposed to singletons, and (5) marked clusters as opposed to unmarked clusters.

Ultimate Outcomes

Efficacy research for phonological disorders in children has demonstrated the ecological validity of intervention from clinical and functional perspectives. We know, for example, that phonological treatment enhances sound production and use in spontaneous connected speech, and that treatment improves overall intelligibility of speech. We also know that the effects of clinical treatment, typically conducted in a carefully controlled environment, will extend to other less structured and nonteaching situations. Other intervention outcomes that bear on administrative issues, related to time in treatment, or financial issues, related to cost of treatment, have not received adequate evaluation in the efficacy literature. Social and client-defined outcomes of phonological treatment also have not been widely explored. These are areas that warrant consideration in continuing evaluations of treatment efficacy.

Research Directions

Treatment of functional phonological disorders in children is an established, well-documented form of clinical intervention. To date, the available research has clearly demonstrated the positive effects of such treatment. Children who receive phonological treatment exhibit improved intelligibility and general communicative functioning. There are no known risks involved in the treatment, and the long-term benefits for continued communicative, educational, and social success are beginning to be documented (Shriberg & Kwiatkowski, 1994).

The direction of clinical research for treatment of functional phonological disorders will likely emphasize an integration of measurement tools used in diagnosis with specific methods of treatment and their success. Research priorities include prospective studies that take into account the intensity of treatment needed to facilitate change in disordered sound systems. Development of novel and improved teaching methods is also called for, with maximum utilization of computer technologies. Continued evaluation of relative treatment efficiency is also an important research goal. The direct comparison of different treatment methods, the time it takes to successfully complete these treatments, and the appropriateness of these for different children are all topics to be addressed. Importantly, research that systematically examines the etiology, course, and remediation of functional phonological disorders will ultimately bring us closer to the prevention, diagnosis, and treatment of this communicative disorder that is so prevalent among children.

Child Language Intervention

Intermediate Outcomes

Much of the language intervention literature has sought to determine whether instructional procedures are responsible for improving language performance (see Goldstein & Hockenberger, 1991 for review). The large number of single-subject experimental design studies in the language intervention literature explore treatment outcomes on a session-by-session basis. Outcomes usually are monitored by observing daily in consistent situations and recording the percentage of opportunities or the frequency with which a child uses a targeted language skill. Thus, a large body of literature documents intermediate outcomes of language intervention programs.

The instructional procedures that are thought to be responsible for improved language performance are packaged into treatments with multiple components, which are sometimes difficult to discern. For example, Hepting and Goldstein (1996) sought to analyze the components of 34 studies characterized as "naturalistic language interventions." They identified eight teaching techniques that manipulate antecedent stimuli to set the occasion for, model, or prompt language performance and three teaching techniques that manipulate consequent stimuli to reinforce performance. Their analysis illustrates the difficulty in comparing the outcomes associated with different treatments. They found that even well-established treatment approaches, such as "incidental language teaching," may differ considerably in the instructional techniques included (cf. Hart & Risley, 1968 vs. McGee, Krantz, & McClannahan, 1985). Likewise, interventions may be referred to differently, for example, "environmental language intervention" and "embedded instruction," but are procedurally similar (cf. MacDonald, Blott, Gordon, Spiegel, & Hartmann, 1974 vs. Neef, Walters, & Egel, 1984). So, while numerous studies present evidence of positive outcomes associated with treatment, it is quite difficult to draw conclusions about what treatment approaches are most effective. Treatment comparisons can be costly and counterproductive, unless alternative approaches previously have undergone extensive development, testing, and refinement.

Of the 34 studies Hepting and Goldstein (1996) reviewed, 31 reported specific data on the goals targeted in the intervention; 26 did not assess overall changes in language development, however. The three studies that used only standardized testing to evaluate changes in language abilities before and after intervention apparently assume instrumental or generalized outcomes associated with intervention. They do not document intermediate outcomes and leave us wondering how differently children functioned after intervention. Other reviews of child language intervention approaches (e.g., Kaiser, Yoder, & Keetz, 1992; Tannock & Giralometto, 1992; Reichle, Mirenda, Locke, Piche, & Johnson, 1992) conclude that positive intermediate outcomes are associated with a variety of treatments, namely milieu language teaching, parent-focused language interventions, and augmentative communication system interventions. These authors point out the challenges associated with evaluating instrumental outcomes in particular.

Instrumental Outcomes

Kaiser, Yoder, and Keetz (1992) distinguish between linguistic performance, knowledge, and development as outcomes of intervention. Performance measures should go beyond intermediate outcomes to determine the extent to which changes in child performance persist outside the context of intervention. The majority of language intervention studies include measures that address the issue of generalized performance (Goldstein & Hockenberger, 1991). Generalization might be assessed across tasks, across settings, across trainers (or interaction partners), and across time. Much progress has been made in developing a technology to facilitate generalized performance since Stokes and Baer's (1977) landmark paper admonished interventionists for the "train and hope" strategy. Despite this progress, it is not surprising to find that language intervention appears to produce less impressive generalized performance depending on the number of dimensions that are varied from the training context. When generalization is probed across tasks, settings, *or* trainers it tends to be demonstrated more consistently than if generalization probes vary tasks, settings, *and* trainers (Kaiser et al., 1992).

Changes in generalized knowledge have been assessed in the language intervention literature less frequently. Kaiser et al. (1992) propose three types of evidence of generalized knowledge that might testify to the learning of a new linguistic rule, concept, or response class. Children could demonstrate new knowledge by extending their responses to words not introduced in training, by applying words or concepts to novel stimuli, by demonstrating transfer between comprehension and production, or by generating novel word combinations (recombinative generalization) to fit the communicative context. Development of procedures for promoting these types of outcomes has been a prime focus of independent programs of research (see Goldstein, 1993). In their review of the literature on milieu language teaching, Kaiser et al. (1992) found limited evidence of these types of instrumental outcomes.

Finally, Kaiser et al. (1992) suggest that acquisition of specific skills may be clinically important and may affect the child's functional use of language, but not necessarily affect a child's global language abilities (e.g., MLU). They caution that global measures, such as standardized tests, may not be sensitive to changes in development. They conclude that there is modest evidence that milieu language teaching facilitates children's language development, but none of the studies reviewed were designed specifically to evaluate whether changes in global development would result from milieu teaching.

Ultimate Outcomes

Measures of ultimate outcomes have taken two forms in the child language intervention literature. First, the retrospective studies have assessed long-term outcomes of individuals with language disorders using the type of measures applied to the handicap level of classification described above. One need not look at such long-term sequelae to find evidence of ultimate outcomes. For example, a number of interventions have been successful in facilitating improved interactions among socially withdrawn children with various impairments and their typical peers (e.g., Gallagher & Craig, 1984; Goldstein & Cisar, 1992; Goldstein, English, Shafer, & Kaczmarek, 1997; Haring, Blair, Lee, Breen, & Gaylord-Ross, 1986). Clearly, the development of competent language skills is pivotal to success in school and eventually in the workplace. It is difficult, however, to relate these ultimate outcomes to specific language intervention efforts, because of the variety of teaching and learning experiences to which American children are exposed. There is no doubt that differences in language learning experiences do predict later outcomes. Hart and Risley (1995) and Walker, Greenwood, Hart, and Carta (1994) provide striking evidence of how large disparities in the amount of language stimulation experienced by *typical* children in American homes predict vocabulary growth and later school achievement.

Second, measurement of the social validity of outcomes is becoming increasingly commonplace in the language intervention literature, especially among behavior analysts. Schwartz and Baer (1991) argue that social validity assessment entails obtaining relevant consumers' opinions about "the acceptability of the program goals, methods, personnel, outcomes, and ease of integration of program components into the consumers' current life-style" (p. 190). This view of social validity is perhaps more encompassing than the typical idea of assessing consumer satisfaction.

The first question to address through social validity assessments is what behavior changes are most relevant to the desired outcome of assisting children to communicate more effectively and more independently. Consumers or competent communicators might be asked to list the most desirable behaviors for a particular situation. For example, Runco and Schreibman (1987) asked schoolchildren to view videotapes of children with autism and to identify "unusual behaviors." They used this information to select especially relevant target behaviors. This approach is a worthwhile adjunct to the typical assessment conducted only after intervention. In this case, consumers are asked to view recorded examples sampled from before and after treatment, to judge what behaviors have changed, and to rate the importance of the apparent changes to improvements in the communicative situation.

The question that usually attracts most interest among applied researchers is: What is the social importance of a treatment effect? Likewise, clinicians as well as payers want to know whether consumers are satisfied with behavior changes. These behavior changes include those targeted as part of intervention, as well as those side effects (be they positive or negative) that may not have been anticipated. A common way to assess social validity is to ask parents and teachers to rate improvement. General measures are more likely than specific measures to reflect bias, however. Consumers are especially prone to rate behavior as improved when they are led to believe that performance will improve with training (Garfield, 1983). Therefore, care should be taken to ensure that consumers are basing their judgments on therapeutic effects, rather than on preconceived notions. To obtain "blind" judgments, one might want to select representative samples of several children's performance before and after treatment, to randomize the ordering so that posttreatment recordings do not always follow pretreatment recordings, and to obtain independent judgments of each sample from consumers.

Perhaps the most perplexing question for social validity assessments is: Who should be making such judgments? There are many potential consumers. They include: the children themselves; their family members; their peers; the referral agents, such as teachers, doctors, other professionals; members of the extended community, such as prospective teachers, peers, neighbors; SLPs or other professionals who are familiar with the population and knowledgeable about communication skills. Of course, if our treatment efforts are successful then one would hope that positive outcomes would be readily perceptible to a variety of consumers. Indeed, involving a broad spectrum of consumers in social validity assessments might facilitate higher rates of adoption of our treatment approaches and perhaps help to mobilize community support for effective treatment programs.

Goldstein (1990) presents an alternative approach to assessing clinical significance. A normative comparison approach could be used to determine whether outcomes of intervention are sufficient for the child to be characterized as "within normal limits" (Jacobson & Revenstorf, 1988). This is a strict test of treatment efficacy. In order to argue convincingly that treatment outcomes are clinically significant, the client must appear essentially normal on some relevant outcome measure(s). For example, Osnes, Guevremont, and Stokes (1986) established norms specific to their preschool freeplay setting by recording the amount of talking demonstrated by seven classmates of two socially withdrawn target children. We should consider that many of our clients and their families would be satisfied with improvements in communicative functioning that fall short of normal functioning, however. This may imply the need to be especially cognizant of the appropriate normative population to be used for comparison purposes. For example, what peer comparison group should be applied to judge the outcome of intervention for communication board users? Perhaps it would be appropriate to identify individuals who are functioning satisfactorily (based on disability-level outcomes) and who despite certain impairments are judged not to be in need of treatment.

Currently, researchers lack established conventions for assessing ultimate outcomes of language intervention programs. There is a recognition, however, that good treatment efficacy research includes assessments of clinical significance or social validity. Such measures are important supplements to our primary means of experimental analysis using statistical models or visual inspection of intermediate and instrumental outcomes data.

Research Directions

There is ample evidence of effective treatments for child language disorders. In fact, the bulk of the intervention research has focused on challenging cases, children who are developmentally disabled with quite limited communication systems. Language intervention of various forms has repeatedly resulted in accelerated development of language skills that permit children to function more effectively in a variety of situations. It is reasonable to expect that the most convincing cases for adopting specific treatment procedures require empirical evidence of intermediate, instrumental, and ultimate outcomes. It is not reasonable, however, to expect single studies to accomplish such an ambitious undertaking. Programmatic research is needed to develop effective treatment programs and to evaluate outcomes thoroughly.

Numerous potential themes for future research can be identified. First, research is needed to optimize the efficiency of intervention efforts. We need (1) to clarify what components of treatment packages are most effective; and (2) to learn to take better advantage of procedures that maximize generalized effects of training such as observational learning, recombinative generalization, stimulus equivalence, and crossmodal transfer. Second, research is needed to learn how to incorporate more high quality learning opportunities and effective teaching strategies into children's everyday social circumstances. We need (1) to learn to enhance motivation and avoid generalization problems; (2) to learn how to involve parents, teachers, and peers in language intervention across the day more effectively; (3) to develop alternative modes of communication that are not so slow and cumbersome to be used effectively in everyday situations; and (4) to develop effective procedures to help parents optimize language and literacy stimulation early in development. Third, research is needed to enable SLPs to select relevant target behaviors more effectively. We need (1) to learn how to adapt goals and teaching procedures to the particular needs of children in their social milieu; (2) to develop strategies for addressing the broad range of communicative functions and content that are typical of children; (3) to develop a better understanding of the relationships among different aspects of language as well as other developmental domains; (4) to teach communication skills that help prevent problem behavior, violence, and aggression; and (5) to teach children to use language to mediate self-control and learning. Finally, we need to merge our knowledge of language intervention to develop comprehensive treatments and to evaluate empirically whether we can indeed produce robust effects using outcomes that are relevant to consumers and payers.

CONCLUSION

Despite great strides in the development of evaluation and management strategies for individuals with language and phonological disorders, those developments do not appear to acknowledge different levels of classifying consequences of those disorders. Traditional diagnostic methods and target behavior selection have focused primarily on impairments in phonological and language processes. Treatment researchers have begun to evaluate outcomes with an eye toward functional contexts. Although this approach shifts the focus to disability level outcomes, it still falls short of an assessment of the functional consequences of disorders and associated treatment efforts. Instead of assessing the extent to which a child uses appropriate or newly learned behaviors in functional contexts, one might assess the extent to which the child operates more fully, more effectively, more efficiently, or more independently as a result of treatment. New evaluation procedures (e.g., ecological inventories or social validity assessments) offer strategies for identifying target behaviors as well as social and educational supports that may relate more directly to disability outcomes. Keep in mind that well-developed evaluation tools are not yet available. Therefore, clinicians will need to develop them and/or to tailor them to their clients' particular circumstances. The nature of disability level assessments should make this feasible. However, generating data for comparison purposes using valid and reliable measurement techniques will require further research and development. Perhaps the most difficult challenge is selecting contexts to sample that are sufficiently representative of functional consequences; reaching consensus may be difficult, especially when it is not clear who should be considered "consumers."

The issue that has perhaps received the least attention is the examination of effects of disorders and associated treatments on social outcomes as reflected by quality of life and lifelong achievements. That is not to say that such outcomes have not been produced, but that the target behaviors identified do not always consider such outcomes or goals. More importantly, such outcomes and goals rarely are assessed. Certainly, evaluating social consequences associated with language and phonological disorders is tricky. One would expect the integrity of treatments and their actual and perceived results to vary depending on numerous social factors, for example, the client's family circumstances, their expectations, prevailing cultural values, social supports in the community, and so on. One dilemma is to determine whose assessments of social consequences should be solicited and how much the input from different consumers and stakeholders should be weighed. One might hope that family-centered and culturally sensitive practices would dictate certain evaluation strategies. However, agencies and companies with direct involvement in reimbursement and payment for services are more prone toward more distal or population-based assessments of social consequences of language and phonological disorders. Thus, evaluation and management strategies may differ considerably based on who is asked to judge the extent to which handicaps exist or persist.

Targeting and evaluating outcomes at different levels of classification is an important advance as the field of communication sciences and disorders implements and promotes its services, but it is not sufficient. Much is to be learned about existing treatments. It is doubtful that many treatments have been so well-refined and well-researched to argue that they have been optimized. For example, little is known about how long and with what intensity treatments should be administered to optimize their benefits.

Many new treatment approaches are under investigation and more are ripe for development. For example, powerful computers are becoming increasingly accessible, but their potential as teaching tools has not been realized. Presently, the development of appropriate and sophisticated instructional technology and software continues to lag behind hardware capabilities. Likewise, rich opportunities exist for evaluating how speech and language treatments can best be incorporated within a child's everyday life. We need to explore the effectiveness of interventions to promote language and literacy development in the home long before children reach preschool age (cf. Hart & Risley, 1995). Recent advances have shown the potential for parents, siblings, peers, and teachers as well as SLPs to serve as intervention agents. We need to explore ways to optimize the effectiveness of their efforts focusing on different levels of outcomes. Once treatment strategies have been developed to address important target behaviors and generalization can be achieved across tasks, settings, and persons, it would make sense to compare outcomes associated with different treatments.

The focus on outcomes provided in this volume reinforces the need for programmatic research on the evaluation and management of language and phonological disorders in children. We have reviewed a number of approaches to the development of outcome measures. Not only will groundwork in assessment techniques better enable clinicians and researchers to assess the effects of treatment, but it will influence the development of treatment approaches as well. Sensitizing clinicians to disability level outcomes, for example, is likely to yield new perspectives on goal selection. It would be a mistake to think that single studies can develop new treatments, produce robust effects, and assess a full continuum of possible outcomes, however. These needs would be better addressed by investigative teams who conduct a series of studies through programs of research. Furthermore, a premature rush to compare treatments may be ill-advised. A broader conceptualization of clinical outcomes and outcomes research may help us realize the need to generate important new knowledge in the field. Hence, an infusion of clinical research training in the field and a larger pool of clinical scientists is needed to produce programs of research that maximize outcomes along the continuum of impairment, disability, and handicap in children with language and phonological disorders.

ACKNOWLEDGMENTS

Preparation of this chapter was supported in part by grants from the U.S. Department of Education (H023C10167 and H086R3011) to the University of Pittsburgh, Howard

Goldstein, Principal Investigator. The authors are grateful to Nancy Hepting for her assistance in preparing this chapter. Preparation of the sections on phonological disorders was supported in part by grants from the National Institutes of Health (R01 DC01694, K04 DC00076) to Indiana University, Judith A. Gierut, Principal Investigator. Jessica Barlow provided invaluable editorial assistance and commentary.

REFERENCES

Aram, D., Ekelman, B., & Nation, J. (1984). Preschoolers with language disorders: 10 years later. *Journal of Speech and Hearing Research, 27,* 232–244.

Aram, D. M., & Hall, N. E. (1989). Longitudinal follow-up of children with preschool communication disorders: Treatment implications. *School Psychology Review, 18,* 487–501.

Aram, D. M., & Nation, J. E. (1980). Preschool language disorders and subsequent language and academic difficulties. *Journal of Communication Disorders, 13,* 159–170.

Asher, S. R., Singleton, L. C., Tinsley, B. R., & Hymel, S. (1979). A reliable sociometric measure for preschool children. *Developmental Psychology, 15,* 443–444.

Bailey, D., & Roberts, J. E. (1987). *Teacher-child communication scale.* Chapel Hill, NC: University of North Carolina.

Bain, B., Olswang, L. B., & Johnson, G. A. (1992). *Topics in Language Disorders, 12*(2), 13–27.

Bankson, N. W., & Bernthal, J. E. (1990). *Bankson-Bernthal Test of Phonology.* San Antonio, TX: Special Press.

Bashir, A. S., Wiig, E. H., & Abrams, J. C. (1987). Language disorders in childhood and adolescence: Implications for learning and socialization. *Pediatric Annals, 16,* 145–156.

Bebout, L., & Arthur, B. (1992). Cross-cultural attitudes toward speech disorders. *Journal of Speech and Hearing Research, 35,* 45–52.

Bernhardt, B. (1992a). The application of nonlinear phonological theory to intervention with one phonologically disordered child. *Clinical Linguistics & Phonetics, 6,* 283–316.

Bernhardt, B. (1992b). Developmental implications of nonlinear phonological theory. *Clinical Linguistics & Phonetics, 6,* 259–281.

Bernhardt, B., & Stoel-Gammon, C. (1994). Nonlinear phonology: Introduction and clinical application. *Journal of Speech and Hearing Research, 37,* 123–143.

Bernthal, J. E., & Bankson, N. W. (1993). *Articulation and phonological disorders* (3rd ed.). Englewood Cliffs, NJ: Prentice Hall.

Bird, J., Bishop, D. V. M., & Freeman, N. H. (1995). Phonological awareness and literacy development in children with expressive phonological impairments. *Journal of Speech and Hearing Research, 38,* 446–462.

Bishop, D. V. M., & Edmundson, A. (1987). Language-impaired 4-year-olds: Distinguishing transient from persistent impairment. *Journal of Speech and Hearing Disorders, 52,* 156–173.

Bradburn, N. M. (1969). *The structure of psychological well-being.* Chicago: Aldine.

Braun, S. L., & Granger, C. V. (1991). A practical approach to functional assessment in pediatrics. *Occupational Therapy Practice, 2,* 46–51.

Bricker, D. (1992). *Assessment, evaluation, and programming system (AEPS) for infants and children: Vol 1, AEPS measurement for birth to three years.* Baltimore: Paul Brookes.

Broen, P. A., Strange, W., Doyle, S. S., & Heller, J. H. (1983). Perception and production of approximant consonants by normal and articulation-delayed preschool children. *Journal of Speech and Hearing Research, 26,* 601–608.

Browder, D. (1991). *Assessment of individuals with severe disabilities: An applied behavior approach to life skills assessment* (2nd Ed.). Baltimore: Paul Brookes.

Camarata, S. M., & Schwartz, R. G. (1985). Production of object words and action words: Evidence for a relationship between phonology and semantics. *Journal of Speech and Hearing Research, 28*, 323–330.

Campbell, A., Converse, P.E., & Rodgers, W. L. (1976). *The quality of life of American life.* New York: Russell Sage Foundation.

Campbell, T. F., & Shriberg, L. D. (1982). Associations among pragmatic functions, linguistic stress, and natural phonological processes in speech-delayed children. *Journal of Speech and Hearing Research, 25*, 547–553.

Carr, E. G., & Durand, V. M. (1985). Reducing behavior problems through functional communication training. *Journal of Applied Behavior Analysis, 18*, 111–126.

Catts, H. W. (1993). The relationship between speech-language impairments and reading disabilities. *Journal of Speech and Hearing Research, 36*, 948–958.

Catts, H. W., & Kamhi, A. G. (1986). The linguistic basis of reading disorders: Implications for the speech-language pathologist. *Language, Speech, and Hearing Services in Schools, 17*, 329–341.

Chiat, S. (1994). From lexical access to lexical output: What is the problem for children with impaired phonology? In M. Yavas (Ed.), *First and second language phonology* (pp. 107–133). San Diego, CA: Singular.

Churchill, J. D., Hodson, B. W., Jones, B. W., & Novak, R. E. (1988). Phonological systems of speech-disordered clients with positive/negative histories of otitis media. *Language, Speech, and Hearing Services in Schools, 19*, 100–107.

Clarke-Klein, S., & Hodson, B. W. (1995). A phonologically based analysis of misspellings by third graders with disordered-phonology histories. *Journal of Speech and Hearing Research, 38*, 839–849.

Cole, K. N., Schwartz, I. S., Notari, A. R., Dale, P. S., & Mills, P. E. (1995). Examination of the stability of two methods of defining specific language impairment. *Applied Psycholinguistics, 16*, 103–123.

Conture, E. G., Louko, L. J., & Edwards, M. L. (1993). Simultaneously treating stuttering and disordered phonology in children: Experimental treatment, preliminary findings. *American Journal of Speech-Language Pathology, 2*, 72–81.

Costello, J., & Onstine, J. (1976). The modification of multiple articulation errors based on distinctive feature theory. *Journal of Speech and Hearing Disorders, 41*, 199–215.

Dean, E. C., Howell, J., Waters, D., & Reid, J. (1995). Metaphon: A metalinguistic approach to the treatment of phonological disorder in children. *Clinical Linguistics & Phonetics, 9*, 1–19.

Diener, E., Emmons, R. A., Larsen, R. J., & Griffin, S. (1985). The Satisfaction With Life Scale. *Journal of Personality Assessment, 49*, 71–75.

Dinnsen, D. A. (1984). Methods and empirical issues in analyzing functional misarticulation. In M. Elbert, D. A. Dinnsen, & G. Weismer (Eds.), *Phonological theory and the misarticulating child (ASHA Monographs No. 22)* (pp. 5–17). Rockville, MD: ASHA.

Dodd, B., Leahy, J., & Hambly, G. (1989). Phonological disorders in children: Underlying cognitive deficits. *British Journal of Developmental Psychology, 7*, 55–71.

Donnellan, A. M., Mirenda, P. L., Mesaros, R. A., & Fassbender, L. L. (1984). Analyzing the communicative functions of aberrant behavior. *Journal of the Association for Persons with Severe Handicaps, 9*, 201–212.

Dunn L., & Dunn, L. (1981). *Peabody picture vocabulary test—Revised.* Circle Pines, MN: American Guidance Service.

Edwards, M. L., & Shriberg, L. D. (1983). *Phonology: Applications in communicative disorders.* San Diego, CA: College-Hill.

Elbert, M. (1992). Consideration of error types: A response to Fey. *Language, Speech, and Hearing Services in Schools, 23*, 241–246.

Elbert, M., Powell, T. W., & Swartzlander, P. (1991). Toward a technology of generalization: How many exemplars are sufficient? *Journal of Speech and Hearing Research, 34*, 81–87.

Falvey, M. (1989). *Community-based curriculum: Instructional strategies for students with severe handicaps* (2nd Ed.). Baltimore: Paul Brookes.

Fazio, B. B., Naremore, R. C., & Connell, P. J. (1996). Tracking children from poverty at risk for specific language impairment: A 3-year longitudinal study. *Journal of Speech and Hearing Research, 39,* 611–624.

Felsenfeld, S., Broen, P. A., & McGue, M. (1992). A 28-year follow-up of adults with a history of moderate phonological disorder: Linguistic and personality results. *Journal of Speech and Hearing Research, 35,* 1114–1125.

Felsenfeld, S., Broen, P. A., & McGue, M. (1994). A 28-year follow-up of adults with a history of moderate phonological disorder: Educational and occupational results. *Journal of Speech and Hearing Research, 37,* 1341–1353.

Felsenfeld, S., McGue, M., & Broen, P. A. (1995). Familial aggregation of phonological disorders: Results from a 28-year follow-up. *Journal of Speech and Hearing Research, 38,* 1091–1107.

Ferguson, C. A., Menn, L., & Stoel-Gammon, C. (Eds.). (1992). *Phonological development: Models, research, implications.* Timonium, MD: York.

Fey, M. E. (1992). Articulation and phonology: Inextricable constructs in speech pathology. *Language, Speech, and Hearing Services in the Schools, 23,* 225–232.

Fey, M. E., Cleave, P. L., Ravida, A. I., Long, S. H., Dejmal, A. E., & Easton, D. L. (1994). Effects of grammar facilitation on the phonological performance of children with speech and language impairments. *Journal of Speech and Hearing Research, 37,* 594–607.

Folkins, J. W., & Bleile, K. M. (1990). Taxonomies in biology, phonetics, phonology, and speech motor control. *Journal of Speech and Hearing Disorders, 55,* 596–611.

Freeby, N., & Madison, C. L. (1989). Children's perceptions of peers with articulation disorders. *Child Study Journal, 19,* 133–144.

Feuerstein, R. (1979). *The dynamic assessment of retarded performers.* Baltimore: University Park Press.

Gallagher, T. M., & Craig, H. K. (1984). Pragmatic assessment: Analysis of a highly frequent repeated utterance. *Journal of Speech and Hearing Disorders, 49,* 368–377.

Garfield, S. (1983). Some comments on consumer satisfaction in behavior therapy. *Behavior Therapy, 14,* 237–241.

Gierut, J. A. (1989). Maximal opposition approach to phonological treatment. *Journal of Speech and Hearing Disorders, 54,* 9–19.

Gierut, J. A. (1990a). Differential learning of phonological oppositions. *Journal of Speech and Hearing Research, 33,* 540–549.

Gierut, J. A. (1990b). Linguistic foundations of language teaching: Phonology. *Journal of Speech-Language Pathology and Audiology, 14,* 5–21.

Gierut, J. A. (1991). Homonymy in phonological change. *Clinical Linguistics & Phonetics, 5,* 119–137.

Gierut, J. A. (1992). The conditions and course of clinically-induced phonological change. *Journal of Speech and Hearing Research, 35,* 1049–1063.

Gierut, J. A. (in press). Treatment efficacy for functional phonological disorders in children. *Journal of Speech and Hearing Research.*

Gierut, J. A., & Neumann, H. J. (1991). Teaching and learning /θ/: A nonconfound. *Clinical Linguistics & Phonetics, 6,* 191–200.

Goldman, R., & Fristoe, M. (1986). *Goldman-Fristoe Test of Articulation.* Circles Pines, MN: American Guidance Service.

Goldstein, H. (1990). Assessing clinical significance. In L. B. Olswang, C. K. Thompson, S. F. Warren, & N. J. Minghetti (Eds.), *Treatment efficacy research in communication disorders* (pp. 91–98). Rockville, MD: American Speech-Language-Hearing Foundation.

Goldstein, H. (1993). Structuring environmental input to facilitate generalized language learning by children with mental retardation. In A. Kaiser & D. Gray (Eds)., *Enhancing Children's Communication: Research foundations for intervention* (pp. 317–334). Baltimore, MD: Paul Brookes.

Goldstein, H., & Cisar, C. L. (1992). Promoting interaction during sociodramatic play: Teaching scripts to typical preschoolers and classmates with handicaps. *Journal of Applied Behavior Analysis, 25,* 265–280.

Goldstein, H., English, K., Shafer, K., & Kaczmarek, L. (1997). Interaction among preschoolers with and without disabilities: Effects of across-the-day peer intervention. *Journal of Speech, Language, and Hearing Research; 40,* 33–48.

Goldstein, H., & Gallagher, T. M. (1992). Strategies for promoting the social-communicative competence of young children with specific language impairment. In S. L. Odom, S. R. McConnell, & M. A. McEvoy (Eds.), *Social competence of young children with disabilities* (pp. 189–213). Baltimore: Paul H. Brookes.

Goldstein, H., & Hockenberger, E. H. (1991). Significant progress in child language intervention: An 11-year retrospective. *Research in Developmental Disabilities, 12,* 401–424.

Goldstein, H., & Kaczmarek, L. (1991). Promoting communicative interaction among children in integrated intervention settings. In S. Warren & J. Reichle (Eds.), *Causes and effects in communication and language intervention* (pp. 81–111). Baltimore: Paul Brookes.

Haley, S. M., Coster, W. J., Ludlow, L. H., Haltiwanger, J. T., & Andrellos, P. J. (1992). *Pediatric evaluation of disability inventory, Version 1.0.* Boston, MA: New England Medical Center Hospitals, Inc.

Hall, P. K., & Tomblin, J. B. (1978). A follow-up study of children with articulation and language disorders. *Journal of Speech and Hearing Disorders, 52,* 227–241.

Haring, T. G., Blair, R., Lee, M., Breen, C., & Gaylord-Ross, R. (1986). Teaching social language to moderately handicapped students. *Journal of Applied Behavior Analysis, 19,* 159–171.

Hart, B. M., & Risley, T. R. (1968). Establishing the use of descriptive adjectives in the spontaneous speech of disadvantaged preschool children. *Journal of Applied Behavior Analysis, 1,* 109–120.

Hart, B., & Risley, T.R. (1995). *Meaningful Differences in the Everyday Experience of Young American Children.* Baltimore: Paul H. Brookes.

Hedrick, D., Prather, E., & Tobin, A. (1984). *Sequenced inventory of communicative development—Revised.* Seattle, WA: University of Washington Press.

Hepting, N. H., & Goldstein, H. (1996). What's "natural" about naturalistic language intervention? *Journal of Early Intervention, 20,* 250–264.

Himmelwright-Gross, G., St. Louis, K., Ruscello, D., & Hull, F. (1985). Language abilities of articulatory-disordered school children with multiple or residual errors. *Language, Speech, and Hearing Services in Schools, 16,* 171–186.

Hodson, B. W. (1986). *The Assessment of Phonological Processes—Revised.* Austin, TX: Pro-Ed.

Hoffman, P. R. (1990). Spelling, phonology, and the speech-language pathologist: A whole language perspective. *Language, Speech, and Hearing Services in Schools, 21,* 238–243.

Hoffman, P. R. (1992). Synergistic development of phonetic skill. *Language, Speech, and Hearing Services in Schools, 23,* 254–260.

Hoffman, P. R., & Daniloff, R. G. (1990). Evolving views of children's disordered speech sound production: From motoric to phonological. *Journal of Speech Language Pathology and Audiology, 14,* 13–22.

Hoffman, P. R., & Norris, J. A. (1989). On the nature of phonological development: Evidence from normal children's spelling errors. *Journal of Speech and Hearing Research, 32,* 787–794.

Hoffman, P., Schuckers, G., & Daniloff, R. (1989). *Children's phonetic disorders: Theory and treatment.* Austin, TX: Pro-Ed.

Horstmeister, D.S., & MacDonald, J.M.. (1978). *Environmental Prelanguage Battery.* Columbus, OH: Charles Merrill.

Hresko, W.P., Reid, D.K., & Hammill, D. (1981). *Test of early language development.* Austin, TX: Pro-Ed.

Ingram, D. (1981). *Procedures for the phonological analysis of children's language.* Baltimore: University Park.

Ingram, D. (1989). *Phonological disability in children* (2nd ed.). San Diego, CA: Singular.

Jacobson, N., & Revenstorf, D. (1988). Statistics for assessing the clinical significance of psychotherapy techniques: Issues problems, and new developments. *Behavioral Assessment, 10,* 133–145.

Johnson, A. F., Shelton, R. L., & Arndt, W. B. (1982). A technique for identifying the subgroup membership of certain misarticulating children. *Journal of Speech and Hearing Research, 25,* 162–166.

Kaiser, A. P., Yoder, P. J., & Keetz, A. (1992). Evaluating milieu teaching. In S. F. Warren & J. Reichle (Eds.), *Causes and effects in communication and language intervention* (pp. 9–47). Baltimore: Paul H. Brookes.

Kamhi, A. G. (1992). The need for a broad-based model of phonological disorders. *Language, Speech, and Hearing Services in Schools, 23,* 261–268.

King, R. R., Jones, C., & Lasky, E. (1982). In retrospect: A fifteen-year follow-up report of speech-language-disordered children. *Language, Speech, and Hearing Services in Schools, 13,* 24–32.

Klee, T. (1992a). Measuring children's conversational language. In S. F. Warren & J. Reichle (Eds.), *Causes and effects in communication and language intervention* (pp. 315–330). Baltimore: Paul H. Brookes.

Klee, T. (1992b). Developmental and diagnostic characteristics of quantitative measures of children's language production. *Topics in Language Disorders, 12*(2), 28–41.

Klein, M. D., Wulz, S. V., Hall, M., Waldo, L., Carpenter, S., Lathan, D., Myers, S., Fox, T., & Marshall, A. (1981). *Comprehensive communication curriculum guide.* Lawrence, KS: Early Childhood Institute, University of Kansas.

Kwiatkowski, J., & Shriberg, L. D. (1993). Speech normalization in developmental phonological disorders: A retrospective study of capability-focus theory. *Language, Speech, and Hearing Services in Schools, 24,* 10–18.

Leonard, L. B. (1973). The nature of disordered articulation. *Journal of Speech and Hearing Disorders, 38,* 156–161.

Leonard, L. B., Schwartz, R. G., Swanson, L., & Loeb, D. (1987). Some conditions that promote unusual phonological behavior in children. *Clinical Linguistics & Phonetics, 1,* 23–34.

Lewis, B. A. (1990). Familial phonological disorders: Four pedigrees. *Journal of Speech and Hearing Disorders, 55,* 160–170.

Lewis, B. A., Ekelman, B. L., & Aram, D. M. (1989). A familial study of severe phonological disorders. *Journal of Speech and Hearing Research, 32,* 713–724.

Lewis, B. A., & Freebairn, L. (1992). Residual effects of preschool phonology disorders in grade school, adolescence, and adulthood. *Journal of Speech and Hearing Research, 35,* 819–831.

Lewis, B. A., & Freebairn, L. (1993). A clinical tool for evaluating the familial basis of speech and language disorders. *American Journal of Speech-Language Pathology, 2,* 38–43.

Linder, T. (1992). *Transdisciplinary play-based assessment: A functional approach to working with young children.* Baltimore: Paul Brookes.

Locke, J. L. (1980a). The inference of speech perception in the phonologically disordered child. Part I: A rationale, some criteria, the conventional tests. *Journal of Speech and Hearing Disorders, 45,* 431–444.

Locke, J. L. (1980b). The inference of speech perception in the phonologically disordered child. Part II: Some clinically novel procedures, their use, some findings. *Journal of Speech and Hearing Disorders, 45,* 445–468.

Locke, J. L. (1983). Clinical phonology: The explanation and treatment of speech sound disorders. *Journal of Speech and Hearing Disorders, 48,* 339–341.

Louko, L. J., Edwards, M. L., & Conture, E. G. (1990). Phonological characteristics of young stutterers and their normally fluent peers: Preliminary observations. *Journal of Fluency Disorders, 15,* 191–210.

Lund, N. J., & Duchan, J. F. (1993). *Assessing children's language in naturalistic contexts*. Englewood Cliffs, NJ: Prentice Hall.

MacDonald, J. (1978). *Environmental language intervention program*. Columbus, OH: Charles Merrill.

MacDonald, J. D., Blott, J. P., Gordon, K., Spiegel, B., & Hartmann, M. (1974). An experimental parent-assisted treatment program for preschool language-delayed children. *Journal of Speech and Hearing Disorders, 39*, 395–415.

Macdonald, C., & York, J. (1992). An assessment of student participation in general education classes. In B. Rainforth, J. York, & C. Macdonald (Eds.), *Collaborative teams for students with severe disabilities* (pp. 256–257). Baltimore: Paul Brookes.

MacWhinney, B. (1991). *The CHILDES Project: Tools for analyzing talk*. Hilsdale, NJ: Erlbaum.

Mahoney, G., & Powell, A. (1988). Modifying parent-child interaction: Enhancing the development of handicapped children. *Journal of Special Education, 22*, 82–96.

McCabe, M. A., & Granger, C. V. (1990). Content validity of a pediatric functional independence measure. *Applied Nursing Research, 3*, 120–122.

McCauley, R. J., & Demetras, M. J. (1990). The identification of language impairment in the selection of specifically language-impaired subjects. *Journal of Speech and Hearing Disorders, 55*, 468–475.

McCauley, R. J., & Swisher, L. (1984). Psychometric review of language and articulation tests for preschool children. *Journal of Speech and Hearing Disorders, 49*, 34–42.

McGee, G. G., Krantz, P. J., & McClannahan, L. E. (1985). The facilitative effects of incidental teaching on preposition use by autistic children. *Journal of Applied Behavior Analysis, 18*, 17–31.

McGregor, K. K., & Schwartz, R. G. (1992). Converging evidence for underlying phonological representations in a child who misarticulates. *Journal of Speech and Hearing Research, 35*, 596–603.

Miller, J. F. (1981). *Assessing language production in children: Experimental Procedures*. Austin, TX: Pro-Ed.

Miller, J., & Chapman, R. (1986). *Systematic analysis of language transcripts (SALT1)* [Computer software]. Madison, WI: University of Wisconsin, Language Analysis Lab.

Minick, N. (1987). Implications of Vygotsky's theories for dynamic assessment. In C. Lidz (Ed.). *Dynamic assessment: An interactional approach to evaluating learning potential* (pp. 116–140). New York: Guilford Press.

Mirenda, P. L., & Donnellan, A. M. (1986). Effects of adult interactive style on conversational behavior in students with severe communication problems. *Language, Speech and hearing Services in the Schools, 17*, 126–141.

National Institute on Deafness and Other Communication Disorders. (1991). *National strategic research plan for balance and the vestibular system and language and language impairments* (NIH Publication No. 91–3217). Bethesda, MD: Author.

National Institute on Deafness and Other Communication Disorders (1994). *National strategic research plan*. Bethesda, MD: Department of Health and Human Services.

National Institutes of Health, National Advisory Neurological Disorders and Stroke Council. (1990, June). Decade of the brain: Implementation plan. Bethesda, MD: Author.

Neef, N. A., Walters, J., & Egel, A. L. (1984). Establishing generative yes/no responses in developmentally disabled children. *Journal of Applied Behavior Analysis, 17*, 453–460.

Newborg, J., Stock, J. R., Wnek, L., Guidubaldi, J., & Svinicki, J. (1984). *Battelle developmental inventory*. Allen, TX: DLM Resources.

Nicolosi, L., Harryman, E., & Kresheck, J. (1989). *Terminology of communication disorders*. Baltimore: Williams & Wilkins.

Olswang, L. B., Bain, B. A., & Johnson, G. A. (1992). Using dynamic assessment with children with language disorders. In S. F. Warren & J. Reichle (Eds.), *Causes and effects in communication and language intervention* (pp. 187–215). Baltimore: Paul H. Brookes.

O'Neill, R., Horner, R., Albin, R., Storey, K., & Sprague, J. (1990). *Functional analysis of problem behavior: A practical assessment guide.* Sycamore, IL: Sycamore Publishing.

Osnes, P. G., Guevremont, D. C., & Stokes, T. F. (1986). If I say I'll talk more, then I will: Correspondence training to increase peer-directed talk by socially withdrawn children. *Behavior Modification, 10,* 287–299.

Owens, R. E. (1995). *Language disorders: A functional approach to assessment and intervention.* Boston: Allyn & Bacon.

Paden, E. P., Matthies, M. L., & Novak, M. A. (1989). Recovery from OME-related phonologic delay following tube placement. *Journal of Speech and Hearing Disorders, 54,* 94–100.

Paden, E. P., Novak, M. A., & Beiter, A. L. (1987). Predictors of phonological inadequacy in young children prone to otitis media. *Journal of Speech and Hearing Disorders, 52,* 232–241.

Panagos, J. M., & Prelock, P. A. (1982). Phonological constraints on the sentence production of language-disordered children. *Journal of Speech and Hearing Research, 25,* 171–177.

Paul, R., & Jennings, P. (1992). Phonological behavior in toddlers with slow expressive language development. *Journal of Speech and Hearing Research, 35,* 99–107.

Paul, R., & Shriberg, L. D. (1982). Associations between phonology and syntax in speech-delayed children. *Journal of Speech and Hearing Research, 25,* 536–547.

Rainforth, B., York, J., & Macdonald, C. (1992). *Collaborative teams for students with severe disabilities.* Baltimore: Paul Brookes.

Records, N. L., Tomblin, J. B., & Freese, P. R. (1992). The quality of life of young adults with histories of specific language impairment. *American Journal of Speech-Language Pathology, 1,* 44–53.

Reichle, J., Mirenda, P., Locke, P., Piche, L., & Johnson, S. (1992). Beginning augmentative communication systems. In S. F. Warren & J. Reichle (Eds.), *Causes and effects in communication and language intervention* (pp. 131–156). Baltimore: Paul H. Brookes.

Reichle, J., & Wacker, D. (Eds.) (1993). *Communicative alternatives to challenging behavior: Integrating functional assessment and intervention strategies.* Baltimore: Paul Brookes.

Rice, M. L., Sell, M. A., & Hadley, P. A. (1990). The social-interactive coding system (SICS): An on-line clinically-relevant descriptive tool. *Language, Speech, and Hearing Services in Schools, 21,* 2–14.

Roberts, E. J., Burchinal, M. R., Koch, M. A., Footo, M. M., & Henderson, F. W. (1988). Otitis media in early childhood and its relationship to later phonological development. *Journal of Speech and Hearing Disorders, 53,* 424–432.

Rotter, J. B. (1982). *Developmental applications of social learning theory.* New York: Praeger.

Runco, M., & Schreibman, L. (1987). Socially validating behavioral objectives in the treatment of autistic children. *Journal of Autism and Developmental Disorders, 17,* 141–147.

Ruscello, D. M., St. Louis, K. O., & Mason, N. (1991). School-aged children with phonologic disorders: Coexistence with other speech/language disorders. *Journal of Speech and Hearing Research, 34,* 236–242.

Rvachew, S., & Jamieson, D. G. (1989). Perception of voiceless fricatives by children with a functional articulation disorder. *Journal of Speech and Hearing Disorders, 54,* 193–208.

Schery, T. K. (1985). Correlates of language development in language disordered children. *Journal of Speech and Hearing Disorders, 50,* 73–83.

Schwartz, I. S., & Baer, D. M. (1991). Social validity assessments: Is current practice state of the art? *Journal of Applied Behavior Analysis, 24,* 189–204.

Schwartz, R. G. (1992). Clinical applications of recent advances in phonological theory. *Language, Speech, and Hearing Services in Schools, 23,* 269–276.

Schwartz, R. G, Leonard, L., Folger, M., & Wilcox, M. (1980). Evidence for a synergistic view of language disorders: Early phonological behavior in normal and language disordered children. *Journal of Speech and Hearing Disorders, 45,* 357–377.

Shriberg, L. D. (1993). Four new speech and prosody-voice measures for genetics research and other studies in developmental phonological disorders. *Journal of Speech and Hearing Research, 36*, 105–140.

Shriberg, L. D., Gruber, F. A., & Kwiatkowski, J. (1994). Developmental phonological disorders III: Long-term speech-sound normalization. *Journal of Speech and Hearing Research, 37*, 1151–1177.

Shriberg, L. D., & Kwiatkowski, J. (1982a). Phonological disorders I: A diagnostic classification system. *Journal of Speech and Hearing Disorders, 47*, 226–241.

Shriberg, L. D., & Kwiatkowski, J. (1982b). Phonological disorders II: A conceptual framework for management. *Journal of Speech and Hearing Disorders, 47*, 242–256.

Shriberg, L. D., & Kwiatkowski, J. (1982c). Phonological disorders III: A procedure for assessing severity of involvement. *Journal of Speech and Hearing Disorders, 47*, 256–270.

Shriberg, L. D., & Kwiatkowski, J. (1988). A follow-up study of children with phonologic disorders of unknown origin. *Journal of Speech and Hearing Disorders, 53*, 144–155.

Shriberg, L. D., & Kwiatkowski, J. (1994). Developmental phonological disorders I: A clinical profile. *Journal of Speech and Hearing Research, 37*, 1100–1126.

Shriberg, L. D., Kwiatkowski, J., Best, S., Hengst, J., & Terselic-Weber, B. (1986). Characteristics of children with phonological disorders of unknown origin. *Journal of Speech and Hearing Disorders, 51*, 140–161.

Shriberg, L. D., Kwiatkowski, J., & Gruber, F. A. (1994). Developmental phonological disorders II: Short-term speech-sound normalization. *Journal of Speech and Hearing Research, 37*, 1127–1150.

Shriberg, L. D., & Smith, A. J. (1983). Phonological correlates of middle-ear involvement in speech-delayed children: A methodological note. *Journal of Speech and Hearing Research, 26*, 293–297.

Smit, A. B., & Bernthal, J. E. (1983). Voicing contrasts and their phonological implications in the speech of articulation-disordered children. *Journal of Speech and Hearing Research, 26*, 486–500.

Stackhouse, J., & Wells, B. (1993). Psycholinguistic assessment of developmental speech disorders. *European Journal of Disorders of Communication, 28*, 331–348.

Stark, R. E., Bernstein, L. E., Condino, R., Bender, M., Tallal, P., & Catts, H. (1984). Four-year follow-up study of language impaired children. *Annals of Dyslexia, 34*, 49–68.

Stein, R. E. K., & Riessman, C. K. (1980). The development of an Impact-on-Family Scale: Preliminary findings. *Medical Care, 18*, 465–472.

Stoel-Gammon, C. (1985). Phonetic inventories, 15–22 months: A longitudinal study. *Journal of Speech and Hearing Research, 28*, 505–512.

Stokes, T. F., & Baer, D. M. (1977). An implicit technology of generalization. *Journal of Applied Behavior Analysis, 10*, 349–367.

Tannock, R., & Girolametto, L. (1992). Reassessing parent-focused language intervention programs. In S. F. Warren & J. Reichle (Eds.), *Causes and effects in communication and language intervention* (pp. 49–79). Baltimore: Paul H. Brookes.

Terman, D. L., Larner, M. B., Stevenson, C. S. & Behrman, R. E. (1996). Special education for students with disabilities: Analysis and recommendations. *The Future of Children, 6*, 4–24

Throneburg, R. N., Yairi, E., & Paden, E. P. (1994). Relation between phonologic difficulty and the occurrence of disfluencies in the early stage of stuttering. *Journal of Speech and Hearing Research, 37*, 504–509.

Tyler, A. A. (1992). Profiles of the relationship between phonology and language in late talkers. *Child Language Teaching and Therapy, 8*, 246–264.

Tyler, A. A., & Sandoval, K. T. (1994). Preschoolers with phonological and language disorders: Treating different linguistic domains. *Language, Speech, and Hearing Services in Schools, 25*, 215–234.

Tyler, A., & Watterson, K. (1991). Effects of phonological versus language intervention in preschoolers with both phonological and language impairment. *Child Language Teaching and Therapy, 7,* 141–160.

Walker, D., Greenwood, C. R., Hart, B., & Carta, J. (1994). Prediction of school outcomes based on early language production and socioeconomic factors. *Child Development, 65,* 606–621.

Webster, P. E., & Plante, A. S. (1992). Effects of phonological impairment on word, syllable, and phoneme segmentation and reading. *Language, Speech, and Hearing Services in Schools, 23,* 176–182.

Weiner, F. F. (1981). Treatment of phonological disability using the method of meaningful minimal contrast: Two case studies. *Journal of Speech and Hearing Disorders, 46,* 97–103.

Winitz, H. (1975). *From syllable to conversation.* Baltimore: University Park.

Wolk, L., Edwards, M. L., & Conture, E. G. (1993). Coexistence of stuttering and disordered phonology in young children. *Journal of Speech and Hearing Research, 36,* 906–917.

Yoder, P. J., & Davies, B. (1990). Do parental questions and topic continuations elicit developmentally delayed children's replies? A sequential analysis. *Journal of Speech and Hearing Research, 33,* 563–573.

CHAPTER 19

Outcomes Measurement in the Schools

Diane L. Eger

INTRODUCTION

The focus on accountability that is so apparent in business and health care has not bypassed the schools. The public mantra of the 1990s has been "Don't raise our taxes." The parent, the taxpayer, the school board member, the superintendent, and the business manager are demanding that the school system be accountable for the educational results of their students. Further, because the cost of educating students with disabilities is significantly higher than that of students without disabilities, there is even greater pressure on special education providers to demonstrate program effectiveness by looking at outcomes, especially student outcomes. Blackstone (1995) summarizes the state of current outcomes of special education in the United States as follows:

> . . . The current state of special education in the United States is characterized by outcomes that truly are disturbing: (a) differential certification, categorization and placement of racial and language minority students; (b) high drop out rates; (c) post-secondary graduation rates less than half of general education graduates; (d) the highest unemployment rate of any population subgroup (two-third of persons with disabilities are not working) and (e) limited community integration for adults with disabilities. [p. 4]

These types of outcomes have not only pushed the inclusion movement onward, but have focused the public debate on the question, "Was it worth the dollars we spent?" Today, therefore, almost every public school entity finds itself under a financial microscope trying to stretch the ever-decreasing tax dollars further and further. This situation demands that we organize mandated and existing paperwork into measurement outcomes as proof of quality of the programs we provide. In addition, we must use customer surveys to determine how we are doing. The purposes of this chapter are to provide the reader with a history of outcomes measurement in the schools; a summary of outcomes measurement for students with disabilities; a discussion of outcome

indicators for students enrolled in speech and language services; and to advocate for outcomes data to demonstrate educational results.

HISTORY OF OUTCOMES MEASUREMENT IN THE SCHOOLS

Unlike today where education and its accountability constitute a major public agenda item, the schools of yesterday were just assumed to be good. The community, parents, teachers, and students were involved and supportive. Teachers taught, gave grades; students learned and everyone was happy. Law suits were rare. The schools were fairly homogeneous in nature and very few "at-risk" students were enrolled. The costs were manageable and systemwide outcome measurements were the exception, not the rule. Customer satisfaction surveys were not even considered.

Then, in response to parent outcry regarding the treatment of students with disabilities, Congress passed P.L. 94–142 or the *Education of All Handicapped Children Act of 1975* (EAHCA). It was created by Congress to accomplish four main goals:

• all handicapped children were to have a free, appropriate public education;

• their rights and those of their parents or guardians were to be protected;

• states and localities were to be assisted in providing for this education; and

• the effectiveness of efforts to educate handicapped children was to be assessed and assured.

This federal legislation changed the face of public education in the United States and was perhaps the precursor to a formal outcomes measurement system in special education. Later revisions of this law were P.L. 99–457—*Education of the Handicapped Act Amendments of 1986,* which extended the rights and protections to handicapped children ages 0 to 5 years, and the P.L. 101–476, *Education of the Handicapped Act Amendments of 1990,* which renamed the act to *Individuals with Disabilities Education Act (IDEA)* and expanded the definition to encompass instruction in all settings, including the workplace and training centers, and added transition plans to the Individualized Education Program (IEP).

At about the same time as the passage of P.L. 94–142 and its Amendments, a large body of research was accumulating on effective schools and effective teaching. This process-product research was conducted in the late 1970s through the mid 1980s by researchers, (Rankin, 1979; Evertson, 1980; Evertson, Anderson, Anderson, & Brophy, 1980; Edmonds, 1981) who went into schools and classrooms where student achievement was high or beyond expected levels. The researchers observed thousands of teachers and recorded their interactions with students. A consistent set of teacher behaviors dealing with classroom management, instructional delivery, expectations, and general classroom atmosphere was found. Researchers also observed classrooms where student achievement was not at expected levels and found none of the characteristics of the successful teachers. The assumption of this body of research is that there is a correlation between the action of the teacher and the achievement of the student as measured by basic skills tests in math and reading. In a nutshell, effective teachers teach students, not content. The outcome measure was performance on basic skills tests in math and reading as correlated with teacher behaviors.

The next major educational issue where adequate student outcome measures would have significantly changed the debate has become known as the Regular Education Initiative (REI). This initiative examined the effect of "pull-out" models on the education of students with learning problems and sought to limit the use of special placements. The concept received a kind of formal recognition at a 1985 conference when the Assistant Secretary of the U.S. Office of Special Education and Rehabilitation Services, Madeline C. Will, stated that the "so-called 'pull-out' approach to the educational difficulties of students with learning problems has failed in many instances to meet the educational needs of these students and has created, however unwittingly, barriers to their successful education" (Will, 1986, p. 412). She called for a partnership between general and special education. Wang, Reynolds and Walberg (1986) also recommended that practices from special and general education be combined "into a coordinated educational delivery system. This system would combine methods that have a strong research record of effectiveness with comprehensive systems of instruction that have evolved from both general and special education" (p. 28). In other words, this initiative was suggesting that student and system outcomes should determine modifications in the curriculum. It was not as simple as it sounded, largely due to the fact that these outcomes were not readily available.

A good overview of the status of outcomes measurement and accountability in the public schools is garnered from a report entitled *Education Reforms and Special Education: The Era of Change for the Future,* prepared by The Regional Resource and Federal Center Program for the Office of Special Education Programs, April 1993 Leadership Conference. In this document, 58 entities were surveyed; these included the 50 states, 7 U.S. territories, and the Bureau of Indian Affairs. This report was prepared as a way to look to "The Era of Change for the Future" as a response to the considerable attention and discussion that has been devoted to reforming the nation's public schools. Many recent reform efforts have consistently emphasized the results of education and therefore placed emphasis on student outcomes and accountability for achieving these outcomes often through statewide assessments.

Table 19–1 summarizes the results of the survey of the 58 entities on the outcomes and accountability domain. Although 71% of the states and territories have a written policy regarding student outcomes in general education, only 34% have one in special education. This means in about two-thirds of the states and territories, student outcomes for students with disabilities cannot be retrieved at the state level in a consistent fashion. About three-fourths of the states and territories have various options such as diploma, certificate of attendance, and certificate of competency for students with disabilities; and about three-fourths of them are also promoting alternative performance—based assessment, such as portfolio assessment, which is a sample of a student's work over a given period of time. However, only 50% of the states and territories require students to pass a competency test for graduation and/or grade promotion, and only a mere 14% of them have passed state legislation and/or adopted policy to replace the Carnegie units with competence on student outcomes. Carnegie units—the current system used to accumulate the required number of credits in order to graduate—is based on the amount of time a student spends in a class, not on a learner outcome. If you are familiar with the work of William G. Spady, the guru of outcome-based education, (OBE), this statistic of only 14% is appalling.

As Spady (1994) explains . . . "Outcomes are clear learning results that we want stu-

Table 19–1. Summary of Survey of States and Territories
on Outcome and Accountability Domain

OUTCOMES AND ACCOUNTABILITY	YES		NO		DID NOT ANSWER	
	#	%	#	%	#	%
Does general education have written policy regarding student outcomes?	41	7	12	21	5	9
Does special education have written policy regarding student outcomes?	20	34	34	59	4	7
Is there state legislation and/or adopted policy replacing Carnegie units with competence on student outcomes?	8	14	45	78	5	9
Does the state require that students pass a competency test for graduation and/or grade promotion?	29	50	22	38	7	12
Are any of the listed options available to students with disabilities? (e.g., Diploma, Certificate of Attendance, Certificate of Competency).	45	78	6	10	7	12
Does the state publish an annual "report card" describing successes in serving students with disabilities?	22	38	33	57	3	5
Is the state promoting alternative performance-based assessments such as portfolio assessment?	43	74	12	21	3	5

*Total number = 58.

SOURCE: Summarized from data presented in the Regional Resource and Federal Centers Program for the U.S. Department of Education, Office of Special Education Programs (1993). *Education Reforms and Special Education: The Era of Change for the Future.* Plantation, FL: South Atlantic Regional Resource Center, Florida Atlantic University, Appendix A.

dents to demonstrate at the end of significant learning experiences" (p. 2). This means if education is based on outcomes, the time standard or base of twentieth-century education must be completely overruled by the results or ends. It also means that "states and districts must establish a clear framework of learning that students will be able to master successfully at the culminating point in their schooling careers . . ." (p. 3). As the summary data from Table 19–1 clearly show, only 14% of the states have policy replacing the Carnegie units (time) with competence or student outcomes and just 50% of the states require students to pass a competency test for graduation and/or grade promotion. As Spady describes:

> . . . A system based on outcomes gives top priority to ends, purposes, learning accomplishments, and results. Decision making is consistent with these priorities. Often, an outcomes approach requires placing the system's traditional definers and shapers—time, procedures, programs, teaching, and curriculum—in a subordinate position. This essential shift from time to accomplishments often puts actual learning results on a collision course with the clock, schedule, and calendar. If time and accomplishments don't mesh, then the term "outcome-based" directly implies that outcomes must take precedence over time. [pp. 3–4]

The philosophy of OBE is success for all students and staff. Spady explains that OBE has two key purposes based on this philosophy. These two purposes are:

- Ensuring that all students are equipped with the knowledge, competence, and qualities needed to be successful after they exit the educational system, and

- Structuring and operating schools so that those outcomes can be achieved and maximized for all students. [p. 9]

It is not surprising that OBE is based on essentially the same assumptions and premises that the inclusion movement has adopted. Both movements are based on the belief that all students can learn and succeed. This premise is backed by voluminous research and over 30 years of educator's practice (Spady, 1994). If this premise is accepted, then outcomes must be both measured and managed to insure that all students do in fact learn and are successful.

The need for outcomes measurement is expressed throughout the recent educational literature from both regular and special education. It is throughout discussions such as reinventing or restructuring our schools, site-based management, strategic planning, mastery learning, authentic assessment, portfolio assessment, and ecological evaluation. Herman (1992) states:

> Education assessment is in a process of invention. Old models are being seriously questioned: new models are in development. Open-ended questions, exhibits, demonstrations, hands-on experiments, computer simulations and portfolios are a few examples. The promise of the new approaches is alluring and is being effectively advanced at the national, state, and local levels all over the country. [p. 74]

Table 19–1 confirms that 74% of the states are promoting alternative performance-based assessments. An example of a system that has restructured to achieve outcomes for all students is Township High School District 214 in Arlington Heights, Illinois. According to Fitzpatrick (1991), they realigned their curriculum into an outcomes-based model as conceptualized in Figure 19–1. The general learner outcomes serve as the foundation of their curriculum process.

Both restructuring in regular education and poor student outcomes demonstrated in pull-out special education programs created and accelerated the inclusion movement. The growing diversity of the student population in America's schools created yet another challenge in efforts to address a wide variety of student needs.

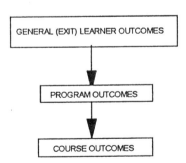

Figure 19-1. Curriculum Alignment

Source: Fitzpatrick (1991) Restructuring to achieve outcomes of significance for all students. *Educational Leadership*, 48 (8), p. 19.

Villa and Thousand (1995) describe inclusive education and school restructuring accordingly:

> The call for restructuring of American education to establish meaningful educational standards (i.e., student outcomes) and to hold schools accountable for accomplishing these outcomes with each and every student, requires great human commitment and effort, individually and collectively. This commitment requires that we believe that each child can learn and succeed, that diversity enriches us all, that students at risk for failure can overcome that risk through involvement in a thoughtful and caring community of learners, that each child has unique contributions to offer to the community of learners, that each child has strengths and needs, and that effective learning results from the collaborative efforts of us all to ensure the success of each student.
>
>   Systems-change initiatives in special education are paralleling similar efforts in general education, often referred to as school restructuring. Educators and researchers are raising fundamental questions regarding the most effective strategies for teaching all students; and many people are designing and implementing numerous innovative and highly effective strategies. [p. 9]

In 1996, Governor Tommy G. Thompson of Wisconsin and IBM Chairman and Chief Executive Officer Louis V. Gerstner, Jr., organized a voluntary 2-day education summit. Most of the governors and many corporate executives attended and focused "on standards assessment, and education technology. . . . the Council of Chief State School Officers urged the governors and state legislatures to provide the money needed to improve standards. In addition, the group said, money is needed to link those standards to assessments that will measure students' progress toward meeting them" (Lawton, 1996, p. 18).

From this brief history of outcomes and outcomes measurement in the schools, we can conclude that the characteristics of both the school restructuring movement and the development of inclusive schools are essentially the same: that *all* students must have a quality education that meets their own educational needs and that the system must be able to demonstrate that this education has outcomes for which the public is willing to pay. Therefore, the need for outcomes measurement in the schools has never been greater.

OUTCOMES FOR STUDENTS WITH DISABILITIES

National Center on Educational Outcomes Model

In the U.S. Department of Education's Sixteenth Annual Report to Congress on the Implementation of Individuals with Disabilities Act (1994), the chapter entitled "Results for Students with Disabilities" (1994) describes the National Center on Educational Outcomes' (NCEO's) conceptual model of outcomes congruent with state-identified goals and national data collection programs, it identifies the educational results data currently collected nationally and by States, and discusses exclusion of students with disabilities in state and national assessments. In 1990, the Office of Special Education Programs (OSEP) funded NCEO to address issues related to assessing educational results for students with disabilities. The NCEO's mission "has been to develop indica-

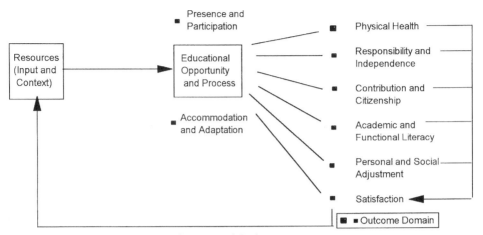

Figure 19–2. NCEO school completion model of outcomes.

Source: National Center on Educational Outcomes (NCEO). U.S. Department of Education (1994). Results for students with disabilities. In *To Assure the Free Appropriate Public Education of All Children With Disabilities-Sixteenth Annual Report to Congress on the Implementation of the individuals with Disabilities Education Act*, p. 133.

tors of educational results for students with disabilities" (U.S. Department of Education, p. 131). Its conceptual model of outcomes at the time of graduation is depicted in Figure 19–2. It is a broader model than the traditional state assessment system that focuses almost entirely on assessing academic achievement. It demonstrates that educational resources (input and context) impact educational opportunity and process, which in turn influence the eight domains. Further, the domains affect both the resources and the opportunity and process.

The NCEO (1994) defined the terms "outcome" and "indicator" as follows:

Outcome: The result of interactions among individuals and educational experiences.

Indicator: A symbolic representation of one or more educational outcomes for infants, children, and youth that enables comparisons to be made. [p. 132]

This model assumes that these outcomes should apply to *all* students. Therefore, indicators of outcomes for students receiving special education services should be related to those identified for students without disabilities. The NCEO definitions of the school completion outcome domains are depicted in Table 19–2.

It is easy to see that school-based speech and language services could and should have a major impact on the academic and functional literacy domain. The domain's outcomes and indicators are listed in Table 19–3. It would be reasonable to write speech-language IEPs using the outcomes noted here. This would allow us to have direct impact on the school's outcomes data in the context of the overall education program.

Many issues are yet to be resolved for including students with disabilities in large-scale assessments of outcomes (Ysseldyke & Thurlow, 1993). It is clear, however, that including *all* students in educational results assessment will be the mandate of the

---

Table 19–2. Definitions of School Completion Outcome Domains

Presence and Participation
> The extent to which an individual is present in a particular setting and the extent to which meaningful participation occurs

Accommodation and Adaptation
> Modifications that must be made for individuals to achieve outcomes

Physical Health
> The extent to which the individual demonstrates healthy behavior, attitudes, and knowledge related to physical well-being

Responsibility and Independence
> The extent to which the individual's behavior reflects the ability to function independently and assume responsibility for oneself

Contribution and Citizenship
> The ways in which or extent to which an individual gives something back to society or participates as a citizen in society

Academic and Functional Literacy
> The use of information to function in society, to achieve goals, and to develop knowledge

Personal and Social Adjustment
> The extent to which the individual demonstrates socially acceptable and healthy behaviors, attitudes, and knowledge regarding mental well-being

Satisfaction
> The extent to which a favorable attitude is held toward education

---

SOURCE: National Center on Education Outcomes (NCEO).
U.S. Department of Education (1994). Results for students with disabilities. In *To Assure the Free Appropriate Public Education of All Children With Disabilities—Sixteenth Annual Report to Congress on the Implementation of The Individuals with Disabilities Education Act,* p. 133.

future. Speech-language pathologists (SLPs), therefore, should prepare to measure their outcomes in this larger context. As the NCEO study summarizes:

> A national shift has occurred from a focus on *process* (what we do) to *results* (what we produce). This trend is very evident in education today. Parents, government agencies, businesses, and the community want to know more than just the number of students in school, the number of teachers and their degrees, the quality of facilities, and the types of books in the school libraries. They want to know how students are affected by school. They want to know whether students are leaving school prepared for work, college, or other post-school experiences. They want to know, in short, if their investment in education has been worth it.
>
> This information is needed for all students, including students with disabilities. Access to special education services remains a critical issue, and educational results are just as important for students who receive special education services as for those who do not. The results are not the sole responsibility of special education, because students with special needs increasingly are part of the general education community. To obtain this information, students with disabilities must be included in the overall system of educational accountability measurement. [U.S. Department of Education, p. 166]

Table 19–3. Academic and Functional Literacy Domain
from NCEO School Completion Model

DOMAIN/OUTCOME	INDICATOR
Academic and Functional Literacy	
Demonstrates competence in communication	Percent of students who use and comprehend language that effectively accomplishes the purpose of the communication
Demonstrates competence in problem-solving strategies and critical thinking skills	Percent of students who demonstrate problem-solving and critical thinking skills
Demonstrates competence in math, reading, and writing skills	Percent of students who demonstrate competence in math necessary to function in their current home, school, work, and community environments
	Percent of students who demonstrate competence in math necessary to function in their next environments
	Percent of students who demonstrate competence in reading necessary to function in their current home, school, work, and community environments
	Percent of students who demonstrate competence in reading necessary to function in their next environments
	Percent of students who demonstrate competence in writing necessary to function in their current home, school, work, and community environments
	Percent of students who demonstrate competence in writing necessary to function in their next environments
Demonstrates competence in other academic and nonacademic skills	Percent of students who demonstrate competence in other academic and nonacademic skills necessary to function in their current home, school, work, and community environments
	Percent of students who demonstrate competence in other academic and nonacademic skills necessary to function in their next environments
Demonstrates competence in using technology	Percent of students who currently apply technology to enhance functioning in home, school, work, and community environments
	Percent of students who demonstrate competence in using technology to function in their next environments

SOURCE: U.S. Department of Education (1994). Results for students with disabilities. In *To Assure the Free Appropriate Public Education of All Children With Disabilities—Sixteenth Annual Report to Congress on the Implementation of The Individuals with Disabilities Education Act,* p 133.

OUTCOME INDICATORS FOR STUDENTS ENROLLED IN SPEECH AND LANGUAGE SERVICES

IEPs

An IEP for each student enrolled in special education has been the mandate since the enactment of P.L. 94–142, the EAHCA. As Smith (1990) explains, there is no document more significant than the IEP to the school community. It is a cornerstone of the federal legislation, P.L. 94–142, which forever changed public education for students with disabilities in the United States. Smith (1990) analyzed IEPs over the past decade and found them inoperative in the IEP process. The process generated both questionable documents and passive compliance. His recommendations included a reexamination of the IEP in the context of the current special education reform debate. Specifically he suggests that we should move from analyzing the IEP process to identifying a system that allows practitioners to prescribe individualized education. In other words, we should move from process to outcomes. Smith suggests we should utilize the school reform discussions to reexamine the impact of the IEP.

I do not disagree with Smith (1990). I would argue, however, for a much simpler solution that would allow for outcome measurements of students enrolled in special education. I believe long-and short-term goals/objectives in the IEP should be written as outcomes in the context of learning. For example, instead of writing a language goal that states: "The student will improve expressive language skills", the goal would be written in one of the following ways:

The student will apply problem-solving and decision making skills in Math and English classes.

The student will use language to create dialogues with teachers and peers to facilitate learning.

The student will be able to follow written directions on objective tests.

The same approach could be used across the range of communication and related disorders. For example, fluency goals can be written as:

The student will demonstrate a reduction of observed fear of speaking situations in the classroom and lunchroom.

The student will utilize a range of effective strategies when confronted with a stuttering episode in the classroom.

The beauty of this approach is that it does not add additional paperwork to an already overburdened clinician. IEPs, for better or worse, are mandated and must be revised at least annually. If IEP goals were written as outcomes, there would be rich outcomes data available from our school speech-language programs that would be relevant to the learning process.

Dismissal Criteria

Another outcome indicator for school-based therapy programs is dismissal criteria. In 1986, I conducted a large clinical study with my colleagues (Eger, Chabon, Mient, and

Cushman, 1986) to provide data to determine when to dismiss a school-aged child from articulation therapy. In this study we determined that clinicians were requiring a high level of articulation performance before recommending dismissal from therapy. In addition, about half of the students continued in therapy for 5 to 8 weeks after the 95% accuracy in conversational speech criterion was reached. We noted in that article, "It may be time for speech and language clinicians to reconsider the dismissal criteria used and base future decisions on empirically based standards of quality rather than apriori notions of acceptability" (p. 25). In other words, we must initiate and analyze outcome studies to determine what the most efficient dismissal criteria for particular communication disorders should be. This need has only grown as fiscal concerns have driven philosophy and practice in the schools. In essence, our school services are being rationed no differently than health care services under managed care plans. The frightening aspect, however, is that we are not using data-based decisions (i.e., outcomes studies) to determine how to ration.

Service Delivery Model Effectiveness

Another type of indicator to demonstrate educational outcomes for students enrolled in speech and language services is the effectiveness of various service delivery models. Changing speech-language service delivery models in the schools have been discussed in the literature for at least a decade (Nieptupski, Scheutz, and Ockwood, 1980; Frasinelli, Superior, and Myers, 1983). As I stated in 1992 (Eger, 1992), there is too much information for one professional to know, and therefore we must use the consultative team model. This consultation/collaborative model is not unique to speech-language pathology, but is being used across many professions. "We must know how and when to use the consultation (indirect) service model as the only and most appropriate service for given students as well as in conjunction with direct service models for other students" (Eger, p. 41).

Collaborative Consultation/Classroom-Based Communication Skills Intervention

Much discussion over the past decade has focused on the collaborative consultation service delivery model of school-based speech and language services. The American Speech-Language-Hearing Association (1991) developed a guideline titled, "A Model for Collaborative Service Delivery for Students with Language-Learning Disorders in the Public Schools." The collaborative service delivery model is described in this document as follows:

> From the perspective of speech-language pathology, collaborative service delivery is designed to assess and treat communication impairments within natural settings and, on a more global level, to enhance the learning experiences of children with and without handicaps. Collaborative service delivery does not necessarily replace the services provided to students under traditional models. Rather, collaborative service delivery can supplement or extend the services that are provided in the isolated intervention context to the classroom, where students are expected to "play the school game" both on an academic performance level and on a social communication level. The collaborative service delivery model affords the speech-language pathologist the opportunity to

(1) observe and assess how the student functions communicatively and socially in the regular classroom, (2) describe the student's communicative strengths and weaknesses in varied educational contexts, and (3) identify which curricular demands enhance or interfere with the student's ability to function communicatively, linguistically, and socially. [p. 45]

This document further describes several of the accountability issues involved in this model. It states:

Accountability requires that educators be responsible for ensuring that appropriate educational programs are provided to meet the individual needs of students. Accountability for special educational services is an issue whose importance looms ever greater as educational costs rise and expenditures are scrutinized. The general efficacy of special educational programs must be demonstrated to ensure continuing support for them. The efficacy of intervention programs can be verified by illustrating student levels of functioning and documenting student progress toward educational goals over time. Collaborative service delivery is well suited to demonstrating the effectiveness of general programs by documenting and summarizing the progress shown by individual students. [p. 48]

It is clear that this model encourages outcome measures that are aligned within regular education. The model also allows equity in assessment between students with disabilities and students without disabilities. Kaufman, Prelock, Weiler, Creaghead, and Donnelly (1994) examined the effect of an intervention program on typically developing third-grade students' ability to improve their understanding of explanation adequacy. The results of this study indicated that students who participated in the Communication Skills Unit improved their metapragmatic awareness of explanation adequacy by increasing their awareness of the need to provide effective explanations of math problems and by increasing their understanding that a goal of explanation is to help another person apply information in contexts other than the present.

A study by Ebert and Prelock (1994) demonstrated another positive outcome of the collaborative training model. They found that teachers who were trained in a collaborative model of service delivery were more accurate in their perceptions of ability levels for students with communication impairments than were teachers who were not trained. Although there have been few published studies that provide actual outcomes data to demonstrate the effectiveness of the consultative model, these data can and should be collected to support the effectiveness of our services.

Early Primary Self-Contained Language Classrooms

Another model that provides powerful outcomes data in terms of impact on academic performance is the early primary self-contained language classroom. This model has fallen out of political favor due to the recent push for inclusionary programs and the elimination of self-contained models. It is, however, an effective model for a select group of students at the kindergarten and first-grade level. These students would demonstrate normal intellectual potential with severe communication deficits not due to hearing or vision loss, emotional disturbance, or physical handicap. These communication deficits would have significant negative impact on these students' educational performance. I have observed this impact personally. A likely scenario might be as follows: the student enters kindergarten, and once in the school system begins to receive "intensive" speech treatment. Although the student makes continual progress in communication skills throughout the primary school years, the student is academically unsuccessful. The reason is that the school curriculum does not wait for the development of functional communication skills. Data from several such programs demonstrate the positive impact on educational performance in the regular education environment (Mrockowski, 1988; Frattali, Eger, Harrison, Jacobson, & Rassi, 1995).

The outcomes data from the kindergarten and first grade self-contained language classroom program at the Allegheny Intermediate Unit serving the 42 suburban school districts surrounding Pittsburgh, Pennsylvania included a teacher survey of the students who returned to their home schools in the fall of 1994. Although we were unable to "cure" severe language disorder or severe apraxia, we were able to teach strategies and compensations that allowed these students to return to their home school districts and perform successfully. Eighty % of our students who returned to mainstream during the 1994–95 school year were reported by their teachers to be either the same as, better than, or significantly better than the other students in the class in terms of *academic readiness*. In addition, 80% of the students were reported by their teachers to be either the same as, better than, or significantly better than the other students in the class in the *understanding of language;* 60% of the students were reported by their teachers to be either the same as, better than, or significantly better than the other students in the class in *attending skills, following directions, play skills, language use,* and *independent work skills.* Seventy percent of these students were reported by their teachers to be at or above grade level in science and 80% in social studies. Further, 50% of the students were reported by their teachers to be either at or above grade level in reading, math, and language arts. The teachers were also asked whether or not the returning students could comprehend language used for the following and responded accordingly:

Small group instruction	Yes: 100%	No:	0%
Large group instruction	Yes: 90%	No:	10%
Workbooks	Yes: 70%	No:	30%
Social interaction	Yes: 80%	No:	20%

These data support the impact our service delivery model has had on the returning students' educational performance. We have always been able to demonstrate growth in the speech and language areas as a result of direct intervention. But the current climate requires that we demonstrate far more than this. In other words, we need to demonstate the impact our services have on the student's ability to achieve academically in the regular or adapted curriculum. From the reports of our students' teachers, our intensive early primary services have had a positive impact on the students' ability to achieve academically in the curriculum.

CONCLUSION

The time has never been better for school-based SLPs to demonstrate the effectiveness of their services by generating outcomes data to describe the service delivery provided. A proportion of these data should be customer surveys, which generate data from administrators, teachers, parents, and the students themselves.

With education on the public agenda and viewed as the key to economic growth in the twenty-first century, the time has never been more critical for the generation of outcomes data to demonstrate educational results. It has been said that if you don't know where you're going, you won't know when you get there. It is time that we know where we are going in school-based speech and language services, produce the outcomes data to prove when we get there, and use the data to demonstrate that it made a difference.

REFERENCES

American Speech-Language-Hearing Association. (1991). A model for collaborative service delivery for students with language-learning disorders in the public schools. *Asha, 33* (Suppl. 5), 44–50.

Blackstone, S.W. (1995). For consumers: Supporting parents and family members. *Augmentative Communication News, 8*(6), 4–5.

Ebert, K.A., & Prelock, P.A. (1994). Teachers' perceptions of their students with communication impairments. *Language, Speech and Hearing Services in the Schools, 25*(4), 211–214.

Edmonds, R. (1981, October). The characteristics of effective schools: research and implementation. *Unpublished article from Michigan State University.*

Eger, D.L. (1992). Why now? Changing school speech-language service delivery. *Asha, 34,* 40–41.

Eger, D.L., Chabon, S.S., Mient, M.G., & Cushman, B.B. (1986). When is enough enough? Articulation therapy dismissal considerations in public schools. *Asha, 28,* 23–25.

Evertson, C.M. (1980). An overview of research: Classroom organization and effective teaching project. Austin, TX: Research and Development Center.

Everston, C., Anderson, C., Anderson, L., & Brophy, J. (1980). Relationships between classroom behaviors and student outcomes in junior high mathematics and English classes. *American Educational Research Journal, 17(1),* 43–60.

Fitzpatrick, K.A. (1991). Restructuring to achieve outcomes of significance for all students. *Educational Leadership, 48*(8), 18–22.

Frasinelli, L., Superior, K., & Myers. J. (1983). A consultation model for speech and language intervention. *Asha, 25,* 25–30.

Frattali, C., Eger, D.L., Harrison, M., Jacobson, B., & Rassi, J.A. (1995). *Measuring Outcomes As Proof of Quality.* ASHA Convention Short Course. Orlando, Florida: ASHA Convention.

Herman, J.L. (1992). What research tells us about good assessment. *Educational Leadership, 49*(8), 74–78.

Kaufman, S.S., Prelock, P.A., Weiler, E., Creaghead, N.A., & Donnelly, A. (1994). Metapragmatic awareness of explanation adequacy: Developing skills for academic success from a collaborative communication skills unit. *Language, Speech and Hearing Services in Schools, 25*(3), 174–180.

Lawton, M. (1996). Chiefs seek summit call for standards review. *Education Week, 15*(27), 18.

Mrockowski, M.M. (1988). Self-contained language classes for kindergartens—nine years of data. In D.L. Eger & Van Hattum (Eds.), *Variations in School Programming. Seminars in Speech and Language, 9*(4), 329–337.

Nieptupski, J., Scheutz, G., & Ockwood, L. (1980). The delivery of communication therapy services to severely handicapped students: A plan for change. *Journal of Association of Severely Handicapped, 45*(1), 13–23.

P.L. 94–142, *The Education for All Handicapped Children Act of 1975.*

P.L. 99–457, *Education of the Handicapped Act Amendments of 1986.*

P.L. 101–476, *Education of the Handicapped Act Amendments of 1990.*

Rankin, S. (1979). A conversation with Stuart Rankin. *Educational Leadership, 1979, 37*(1), 74–77.

Regional Resource and Federal Centers Program (1993). *Education Reforms and Special Education: The Era of Change for the Future.* Plantation, FL: South Atlantic Regional Resource Center, Florida Atlantic University.

Smith, S.W. (1990). Individualized education programs (IEPs) in special education—from intent to acquiescence. *Exceptional Children, 57*(1), 6–14.

Spady, W.G. (1994). *Outcome-Based Education: Critical Issues and Answers.* Arlington, VA: The American Association of School Administrators.

U.S. Department of Education (1994). Results for students with disabilities. In *To Assure the Free Appropriate Public Education of All Children with Disabilities—Sixteenth Annual Report to Congress on the Implementation of The Individuals with Disabilities Education Act,* 131–172.

Villa, R.A., & Thousand, J.S. (Eds.) (1995). *Creating An Inclusive School.* Alexandria, VA: Association and Curriculum Development.

Wang, M.C., Reynolds, M.C., & Walberg, H.J. (1986). Rethinking special education. *Educational Leadership, 44*(1), 26–31.

Wiederholt, J.L. (Ed.) (1988). Regular education initiative. *Journal of Learning Disabilities, 21*(1).

Will, M.C. (1986). Educating children with learning problems: A shared responsibility. *Exceptional Children, 52,* 411–415.

Ysseldyke, J., & Thurlow, M. (1993). *Views on inclusion and testing accommodations for students with disabilities* (Synthesis Report 7). Minneapolis, MN: University of Minnesota, National Center on Educational Outcomes.

CHAPTER 20

Outcomes Measurement in Health Care Settings

BECKY SUTHERLAND CORNETT

INTRODUCTION

Those of us who work in health care settings are frightened by the term "outcome." We struggle with understanding definitions, dimensions, philosophies, and measurement methods. We are not sure what we should do about outcomes. Yet, we are compelled by health care reform and the demands of managed care organizations to concentrate on reducing costs, improving efficiency, and demonstrating our effectiveness. In the future, we may not be paid for our services unless we produce specific outcomes. As health professionals scramble to learn about outcomes, we must ask ourselves—is the "new" focus on outcomes really new?

Frattali told us in Chapter 1 about the historical precedent for measuring outcomes set by Codman and Nightingale, and the modern-day parameters suggested by Deming, Donabedian, and Ellwood. These and other persons have long tried to help health professionals link what they do (the process of care), to the results (outcomes) of care. Certain health care outcomes, such as mortality, morbidity, infection rates, and severity-of-illness have been measured for many years. Only recently have we begun to use health outcomes as performance measures, to determine the value of services rendered (Schyve, 1995).

Although we know health care outcomes are often influenced by many other factors, clinical accountability is a primary driving force of outcomes measurement efforts. Bob Douglass, former ASHA president, wrote an article over a decade ago titled "Defining and Describing Clinical Accountability" (Douglass, 1983). I've used his last paragraph many times in presentations. I can't find anything more direct, or more powerful, to help us focus our discussion here:

> The scientific study of client satisfaction with therapy, the impact that improved communication has on the client and those closest to him, the changes that occur in therapy, the interrelated variables of client, clinician, and the continuing interaction between

them pose tremendous problems in research design. Yet, it is in this domain that the effectiveness and efficiency of clinical services should properly be studied. It is here that answers can be found to the real question behind accountability, "How do we know and how can we show that what we do in therapy really makes a difference?" [p. 117]

The focus of this chapter will be on "making a difference" in health care settings. I will try to help you know, and show, what role health care providers, professionals, organizations, and health plans play in facilitating outcomes.

DESCRIBING AND DETERMINING HEALTH CARE OUTCOMES

I like the generic equation Kane (1994) used to illustrate how health care outcomes are determined: "outcomes = f (baseline, patient factors, environment, treatment)" (p.57). This equation presents simply the framework for examining outcomes measurement in health care settings. Donabedian (1992) has said, "any consequence of health care is an outcome" (p. 356), but *outcomes measurement* considers the states of individuals or populations that are *attributable to antecedent health care.* Considerations include changes in health status, knowledge, or behavior, and satisfaction with care. These outcomes can be classified as clinical, physiologic-biochemical, physical, psychologic, social/psychosocial, integrative, or evaluative. Donabedian's outcomes classification and listing is presented in Table 20–1.

Piccirillo (1993), reporting on the work of Fries and Spitz (1990), describes health care outcomes in a hierarchy of ascending order: morbidity and mortality are the first two levels. Health status (including the physical, functional, and emotional aspects of the individual) and HRQL form the next two levels, and patient satisfaction tops the hierarchy. In this model, patient perceptions and satisfaction (types of service outcomes) are at least as important as technical outcome.

Wilkerson's outcome targets for rehabilitation services (1995) are similar to Piccirillo's when she contends that we must define rehabilitation outcomes in ways that respond to the demands and trends associated with health care reform, managed care, and the age of consumerism. Wilkerson stressed that we focus on the "new" rehabilitation outcome targets: the reduction of handicap, community integration, quality of life, and consumer satisfaction. She also emphasized the importance of benefit retention; that is, how long the functional gains achieved during treatment are sustained.

All inputs must be considered in determining outcomes, some of which make it more difficult to attribute outcomes specifically to processes of care, and to measure provider performance. The complexity of tracking and measuring health care outcomes was discussed by the Health Care Advisory Board (1993) in its publication *Line of Fire: The Coming Public Scrutiny of Hospital and Health System Quality.* The Board presented eight recurring problems with outcomes measurement methods:

1. measures are not statistically meaningful;
2. results are not comparable across institutions;
3. measures are not severity-adjusted;
4. measures are not risk-adjusted;

Table 20–1. A Classification and Listing of Some Outcomes of Health Care

---

A. Clinical
  1. Reported symptoms that have clinical significance.
  2. Diagnostic categorization as an indication of morbidity.
  3. Disease staging relevant to functional encroachment and prognosis.
  4. Diagnostic performance—the frequency of false positives and false negatives as indicators of diagnostic or casefinding performance.

B. Physiologic-biochemical
  1. Abnormalities
  2. Functions
    a. Loss of function.
    b. Functional reserve-includes performance in test situations under various degrees of stress.

C. Physical
  1. Loss or impairment of structural form or integrity-includes abnormalities, defects, and disfigurement.
  2. Functional performance of physical activities and tasks:
    a. Under the circumstances of daily living;
    b. Under test conditions that involve various degrees of stress.

D. Psychologic, mental
  1. Feelings—includes discomfort, pain, fear, anxiety (or their opposites, including satisfaction).
  2. Beliefs that are relevant to health and health care.
  3. Knowledge that is relevant to healthful living, health care, and coping with illness.
  4. Impairments of discrete psychologic or mental functions:
    a. Under the circumstances of daily living;
    b. Under test conditions that involve various degrees of stress.

E. Social and psychosocial
  1. Behaviors relevant to coping with current illness or affecting future health, including adherence to health care regimens and changes in health-related habits.
  2. Role performance
    a. Marital
    b. Familial
    c. Occupational
    d. Other interpersonal
  3. Performance under test conditions involving varying degrees of stress.

F. Integrative outcomes
  1. Mortality
  2. Longevity
  3. Longevity, with adjustments made to take account of impairments of physical, psychologic, or psychosocial function: "full-function equivalents."
  4. Monetary value of the above.

G. Evaluation outcomes
  1. Client opinions about and satisfaction with various aspects of care, including accessibility, continuity, thoroughness, humaneness, informativeness, effectiveness, cost.

SOURCE: From: *Explorations in Quality Assessment and Monitoring, Volume 2, The Criteria and Standards of Quality* by A. Donabedian, 1982, pp. 367–368. MI: Health Adminstration Press. Reprinted by permission.

5. indicator has no direct link to provider action;

6. data cannot be collected due to technological restraints;

7. data is prohibitively expensive to collect;

8. results are easily manipulated. (p. 47)

A comprehensive listing of measurement complexities and associated examples is found in Table 20–2.

Schyve (1995) further expands upon concerns raised about the links between processes of care and outcomes, suggesting that the temporal relationship between care and outcomes is very important in determining practitioner performance. He classifies outcomes into three groups:

- *immediate outcomes* emerge during or directly after a procedure.

- *intermediate outcomes* occur when an episode of care is completed.

- *long-term outcomes* refer to the end-point of treatment for a particular disease, condition, or disorder, and are usually measured at follow-up periods, months, or years after completion.

(For another version of temporal outcomes, see Chapters 1 and 6 of this text.) Schyve cautions that specific links between outcomes and processes become more difficult to determine as time passes. Yet, it is precisely the durability of outcomes achieved (see Wilkerson, 1995) about which we who work in the rehabilitation field are most concerned.

Outcomes desired vary with model of health care used and the setting in which care occurs. Technical outcomes associated with the medical model, in which disease predicts the need for care, are different from technical outcomes associated with the functional or consequence model of care familiar to rehabilitation professionals. The consequence model follows the now-familiar impairment-disability-handicap continuum presented in the *International Classification of Impairments, Disabilities, and Handicaps* (WHO, 1980). Swanson (1995) depicted the relationships between health care model and technical outcome in Table 20–3.

Clearly, the demand for health care outcomes data is driven by health care reform—essentially managed care—but accrediting bodies and consumers of all types are asking questions about the results of health care services and programs. The Health Care Advisory Board has listed the types of outcome indicators requested currently through predictions of demands for the year 2003 and beyond in Table 20–4. It is interesting that the concepts of severity adjustment and risk adjustment are just beginning to become very important components of outcomes measurement and reporting.

Risk Adjustment Issues

The concept of *risk* is now very familiar to many health professionals as managed care contracts require that providers assume financial risk under per diem, case rate, and capitated arrangements. As health professionals are also held more accountable for specific patient outcomes as part of health reform and managed care trends, *risk adjustment* as part of outcomes measurement and outcomes studies becomes imperative. Risk adjustment methodologies were brought to the forefront after the now-famous HCFA debacle in 1986, in which hospital mortality data for Medicare patients were

Table 20–2. The Enormous Complexity of True Outcomes Tracking

COMPLEXITY	EXAMPLES
Indicators not Meaningful	
#1 Indicators not equally relevant to all procedures; critical indicator for one procedure may be meaningless for another	Mortality a primary outcome for bypass patients because a meaningful chance of death exists, but it is irrelevant for tonsillectomy because patients rarely die
#2 Though potentially relevant, some indicators' frequency may not be sufficient to generate statistically significant comparisons.	Blood loss in transurethral resection of the prostate (TURP) patients occurs infrequently.
#3 Imprecisely defining the population to be measured can lead to biased, less meaningful statistics	Primary C-section rate more meaningful than a rate which tracks both primary and repeat C-sections.
#4 Relevance of indicators varies due to differing treatment goals of patients; one patient may prefer to maximize length of life, another quality of life, yet another quality of life on a different index	One woman chooses radical mastectomy to eliminate fear of recurrence of cancer; another chooses lumpectomy to minimize disfigurement.
#5 Clinical outcomes measures potentially at odds with desired patient outcomes	Hypertension treatment may improve a patient's "numbers," but side-effects lower quality of life significantly.
#6 Clinical outcomes measures for a given procedure might be too detailed (and too numerous) to be useful for purchaser evaluation	Percentage of colectomy patients requiring treatment due to respiratory compromise is not an indicator payers will be able to utilize for broad evaluations.
#7 Aggregate institutional measures may be too broad to be useful for clinical process improvement	Higher-than-expected morbidity rate not as telling as high urinary tract infection (UTI) rate in prostate surgery cases.
#8 Some DRGs or even smaller units of analysis unlikely to generate enough cases to calculate statistically significant variations in outcomes	Heart-lung transplant procedures occur so infrequently that indicators hard pressed to achieve statistical significance.
#9 Some indicators may have inverse relationships; optimizing one indicator may negatively impact another indicator	Minimizing mortality may actually increase morbidity rates as those patients who otherwise would have died have major complications.
Issues with Risk Adjustment	
#10 Risk factors necessary to adjust for mortality different than factors necessary to adjust for major complications	Surgery patients' comorbidity may create risk of a complication, but not greater risk of death.
#11 Many risk factors that can affect the success of critical procedures not captured systematically anywhere in a patient record	Cardiac surgeons can predict the success of surgery based upon condition of vessels (whose description is not necessarily captured on the record).
Linking Outcomes to Providers' Actions	
#12 Outcomes act as a flag for further investigation; outcomes often do not point to specific processes of care that require modification	Mortality rate does not tell provider which aspect of care should be improved (or how it should be improved)

(continued)

Table 20–2. The Enormous Complexity of True Outcomes Tracking *(continued)*

COMPLEXITY	EXAMPLES
Linking Outcomes tp Providers' Actions (cont.)	
#13 Outcomes tracked after a long period of time may be result of treatment or just the natural progression of disease	If a congestive heart failure patient ultimately has a MI, it is difficult to gauge whether the MI is a result of poor management or just the natural course of the disease.
#14 Positive outcomes of treatment (e.g., functional status) often correlate with patient compliance with physicians' recommendations; patient compliance often a difficult variable to capture	Success of managing diabetes depends upon patient maintaining insulin regimen. Bypass patient recovery depends on willingness to quit smoking, change diet, and minimize stress; patient who refuses could ultimately require a repeat procedure.
#15 Family history, environmental conditions important variables in assessing potential outcome of treating a disease; patient may withhold or not know relevant facts	Family history of heart disease is potentially more telling of patients' likelihood of coronary disease than is patient management.
#16 Without controlled trials, "true" effect of a specific process of care muddled by other procedures, treatments patient may receive	Effectiveness of angioplasty one year after the treatment is affected by other treatments received (e.g., thrombolytic therapy and medical therapy).
Indicators not Comparable	
#17 Differences in how indicators are defined render comparisons across institutions impossible	Infection rates may vary across institutions due to nonstandard definitions of infections.
#18 Comparisons hampered by a lack of trending data (in the short term)	One-year mortality may not be necessarily representative of a true average for the institution.
Issues with Data Collection	
#19 Critical data often difficult to track without linked data systems in facility; inconsistent patient identification numbers, insufficient system linkages hamper flow of information	An unanticipated return to emergency department (ED) is a valuable indicator but can only be tracked if ED visit is captured on central data source.
#20 Some indicators impossible to track without linked community data base	Repeat procedures, readmissions valuable indicators but easily undercounted is patient goes to different hospital, physician.
#21 Some events (e.g., complications) might be difficult to identify, thus affecting the consistency of data collection	Some incidences of stroke may be so short-lived that they are missed by physician.
Issues with Administrative Data	
#22 Widespread miscoding calls into question the accuracy of information	Any number of events or indicators may be miscoded.
#23 Inconsistent definitions applied to coding of certain medical conditions minimizes the comparability of data	One hospital may code a lower level of infection as a major complication.

(continued)

Table 20–2. The Enormous Complexity of True Outcomes Tracking *(continued)*

COMPLEXITY	EXAMPLES
Issues with Administrative Data (cont.)	
#24 Coding "upgrades" to maximize reimbursement may overstate any "negative" clinical outcomes	Patient monitored for possible renal failure that never transpires may be coded as having mild renal failure to cover cost of monitoring.
#25 Outcomes data tracked limited to major complications and mortality	Many clinically meaningful variables and outcomes like lab test results and procedure-specific complications not captured.
Issues with Patient-Reported Data	
#26 Different patients will respond differently to the same data requests, potentially affecting consistency of information	Patients tolerate pain differently and will report different pain scores.
#27 Patient may not apply consistent parameters to same question over time	Recorded health status score changes but patient does not communicate any real change in status during follow-up visit.
#28 Large sample size is required for statistical significance, increasing expense of collection.	If mailed, health status questionnaires cost $7–$8 per patient surveyed; Reason: Aggressive follow-up work is necessary to achieve high return rate.
Issue with Medical Abstraction	
#29 Abstractors may apply different definitions when coding medical records due to varying degrees of clinical experience	A clinically experienced coder may recognize relevant drugs and treatments outside system's prescribed parameters that less experienced coders will miss
Indicator Manipulation (e.g., "Gaming")	
#30 Indicators may inadvertently create incentives to "artificially" inflate measure	A measure that tracks "admissions to hospital after ambulatory surgery" encourages provider to perform potential outpatient cases as inpatients or (worse yet) to send patients home who should be admitted.
	Physician may be encouraged to treat less severe patients if a penalty exists for treating higher risk patients.
#31 An indicator is only as good as measurement instrument; if the measurement instrument is incorrect or poorly executed, indicator is meaningless	The number of Pap smears performed is meaningless if the quality of lab process is poor.
#32 Focusing on the quality of a few procedures can create incentives to ignore other indicators, processes not being tracked	If measuring C-section rates, physician and hospital staff may focus all attention on C-sections, ignoring quality indicators for vaginal deliveries.

SOURCE: From: *Line of Fire: The Coming Public Scrutiny of Hospital and Health Care System Quality,* by the Health Care Advisory Board, 1993. The Advisory Company, Washington, D.C. Reprinted by permission.

released without accounting for patient risk of death in particular types of facilities, such as a hospice.

According to Iezzoni (1994), who has edited what may be the definitive book on the topic, meaningful evaluation of patient outcomes requires two things: a measure of the outcome itself, and a way to adjust for patients' risks for various outcomes (particularly adverse outcomes). The goal of risk adjustment is to "level the playing field—to control for those factors that patients bring to a health care encounter that could affect their outcomes . . . risk adjustment facilitates comparisons with 'apples to apples' (p. xi)."

We cannot make inferences about the effectiveness of patient care without first accounting for certain patient characteristics which may adversely, or positively, affect outcome. These patient characteristics, or dimensions of risk, include: age, sex, clinical stability, diagnosis, severity of illness, comorbidities, complications, physical and cognitive/psychologic functional status, socioeconomic status, cultural/social behaviors, patient attitudes, and preferences (Iezzoni, 1994, p. 31).

Consideration of risk factors also raises fundamental conceptual questions. Iezzoni asks simply "risk of what?" Schwartz and Ash (1994) present the following list of questions to guide our discussion:

- Risk of what outcome (e.g., death, long length of stay, unusual consumption of resources)?

- Risk for whom (older vs. younger persons, patients with particular diagnoses)?

- Risk during what time period (during ICU stay, 30 days following discharge, 2 years postsurgery)?

- Risk attributable to what factors (e.g., a particular procedure, therapeutic approach, or provider)? (p. 288)

Table 20–3. Relationships Between Health Care Model and Technical Outcomes

MODEL OF HEALTH CARE	ASSESSMENT	TECHNICAL OUTCOME
Medical—Disease predicts need for care (ICD-9)	Etiology	Preventon/Reduction of Risk *Example:* prevention of breast cancer
	Pathology	Cure *Example:* cure AIDS
	Manifestations	Control of Symptoms *Example:* reduce hypertension
Functional—The consequence of disease predicts the need for care (ICIDH)	Loss of Body System Function	Eliminate Impairments *Example:* eliminate musculoskeletal pain, or restore normal range of motion
	Loss of Ability to Perform Tasks/Activities	Eliminate or Reduce Disability *Example:* reduce walking disability or eliminate lifting problem
	Resulting Disadvantage	Eliminate or Reduce the Handicap *Example:* return to work

SOURCE: From "Predicting and Managing Functional Outcomes," *Rehab '95 Symposium by* Gretchen Swanson, June 2, 1995, Mt. Carmel Hospital, Columbus, OH. Used by permission.

Table 20–4. Growing Demand for Outcomes Data*

CURRENT	1993–1998	1998–2003	2003 AND BEYOND*
Mortality	Severity-adjusted average charge	Longevity of specific clinical programs	Risk-adjusted mortality and morbidity
Morbidity			
Length of Stay	Severity-adjusted length of stay	Severity-adjusted mortality	Other risk-adjusted clinical indicators (number and type of indicator will vary by DRG)
Average Charge		Severity-adjusted morbidity	
Patient Satisfaction	Functional status (for specific DRGs)	Severity-adjusted length of stay	
Number of active medical staff	Patient satisfaction	Severity-adjusted average charge	Risk-adjusted average charges
Percentage of active medical staff board-certified	C-section rates	Functional status (for specific DRGs)	Patient satisfaction
	DRG-specific mortality and morbidity	Patient satisfaction overall quality of care skill of physicians, nurses length of time in hospital explanation of care processes and medications	Functional status (for specific DRGs)
ED and tertiary care facilities	Major complication rates		
JCAHO accreditation	Average rates of increase of hospital charges		
Procedure volume			
Severity-adjusted mortality	Inpatient admission rates for ambulatory care sensitive conditions	C-section rates	
Severity-adjusted morbidity		DRG-specific mortality and morbidity	
	Strength of hospital-physician relationship	Unplanned return to ED	
		Unplanned return to OR	
	Existence of and compliance with clinical pathways	Unplanned readmissions	
		Surgical wound infection rates	
	Documented results from quality improvement program	Unplanned transfer to special unit	
		Overall infection rates	
		Perioperative mortality	
		Unplanned admission following outpatient procedure	
		Surgical complication rates	
		Adverse drug reactions	
		Hospital-acquired adverse events	
		Low birth weight rates	
		Frequency of preventable acute episodes for chronic conditions.	

*When science catches up with the demand for data, measures will be fewer, but more powerful and more precise

It is important to remember that risk adjustment is used to calculate what Iezzoni calls the "algebra of effectiveness"—the concept that measuring outcomes involves a complex web of clinical and nonclinical patient attributes as well as determining the effectiveness and efficiency of services provided.

Currently, severity-of-illness measurement systems are the primary means used to adjust patient population statistics according to risk factors, although risk adjustment systems for many other purposes are being developed (see Iezzoni & Greenberg, 1994). These systems focus on short-term outcomes for hospitalized patients, viewing acute-care hospitalization as the episode of illness.

Severity measures are typically divided into those that define severity based on resource use (cost, LOS), or clinical issues. Some systems are population-specific (e.g, pediatric or Medicare patients only), diagnosis-specific (e.g., cancer, cardiology, or surgery patients), or subgroup specific [e.g., patients in an intensive care unit (ICU)].

Of the many measurement systems I could list here, I have selected several of the most well known for brief discussion. Diagnosis-related groups (DRGs) (Fetter, Shin, Freeman, Averill, & Thompson, 1980) were first used in 1983 to establish the Medicare Prospective Payment System (PPS). The DRG system uses over 470 diagnostic categories, which are assigned relative weights to determine payment based on examination of discharge abstracts. Severity is defined by total hospital charges or LOS.

MedisGroups (see Steen, Brewster, Bradbury, Estabrook, & Young, 1993), classifies severity according to in-hospital mortality and considers all hospitalized patients. Probability of in-hospital death is calculated according to key clinical findings. Acute Physiology, Age, and Chronic Health Evaluation-III (APACHE) (Knaus, Wagner, Zimmerman, & Draper, 1993) also defines severity by probability of in-hospital mortality, but focuses on adult ICU patients.

Function-related groups (FRGs) have been discussed for several years as the basis for a Medicare prospective payment system for rehabilitation. The RAND Corporation is currently designing such a system under contract to the Health Care Financing Administration. FRGs classify patients by functional status, and are based on the concept that functional status is the best predictor of the need for and use of rehabilitation services. The RAND Corporation is testing FRGs as a risk-adjustment strategy in that the groupings (considering age, impairment group, and functional status at admission) may be predictive of duration and intensity of rehabilitation services (Fleming, 1996).

It is beyond the scope of this chapter to present detailed information about risk adjustment methodologies, data requirements, or approaches. Please see Iezzoni (1994) for a complete discussion.

OUTCOMES ACROSS THE HEALTH CARE CONTINUUM

We have discussed a number of issues related to outcomes: definitions, parameters, complexities of measurements, risk, and severity issues. Now we turn to the health care continuum and the types and levels of outcomes associated with various venues of care. Acceptable or desired outcomes are usually quite different among the different components of the continuum.

Outcomes or results for many persons may be simply a report of "no problems identified" at their annual check-up. Another simple outcome might be a report of "no cavities" at the 6-month visit to the dentist. On the other hand, desired outcomes of an acute-care hospitalization of a person who has had a stroke might be that the SLP has completed brief communication and swallowing assessments, other appropriate initial diagnoses were made by other health professionals, and the patient has been accepted for the next level of care at an acute-inpatient rehabilitation facility. A "good" outcome of an ICU stay might be that the patient has now stabilized and may now be moved to the hospital's medical-surgical unit. Obviously, types of and expectations for outcomes vary widely.

Acute Inpatient Rehabilitation Outcomes

In the rehabilitation field, the focus of outcomes measurement for many years has been on acute inpatient rehabilitation, but is now expanding quickly to other venues as the result of shortened LOS. Most of the widely used functional assessment instruments in rehabilitation were developed for the inpatient rehabilitation population, primarily the FIM, developed by the UDSMR (State University of New York, 1993), and the WeeFIM (State University of New York, 1993) for use in children's hospitals (see Resources section). Other well-known instruments include the RICFAS-IV (Cichowski, 1996), the LORS-III (owned by Formations in Health Care; see Resources), and the PECS (owned by Marianjoy Rehabilitation Hospitals & Clinics; see Resources). Both UDS and Formations in Health Care offer participation in national databases of outcomes measurement and management information. Typically, health providers use a combination of global and specific assessment tools. The Functional Assessment Measure (FAM) (see Hall, 1992) intended for use with the brain injury population, is a 12-item expansion of the 18-item FIM, and focuses on cognition, psychosocial adjustment, and communication. For complete information about comprehensive and population-specific functional assessment measures, see Chapters 3 and 11 through 18 in this book.

Just as Burgess (1996b) cautioned that "home is a destination, not a discharge plan," (p. 27) a score on any of the available or developing global or specific functional assessment instruments is not the outcome itself. Scale scores, whether paper/pencil or automated, are tools that help professionals, considering also a number of other factors (e.g., LOS, costs), to determine whether they are, indeed, making a difference. According to Royal (in Breske, 1995a):

> If a patient is discharged from inpatient rehab, then clinicians must determine what resources the patient will consume later. The real outcome . . . is determined by measuring a reduction in potential future resources. If we want to justify our services, the outcome needs to measure what the cost is after discharge. [p. 17]

Subacute and Long-term Care Outcomes

The market for what is called "subacute" care facilities and programs has expanded rapidly in the last 5 years as this type of care has been identified as perhaps a less expensive alternative to acute inpatient care. *Subacute care* has been variously defined by associations and accrediting organizations, and encompasses both medical subacute care and rehabilitation subacute care. According to Manard (1995), subacute care as used in practice "nearly always refers to patients whose needs fall somewhere between acute hospital care and 'traditional' longer-term nursing facility care" (p. 2–9). Subacute care accreditation standards for rehabilitation, established on January 1, 1995, are listed in Categories II and III of The Rehabilitation Accreditation Commission's *Standards Manual & Interpretive Guidelines for Medical Rehabilitation* (CARF, 1996). JCAHO has also accredited subacute facilities since January, 1995.

Specific outcome measures for subacute care are currently limited, but several proprietary systems have become available recently or are in development (Manard, 1995). In contrast to acute rehabilitation programs, many subacute programs appear to be using their own customized measures. Manard (1995) recommends that subacute providers use a national measure to allow comparisons of outcomes across the subacute industry and also between acute-rehabilitation and subacute care.

According to Moore and Salcido (1996) and Manard (1995), the FIM of the UDSMR, initially developed for use in acute-rehabilitation facilities, is still the most widely used tool for assessing patient outcomes in subacute facilities offering rehabilitation services. UDS has begun collecting data from self-identified subacute facilities in an effort to establish the recommended national data base of outcomes information for subacute care.

Formations in Health Care, Inc. (which merged with Medirisk, Inc., in January, 1996), offers outcomes measurement systems across the continuum of care, and includes both medical subacute and subacute rehabilitation factors in their "Medical Outcomes System." A national data base is offered to compare subacute outcomes across facilities and programs.

Forer (1995) cautioned subacute providers not to use their own modified versions of the FIM as an outcomes measurement tool, but recommended that subacute programs use the following outcome indicators:

- selected elements of the Minimum Data Set (MDS) for Nursing Home Resident Assessment & Care Screening;
- FIM;
- diagnosis/impairment-specific measures;
- severity/acuity indices;
- medical outcomes;
- discharge destination;
- program interruptions (transfers to acute-care facilities);
- medical complications;
- patient/family satisfaction;
- follow-up status;
- health-related quality of life measures. (p. 139)

Although global measures can provide general outcomes across impairment groups, no single measure appears to be appropriate for all individuals served in subacute facilities. It is important to identify case-mix, diagnostic, and impairment groups before selecting specific measures (Forer, 1995).

I listed the MDS in the previous paragraphs about subacute care. Although elements of the MDS are used for subacute outcomes measurement, use of the MDS was mandated by the Nursing Home Reform Act (part of the OBRA of 1987) for nursing facility certification by the HCFA. The MDS is a comprehensive measure that assesses key indicators of long-term care (LTC) resident functioning (e.g., cognitive patterns, communication/hearing patterns, vision, psychosocial well-being, continence, physical functioning, activity pursuit patterns, skin, health conditions, nutritional status, medication use).

Although in practice referred to as the "MDS," the official name of the required measure is the RAI, developed by HCFA's Health Standards and Quality Bureau. The RAI is comprised of the MDS (based on an early version of the FIM) and the Resident Assessment Protocols (RAPs). The purpose of the RAI is to provide a comprehensive assessment upon a resident's admission, upon a significant change in status, and annually thereafter. The RAPs assess specific areas of an individual's strengths, preferences, and needs and provide guidelines for in-depth evaluation of particular areas of concern, such as use of restraints and risk of falls. In addition, LTC residents are assessed quarterly on a subset of the MDS. The purpose of these assessments is to promote individualized care planning focusing on improving, maintaining, or minimizing decline of a resident's functional status, and to facilitate problem identification, care planning, and problem resolution (Hawes, Morris, et al., 1995). Computerization of the MDS is planned to provide a national data base for comparison across all facilities.

Outcomes associated with LTC facilities, unlike subacute programs, are not focused primarily on moving patients elsewhere; rather, persons in LTC facilities are residents for whom LTC may be the best life situation. Therefore, outcomes measurement more often considers quality of life and functioning within the care setting, not necessarily placement in another discharge environment. Burgess (1996a) admonished therapists who believe that patients should not be admitted to acute rehabilitation facilities if they are being discharged to "nursing homes." She stressed the importance of identifying factors that will help patients make a successful transition to the LTC. Burgess listed four key functions she contends are basic to a LTC resident's quality of life: (1) getting out of bed; (2) eating; (3) communicating needs and desires; (4) toileting. The patient's discharge to the LTC facility may be considered a positive outcome if acute rehabilitation professionals can facilitate the patient's ability to do those four things independently, or with little assistance, in that environment.

Outcomes Associated with Home Care and Outpatient Services

As patient LOS in acute inpatient rehabilitation hospitals and units has decreased, outpatient services have grown. "Community reintegration" was once an outcome goal in inpatient settings. Now, health professionals who work in outpatient settings focus on home, school, work, and community reintegration activities. They also continue many goals related to both basic and instrumental activities of daily living skills begun as part of an individual's short inpatient stay. Thus, outcomes expectations have adjusted along the continuum of care.

Comprehensive outcomes measurement tools for outpatient services are somewhat limited, but local and national initiatives to develop and refine existing tools are underway. Currently, Formations in Health Care, Inc. offers neurologic, orthopedic, and occupational outcomes measurement scales. Focus on Therapeutic Outcomes, Inc. (FOTO), also offers outpatient outcomes measurement and outcomes management systems, but these focus on physical and occupational therapy services. In March, 1996, the American Physical Therapy Association (APTA) and FOTO announced a collaborative research effort on functional outcomes of physical therapy. FOTO is currently expanding its focus by developing a Rehabilitation Outcome Measurement Scale for neurologic disorders. Finally, the UDSmr is also developing an FIM for adult outpatient services. UDS published the *Guide for the Uniform Data Set for*

Medical Rehabilitation for Children (WeeFIM) Version 4.0—Community/Outpatient in 1993 (State University of New York, 1993).

SLPs who offer outpatient services also use a wide variety of functional assessment tools designed to evaluate communication and swallowing progress and outcomes. See Chapters 3 and 11 through 18 in this book for detailed information.

Like outpatient services, home care is expanding rapidly. In fact, home care is the fastest growing component of the health care continuum. Over 17,000 providers offered home care services to about 7 million persons in 1995. Proponents contend that home care is a low-cost alternative to inpatient care (National Association for Home Care, 1995). HCFA eligibility rules for home care require patients to be "homebound." Therefore, a primary goal of home care may be to help patients disqualify themselves by achieving the ability to return to community activities. Professionals also focus on: family/caregiver education about safety, community resources, medical and rehabilitation techniques and procedures; prevention of medical complications, and further impairment; environmental modifications; and other aspects of reintegration of patients into the home environment.

CARF requires that home- and community-based rehabilitation programs track the following outcomes as part of program evaluation activities: persons served who return to the acute hospital or other institutional care settings; persons served who remain in the community; persons served who have medical interventions that interrupt the delivery of rehabilitation services; and persons served who meet discharge goals and maintain or improve their discharge level of function (CARF, 1995, p. 157).

Unlike the majority of acute inpatient rehabilitation programs who use the FIM to track outcomes, there is no comprehensive national functional assessment or outcome scale that most home care agencies or programs use. However, home care programs do use FIM, like many subacute care organizations, because specific global tools for home care and subacute care are now in the developmental stages. Formations in Health Care offers a home-care outcomes assessment tool, available by subscription (see Resources section). Home care companies such as Olsten Kimberly Quality Care have also built databases of outcomes information (Breske, 1995b). Home care professionals also use a variety of diagnosis-specific or specific function tools (e.g., mobility, transfers, communication) to assess outcomes (Moffa-Trotter & Anemaet, 1995).

Clearly, many opportunities exist for developing comprehensive outcomes assessment tools targeted for home care and outpatient services. The emphasis will be upon building national databases for comparison across programs. These databases will be important to meet the data demands of payors and referral sources, particularly managed care organizations.

Managed Care Organizations and Outcomes

Many of us have associated the concept of managed care and the practices of managed care organizations only with cost reductions and limitations on speech-language pathology and other services. However, managed care plans have also developed outcomes measurement systems. The primary force behind outcomes measurement and managed care is the NCQA, a Washington, D.C.-based non-profit organization, which accredits health plans and develops performance criteria, including "report cards" based on standard performance measures. Several states and a number of large companies and major health plans require NCQA accreditation as a contract provision (Cohen, 1995).

The JCAHO developed accreditation standards for health plans and integrated health systems, which were effective July, 1994. The standards are published in the *Accreditation Manual for Health Care Networks* (JCAHO, 1996). JCAHO is currently focusing on integrating performance measures with the survey process. A large set of health care indicators has been developed, to be incorporated into JCAHO's Indicator Measurement System (IMS). "Health Plan and Network Indicators" will be the first segment available (August, 1996) of a National Library of Health Care Indicators (NLHI). Publication of the full complement of indicators, for all health care phases, is expected in 1998 (Hanold, 1996).

The primary tool used for reporting a range of outcomes information by managed care plans is the HEDIS-2.5, developed by NCQA. HEDIS includes over 60 measures used to report managed health plan performance in a standard manner to purchasers of health care services. HEDIS 2.0 was first published in November, 1993. HEDIS 2.5 was issued in January, 1995 as a comprehensive technical update. A third revision, HEDIS 3.0, still in the planning stages, includes risk-adjusted data. HEDIS measures are used by health plans to focus their quality improvement activities; employers use the data to evaluate the value of plans purchased and to compare trends among plans with whom they contract across regions (Cohen, 1995). Categories of indicators include: clinical quality—prevention/screening, disease management, appropriateness, access and member satisfaction, membership and utilization, and financial performance.

An integral part of outcomes measurement for managed care health plans involves health status versus disease-related measures. One of the selling points of managed care has been a focus on prevention and wellness. Employers are beginning to demand data demonstrating health status of enrollees. Enrollees' perceptions of well-being and functionality are also considered important indicators of health plan value (Health Care Advisory Board, 1994; Kenkel, 1995).

SLPs and other practitioners who are employees of or contractors with managed health plans are involved in managed care accreditation and outcomes measurement and management processes. Just as managed care plans are scrutinized by NCQA and JCAHO, these health plans scrutinize the providers with whom they are associated. Increasingly, MCOs are requiring health providers to present extensive quality and outcomes management data before inclusion in the provider panel, and as a condition of continuation. For more information about participating in managed care, see Ad Hoc Committee on Managed Care, ASHA (1995).

OUTCOMES MANAGEMENT

In the first chapter of this book, Frattali stated "once outcomes are measured, they must be managed if they are to have any purpose at all" (p. 32). That is, we must engage in the process of collecting, analyzing, and using patient care and related data to determine if what we do in health care makes a difference and to continually improve what we do. *Outcomes management* is the term for this process, coined by Paul Ellwood in the landmark Shattuck Lecture to the Massachusetts Medical Society (1988). Ellwood proposed that we "adopt a technology of collaborative action . . . to help patients, providers, and payers make rational medical care-related choices based on better insight into the effect of these choices on the patient's life" (p. 1551). Ellwood suggested the use of four outcomes management techniques:

- development of clinical standards and guidelines;
- systematic measurement of patient functioning and well-being at appropriate time intervals;
- pooling clinical and outcome data on a massive scale;
- analysis and dissemination of results from the data base targeted to the concerns of each decision maker.

It seems that all health care organizations, professional associations, and practitioners have developed or are currently developing patient care guidelines. These guidelines have many names and various definitions: critical/clinical pathways, practice guidelines, care maps, preferred practice patterns, practice parameters, treatment protocols, and algorithms. Although there are important distinctions among the different types, Merry (1995) refers to these tools generically as "structured care methodologies" (p. 1). According to Merry, the purpose of structured care methodologies (SCMs) is to minimize variation in patient care, thus improving quality, reducing costs, and enhancing value (Merry, 1995). All forms of SCMs are integral to outcomes management in that such structure enhances our ability to quantify, standardize, and coordinate the processes of care. A burgeoning literature is available on the development and use of clinical guidelines. I suggest these references: ASHA (1993); ASHA (1996); Field and Lohr (1992); Hoffman (1993); Horn and Hopkins (1994); McDermott and Toerge (1994); Mozena, Emerick, and Black (1996); Schoenbaum and Sundwall (1995); and Shekim (1994).

At this point, I would like to leave our discussion of outcomes management in the "scientific" sense described by Ellwood, and refer you to Chapters 3, 5, 7, and 9 in this book for further information on technologies and methods, as well as Bianchi (1995), Framroze (1995), Reinertsen (1993), and Wilkerson (1995). However, before turning to a discussion of outcomes management as predicting and controlling (or at least facilitating) outcomes in clinical practice, I would like to quote Byron Hamilton's delightful statement in an interview with Framroze (1995) about using outcomes data:

> The other thing that indicates the importance and growth of outcomes management is that more and more facilities are using this kind of information. Many facilities may not know that they're actually involved in outcomes management when they get their reports back, but when they use the reports to compare themselves to the region or nation, and begin to examine why and how they're different, then begin to look at those outcomes and try to improve those areas, then they're in the process of outcomes management. [p. 61]

I told you that many of us in health care are afraid of outcomes. We make it something too lofty and difficult to understand and use.

In their book, *Outcome-Oriented Rehabilitation,* Landrum, Schmidt and McLean (1995) present a new approach to rehabilitation care, which is both a model for reengineering rehabilitation services and a tightly woven outcomes management strategy. This model is based upon the reality in today's reform environment that we can no longer admit patients to a rehabilitation hospital and "wait and see" what improvements can be made over time. Our goal for patients can no longer be to "maximize independence."

Outcome-oriented rehabilitation services requires a shift in thinking from service-based to outcome-based rehabilitation. Clinicians become "managers of outcome" as well as "caregivers" (Schmidt, 1995). The service-based sequence of assess/diagnose, treat, wait for result, and discharge is replaced by the following sequence: assess/identify skill requirement for success in the discharge setting, project outcome, define barriers, define resources available, and manage for results (Schmidt, 1995, p. 151). Table 20–5 differentiates service-based from outcome-based rehabilitation.

Gretchen Swanson, PT, a health-care consultant, advocates a "predict and manage" model of rehabilitation care, using an outcomes-oriented approach. She suggests the development of a clinical management plan based upon patient risk factors and medical and functional requirements for discharge. Medical and functional outcomes are predicted and patients are classified (by diagnosis, payment, utilization groups, severity, and World Health Organization disability scales). Services provided are based upon protocols. Swanson has also developed a documentation tool "functional outcome report" (1993) that follows the "predict and manage" model. The report method was developed for physical therapy, but can be adapted for speech-language pathology.

The "salient factors" approach to rehabilitation care, developed by consultant Connie Burgess, RN, is also aligned with the tenets of outcome-oriented rehabilitation. This approach manages care, costs, and outcomes in a single process, and is based upon patient-specific consequences of the injury or illness, not the diagnosis. Salient care planning considers first the discharge environment, and plans care around what the

Table 20–5.

SERVICE-BASED REHABILITATION	OUTCOME-BASED REHABILITATION
Assesses the patient's impairments	Utilizes a patient-centered assessment
Defines assessment parameters according to the discipline	Defines assessment parameters by the discharge environment; focuses on skill requirements of discharge environment
Organizes the treatment plan around patient limitations	Organizes treatment plan around skill requirements of the discharge setting
Focuses treatment on reduction of impairments that underlie skill; remediates first and compensates as last resort	Focuses treatment on functional skills reacquisition; considers compensation first
Sets discipline-based goals	Sets functional goals based on the outcome result to be achieved
Provides family teaching at the time of discharge	Begins family teaching at admission and continues throughout duration of the treatment (first item taught to family is what an outcome is)
Assumes skills generalization	Builds skills generalization into the treatment plan

SOURCE: From *Outcome-Oriented Rehabilitation* by P. Landrum, N. Schmidt & A. McLean, 1995, p. 156. Gaithersburg, MD: Aspen. Copyright 1995 by Aspen Publishers, Inc. Reprinted by permission.

patient needs to move to the next level of care, including identifying barriers to discharge (see Burgess, 1996a, 1996b).

I said in the preceding paragraphs that outcome-oriented rehabilitation is a model for reengineering rehabilitation services. I would like now to discuss the relationships among outcomes, reengineering, and resources management.

Outcomes, Reengineering and Resources Management

We typically think of health care reengineering as today's solution to overstaffing, overspecialization, fragmentation of care, and service inefficiencies, driven by the forces of managed care. We do not immediately associate outcomes management with reengineering. Yet, reengineering our organizations and programs to improve effectiveness and efficiency positions us to manage outcomes. We reorganize, reconfigure and reorient our structure and process in order to offer "outcomes-oriented" services. See Cornett (1995), Freeda and Rao (1995) and Zimmerman and Skalko (1994) for more information about reengineering health care.

A focus on resources management is a large part of reengineering efforts, and also a cornerstone of managed care. According to Frattali and Cornett (1994):

> the success of 'managed care' depends on the careful monitoring and control of services rendered. Managed care *is* resources management. This focus . . . relates directly to quality of care because the purpose is to manage services to achieve optimal efficiency and effectiveness through the coordination of patient care and the integration of information. [p. 38]

Resources management is an outgrowth of the old "utilization review" method of determining appropriateness of hospitalization, tests and procedures ordered, and ancillary services used. Resources management has many components, including:

- admission and discharge planning
- utilization management
- clinical productivity studies
- cost-benefit analyses
- quality improvement activities
- use of clinical practice guidelines
- risk management

(See Frattali & Cornett, 1994 and Malkmus & Johnson, 1992 for more information about quality and resources management issues.) It is obvious now that resources management is also outcomes management.

CONCLUSION

This is the best and worst of times for health care, for rehabilitation professionals, and for SLPs. We are discouraged by criticism, but also challenged and encouraged to participate in exciting efforts to quantify, qualify, improve, and expand what we do. There is nothing wrong with being asked to demonstrate effectiveness and efficiency. As Whiteneck (1994) contends, "more attention should be given to measuring what matters: the full breadth of rehab outcomes, including successes achieved in the community as well as skills mastered in the rehabilitation hospitals" (p. 1073). Measures of handicap and health-related quality of life over the long term are becoming hallmarks of outcomes measurement in the rehabilitation field.

The three principles of rehabilitation articulated by Alexander and Fuhrer (in Frey, 1988), although 8 years old, explain the importance of viewing rehabilitation outcomes within context:

1. The primary concern of rehabilitation is the disadvantage (handicap) placed on the person by society.

2. Rehabilitation should be an educational process, providing assistance to people in adapting to their own environments.

3. Rehabilitation efforts should be directed at improving opportunities to pursue activities consistent with the person's goals. (p. 162)

We will be spending many more years redefining, revising, demonstrating, investigating, and improving health care outcomes. It will be both frustrating and satisfying. More importantly, it will help us focus on why we do what we do: to help other human beings enjoy their lives.

REFERENCES

Ad Hoc Committee on Managed Care (1994). *Managing managed care: A practical guide for audiologists & speech-language pathologists.* Rockville, MD: American Speech-Language-Hearing Association.

American Speech-Language-Hearing Association (1993, March). Preferred practice patterns for the professions of speech-language pathology and audiology. *Asha, 35*(Suppl. 11).

American Speech-Language-Hearing Association (1995). *ASHA Desk Reference.* Rockville, MD: Author.

Bianchi, B. (1995). Pragmatic outcomes. *Rehab Management, 8*(5), 112–132.

Breske, S. (1995a, April). Outcomes. *Advance for Directors in Rehabilitation, 4*(4), 15–18.

Breske, S. (1995b, November). No place like home. *Advance for Directors in Rehabilitation, 4*(10), 25–29.

Burgess, C. (1996a, February 13). *Who really cares about outcome measurement and management?* Paper presented at the CARF National Medical Conference, 1996 Standards and Best Practices, Tucson, AZ.

Burgess, C. (1996b, February/March). Hitting the wall. *Rehab Management, 9*(2), 25–27.

CARF—The Rehabilitation Accreditation Commission (1996). *Standards manual and interpretive guidelines for medical rehabilitation.* Tucson: Author.

Cichowski, K. (Ed.) (1996). *RIC-FAS-IV—Rehabilitation Institute of Chicago Functional Assessment Scale.* Chicago: Rehabilitation Institute of Chicago.

Cohen, S. (1995). National Committee for Quality Assurance. *Rehab Management, 8*(6), 13–109.

Cornett, B. (1995, December). Reengineering: Changing the focus of health care services. *Quality Improvement Digest.* Rockville, MD: The American Speech-Language-Hearing Association.

Donabedian, A. (1992, November). The role of outcomes in quality assessment & assurance. *Quality Review Bulletin,* 356–360.

Donabedian, A. (1982). *Explorations in quality assessment & monitoring, Volume 2, The criteria & standards of quality.* Ann Arbor: Health Administration Press.

Douglass, R. (1983). Defining and describing clinical accountability. *Seminars in Speech & Language, 4*(2), 107–118.

Ellwood, P. (1988). Shattuck lecture—outcomes managment: A technology of patient experience. *New England Journal of Medicine, 318*(23), 1549–1956.

Fetter, R., Shin, Y., Freeman, R., et al. (1980). Case mix definition by diagnosis related groups. *Medical Care, 18*(Suppl. 2), 1–53.

Field, M., & Lohr, K. (Eds.) (1992). *Guidelines for clinical practice.* Washington, DC.: Institute of Medicine, National Academy Press.

Fleming, J. (1996, April). Current issues in rehabilitation: The RAND study. *Medical Rehab Report #21.* Washington, DC: American Rehab Association.

Forer, S. (1995, June/July). Outcomes evaluation in subacute care. *Rehab Management, 8*(4), 138–164.

Framroze, A. (1995, June/July). A look at Rehab outcomes. *Rehab Management, 8*(4), 60–65.

Frattali, C., & Cornett, B. (1994). Improving quality in the context of managed care. In Ad Hoc Committee on Managed Care (Eds.), *Managing managed care: A practical guide for audiologists and speech-language pathologists* (pp. 33–42). Rockville, MD: The American Speech-Language-Hearing Association.

Freeda, M., & Rao, P. (1995, October/November). Rehab's sea change. *Rehab Management, 8*(6), 62–67.

Frey, W. (1988). Functional outcome: Assessment and evaluation. In J. DeLisa (Ed.), *Rehabilitation medicine: Principles and Practice* (pp. 158–172). Philadelphia: Lippincott.

Fries, J., & Spitz, P. (1990). The hierarchy of patient outcome. In B. Spilker (Ed.), *Quality of life assessments in clinical trials* (pp. 25–35). New York: Raven.

Hall, K. (1992). Overview of functional assessment scales in brain injury rehabilitation. *NeuroRehabilitation, 2*(4), 98–113.

Hanold, L. (1996, May 13). Personal communication. Oakbrook, IL: The Joint Commission on Accreditation of Healthcare Organizations.

Hawes, C., Morris, J., Phillips, C., et al. (1995). Reliability estimates for the Minimum Data Set for Nursing Home Resident Assessment and Care Screening. *The Gerontologist, 35*(2), 172–178.

Health Care Advisory Board (1994). *Next generation of outcomes tracking.* Washington, D.C.: The Advisory Board Company.

Health Care Advisory Board (1993). *Line of fire: The coming public scrutiny of hospital and health system quality.* Washington, DC: The Advisory Board Company.

Hoffman, P. (1993, July). Critical path method: An important tool for coordinating care. *Journal on Quality Improvement, 19*(7), 235–246.

Horn, S., & Hopkins, D. (1994). *Clinical practice improvement: A new technology for developing cost-effective quality health care.* New York: Faulkner & Gray.

Iezzoni, L. (1994). *Risk adjustment for measuring health care outcomes.* Ann Arbor: Health Administration Press.

Iezzoni, L., & Greenberg, L. (1994). Widespread assessment of risk-adjustment outcomes: Lessons from local initiatives. *Journal on Quality Improvement, 20*(6), 305–316.

Joint Commission on Accreditation of Healthcare Organizations (1996). *Accreditation manual for healthcare networks.* Oakbrook Terrace, IL: Author.

Kane, R. (1994, May). Looking for physical therapy outcomes. *Physical Therapy, 74*(5), 56–60.

Kenkel, P. (1995). *Report cards: what every health care provider needs to know about HEDIS and other performance measures.* Gaithersburg, MD: Aspen.

Knaus, W., Wagner, D., Zimmerman, J., & Draper, E. (1993). Variations in mortality and length of stay in intensive care units. *Annals of Internal Medicine, 118*(10), 753–761.

Landrum, P., Schmidt, N. & McLean, A. (1995). *Outcome-oriented rehabilitation.* Gaithersburg, MD: Aspen.

Malkmus, D., & Johnson, P. (1992). Dedicated management of outcome, quality, and value: Internal case management. *Journal of Head Trauma Rehabilitation, 7*(4), 57–67.

Manard, B. (1995). *Subacute care: Policy synthesis and market area analysis.* Washington, DC: Dept. of Health & Human Services, Office of Disability, Aging & Long-term Care Policy (prepared under task order contract by Lewin-VHI, Inc.).

McDermott, M., & Toerge, J. (1994). *Developing critical paths of rehabilitation care: An instruction manual.* Washington, DC: The National Rehabilitation Hospital.

Merry, M. (1995, November). Guidelines & pathways: Where do they fit in? *Inside case management, 2*(8), 1–3.

Moffa-Trotter, M. & Anemaet, W. (1995, July/August). Measuring up in home health. *Advance for Directors in Rehabilitation, 4*(7), 23–27.

Moore, R., & Salcido, R. (1996, December/January). Rehabilitation outcomes in subacute care. *Rehab Management, 9*(1), 97–111.

Mozena, J., Emerick, C., & Black, S. (1996). *Clinical guideline development: An algorithm approach.* Gaithersburg, MD: Aspen.

National Association for Home Care (1995). *Basic statistics about home care 1995.* Washington, DC: Author.

Piccirillo, J. (1993). Outcomes research in clinical practice. *Insights in Otolaryngology, 8*(5), 1–8.

Reinertsen, J. (1993, January). Outcomes management and continuous quality improvement: The compass and the rudder. *Quality Review Bulletin, 19*(1), 5–7.

Schmidt, N. (1995). Preparing rehabilitation teams for outcome-based rehabilitation. In P. Landrum, N. Schmidt, & A. McLean (Eds.), *Outcome-oriented rehabilitation* (pp. 147–185). Gaithersburg, MD: Aspen.

Schoenbaum, S., & Sundwall, D. (Eds.) (1995). *Using clinical practice guidelines to evaluate quality of care, Volume 2: Methods.* Washington, DC: U.S. Dept. of Health & Human Services, Agency for Health Care Policy & Research (Pub. #95–0046).

Schyve, P. (1995). Outcomes as performance measures. In Schoenbaum, S., & Sundwall, D. (Eds.), *Using clinical practice guidelines to evaluate quality of care, Volume 1: Issues.* Washington, DC: U.S. Dept. of Health & Human Services, Agency for Health Care Policy & Research (Pub. #95–0045).

Shekim, L. (1994, Fall). Critical pathways. *Quality improvement digest.* Rockville, MD: The American Speech-Language-Hearing Association.

Schwartz, M., & Ash, A. (1994). Evaluating the performance of risk-adjustment methods: Continuous measures. In L. Iezzoni (Ed.), *Risk adjustment for measuring health care outcomes* (pp. 287–311). Ann Arbor: Health Administration Press.

State University of New York at Buffalo, Research Foundation (1993). *Guide for use of the Uniform Data Set for Medical Rehabilitation: Functional Independence Measure.* Buffalo: Author.

Steen, P., Brewster, A., Bradbury, R., Estabrook, E., & J. Young, (1993). Predicted probabilities of hospital death as a measure of admission severity of illness. *Inquiry, 30*(2) 128–141.

Swanson, G. (1993). Functional outcome report: The next generation in physical therapy reporting. In D. Stewart & S. Abeln (Eds.), *Documenting functional outcomes in physical therapy* (pp. 101–134). St. Louis: Mosby.

Swanson, G. (1995, June 2). *Predicting and managing functional outcomes.* Article presented at the Rehab '95 Symposium. Mt. Carmel Medical Center, Columbus, OH.

Whiteneck, G. (1994). Measuring what matters: Key rehabilitation outcomes. *Archives of Physical Medicine & Rehabilitation, 75*(10), 1073–1076.

Wilkerson, D. (1995, December/January). Developing outcomes management tools. *Rehab Management, 8*(1), 114–129.

World Health Organization (1980). *International classification of impairments, disabilities, and handicaps.* Geneva: Author.

Zimmerman, D., & Skalko, J. (1994). *Reengineering health care.* Franklin, WI: Eagle Press.

Resources

Long-term Care

Resident Assessment Instrument
    Minimum Data Set (MDS)

MDS Coordinator
Health Care Financing Administration
Office of Survey & Certification
Division of Long-term Care Services
6325 Security Blvd.
Meadows East Bldg., Rm. 2-D-2
Baltimore, MD 21207
(410) 786–3000

Continuum of Care Outcome Measures

Functional Independence Measure (FIM)

(intended primarily for acute inpatient rehabilitation, many subacute providers also use FIM)

Director, Subscriber Services
UDSMR
232 Parker Hall
3435 Main St.
Buffalo, NY 14214
(716) 829–2076

Functional Assessment Measure (FIM+FAM)
Santa Clara Valley Medical Center
751 S. Bascom Ave., Box A421
San Jose, CA 95128
(408) 295–9896

LORS-III, home care, acute care, acute rehabilitation, medical outcomes system, and neurological, orthopedic, and occupational outcomes scales for outpatient services.

Formations in Health Care, Inc. (Medirisk)
155 N. Wacker Drive
Suite 725
Chicago, IL 60606
(312) 849–4200

Medirisk Corp. Headquarters
Two Piedmont Center, Suite 400
3565 Piedmont Rd.
Atlanta, GA 30305–1502

Patient Evaluation and Conference System (PECS)
Rehabilitation Outcome Reporting System
Marianjoy Rehabilitation Hospital & Clinics
P.O. Box 795
Wheaton, IL 60189
(708) 462–4403

Focus on Therapeutic Outcomes, Inc. (FOTO)
P.O. Box 11444
Knoxville, TN 37939
(800) 482–FOTO
(423) 450–9699

Managed Health Plan/Network Accreditation

National Committee for Quality Assurance
1350 New York Ave., NW
Suite 700
Washington, DC 20005
(202) 955–3500

Joint Commission on Accreditation of Healthcare Organizations
Provider Network Accreditation
One Renaissance Blvd.
Oakbrook Terrace, IL 60181
(708) 916–5721

Rehabilitation Services Accreditation

CARF . . . The Rehabilitation Accreditation Commission
4891 East Grant Road
Tucson, AZ 85712
(520) 325–1044

Outcome-Oriented Rehabilitation Principles/Methods

Connie Burgess
Connie Burgess & Associates
5505 E. Carson St., Suite 345
Lakewood, CA 90713
(310) 497–2050

Gretchen Swanson
Swanson & Company
2734 E. Broadway, Suite 7
Long Beach, CA 90803
(310) 438–5799

Home Care Services
National Association for Home Care
228 Seventh St., SE
Washington, DC 20003–4306
(202) 547–7424

CHAPTER 21

Outcomes Measurement in Universities

JUDITH A. RASSI

INTRODUCTION

Outcomes measurement,[1] in one form or another, has been an integral part of most university[2] educational programs throughout their existence. In traditional higher education, like secondary and elementary education, student learning is typically assessed via standardized and nonstandardized examinations. Evaluating the effectiveness of classroom instruction and curriculum design is not uncommon. Accrediting bodies set standards that require universities not only to maintain adequate resources and personnel but also to engage regularly in program self-study and obtain outcomes measures as part of their program planning and evaluation (ASHA, 1994a; ASHA, 1995).

Educators and administrators have thus participated in different types of evaluative efforts. Many of these, however, have been based on measuring inputs or processes rather than outcomes. Moreover, as general higher education is subject to increasing scrutiny by government officials, accreditation agencies, reform commissions, and the public, so, too, are the appropriateness and quality of assessment methods (Erwin, 1991). Demands for health care reform have also led to new demands for substantial educational reform, especially in entry-level programs for allied health professionals (Markus, 1995). At the same time, professional communities and employers are calling for greater accountability by university preparation programs. Their main concern is the preparedness of graduates for independent, efficient, and competent service delivery in today's work force (Spahr, 1995).

Complicating the conditions imposed by external forces are other related factors such as: diminishing and unpredictable financial support (Davis, 1995); expanding knowledge bases and scopes of professional practice; restricted faculty size and increasing student enrollment; and organizational restructuring of departments, universities,

---

[1]For the purposes of this chapter, the words *measure(ment)* and *assess(ment)* are used interchangeably.
[2]The word *university*, as used in this chapter, refers to colleges as well as universities.

and university systems. The uncertain climate created by these circumstances is pervading institutions of higher learning, much like that which has already affected health care organizations as well as businesses, corporations, and industries nationwide. Communication sciences and disorders (CSD) educational programs, whose viability hinges on their strength within the arenas of both health care and higher education, are clearly vulnerable to the consequences of such sweeping systemic change.

The reasons for educators to rethink and reexamine are compelling. Cost containment has become as important in education delivery as it is in health care delivery. Academic accountability requirements have increased accordingly. University downsizing initiatives to streamline or even eliminate departments, some of them in our field, have taken place. Meanwhile, educational quality at all levels has emerged as a major national issue.

The message is clear. Unless we can prove that the ways in which we educate are the most effective and efficient possible, it will be difficult to justify the continuation of our positions or our programs. Neither can we reasonably expect to receive the kind of financial, administrative, or public support necessary to sustain our work. To survive in this changing academic environment, CSD educators must incorporate programmatic, curricular, and teaching innovations into their programs. Then they must continually prove the worth of their efforts by providing irrefutable evidence of positive educational outcomes.

This chapter familiarizes you with the purposes, goals, and types of educational outcomes measurement. Because of the scope of the topic—entire books and journals are devoted to it—discussion is necessarily limited. Noticeably, the extensive topic of graded student examinations is presented only in general terms. However, samples of other measurements known and used by educators across disciplines, are described, and some ways of implementing them suggested. A dissection of instrument elements and design considerations follows. Classroom assessment techniques, not as widely applied as traditional measures and often experimental in nature, are discussed in a separate section because of their great potential for application in CSD education. Together, these topics should provide you with a framework for thinking about possible measurement variations that might be suitable for yourself or your university program. The concluding sections of this chapter look at the status of CSD outcomes studies and applications, then explore needs and future directions.

PURPOSES OF OUTCOMES MEASUREMENT

A major purpose of educational outcomes measurement is quality improvement. This basic concept, if not its multiple procedural variations, is now familiar to virtually every organization or individual who has been involved in the national quest for efficacy and efficiency. Still, quality in higher education has a different connotation than does quality in other sectors. Frazer (1992) captures it in these words:

> . . . quality in higher education is a pervasive, but elusive concept, is multifaceted, requires judgments by people with experience, and cannot simply be equated with excellence. Whereas standards refer to the intentions of a program and the achievements of graduates who follow it, quality is much broader and includes standards as well as the processes of teaching and learning, the activities of departments and institu-

tions and the congruence between the goals of a program and the competences of its graduates. [p. 15]

Even though this view of quality has a unique set of defining characteristics, widely used quality improvement principles readily lend themselves to application in the higher education arena (Whittington & Ellis, 1993). Among these are continuous improvement, process thinking, customer focus, team decision making, and data collection (Scholtes, 1994). Mission and vision statements and constancy of purpose (Hospital Corporation of America et al., 1991) are other quality improvement elements consistent with a rationale for measuring outcomes.

As implied in the chapter introduction, accountability is also a primary reason for and purpose of educational outcomes measurement. Depending on the circumstances of a given CSD program, mandates may be emerging or already in place. Whatever the urgency of current accountability requirements, professionals need to seize the initiative to determine their own assessment directions. Delay in doing so makes it possible for others to choose specific assessment methods or impose certain directions that might be inappropriate or undesirable for a particular program or institution (Erwin, 1991). Adopting a proactive rather than reactive stance, however, allows educators the opportunity to manage their own accountability.

The relationship between these two major purposes of educational outcomes measurement—quality improvement and accountability—is apparent. Accountability follows, and depends on, quality improvement: we account for the quality of our work by providing evidence that we are continually striving to improve that quality. Quality improvement, on the other hand, is driven by accountability: we seek to improve quality because we, as well as others, hold ourselves accountable for what we do. The essential connection between these two purposes is outcomes measurement. Without it, qualities such as educational effectiveness and customer satisfaction can only be assumed, not proven. Without it, accountability has no basis.

GOALS OF OUTCOMES MEASUREMENT

What are the goals of outcomes measurement in universities? What is it that we are trying to measure, and why? The answers to these questions can be broad, covering the entire range of university operations, or narrow, focusing on individual performance in a particular situation. In keeping with the aim of this chapter, general areas that are commonly selected for university evaluation are mentioned briefly, whereas specific classroom measures are examined in greater detail.

Institutional and Programmatic Measurement Goals

Universities are held accountable by accreditors and standards-setting groups for meeting specified criteria. Public institutions answer directly to state governments and/or federal government, while universities in the private sector must do the same where governmental funding of research or other programs is concerned. Governing boards of trustees and directors, alumni, and other stakeholders also hold universities responsible for certain policies and actions.

To satisfy the various compliance requirements, universities engage in many different kinds of evaluation or information-gathering activities. As alluded to earlier, descriptions of input or process variables (for example, library size or faculty qualifications) have been used traditionally (Jordan, 1989). General self-study efforts, meanwhile, have concentrated on the areas of mission, teaching, curriculum, research, and service. Table 21–1 lists these and other areas, as well as some of the subcategories, which are considered to be quality indicators and thus are typically targeted for data collection.

As is apparent, these kinds of data are important for carrying out such important tasks as administrative planning, allocation of funds, and program development. Their contribution to effective institutional operation is unquestionable. And they do meet logical accountability requirements. However, with a few notable exceptions, such information is neither outcome-based nor does it necessarily offer proof of educational quality.

Table 21–1. Sample Targeted Data-Collection Areas in Universities

ADMISSIONS
    Applicants: demographic distribution, characteristics, entry qualifications
    Process: criteria, procedural steps, timelines

ALUMNI
    Gift support

BUDGET
    Funds for equipment, maintenance
    External funding
    Salary schedules

CAMPUS
    Campus life: dormitory life, faculty availability; student housing
    Campus size
    Coordination and management of campus services: business office; campus police; building maintenance; parking; registration
    Staff views: library; computer center; research office

CURRICULUM
    Design, development, planning
    Scope: topic coverage

FACILITIES
    Classrooms
    Laboratories
    Space availability

FACULTY
    Characteristics: age; gender; rank; tenure status

Individual teaching loads
Qualifications: teaching, publication, research accomplishments
Size of faculty, number of full-time equivalents (FTEs)

FINANCIAL ASSISTANCE FOR STUDENTS

MISSION
    Adherence to university mission
    Adherence to program mission

RESEARCH
    Research grants funded
    Research funding for doctoral programs

RESOURCES: FINANCIAL, PHYSICAL

SERVICE
    Service activities of university in community
    University relations with the community

STUDENTS
    Enrollment: full-time vs part-time students
    Grades
    Graduate employment rates
    Retention rates

TEACHING
    Class size
    Course design

Classroom Measurement Goals

At the classroom level, measurement goals can concentrate specifically on the two fundamental areas that most challenge today's educational reformers: student learning and teacher effectiveness. Indeed, these have been the actual target areas of external groups who demand that universities "explain what they are trying to do and . . . demonstrate how well they are doing it" (Angelo & Cross, 1993, p. xiii).

Higher education has begun to respond to such demands by renewing and redirecting its efforts in classroom as well as institutional assessment and in instructional improvement. These efforts have been reflected in classroom research, which is seeking ways to help instructors better understand the teaching-learning process and how their own teaching can be more effective. Many university campuses now have teacher support centers where special programs and resources on classroom teaching methods are available to instructors (McElroy & Rassi, 1992b).

Classroom assessment, a major component of classroom research and widely applied in universities throughout the country (Angelo, 1995), focuses on the direct involvement of both students and teachers in continuously monitoring the learning that takes place. This dual involvement brings out important feedback—feedback to teachers on the effectiveness of their teaching and feedback to students on the progress of their learning (Angelo & Cross, 1993). Moreover, the ongoing sampling of learning outcomes in an actual classroom can be particularly meaningful and useful, as both teachers and students stand to benefit from immediate action on the results. In other words, classroom assessment, when appropriately executed and applied, incorporates functional measures.

Clinical Practicum Measurement Goals

As with measurement goals in the classroom, outcomes of student learning and teacher effectiveness in clinical practicum endeavors are also critical to the quality of educational programs. Requiring students to demonstrate evidence of their knowledge and skill in carrying out clinical activities is one way for educators to address employers' concerns about the preparedness of CSD graduates to function as independent, competent clinicians. Likewise, continuous assessment of clinical teaching (supervision) effectiveness by participants allows and encourages ongoing adjustments to accommodate the teaching-learning process. The parallel between classroom and practicum assessment is thus apparent.

Laboratory Measurement Goals

Laboratory instruction, when offered as an adjunct to classroom and clinical teaching, comprises another instructional area in CSD education that warrants the scrutiny of outcomes measurement. Typically designed to provide students with opportunities to learn, demonstrate, and practice clinical, research, and related problem-solving skills, educational "labs" often serve as an essential link between classroom and clinical instruction (McElroy & Rassi, 1992a). Lab instructors or facilitators are in a position, like their counterparts in the classroom and clinic, to measure learning outcomes and instructional effectiveness. The means commonly used to accomplish lab teaching objectives—computer-assisted instruction (CAI), learning modules, videotapes and audiotapes, clinical and research equipment—as well as the skills and knowledge to be acquired, are especially conducive to discrete measurement of learning outcomes.

TYPES OF OUTCOMES MEASUREMENT

As implied in the preceding sections, measurements of educational outcomes vary according to their primary purpose and specific goals. They also may be as different and individualized as the universities, programs, or persons who design them. Except in those instances where uniform, standardized assessment across institutions is desirable for comparative purposes, such variation is appropriate. In effect, it renders outcome data more usable and useful.

Variation Types

For CSD educational programs, the various individuals and groups called upon to provide input into measurement activities may include, but are not limited to: students; graduates; course instructors; practicum internship (on-campus) supervisors; practicum externship (off-campus) supervisors; clinical fellowship supervisors; and other employers of graduates. Individually and collectively, these persons bring different perspectives to the process, thereby allowing important cross-checks of information.

Data collection methods and instruments also vary. These might be administered in the form of practical examinations, nonstandardized written examinations, standardized written examinations, surveys, or interviews. As will be discussed later, classroom assessment techniques employ multiple variations that are even more specific. Regardless of the means used to gather information, it is essential that the questions asked be purposeful and relevant.

Sampling time points along the educational continuum constitute another set of variables. Students' views, skills, and learning can and should be sampled at various stages of their undergraduate and graduate study—during and after courses, during and after practicum assignments. Formative assessment, conducted while an educational event or procedure is ongoing, yields information substantially different from that obtained in summative assessment, which is administered at the time of term completion. Likewise, pre- and postgraduation measures can reveal significantly different outcomes for students, as can samplings of recent and previous graduates. Time factors may also influence the responses of course instructors, practicum supervisors, and other contributors of measurement information.

Commonly Used Approaches

Given the types of variations in outcomes measurement, there are many possible combinations, hence many feasible designs. A number of the approaches commonly used in higher education and health professions education are applicable in CSD programs (Rassi, 1995b). Representative procedures are delineated in Tables 21–2 and 21–3 according to these parameters: (1) the person(s) providing input; (2) the person(s), process(es), or procedure(s) being measured; (3) the medium or tool being used; (4)

Table 21–2. Representative Learning Outcomes Measurement Procedures Applicable in CSD Programs, According to Parameter Combinations

(1) BY WHOM	(2) OF WHOM/WHAT	(3) MEDIUM	(4) MODE	(5) OUTCOME(S) MEASURED
clinical supervisors	students	examination	practical/ oral	clinical performance
course instructors	students	examination	written	theoretical knowledge/ applied knowledge
lab instructors	students	examination	practical	applied knowledge/ demonstrated skills
employers	graduates	survey	written	on-the-job performance
*professional certification body	certificate applicants	standardized examination	written	theoretical knowledge/ applied knowledge
*licensure board	licensure applicants	standardized/ nonstandardized examination	written practical/ oral	theoretical knowledge/ applied knowledge

*Outside the purview of the university, but pertinent to an educational program's targeted learning outcomes.

the mode or method of administration; and (5) the outcome(s) being measured. Table 21–2 identifies learning outcomes measures, and therefore is product-oriented. Table 21–3 lists measures of educational outcomes, and thus is process-oriented.

SAMPLE CSD OUTCOMES MEASUREMENTS

It has already been suggested that outcomes measurements are most useful if tailored to the specific requirements and goals of a particular educational program or of the learning units and individuals within it. Even so, for purposes of highlighting content and format features, this section presents excerpted, summarized material from sample CSD instruments.[3] Each illustrative figure contains information on instrument use and instructions, as well as the rating scale and descriptors, sample items, and scoring, where these are applicable. A brief discussion follows each figure.

The Student Performance Review in Speech-Language Pathology Clinical Practicum, whose features are presented in Figure 21–1, was developed to achieve certain objectives of an overall clinical instruction system (Rassi & Hancock, 1993). Based on the premise that competency-based education offers a logical approach to the preparation of CSD practitioners and that a continuum framework for clinical supervision is conducive to competency/skill development and professional growth, the system design merges these two concepts. Along with goal-setting, progress-monitoring, evalu-

[3]These abridged versions are based on some of the educational assessment documents designed, adapted, and/or refined by faculty and staff members of the Division of Hearing and Speech Sciences, Vanderbilt University School of Medicine.

ation, and grading elements, there are provisions for planning, skill development, feedback, and self-supervision incorporated into the design.

The instrument itself serves as the basis for ongoing discussion between a clinical teacher and practicum student about the student's clinical development. Both parties are involved in setting goals, monitoring progress, and assessing final outcomes. In other words, skill development and movement toward independence, that is, the student's attainment of jointly-established goals, are the focus of such discussion. Importantly, the appropriateness of the clinical teacher's supervision for the student's clinical competency levels is also subject to monitoring by both parties. In either case, at the conclusion of a practicum placement, these individuals' separate or collective perceptions of goal attainment are recorded as the documented outcomes.

Table 21–3. Representative Educational Outcomes Measurement Procedures Applicable in CSD Programs, According to Parameter Combinations

(1)	(2)	(3)	(4)	(5)
BY WHOM	OF WHOM/WHAT	MEDIUM	MODE	OUTCOME(S) MEASURED
students	course instructors/ course design	questionnaire	written	teaching effectiveness/ attainment of course objectives
students	course instructors/ course design	individual interview/ class discussion	oral	teaching effectiveness/ attainment of course objectives
students	program curriculum	questionnaire	written	curriculum design/ attainment of program objectives
students	program curriculum	interview	oral	curriculum design/ attainment of program objectives
students	clinical supervisors/ practicum placement	questionnaire	written	supervisory effectiveness/ attainment of practicum objectives
students	clinical supervisors/ practicum placement	interview	oral	supervisory effectiveness/ attainment of practicum objectives
graduates	aspects of educational program	exit interview	oral	attainment of program objectives
graduates	aspects of educational program	retrospective analysis	written	attainment of program objectives
professional accreditation body	aspects of educational program	self analysis/ site visit review	written/ oral	attainment of accreditation standards

Figure 21–1. Sample student performance review in speech-language pathology clinical practicum (excerpted, summarized).

The competency statements that comprise this document were designed for purposes of practicum goal-setting and the monitoring and evaluating of students' clinical performance. Supervisors and students use the scale and descriptors shown on the dual-movement (supervisor and student) supervision continuum.

INSTRUCTIONS WITH RATING SCALE AND DESCRIPTORS

STUDENT

ABSENT	EMERGING	PRESENT	DEVELOPED	CONSISTENT
Competency/skill not evident	Competency/skill emerging	Competency/skill present but needs further development	Competency/skill developed but needs refinement and/or consistency	Competency/skill well-developed and consistent

SUPERVISOR

MODELING/ INTERVENTION	FREQUENT INSTRUCTION	FREQUENT MONITORING	INFREQUENT MONITORING	GUIDANCE
Requires constant supervisory modeling/ intervention	Requires frequent supervisory instruction	Requires frequent supervisory monitoring	Requires infrequent supervisory monitoring	Requires guidance/ consultation only

Supervisors: Using the following key, circle the appropriate descriptor in the first column to indicate the student's initial goal for each competency statement being reviewed. Then, record midterm status and final level of competency/skill development, respectively, in the second and third columns.

$$
\begin{array}{rcl}
\text{CONS} & = & \text{CONSISTENT} \\
\text{DEVEL} & = & \text{DEVELOPED} \\
\text{PRES} & = & \text{PRESENT} \\
\text{EMERG} & = & \text{EMERGING} \\
\text{ABS} & = & \text{ABSENT}
\end{array}
$$

After the final competency level has been determined for each item under review, indicate in the last column the status of goal attainment, where—

- − (minus) means goal not attained
- = (equal) means goal attained
- + (plus) means goal surpassed

SAMPLE ITEMS

PLANNING	Goal					Mid	Final	Attain
Reviews file for each individual to obtain information	ABS	EMERG	PRES	DEVEL	CONS	___	___	___
Develops appropriate long-term goals for clients	ABS	EMERG	PRES	DEVEL	CONS	___	___	___

(continued)

485

Figure 21–1. Sample student performance review in speech-language pathology clinical practicum (excerpted, summarized). *(continued)*

IMPLEMENTATION	Goal		Mid	Final	Attain
Elicits relevant information in an organized manner and pursues pertinent points	ABS EMERG PRES DEVEL CONS		_____	_____	_____
Uses appropriate verbal and nonverbal reinforcers effectively	ABS EMERG PRES DEVEL CONS		_____	_____	_____
INTERPRETATION					
Recognizes client's goal attainment or client's need for goal adjustment	ABS EMERG PRES DEVEL CONS		_____	_____	_____
CASE MANAGEMENT					
Demonstrates sensitivity to client and family members	ABS EMERG PRES DEVEL CONS		_____	_____	_____
REPORT WRITING					
Incorporates appropriate information into report content	ABS EMERG PRES DEVEL CONS		_____	_____	_____
SUPERVISORY CONFERENCES					
Takes initiative to make suggestions regarding own clinical development	ABS EMERG PRES DEVEL CONS		_____	_____	_____

SCORING INFORMATION SUMMARY

Grade calculation is based on goal attainment. Total number of goals attained/surpassed is divided by total number of competency items scored, then multiplied by 100, resulting in the BASIC PERFORMANCE PERCENTAGE. Percentage points may be added for extraordinary performance or subtracted for absent professionalism skills, resulting in an ADJUSTED PERFORMANCE PERCENTAGE. The final performance percentage, whether basic or adjusted, is then converted into a letter grade on the basis of this table:

If FINAL PERFORMANCE is	Then letter grade is
90% or higher	A+ or A or A–
80% to 89%	B+ or B or B–
70% to 79%	C+ or C or C–
60% to 69%	D+ or D or D–
lower than 69%	F

As shown in Figure 21–2, the Evaluation of Externship Experience is designed to elicit feedback from students on their culminating clinical practicum experience, a full-time 10-week placement typically located at a distant site. This review mechanism brings to the university educational program important insight as well as factual information for consideration in future educational planning. To the extent that university

Figure 21–2. Sample evaluation of externship experience (excerpted, summarized).

USE OF INSTRUMENT

At the conclusion of their final externship, students give feedback on their experience, providing a description of the facility, patient population, clinical services, and staff composition, as well as their assessment of the placement.

INSTRUCTIONS

Extern: On the reverse side of this page, and on continuation pages, if needed, summarize your assessment of this externship placement. Consider the following:

- Its contribution to your total graduate education experience
- The appropriateness of the clinical activities for your needs and interests
- The influence of this placement on your professional goals
- The quality of supervision provided
- The advisability of using this site again for externships
- Any other feedback you deem important

RATING SCALE AND DESCRIPTORS

No rating scale used. Narrative description only.

SAMPLE ITEMS

Response to specific items not required. Topics suggested in instructions.

SCORING INFORMATION SUMMARY

Not applicable.

---

coordinators can gauge the results of their externship placement efforts through students' perceptions, this tool yields critical outcomes data.

The Curriculum Evaluation, capsulized in Figure 21–3, affords students an opportunity to engage in a retrospective comprehensive review of the academic program. The detailed information sought in this measure provides administrators and other faculty and staff members with students' reactions to the program as a whole and as an aggregation of its component parts. Program strengths and weaknesses become apparent when individual responses are compared within a particular class of students and between classes from year to year. This is particularly helpful in tracking outcomes for quality improvement purposes and in checking the program's adherence to its mission.

The Supervisor/Employer Evaluation of Graduate, excerpted in Figure 21–4, represents what some might consider to be the truest kind of outcomes measure. That is, employers of graduates provide feedback for the university program, commenting on the products (outcomes) of educational preparation and reporting on whether or not graduates met employers' expectations for job performance. Moreover, these employers' observations are not based on what they think a graduate should be able to do, but rather on what they actually find a graduate is able to do. In a quality improvement paradigm, this kind of outcomes measurement determines if the needs of an educational program's external customers—employers of its graduates—are being met. As with the retrospective curriculum evaluation, employers' evaluations of graduates may

Figure 21–3. Sample curriculum evaluation (excerpted, summarized).

USE OF INSTRUMENT

At the conclusion of their master's degree program, students are asked to provide thoughtful and candid input concerning curriculum and related academic issues. This information is used for curriculum planning.

INSTRUCTIONS

Students: For each of the courses listed below, please indicate the extent of your disagreement or agreement with these statements:

1. I found this course/seminar to be an important part of my master's curriculum.
2. The order of this course/seminar in the master's curriculum sequence met my learning needs.
3. The number of credit hours, that is, the amount of weekly class time allocated for this course is appropriate for the amount of material and importance of the topic in clinical practice.
4. Where relevant, the content of this course was consistent with (that is, not contradicted by) my related clinical practicum experience.

Circle the appropriate indicator for each statement.

RATING SCALE AND DESCRIPTORS

$$X = \text{Did Not Take Course}$$
$$SD = \text{Strongly Disagree}$$
$$D = \text{Disagree}$$
$$N = \text{Neutral}$$
$$A = \text{Agree}$$
$$SA = \text{Strongly Agree}$$

SAMPLE ITEMS

COURSE NUMBER/ TITLE		1. IMPORTANT PART OF CURRICULUM	2. SEQUENCE MET LEARNING NEEDS	3. CREDIT HOURS APPROPRIATE	4. CONTENT CONSIST W/ CLIN PRACT
206/Intro to Speech Science	X	SD D N A SA	SD D N A SA	SD D N A SA	SD D N A SA
304/Child Lang Acquisition	X	SD D N A SA	SD D N A SA	SD D N A SA	SD D N A SA
314/Artic Dis and Phonetics	X	SD D N A SA	SD D N A SA	SD D N A SA	SD D N A SA
331/Aphasia	X	SD D N A SA	SD D N A SA	SD D N A SA	SD D N A SA
335/Augment Communication	X	SD D N A SA	SD D N A SA	SD D N A SA	SD D N A SA

ADDITIONAL INSTRUCTIONS FOR ADDITIONAL SECTIONS

In the space below (or on an attached page), please indicate other course or curriculum changes that you think would be beneficial to master's level students. Specify reasons for any suggestions. Consider these possibilities:

- Expanding or reducing topic coverage within a specific course. Combining two or more courses.
- Adding or deleting specific course labs.

488

Figure 21–3. Sample curriculum evaluation (excerpted, summarized). *(continued)*

- Eliminating or adding a particular course or seminar.
- Shortening or extending the master's program.
- Providing the means for combining a master's and doctoral program of study.
- Changing a required course to an elective course, or vice-versa.
- Changing the required status of a course, e.g., for audiology students only, for speech-language pathology students only, or for students without undergraduate speech/hearing background only.

In the space below (or on an attached page), please indicate the kinds of changes in clinical practicum assignments that you think would be beneficial to master's level students. Specify reasons for any suggestions. Consider these possibilities:

- Rearranging practicum and class schedules to accommodate different clinical assignment times.
- Providing more practicum opportunities in specific settings or with specific populations.
- Adding more off-campus practicum opportunities.
- Scheduling more practicum hours or fewer practicum hours within a particular semester.
- Extending, shortening, or eliminating the externship.

ADDITIONAL SAMPLE ITEMS

From your perspective, what are the major *strengths* of the master's program?
From your perspective, what are the major *needs* of the master's program?
Please offer your comments about this program evaluation tool. Indicate any changes that might be made to increase its effectiveness.

SCORING INFORMATION SUMMARY

Not applicable.

also provide useful information about program strengths and weaknesses when the results show certain patterns.

The Course Evaluation features shown in Figure 21–5 are typical of those for many educational programs within or outside CSD. In that students provide feedback concerning course design and instruction, the information gathered in this manner can be used to determine what modifications might be indicated for a teacher's future classes. On the other hand, any review of outcomes at the end of a course cannot effect change for the students who just completed the course and yet were the ones who provided the input—a major drawback and strong argument for ongoing classroom assessment, as discussed elsewhere in this chapter.

The results of course evaluations are often included in university administrators' appraisals of faculty and staff performance. When applied in this way, student feedback can have a powerful impact on individual instructors' career development and thus the direction of an educational program. In a quality improvement context, where students are seen as the educational program's primary internal customers, it is logical that course outcomes should be analyzed from a student perspective. This also gives students the opportunity to participate in program decision making. Finally, if the course evaluation instrument is so designed, valuable information regarding students' self-perceived learning can be obtained.

Figure 21–4. Sample supervisor/employer evaluation of graduate (excerpted, summarized).

USE OF INSTRUMENT

This instrument seeks evaluative feedback on graduates from their on-the-job supervisors or employers.

INSTRUCTIONS

Supervisor/Employer of Graduate: Please evaluate the knowledge and performance of the graduate who gave you this form, then return the completed form in the attached envelope. Rate the graduate's knowledge and/or performance according to the scale by circling the most appropriate number.

RATING SCALE AND DESCRIPTORS

1 = Poor
2 = Less than satisfactory
3 = Satisfactory
4 = Good
5 = Excellent
X = Unable to evaluate/not applicable

SAMPLE ITEMS

CLINICAL COMPETENCY—SPEECH-LANGUAGE PATHOLOGY

	Knowledge	*Performance*
Evaluation of speech disorders—adult	1 2 3 4 5 X	1 2 3 4 5 X
Evaluation of speech disorders—child	1 2 3 4 5 X	1 2 3 4 5 X
Evaluation of language disorders—adult	1 2 3 4 5 X	1 2 3 4 5 X
Evaluation of language disorders—child	1 2 3 4 5 X	1 2 3 4 5 X
Treatment of speech disorders—adult	1 2 3 4 5 X	1 2 3 4 5 X
Treatment of speech disorders—child	1 2 3 4 5 X	1 2 3 4 5 X
Treatment of language disorders—adult	1 2 3 4 5 X	1 2 3 4 5 X
Treatment of language disorders—child	1 2 3 4 5 X	1 2 3 4 5 X
Counseling / management	1 2 3 4 5 X	1 2 3 4 5 X
Clinical report writing	1 2 3 4 5 X	1 2 3 4 5 X

OTHER AREAS OF COMPETENCY

	Knowledge	*Performance*
Research competency	1 2 3 4 5 X	1 2 3 4 5 X
Administrative competency	1 2 3 4 5 X	1 2 3 4 5 X
Teaching / supervision competency	1 2 3 4 5 X	1 2 3 4 5 X
Interpersonal communication competency	1 2 3 4 5 X	1 2 3 4 5 X

ADDITIONAL SAMPLE ITEMS

Please comment on any other noteworthy aspects of this graduate's knowledge/performance. In particular, please indicate any specific strengths or needs that you think are a reflection of the graduate's educational preparation.

When the graduate began this position, how did his/her knowledge and performance compare with that of other persons you have supervised/employed in comparable positions?

much poorer		about the same		much better
1	2	3	4	5

Figure 21–4. Sample supervisor/employer evaluation of graduate (excerpted, summarized). *(continued)*

How did the amount/type of on-the-job training required for this person compare with that usually required?

much more		about the same		much less
1	2	3	4	5

If you had appropriate positions available, would you want to employ other graduates of this program?

yes _____   no_____   other_____ (please explain)

Please add any other comments that you think would be helpful in our educational program planning.

SCORING INFORMATION SUMMARY

Not applicable, although mean ratings can be calculated to determine group trends.

ELEMENTS OF MEASUREMENT INSTRUMENTS

As indicated by the instrument features highlighted in Figures 21–1 through 21–5, traditional measurement instruments have several common elements. The discussion here provides a general description of elements and explores related ideas on design and implementation.

Identifying and Introductory Information

Following an appropriate title, which usually heads a formal paper-and-pencil measure, the first section requires the person who is completing the form to supply identifying information, and contains appropriate blanks and/or space for this to be accomplished. Statements of purpose appear next. These statements must be carefully worded because: (1) they are intended to help respondents understand the purpose of the measurement—indeed, clarity of understanding can directly affect an individual's responses; and (2) they must be readily understood by those persons who eventually become involved in the processing and interpretation of data.

Instructions for completing the form usually follow purpose statements. For the same reasons just cited, instructions must be clearly written. They also need to be concise, but procedural steps should be sufficiently detailed for participants to proceed without seeking additional direction.

Measurement Criteria

The method selected for dissecting or examining collected information is logically presented in the section following instructions so that explanatory keys or examples can be shown. Here, the instrument user is familiarized with measurement criteria and other

Figure 21–5. Sample course evaluation (excerpted, summarized).

USE OF INSTRUMENT

At the conclusion of each course, students provide written feedback concerning various aspects of course design and teaching.

INSTRUCTIONS

Use the following rating scale to evaluate this course. Please feel free to add comments, for example, your basis for a given response, within the body of the form as well as in the comments section at the end of the form.

RATING SCALE AND DESCRIPTORS

---

1 = Poor
2 = Below Average
3 = Average
4 = Above Average
5 = Excellent

SAMPLE ITEMS

CONTENT

	Poor				*Excellent*
Instructor has a thorough knowledge of subject matter	1	2	3	4	5
Course meets defined objectives	1	2	3	4	5
Course content is relevant to student's professional needs	1	2	3	4	5

METHODS

Learning experiences are organized to meet objectives	1	2	3	4	5
Material presented is relevant and comprehensive	1	2	3	4	5
Format (e.g., small groups, teacher lecture, student presentations) is appropriate to subject matter	1	2	3	4	5

EVALUATION AND GRADING

Course requirements are clearly delineated in advance	1	2	3	4	5
Evaluation is appropriate to the task	1	2	3	4	5
Adequate and immediate feedback and/or evaluation of performance is provided	1	2	3	4	5

INTERACTION

Instructor is available outside of class for help with course-related problems	1	2	3	4	5
Instructor has respect for individual students	1	2	3	4	5
Instructor has respect for class as a whole	1	2	3	4	5

SCORING INFORMATION SUMMARY

For every class, group mean responses and standard deviations are calculated, item by item. These results, along with typed versions of respondents' written comments, are compiled for each course and given to the course instructor.

ways in which information is to be judged or reported. Common observaton, survey, and questionnaire formats utilize checklists, rating scales, or open-ended questions. Surveys or questionnaires may seek factual information or probe respondents' opinions, interests, or attitudes. Traditional examinations might employ multiple-choice, essay, short-answer, true-false, compare-and-contrast, item-matching, or problem-solving designs. Construction of each is governed by a set of definitive rules (McBeath, 1992).

Most educators are familiar with checklists as being composed of desirable behaviors that can be observed, then marked as present or absent. In CSD education, checklists are frequently used by clinical practicum supervisors and laboratory instructors. Although not shown here, the measurement tool excerpted in Figure 21–1 does have a section addressing professionalism that utilizes a checklist format. Use of rating scales is evident in all four of the sample instruments presented in Figures 21–1, 21–3, 21–4, and 21–5. The remaining instrument, depicted in Figure 21–2, requires narrative description in response to a set of suggested considerations.

Rating scales in these examples vary according to their measurement criteria. The Figure 21–1 sample pairs an unnumbered 5-point developmental scale, where the descriptors reflect a student's clinical skill development, with a parallel supervision scale in which a succession of supervisory styles serve as markers. Although this dual scale is behaviorally anchored, it does not conform to a conventional poorest-to-best interpretation because of the unique way in which it is applied to changing goals over time. A more traditional Likert scale (Likert, 1932) is used in the Figure 21–3 example. Its construction is bipolar, based on the extent of a respondent's agreement or disagreement (relative to a neutral center position) with content statements.

The scales in Figures 21–4 and 21–5 represent the simplest kind of semantic differential rating (Osgood, Suci, & Tannenbaum, 1957) where contrasting adjectives appear at either extreme of the continuum, and adjectives of graduated meaning mark the options within. In these particular scales, ordinary adjective descriptors are sequenced in a negative-to-positive order and given numerical value, or weighted, according to a 1-to-5 scale. Although rating decisions must be considered in the light of an assumed standard ("satisfactory," "average"), they are entirely subjective and based on individual interpretation. Still, the relative values signified by the accompanying numbers do allow raters to make comparative distinctions independent of semantic content.

The measurement components discussed here can be combined in various ways to suit the goals of a particular measurement plan. In addition, there are many other kinds of options available to designers of measurement instruments. Specific information may be found in educational measurement and assessment literature, including that which is specific to allied health professions.

Content Items

The main body of a measurement instrument usually comprises the content items. Whether cast in the form of test questions, competency statements, multiple-choice or rating items, or other types of response items, they are coordinated here with the selected measurement mechanism to meet data-collection objectives. Thus, the actual content derives from the topic being addressed. Items may be expressed in single words, phrases, or sentences.

The selection of content items is as challenging to educators as the decision about measurement criteria. Indeed, as critics of higher education often ask: Are we assessing the right thing? Are we assessing what really matters? Or, as so often phrased by those who would hold us accountable, are we measuring functional outcomes? The probable answer to each: sometimes yes; sometimes no. Importantly, whatever the content decisions being weighed, educators should consider an array of available options and then choose what best accomplishes their actual measurement intention.

In their studies of classroom assessment, Angelo and Cross (1993) discovered that instructors may not know when, or how, to assess a particular area, such as students' thinking skills, because the instructors are not certain exactly when or how they are even teaching such skills. To minimize this kind of uncertainty, instructors need to have a clearer conceptual understanding of assessment content areas (in this case, critical thinking) (Pike, 1996), of general educational objectives, and of individual instructional objectives before proceeding with the "what" of content decisions.

The classic taxonomies of educational objectives for the cognitive domain (Bloom, 1956) and affective domain (Krathwohl, Bloom, & Masia, 1964) can provide guidance in formulating individual objectives and, ultimately, in constructing assessment items. Cognitive domain categories are outlined here:

   1.00 Knowledge
      1.10 Knowledge of specifics
         1.11 Knowledge of terminology
         1.12 Knowledge of specific facts
      1.20 Knowledge of ways and means of dealing with specifics
         1.21 Knowledge of conventions
         1.22 Knowledge of trends and sequences
         1.23 Knowledge of classifications and categories
         1.24 Knowledge of criteria
         1.25 Knowledge of methodology
      1.30 Knowledge of the universals and abstractions in a field
         1.31 Knowledge of principles and generalizations
         1.32 Knowledge of theories and structures
   2.00 Comprehension
      2.10 Translation
      2.20 Interpretation
      2.30 Extrapolation
   3.00 Application
   4.00 Analysis
      4.10 Analysis of elements
      4.20 Analyses of relationships
      4.30 Analysis of organizational principles
   5.00 Synthesis
      5.10 Production of a unique communication
      5.20 Production of a plan, or proposed set of operations
      5.30 Derivation of a set of abstract relations
   6.00 Evaluation
      6.10 Judgments in terms of internal evidence
      6.20 Judgments in terms of external criteria (pp. 201–207)

The outcomes of an educational measurement, whether formative or summative, can be functional if they provide information that is acted upon or changes behavior in accordance with program objectives. In other words, the action or behavior may take place in the context of the educational program or the employment setting of the graduate. Thus, the timing of the measurement does not determine its functional nature. Content selection does. For example, student achievement testing can seek outcomes in certain knowledge acquisition areas that are not necessarily functional, or it can address competencies such as analytical skill, communication effectiveness, and problem solving ability, which have professional applications and are therefore functional. Of course, achievement testing can and should be designed to accomplish both. The point to be made here is that outcomes serve a functional role only if the content area and content items reflect and then accomplish this intent.

Interpretation of Results

The final section of a typical measurement instrument is devoted to an explanation of scoring and its interpretation, where such is applicable. As with the initial purpose statements in a document, an explanation of the significance or intended use of the collected information should be communicated to those who give their input or process the data. Not incidentally, this message also helps to clarify for instrument designers what their own intentions are.

Depending on the goals of a particular measurement, matters of validity and reliability need to be taken into account when tools are developed or results are interpreted. If comparisons are being made, interpretations also need to be referenced—criterion-referenced, norm-referenced, or self-referenced (Erwin, 1991). In other words, when data are being used to make consequential comparisons or programmatic decisions or add to a quantitative research base, statistical treatments are in order. However, if the measurement is less formal, as, for example, in the collection of information on student learning to inform individual teaching, this kind of rigor becomes less important (Gibbs, 1995).

Regardless of the measurement intent, certain steps can be taken to increase reliability even if you are creating the simplest of measurement tools. For instance, the reliability of conventional classroom examinations can be generally strengthened by increasing test length. To combat the common problems of rater (dis)agreement and rater bias, raters can be trained and behavioral descriptors used for rating scales (Erwin, 1991).

Validity, that is, whether or not an instrument is actually measuring what you intended it to measure, poses a different set of concerns. Whereas statistically-based standardized measures usually account for validity as it relates to item content, measurement criteria, and instrument construction, even these instruments may be inappropriate, hence invalid, if selected for an application for which they were not intended. As with reliability, strict adherence to validity rules is difficult when assessment tools are customized for use within a particular course or program. But, again, steps can be taken to minimize problems, such as being clear about the purpose of the assessment and defining measurement criteria carefully (Erwin, 1991).

Because no measure can be completely reliable or valid, some critics believe that assessment should not be pursued (Erwin, 1991). Many educators, however, see great value in this endeavor (Angelo & Cross, 1993; Erwin, 1991; Whittington & Ellis, 1993).

They assert that, while we must seek to achieve as much integrity as possible in our assessment efforts, the constant and consistent collection of data is essential to the improvement of educational programs. We must experiment with new ways, better ways. For instance, it has been shown that teacher effectiveness cannot be assessed adequately by students only, but can be better accomplished through multiple approaches—evaluations by students, peers, and administrators, in combination with self-evaluations (Dilts, Haber, & Bialik, 1994; McElroy & Rassi, 1992b). The result is greater overall validity. More important, perhaps, is the increased likelihood of improved teaching.

CLASSROOM ASSESSMENT

Classroom assessment techniques (CATs) are probably the most contributory kind of educational measurement, certainly the most consequential in their influence on classroom teaching and student learning. They are learner-centered, teacher-directed, formative, context-specific, ongoing, and grounded in effective teaching practice (Angelo & Cross, 1993). Furthermore, the direct involvement of students in decision-making about their own learning is consistent with quality improvement principles. For these reasons, additional information on classroom assessment is presented here.

Assessment Principles

Whatever your individual assessment goals, the use of sound guiding principles will enhance their effectiveness in actual practice (Banta et al., 1996). To this end, a group of assessment experts in higher education, drawing on the experiences of educators throughout the nation, developed a set of nine assessment principles. Subsequently published by the American Association for Higher Education (1992) as *The Principles of Good Practice for Assessing Student Learning,* these principles are as follows:

1. The assessment of student learning begins with educational values.
2. Assessment is most effective when it reflects an understanding of learning as multidimensional, integrated, and revealed in performance over time.
3. Assessment works best when the programs it seeks to improve have clear, explicitly stated purposes.
4. Assessment requires attention to outcomes but also and equally to the experiences that lead to those outcomes.
5. Assessment works best when it is ongoing, not episodic.
6. Assessment fosters wider improvement when representatives across the educational community are involved.
7. Assessment makes a difference when it begins with issues of use and illuminates questions that people really care about.
8. Assessment is most likely to lead to improvement when it is part of a larger set of conditions that promote change.
9. Through assessment, educators meet responsibilities to students and to the public. (pp. 2–3)

Assessment Techniques

As already indicated in the discussion on content items, educators must clarify, by writing appropriate instructional goals or objectives, what they want their students to learn, particularly if the intent is to assess and improve classroom instruction. To this end, Angelo and Cross (1993) developed the Teaching Goals Inventory (TGI), a self-scoring tool for teachers to use in identifying and clarifying their teaching goals. The TGI contains 52 goals, divided into these six clusters: higher-order thinking skills; basic academic success skills; discipline-specific knowledge and skills; liberal arts and academic values; work and career preparation; and personal development. Use of this kind of tool, along with a resource like the earlier-mentioned Bloom taxonomy, can help teachers sort through the content possibilities that might apply to their particular classroom assessment endeavors and, then, through employment of CATs, determine if their instructional goals are being met.

On analyzing the results of CATs—there are dozens of variations—an instructor can adjust teaching accordingly. To illustrate, Angelo and Cross (1993) present in their handbook a number of CATs for assessing the following course-related knowledge and skills: students' prior knowledge, recall, and understanding (CAT example—Memory Matrix); skill in analysis and critical thinking (CAT example—Pro and Con Grid); skill in synthesis and creative thinking (CAT example—One-Sentence Summary); skill in problem solving (CAT example—Documented Problem Solutions); and skill in application and performance (CAT example—Student-Generated Test Questions).

How do CATs relate to traditional classroom tests and course grades? At any time throughout a course or term, and/or at its conclusion, graded assignments or examinations of students' accumulated learning—that is, their learning outcomes—can be used to test the knowledge and skills previously tapped in ungraded formative classroom assessments, or CATs. The two approaches can thus complement one another. In a different configuration, when grading is used to inform and improve teaching, the grading itsef becomes a form of classroom assessment (Walvoord & Anderson, 1995).

CSD OUTCOME STUDIES AND APPLICATIONS

Investigative Studies

Since the 1960s, numerous clinical teaching studies have been presented and published in the field (Rassi, 1994). Some have been outcome-based; others not. Some have explored the application of innovative methods and instruments. These many experiments and analyses have generally increased our understanding of the supervisory process and of clinical practicum. Their impact on actual educational practice across the field has not yet been determined, however, and answers to fundamental efficacy questions are just emerging (Gillam, Strike Roussos, & Anderson, 1990; Shapiro & Anderson, 1989).

In comparison to the ongoing collection and dissemination of clinical supervision data, laboratory and classroom instruction in our field have not been similarly investigated (Rassi & McElroy, 1992b). Small amounts of information, though, have appeared in recent publications and presentations, indicating that these instructional areas are beginning to receive some attention (Fowler & Leonards, 1992; Fowler & Wilson, 1992; Rassi, 1995a; Tharpe, Rassi, & Biswas, 1995).

Outcomes-Based Standards

As stated in the introduction to this chapter, accreditation standards require CSD educational programs to carry out certain kinds of outcome measures. Inasmuch as certificate applicants must successfully complete coursework, practicum, and clinical fellowship requirements, and also obtain a passing score on a national examination (ASHA, 1994b), certification standards also relate to outcomes. Despite this inclusion of outcome elements, however, both academic accreditation standards and certification standards in the field have emphasized input rather than output.

Our standards-setting bodies, the Council on Academic Accreditation (CAA) and the Council on Professional Standards (SC), are now seeking to shift this emphasis. Specific knowledge and skills outcomes, for example, are being incorporated by the SC into its current revision of audiology certification standards. Even the decision to revise these standards was outcome-based, drawing on results of a job analysis study designed and administered by the Educational Testing Service (Tannenbaum & Rosenfeld, 1995). This study compared the views of practitioners, educators, and clinical fellowship supervisors on the importance of clinical activities and knowledge areas, and where they are, and should be, learned. An upcoming review of speech-language pathology certification standards will use this same kind of approach.

CONCLUSION

The need for educational outcomes measurement, in all its permutations, has never been more apparent. For higher education, in general, and CSD education, in particular, the demands for quality improvement and accountability have never been more pressing. And yet, in the midst of this clamor, many educators seem not to know where to turn or what to do. In addressing this problem at a colloquy on challenges and solutions for academia (Goldsmith, Fagan, & Battle, 1995), participants offered the following premise and solutions for just one of several faculty development issues,[4] that of improving instruction:

Issue

Improve Instruction

All levels and stages of instruction should be competency based, integrated, and should be relevant to current needs in the work place. To improve cost-effectiveness, technology must be infused throughout the curriculum, regardless of the instructional environment, including classroom, laboratory, and practicum sites.

Solutions

1. Explore use of case-based and problem-based learning.
2. Promote use of interactive technologies for various instructional experiences (i.e., levels and types).

[4]In addition to several faculty development issues, participants addressed these equally important and interrelated issues: educational structures, mission, and evaluation; managing change; accreditation and certification; and curriculum and instruction.

3. Develop instructional packages that address issues ranging from specific tasks to complete courses.

4. Conduct search for innovative instructional models and materials across disciplines.

5. Establish national clearing house for innovative instructional models and materials.

6. Identify and promote more cost-effective models of supervision, such as sequential, layered, team, distance supervision.

7. Develop a national data base relative to the efficacy of alternate practicum experiences through interactive technologies as an alternative to face-to-face supervision.

8. Develop functional outcome measures of classroom instruction, supervision, and curriculum relative to competencies of graduates. (Appendix A, pp. 1–3)

Also suggested were the types of individuals or groups who might be best prepared to tackle these tasks, and the additional resources needed for implementation. Colloquy participants did emphasize in their deliberations that faculty members from, and within, CSD educational programs across the country would need to take an active role in any innovative educational effort of this magnitude.

All of the cited solutions, not just the eighth one, speak directly to the challenge of outcomes measurement. Indeed, we need comprehensive educational research aimed at every facet of our university preparation programs. As reported earlier in this chapter, classroom research encompasses classroom assessment. Likewise, educational research comprises the entire range of possible educational outcomes measurements. In operational language, this means that we must proceed to collect all sorts of educational data—data on existing educational approaches as well as experimental ones and data on educators and students, teaching and learning, models and methods, effectiveness and efficiency, relevance and efficacy. Unless we can present a reasonable and defensible rationale for what we do, continued program support, financial and otherwise, may no longer be justified. As Logemann (1995) points out, ". . . administrators look hard at our (CSD) programs because they contain a great deal of highly expensive individualized education. What data do we have that support our current educational model as the best way to educate clinicians in our professions?" (p. 19).

Simply collecting data is not enough, of course. We have to act on our findings. And then collect more. The number of investigational possibilities is virtually unlimited. In the abbreviated list of colloquy solutions, for example, several avenues are evident—incorporating innovative teaching methods into our classroom instruction, utilizing new educational technologies, importing educational expertise and information from other disciplines, and experimenting with more cost-effective clinical teaching strategies. Each solution calls for substantial change—change in our ways of thinking about higher education and CSD education. We need to examine our assumptions about traditional ways of teaching, traditional educational models, traditional professorial and supervisory roles, and traditional curricula (Rassi & McElroy, 1992a).

Such an examination of assumptions will require CSD educators' individual and collective thinking—consulting with experts in health professions education, higher education, educational measurement, and classroom assessment; reading and discussing the literature in these and other related areas; and insisting that education become and remain a top priority for systematic study and experimentation in our field. Together, these kinds of initiatives can lay the foundation for CSD-specific educational research, including the study and application of outcomes measurement. It is important to note that ASHA, in addition to sponsoring the aforementioned colloquy, has made impressive strides over the past few years in mobilizing CSD educational resources. Involvement of this and other related professional organizations will continue to be critical to educational reform efforts.

A final observation: the selection and use of measurements is ultimately related, either directly or indirectly, to the educational philosophies and practices espoused by the universities, programs, or individuals who adopt them. Similarly, the extent to which measurements are carried out and outcomes data are actually used to effect change is a reflection of commitment to quality.

REFERENCES

American Association for Higher Education (1992). *Principles of good practice for assessing student learning.* Washington, DC: Author.

American Speech-Language-Hearing Association (1994a). *ESB. Educational Standards Board Accreditation Manual.* Rockville, MD: Author.

American Speech-Language-Hearing Association (1994b). *Membership and Certification Handbook. Speech-Language Pathology. 1995.* Rockville, MD: Author.

American Speech-Language-Hearing Assocation (1995). ASHA Academic Accreditation Transition Team. *Resource manual. Academic accreditation standards: Comparison of the standards of eighteen accreditation agencies.* Internal document.

Angelo, T.A. (1995). Improving classroom assessment to improve learning: Guidelines from research and practice. *Assessment Update, 7*(6), 1,2, 12,13.

Angelo, T.A., & Cross, K.P. (1993). *Classroom assessment techniques. A handbook for college teachers.* (2nd ed.) San Francisco: Jossey-Bass Publishers.

Banta, T.W., Lund, J.P., Black, K.E., & Oblander, F.W. (1996). *Assessment in practice.* San Francisco: Jossey-Bass Publishers.

Bloom, B.S. (1956). (Ed.). *Taxonomy of educational objectives. Handbook I: Cognitive domain.* New York: Longman, Inc.

Davis, J.M. (1995). Looking at the big picture: Changing fiscal, policy, demographic, and technological environments in higher education. In S.C. Goldsmith, E. Fagan, & D.E. Battle (Eds.), *Educating Future Professionals: Challenges and Solutions for Academia. Blueprint for a New Academic Agenda: A compilation of articles inspired by the December 1994 ASHA Colloquy* (pp. 7–14). Rockville, MD: American Speech-Language-Hearing Association.

Dilts, D.A., Haber, L.J., & Bialik, D. (1994). *Assessing what professors do. An introduction to academic performance appraisal in higher education.* Westport, CT: Greenwood Press.

Erwin, T.D. (1991). *Assessing student learning and development. A guide to the principles, goals, and methods of determining college outcomes.* San Francisco: Jossey-Bass Publishers.

Fowler, C.G., & Leonards, J.S. (1992). Research laboratory teaching: Preparing lessons and planning instruction. In J.A. Rassi & M.D. McElroy (Eds.), *The education of audiologists and speech-language pathologists* (pp. 279, 300). Timonium, MD: York Press.

Fowler, C.G., & Wilson, R.H. (1992). Education in the research laboratory. In J.A. Rassi & M.D. McElroy (Eds.), *The education of audiologists and speech-language pathologists* (pp. 159–173). Timonium, MD: York Press.

Frazer, M. (1992). Quality assurance in higher education. In A. Craft, (Ed.), *Quality assurance in higher education* (pp. 9–25). Washington, DC: The Falmer Press.

Gibbs, G. (1995). Research into student learning. In B. Smith & S. Brown (Eds.), *Research, teaching and learning in higher education* (pp. 19–29). London: Kogan Page.

Gillam, R.B., Strike Roussos, C., & Anderson, J.L. (1990). Facilitating changes in supervisees' clinical behaviors: An experimental investigation of supervisory effectiveness. *Journal of Speech and Hearing Disorders, 55*, 729–739.

Goldsmith, S.C., Fagan, E., & Battle, D.E. (Eds.). (1995). *Educating Future Professionals: Challenges and Solutions for Academia. Blueprint for a New Academic Agenda: A compilation of articles inspired by the December 1994 ASHA Colloquy.* Rockville, MD: American Speech-Language-Hearing Association.

Hospital Corporation of America, Quorum Health Resources, Inc., and Executive Learning, Inc. (1991). *Hospitalwide quality: Focus on continuous improvement. Leader workbook, Version 91.1.* Nashville, TN: Author.

Jordan, T.E. (1989). *Measurement and evaluation in higher education: Issues and illustrations.* New York: The Falmer Press.

Krathwohl, D.R., Bloom, B.S., & Masia, B.B. (1964). *Taxonomy of educational objectives. Handbook II: Affective domain.* New York: Longman, Inc.

Likert, R. (1932). A technique for the measurement of attitudes. *Archives of Psychology, 140*, 44–53.

Logemann, J.A. (1995). Forces affecting academic programs. In J.E. Bernthal, E. McNiece, D. Nash, & D. Sorenson (Eds.), *Proceedings of the Annual Conference on Graduate Education: Restructure* (pp. 17–22). Council of Graduate Programs in Communication Sciences and Disorders.

Markus, G.R. (1995). Educating future professionals: The purchaser viewpoint. In S.C. Goldsmith, E. Fagan, & D.E. Battle (Eds.), *Educating Future Professionals: Challenges and Solutions for Academia. Blueprint for a New Academic Agenda: A compilation of articles inspired by the December 1994 ASHA Colloquy* (pp. 15–19). Rockville, MD: American Speech-Language-Hearing Association.

McBeath, R.J. (Ed.). (1992). *Instructing and evaluating in higher education. A guidebook for planning learning outcomes.* Englewood Cliffs, NJ: Educational Technology Publications.

McElroy, M.D., & Rassi, J.A. (1992a). Classroom teaching: Designing and planning courses. In J.A. Rassi & M.D. McElroy (Eds.), *The education of audiologists and speech-language pathologists* (pp. 225–278). Timonium, MD: York Press.

McElroy, M.D., & Rassi, J.A. (1992b). Learning teaching, improving teaching. In J.A. Rassi & M.D. McElroy (Eds.), *The education of audiologists and speech-language pathologists* (pp. 3–30). Timonium, MD: York Press.

Osgood, C.E., Suci, C.J., & Tannenbaum, P.H. (1957). *The measurement of meaning.* Urbana: University of Illinois Press.

Pike, G.R. (1996). Assessment measures. Assessing the critical thinking abilities of college students. *Assessment Update, 8*(2), 10–11.

Rassi, J.A. (1994). Supervision and the supervisory process. In R. Lubinski & C. Frattali (Eds.), *Professional issues in speech-language pathology and audiology: A textbook* (pp. 293–305). San Diego: Singular Publishing Group.

Rassi, J.A. (1995a). *Incorporating problem-based learning into classroom teaching: Experimentation and analysis.* Presentation at the annual meeting of the American-Speech-Language Hearing Association.

Rassi, J.A. (1995b). *Measuring educational outcomes in universities.* Presentation at the annual meeting of the American-Speech-Language Hearing Association.

Rassi, J.A., & Hancock, M.D. (1993). *Competency- and continuum-based clinical instruction: System development and use.* Presentation at the annual meeting of the American Speech-Language-Hearing Association.

Rassi, J.A., & McElroy, M.D. (1992a). Curriculum development. In J.A. Rassi & M.D. McElroy (Eds.), *The education of audiologists and speech-language pathologists* (pp. 63–107). Timonium, MD: York Press.

Rassi, J.A., & McElroy, M.D. (1992b). Preface. In J.A. Rassi & M.D. McElroy (Eds.), *The education of audiologists and speech-language pathologists* (pp. xiii–xv). Timonium, MD: York Press.

Scholtes, P.R. (1994). *The team handbook for educators. How to use teams to improve quality.* Madison, WI: Joiner Associates Inc.

Shapiro, D.A., & Anderson, J.L. (1989). One measure of supervisory effectiveness in speech-language pathology and audiology. *Journal of Speech and Hearing Disorders, 54,* 549–557.

Spahr, F.T. (1995). The impact of external forces on the education of audiologists and speech-language pathologists. In S.C. Goldsmith, E. Fagan, & D.E. Battle (Eds.), *Educating Future Professionals: Challenges and Solutions for Academia. Blueprint for a New Academic Agenda: A compilation of articles inspired by the December 1994 ASHA Colloquy* (pp. 21–27). Rockville, MD: American Speech-Language-Hearing Association.

Tannenbaum, R.J., & Rosenfeld, M. (1995). *The practice of audiology. A study of clinical activities and knowledge areas for the certified audiologist. A job analysis conducted on behalf of the American Speech-Language-Hearing Association.* Princeton, NJ: Educational Testing Service.

Tharpe, A.M., Rassi, J.A., & Biswas, G. (1995). Problem-based learning: An innovative approach to audiology education. *American Journal of Audiology, 4*(1), 19–25.

Walvoord, B.E., & Anderson, V. (1995). An assessment riddle. *Assessment Update, 7*(6), 8,9; 11.

Whittington, D., & Ellis, R. (1993). Quality assurance in health care: The implications for university teaching. In R. Ellis (Ed.), *Quality assurance for university teaching.* Bristol, PA: Open University Press.

CHAPTER 22

Outcomes Measurement in Private Practice

CHRISTIE-ANN M. CONRAD

INTRODUCTION

As the health care and education industries change, so too must private practice. During a time of intense scrutiny of the "why's" and "how's" of service delivery, private practitioners may risk reimbursement from third party payers (as well as from clients themselves) unless accountability for treatment benefit is both defined and demonstrated. With drastic increases in service costs, forced reductions in human and financial resources, growing demands for services, and more educated consumerism, clients and their sponsors (e.g., payers, regulators, employers) want lower costs and greater predictability of results.

This chapter takes primarily the perspective of the private practitioner in solo or small private practice. It covers the three-party system in which private practitioners typically work, the importance of measuring practice patterns, consumer satisfaction, functional outcome reporting, and cost considerations. While skimming only the surface of the outcomes measurement issues facing private practitioners today, these areas are considered vital to the survival of the private practice sector during a time when other service options may seem more attractive as the system braces for yet further restructuring and unprecedented change.

THE THREE-PARTY SERVICE DELIVERY SYSTEM

The discussion of client outcomes as they relate to private practice requires, at the outset, a review of the system that affects us directly and contributes to our financial existence. Generally, we have a three-party system involved in the payment of services to the private practice.

The First Party: Private Practitioner

The private practice is the first party, defined as the provider of service. In order to be the most effective provider possible, it is helpful to subscribe to the adage, "to thine own self be true." In other words, we must first define ourselves as individual practitioners. Our strengths and weaknesses must be identified. Through this knowledge, we will have the ability to understand our limitations and know what we can change. This will enable us to accept the challenge of competing to the best of our individual abilities. This introspective process begins with asking some basic questions (Stewart & Abeln, 1993):

- Am I a good clinician?
- What are my strengths?
- What are my weaknesses?
- What types of cases am I best prepared to assess and treat?
- Which cases do I need to refer to another provider?
- Do I provide "quality" care and how is it defined in the field of speech-language pathology?
- Do I believe this type of care is demonstrated in my practice?
- How do I judge the quality of care I provide?
- Do I routinely provide quality of care as a standard of practice?
- Do I enjoy doing what I am doing?
- Am I in this for the short-term or long-term?
- Am I flexible?
- Does my concept of "quality" guarantee that my clients are satisfied with my treatment?
- Would my clients come to me again for service?
- Do my clients "get better" and/or resolve their problems?
- Does their communicative functioning improve?

All of these questions should be addressed routinely by any private practitioner. In order to carve a niche and define a standard of practice, you must know yourself and your practice. It is through this in-depth knowledge of your own private practice that you will be able to thrive in the present and plan for the future.

The Second Party: Client

The receiver of the service (the client and significant others) is the second party in our third-party system. In this relationship, it is helpful to remember that "perception is reality." Client satisfaction plays an increasingly important role in our delivery of service. Client statements such as, "I'm not any better," and "You didn't do what I thought you said you would" become issues when they capture the attention of payers. The literature supports consumer satisfaction as playing an important role in defining quality (ASHA, 1995a). We have even moved in the direction of renaming our clients as "customers" and following the lead of manufacturers in terms of "product" satisfaction.

Unlike a product, however, an unhappy client cannot be returned. But, as with any unacceptable product, money for payment can be withheld. Shared or agreed-upon expectations by the client and clinician preceding treatment, then, can often minimize dissatisfaction, whether perceived or real. Further queries can adjust these expectations (Stewart & Abeln, 1993):

- How do your clients perceive you?
- How do they define your role?
- What do your clients think is good or "quality" care?
- Why did your clients come to you?
- Would your clients come to you again based upon their experiences?
- Do your clients believe good quality care is consistently being delivered?

Services need to be both consumer friendly and client/family driven. It is recommended that before any treatment, the client and/or significant others state what their goals and expectations are in writing. These goals need to be agreed upon and modified periodically. Certainly, before discharge these written statements should be reviewed, revised, and discussed with all involved parties. Appendix 22–A and 22–B, provide examples of satisfaction surveys that can be used with clients/family and payers/employers at the completion of treatment (see also Chapter 4 in this volume).

Central to the issue of client satisfaction, are estimated cost of services and projected duration of treatment. As stated in the "Model Bill of Rights" (ASHA, 1995b), the client has the right to know in advance the fees for services *regardless of method of payment*. Disclosure prior to treatment enables both the client and clinician to anticipate and resolve many problems that may occur due to an initial lack of agreement or differences in perceived expectations.

The Third Party: Payer

The third party involved in the system of service delivery is the payer, commonly known as the health insurance company, the health plan, Medicare, or Medicaid. In order to flourish in their complex world, we as the practitioners must "know the code." Following an exploration of ourselves and our clients, then, we must explore our payer. Questions the practitioner might ask regarding the funding sources include (Stewart & Abeln, 1993):

- How much of the revenue of your practice, or your income, comes from your client?
- How much revenue comes from other payer sources?
- Who are these other payers?
- What are their expectations of you?
- Do they think you practice good, quality care?
- Are they satisfied with your treatment of the client?
- Do they think you improve your client's well-being?
- Are their members satisfied with your services?

- Is care documented?
- Do the services provided aid the client in returning to the least restrictive environment as quickly as possible?
- And (most importantly) is your care cost effective and does it lead to a quantifiable functional improvement?

Payers are starting to send out questionnaires to the recipients of care to assess both the quality of care and the satisfaction with services rendered.

Demanding provider accountability for services has been an accepted way of containing costs. Based upon the satisfaction of third-party payers and your clients, your practice can grow proportionately. Good definable client care, client satisfaction, and an open communication line with payers all contribute to the present and future success of your practice.

MEASURING PRACTICE PATTERNS

Third-party payers have lifted the shroud of secrecy surrounding the importance of quality management. Payers must not only know how to limit costs, but also how to track underutilization or overutilization, which often leads to poor client outcomes and unnecessary expenses. We, as private practitioners, place equal importance on quality management in our administrative functions. We must compare the *cost* of our services to the amount of *reimbursement* for services. Thus, the collection and reporting of data on quality have become an essential tool used to realistically and quantitatively analyze the impact of the services we provide. While individual case reviews have been the standard of quality assessments by payers, a trend towards identifying acceptable practice patterns has emerged. Consequently, payers are encouraging the assessment of private practices in terms of *practice patterns,* rather than on quality on a case-by-case basis. Stated by one fiscal intermediary, "the insurance companies are holding up a mirror to reflect back to the provider of services exactly what he or she is doing and presenting it as a total picture." So, in addition to physical environment and available equipment and supplies (i.e., the structure of care) quality, satisfaction with services, and acceptable practice patterns (i.e., the process and outcome of care) also need to be assessed.

The following practice patterns should be identified: (1) entry/exit criteria, (2) minimal standards of care; (3) complications of care, (4) preventative screening (i.e., well-baby care) and, (5) under- and overutilization. Exploration of these practice patterns allows us to examine, not just assess, the quality of services that we provide to permit continual improvements.

In essence, the key stakeholders want to have a guarantee of sorts that what we are doing is working at a cost that is commensurate with benefits resulting in functional outcomes. This is why it is so critical that even before treatment begins, expectations of the client, family, payer, physician, and clinician are recorded, reviewed, and revised regularly. It is through this communication that all involved parties unite in these efforts to optimize the benefits of service.

As a part of the initial interview, a survey is recommended that fully discloses:

1. The client's expectation of therapy and results.

2. The family's or significant other's expectation of therapy.

3. The payer's expectation and results.

4. The referral source's expectation of therapy and results.

5. The clinician's expectation of therapy and results.

It is only with this information that the treatment plan is developed and modified. The following case example illustrates the benefits of this approach.

A CASE EXAMPLE

A 26-year-old female presents with recurrent bilateral vocal nodules following surgical intervention 2 years earlier. For the past 6 months she presented with hoarseness and harshness affecting her ability to continue teaching her class at the middle school level. The client was referred by the otolaryngologist to the speech-language pathologist (SLP) for evaluation and possible intervention. During the initial interview, the following expectations and goals of function were verbalized by all involved parties (Ladarum, Ketchelds, Schmidt et al., 1993).

Client: "To eliminate my hoarseness so continued teaching and parenting can occur."

Family: "For our wife and mother to decrease depression due to the voice problem and increase social interaction with our friends and family."

Payer: "To remediate problem ASAP through limited sessions and the SLP's participation in the education of the client's family so that extensive costs are not incurred and the client is able to return to work."

Physician: "To remediate suspected abuse so surgery would be avoided."

Clinician: "To develop a plan of treatment focusing on good vocal practices, compensatory movements, and client's family education so that the client can return effectively and safely to work and participate functionally in the home environment as quickly as possible."

Traditionally, as SLPs, our clients are treated until therapy is no longer clinically necessary. Now the availability of reimbursement may be the determining factor in discontinuation of service. More often termination of therapy is dictated by the end of reimbursable services, *not* when the client has reached his/her optimal level of performance.

THE EMERGENCE OF FUNCTIONAL OUTCOMES

Throughout past years, SLPs have struggled to identify their professional boundaries. Our scope of practice was largely dictated and driven by individual practitioners. We continued to expand in the areas of swallowing, cognitive retraining, and dementia management without sufficient hard data to support our interventions. Our services (as others) expanded and costs soared. Today, we no longer have the luxury of pursuing a goal for the client because *we think* it is important without having the data to support its claim. Today we must clearly demonstrate the functional consequences of clinical intervention.

FUNCTIONAL OUTCOME REPORTING

Although functional outcomes are universally demanded, particularly by payers, there is not an accepted standard of reporting. By definition, functional outcome activities must be:

1. Meaningful to the client and/or caregiver.
2. Practical to the client.
3. Sustainable over time.

In order to understand the importance of functional outcomes and their impact, it is helpful to compare and contrast the customary accepted practice of evaluation and treatment with the current method utilizing functional outcomes. Traditionally, clients' impairments were only assessed using standardized diagnostic instruments. Based upon the results, a plan of treatment to remediate the impairment was implemented. Goals, such as "Client will demonstrate 90% fluency at the sentence level in a structured clinical environment" were written. Following a clinician-driven plan, a list of strategies the client could utilize would be instructed by the clinician. The clinician would then begin a series of drills, collecting data, and modifying goals, based upon client performance. If the clinician's goals for the client were achieved (and before funding ended), family education would be provided before discharging the client. Success was measured at this point and the client was expected to generalize the newly acquired skills to everyday life activities. When problems occurred, the process of evaluation and treatment was repeated.

Recently, the concept of functional outcome reporting was introduced in payer guidelines and accreditation standards. If this same client entered with the same impairment, an assessment of strengths and needs (in addition to traditional diagnostic testing) would be completed. During this assessment, discharge plans would be discussed and functional skills and limitations would be defined. Treatment plans would not only focus on functional skill remediation but on instruction in the implementation of compensatory strategies, designed to promote efficient and immediate carry-over into the client's everyday environment. All parties involved with the client's care, and most importantly the client himself/herself, would develop relevant goals. The family would be a part of the intervention process, providing valuable input and feedback as the treatment process continued. Generalization to the discharge environment would not wait until services were discontinued but would be an integral component of each treatment session. Therefore, desired outcomes would be addressed at the outset and treatment would be designed to meet the functional needs of the individual.

Given the current service delivery environment, measurable treatment goals are expected to be achieved in shorter periods of time. Instead of the broad-based goals of rehabilitation, a focus is needed on specific, attainable, and functional outcomes. Because each client is unique, universal functional goals cannot be devised. Instead, goals should be tailored to best suit the personal needs of each client. Functional goals should not be synonymous with basic skill acquisition, but instead should result in meaningful, successful, effective, and relevant outcomes for each client.

MEASURING COST EFFECTIVENESS

Beyond devoting attention to our individual clients, we need to begin to establish a data base of acceptable practice patterns for particular diagnoses. Consider the range of clients with specific speech, language, cognitive, and swallowing disorders. Why would a client choose to receive services in a private practice instead of a hospital, school, home environment, or even a competitor's private practice? Traditionally, our response has been, "Because of our reputation for the provision of good care." However, as financial resources continue to dwindle, a strong factor contributing positively to the selection of private practices as a viable option will be *cost effectiveness.* Payers and employers want the most for their money. With the increasing financial contributions demanded of the client, they too will "shop around." Therefore, private practices should (if not for the future of private practices in general but for our own survival) view the establishment of practice patterns as an indicator of value.

Private practices should be able to calculate the cost per unit to treat the client. Equipment, administrative activities, physical plant, supervisory functions, support staff, marketing, and other overhead expenses should all be assessed in order to calculate the cost per unit of treatment. Overall costs should also include the fee for the evaluation and the prediction of the cost incurred over the length of treatment. Based upon one's previous experiences and the information shared during the assessment, along with a data base of historical data, the clinician should be able to predict the anticipated average number of sessions the client would need to achieve the desired outcome.

It is important, however, that we not lock ourselves into a set of predictions derived from historical data. As with other standards of care, the private practitioner needs to use available data as a base, but based upon individual clients, necessary modifications should be made. If treatment needs to be altered to improve outcomes or decrease costs, the practitioner is obligated to make these modifications and justify them to the attendant parties. Another case example that incorporates these cost considerations is presented.

A CASE EXAMPLE

A 7-year-old child presents with lateralized /s/ with no previous history of treatment and no medical complications reported. The child's parents report that friends and family are "teasing the child" and she is withdrawing from social and school situations.

The clinician assesses the child and finds she is stimulable but inconsistent in production of the target phoneme. Based upon current practice guidelines and in the child's best interest, the clinician might traditionally recommend 2 weeks of treatment daily with a focus on consistent production in the home and school environments. If the parents report the child is unable to attend daily but only 2 times per week, the clinician would modify the treatment to 8 sessions per month for an extended period of 2 months. Also, prior to discharge, psychosocial components (e.g. fear of speaking in class, social withdrawal) and family and school education would also be included in this assessment of treatment goals and expectations before discharge. Early care provided at this level or modifications to treat at the child's current developmental level will ultimately result in reduced cost as the child progresses. The speech-language pathologist might measure the consequences of the impairments manifested in performance of the child's everyday life activities. This combination of tailoring the treatment to the child's needs, providing education, and addressing preventive measures to offset anticipated long-term problems will result in a cost- effective alternative to traditional treatment.

In our experience, we have found clients and family to be agreeable to any modifications in treatment *as long as they were discussed and acknowledged prior to the anticipated end of therapy.* Professional expertise and revision of the plan of care in the client's best interest are respected, not resented. If client and family are informed, they are more likely to comply with the modifications and participate fully and effectively throughout the treatment process.

CONCLUSION

For the solo or small private practice, a frequently asked question is, "Why have I chosen this service option?" The correct answer is, "Because I can offer the kind of personal service, professional direction, and quality care that is in my control and my clients deserve." Certainly, the goal of any private practitioner is to build a self-sustaining practice. This involves the delicate balance of providing quality care in a cost-effective manner. As successful businesses have done for years before us, we too must employ certain tactics in order to survive, including among them:

- Linking costs to clinical and client-defined outcomes (including functional skills and quality of life).
- Making a commitment to lifelong learning to continually update and advance skills and institute new technologies and research-based procedures.
- Seeking routinely the opinions and perspectives of clients and their sponsors (families, payers, regulators, and employers) and integrate them into a sound business philosophy.
- Acquiring broad-based skills (e.g., as clinicians, administrators, counselors, managers, ethicists).

Without employing these and other tactics, the business (and future) of private practice is placed in jeopardy. But as other service entities are faced with change and few are sitting in comfortable strategic seats, we need to regard the changes as opportunities for growth and diversification. Instead of reacting to the change, we are best advised to drive the change. Our professional livelihood may indeed depend on it.

BIBLIOGRAPHY

American Speech-Language-Hearing Association. (1995, November). Task Force on Treatment Outcome and Cost Effectiveness, PPOs: Are they good for ASHA members? *Asha,* p. 39.
American Speech-Language-Hearing Association. (1995, September). Governance, EB Actions. *Asha,* p. 21.

American Speech-Language-Hearing Association. (1995, September). Research, Omnibus Survey: Practice issues for speech-language pathologists. *Asha*, p. 29.

American Speech-Language-Hearing Association. (1995, September). Managed Care 101: Introducing managed care into the curriculum, *Asha*, p. 45.

American Speech-Language-Hearing Association. (1995, June/July). Treatment outcomes: Task Force Update. *Asha*, p. 26.

American Speech-Language-Hearing Association. (1995, May). Treatment Outcome: Our consumers are satisfied. *Asha*, p. 23.

American Speech-Language-Hearing Association Health Care Financing Division. (1996). Resource-based relative value scale (RBRVS): Impact on audiologists and speech-language pathologists including 1996 Medicare fee schedule. Rockville MD: Author.

Berthelette & Lewis, C. (1995, November) Using functional outcome tools. *ADVANCE for Speech-Language Pathologists & Audiologists.*

Cordova, K.B. (1996, June). Whose treatment is this anyway? Navigating the perils of private practice. *ADVANCE for Speech-Language Pathologists & Audiologists, June 3.*

Frattali, C.M. (1993). Perspectives on functional assessment: Its use for policy making. *Disability and Rehabilitation, 15*(1), 1–9.

Frattali, C.M., Thompson, C.K., Holland, A.L., Wohl, C.B., & Ferketic, M.M. (1995). *Functional assessment of communication skills for adults.* Rockville, MD: American Speech-Language-Hearing Association.

Gelman, J. (1995; December 25). Measuring functional outcomes in stroke rehab. *ADVANCE for Speech-Language Pathologists & Audiologists.*

Klontz, B.S., Harriett, A., McCarty, J.P., & White, S.C., *Private health plans handbook for speech-language pathology and audiology services.* Rockville, MD: American Speech-Language-Hearing Association.

Landrum, M.A., Kitchell, P., Schmidt, N.D., & McLean, Jr., A. (1995). *Outcome oriented rehabilitation: Principles, strategies, and tools for effective program management.* Gaithersburg, MD: Aspen Publishers, Inc.

Stewart, D.L., & Abeln, S.H. (1993). *Documenting functional outcomes in physical therapy.* St. Louis, MO: Mosby-Year Book, Inc.

Trace, R. (1995, December 25). Outcome measures lead to increased accountability. *ADVANCE for Speech-Language Pathologists.*

Williams, V. (1996). Becoming a player in the managed care game. *ADVANCE for Speech-Language Pathologists & Audiologists.*

Zarrella, S. (1995, August 14). Outcome measures prove efficacy of dysphagia intervention. *ADVANCE for Speech-Language Pathologists & Audiologists.*

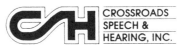

Kathryn L. Rector
Director

205 East McMurray Road
McMurray, PA 15317
(412) 941–4434
FAX: (412) 941–4717

Christie-Ann M. Conrad
Director

Appendix 22–A

Client/Family Satisfaction Survey

We welcome your suggestions for improvement (and your compliments) in refining our office procedures. We wish you to convey in this survey an honest opinion of our services. When completed,
please return this questionnaire in the envelope provided.

Please rate according to the following:

1 = Poor   2 = Fair   3 = Neutral   4 = Good   5 = Excellent
N/A = Not Applicable

Rating

1. Registration and scheduling were completed without delay. _____
2. The staff was friendly and polite. _____
3. Services were performed in a timely manner. _____
4. Only professional conversations were conducted during our visits. _____
5. Staff performed their roles in a highly-skilled manner. _____
6. I was treated with respect at all times. _____
7. Everyone who cared for me introduced themselves. _____
8. Facilities were neat and clean. _____
9. Home assignments were useful. _____
10. During the evaluation, goals and expectations of therapy were discussed.
    a) mine (the client) _____
    b) my family's _____
    c) my clinician's _____
11. Prior to the start of therapy, I was informed of:
    an approximate cost of service. _____
    an approximate duration of service. _____
    expectations of all involved parties. _____
12. Progress and goals were frequently updated and shared with me. _____
13. I would use CSHI services again. _____
14. I would recommend CSHI services to others. _____
15. Overall, the rating of my experience is: _____

Check the type and frequency of service(s) you received.

Speech/Language: ❏   Audiology: ❏

Evaluation: ❏   Treatment: ❏

Frequency: ❏ 1–3x Total   ❏ Daily   ❏ 1x Weekly   ❏ 2–3x Weekly

Additional Comments: _____

_____

_____

Name: _____   Date: _____
                    (Optional)
I am the Client _____
I am the family of the Client _____
I wish this survey to remain confidential: ❏ Yes   ❏ No

Thank You!
CSHI Staff & Friends

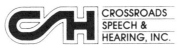

CROSSROADS
SPEECH &
HEARING, INC.

Kathryn L. Rector
Director

205 East McMurray Road
McMurray, PA 15317
(412) 941–4434
FAX: (412) 941–4717

Christie-Ann M. Conrad
Director

Appendix 22–B

Payer/Employer Satisfaction Survey

Re: _____ *(Name)* _____

We are in an ongoing process of refining our office procedures, products and services. We would appreciate your completion of this survey and then returning it in the envelope provided.

Please rate the following:

	Yes	Somewhat	No	N/A
1. Member/Employee was satisfied with care.				
2. Care received was judged as "effective."				
3. Care received was appropriately and fully documented.				
4. Care received was cost-effective.				
5. Clinic staff was responsive to any questions/problems.				
6. I would refer to CSHI again.				

Additional Comments: _____

_____

_____

Name: _____   Date: _____

Position: _____

Thank You!
CSHI Staff

513

CHAPTER 23

State Initiatives in Outcomes Measurement

MELINDA K. HARRISON

INTRODUCTION

As is characteristic of so many political aspects of our profession, it has been difficult for states to identify issues of critical need in a proactive fashion. With most of us involved in politics as volunteers, we end up in a reactive stance, frequently unprepared for the questions, tasks, and requirements of our legislators, regulators, and payers until it is late in the process and we are already behind.

Florida's introduction to the need for outcomes data occurred rather abruptly in the early 1990s. With the passage of the Health Care and Insurance Reform Act of 1993 (Chapter 93–129, Laws of Florida), we were drawn quickly into the debate of what services should be provided when limited funds are available. Stated plainly, the discussion centered on the question "If I have $100 a month for an insurance premium, on what services should it be spent?"

Having never been involved in a discussion of this sort before, the remainder of our year was spent trying to determine how our work and our value to clients fit into this discussion. When reviewing the need for prenatal care, cancer care, vision care, home health, psychiatry and psychology treatment, dialysis, and preventive care (e.g., immunizations, routine blood work, and organ transplants), what claim did we have on a part of that $100? The most difficult aspect of this discussion came to light during testimony given on this very issue. When listening to a 35-year-old mother of two preschoolers argue for the use of health care dollars for her cancer treatment so that she may live to see her children grow up, perspectives change. If the money we charge takes away from the money available for cancer care, emergency care, preventive care, or surgical care, are we better than these fields at using the money well? Are we the ones who deserve it?

We were asked the following questions in formal hearings:

How much did the provision of speech-language pathology services add to the cost of an insurance premium on a monthly basis?

How many of our patients could be helped by 10 visits if that is all they were provided through their insurer?

How many visits would need to be covered by an insurance policy to treat our patients successfully?

When attempting to obtain information that would allow us to answer these questions accurately, we were surprised to learn that there was little good information available. To obtain the insurance premium information, we placed calls to professionals in the state who had worked with an insurance carrier, our own employers' benefits plans, and leaders in other states. The figures we used (we had only 5 days to find them) were obtained through the efforts of the American Speech-Language-Hearing Association (ASHA) National Office staff through the CNA Insurance Company.

When asked how many of our clients would be helped after 10 therapy visits, we had no definitive answers. Our solution was to gather the case load information of the most recent ASHA Omnibus Survey (ASHA, 1992) and extrapolate those "perceptions" of case load content into percentages by diagnostic types. Then, after telephone surveys of clinicians, we "predicted" what percentage of our clients would indeed achieve some level of progress after 10 visits. It was a guess—an educated one, but only a guess. (We had 2 weeks to gather the information.)

When we were asked "If 10 visits are not enough, how many do you need?", we had nothing factual to provide. We did not know how many visits were sufficient for any diagnosis for which we provided treatment.

Later, when hearings became even more data based, we were asked to submit outcomes and efficacy data to the State's Agency for Health Care Administration (AHCA). Again, ASHA staff forwarded the extent of information available. But once again, the information yielded very little usable data. There were no cost figures, estimated number of visits, or consistently measured outcomes. An alarming number of efficacy studies employed single subject designs which unfortunately held no credence with the insurance carriers who wanted data that could be generalized with large client populations. These studies alone did not meet the needs of the payers and legislators who were sitting on a panel struggling with how best to utilize limited health care dollars for maximal client outcomes.

My purposes for this chapter are to give you an example of one states' experience in lobbying, through the use of data, for inclusion in a standard benefit package, summarize two other states' data collection efforts, detail the outcomes initiative launched by the Council of State Association Presidents, and share some thoughts on needed directions for states to take in outcomes measurement activities.

THE FLORIDA EXPERIENCE

The simple questions, "How do we best spend limited health care dollars for maximal client outcome?" drove the Florida Association of Speech-Language Pathologists and Audiologists (FLASHA) into the complicated and politically laden business of outcomes measurement. When we realized the potential impact of the all-encompassing health care law written by an array of national health care experts, we focused on three critical needs:

1. educating our members about shifts in state policy

2. answering the fair questions being asked

3. training our members on what data collection was needed to remain viable as a profession.

We convened a group of speech-language pathologists (SLPs) and audiologists in the state to meet these three critical needs. This group recommended that a series of regional workshops be made available to FLASHA members to review the impending changes and their potential role in supporting the profession. These were accomplished over the next 6 months with seven workshops offered. The second decision made by this group targeted the other two critical needs: answering the questions we were being asked and designing the data collection tool with which to do so. We began by collecting data to answer the questions we were repeatedly asked: How many visits with an SLP or audiologist did our clients need?

Targeting this one question, we designed a *data tracking* form. Because we also wanted to train our members in data collection and wanted maximum participation, we believed that this form, at least at the outset, would need to be brief and user-friendly. The form was designed to collect basic demographic information, primary diagnosis, and length of treatment (see Appendix 23-A). It also tracked a "final disposition" (e.g., patient was discharged, met goals) as a gross outcome measure. In order to collect outcome data regarding client satisfaction, we asked, "Did you benefit from therapy?" and "Are you satisfied with the outcome?"

The data tracking form was piloted in three sites, to be debugged and then distributed with directions for use to the FLASHA membership via an insert in the bimonthly state association newsletter. We asked for voluntary participation and outlined a monthly process for completing forms. We reinforced the need for membership assistance in all subsequent newsletters.

At the time of this writing, we had collected over 4,000 data tracking forms from 51 clinical sites. The sites producing the highest percentage of usable forms were inpatient acute hospital sites; the least, home health. Sixty percent of the forms collected were evenly distributed among outpatient clinics, skilled nursing facilities, and inpatient rehabilitation hospitals. The mean age was 66 years with a range of 1 to 98 years of age. Collecting data from minority groups was identified as a problem with only 10% of data collected from African-American clients and 5% from Hispanic clients, which is not representative of Florida demographics. By far, the most frequently reported diagnoses were dysphagia (26%) and aphasia (27%), constituting half of all forms collected, and cognitive communication (18%) and dysarthria (9%) as the other largely reported disorders. The remaining 20% were divided among 18 different diagnostic groups. We found that roughly 38% of the clients from whom data were collected were discharged to other sites, making their data collection incomplete. Another one-third were felt to have met their goals. Very few (less than 2%) appeared to be discharged due to lack of funding.

The survey asked therapists to predict, prior to the onset of therapy, the number of sessions they anticipated it would take to successfully work with each client. Consistently, therapists predicted it would take them twice as long as they actually worked with that client. Relative to judgements of benefit, over 90% of clients felt they did benefit from therapy and just under 90% were satisfied with the outcome.

In retrospect, our training should have been more formal. Questions arose after forms were returned and we would have roughly 25% more forms had these been addressed at the outset. We also have struggled with evaluating the content of these forms. We identified the need to focus data collection efforts on pediatric communication disorders and minority populations. Approximately one year after utilizing the form, members of the original design team met with other FLASHA members at our State Convention. The meeting did not result in any recommendations for change in the form's structure and is continuing to be used.

THE ISSUE OF PRACTICE GUIDELINES

In Florida, we grappled with the development of practice guidelines and how they could be designed using outcomes data. We have followed the "definition" of practice guideline as it evolved into a medical algorithm, an equation of how many sessions, tests, and professionals it will take to achieve a predefined level of functioning. The Florida law provides guidance on the process of developing algorithms (defined in the law as practice parameters).

Practice Parameters

(1) The Agency for Health Care Administration shall coordinate the development, endorsement, implementation, and evaluation of scientifically sound, clinically relevant practice parameters in order to reduce unwarranted variation in the delivery of medical treatment, improve the quality of medical care, and promote the appropriate utilization of health care services. "Practice parameters" or "practice guidelines" are defined to mean strategies for patient management that are developed to assist physicians in clinical decision making.

(2) The agency shall establish a work group of appropriate medical and technical professional and agency personnel to develop uniform standards and methods for the collection and analysis of patient outcomes data. The work group shall focus on collecting data which measures both the efficient utilization of medical resources and the effectiveness of medical care, and shall include such factors as patient diagnosis, the severity of the patient's condition, patient length of stay, number of diagnostic tests and scans performed, procedures performed, medications prescribed, number of consultations, patient mortality, source and date of patient admission and readmission, total patient charges and source of payment, and patient discharge status. . . .

(4) The agency shall summarize the effectiveness and cost of care outcomes for each diagnosis by hospital, by district, by region, and across the state as well as by any other grouping which will facilitate the development of clinically relevant practice parameters.

(5) The agency, in conjunction with the Florida Medical Association . . . and other health professional associations . . . shall develop and may adopt by rule state practice parameters based on the data received under subsection (4) as well as on nationally developed practice guidelines. . . . The agency shall prioritize the development of those

practice parameters which involve the greatest utilization of resources either because they are the most costly or because they are the most frequently performed.

(6) The agency, in conjunction with the appropriate health professional associations shall develop and may adopt by rule practice parameters for services provided by . . . and comprehensive rehabilitative services. [Speech-language pathology implied]. [Florida Health Care and Insurance Reform Act of 1993, Section 408.02 Florida Statutes]

Initially, with the support of an ASHA grant, we pursued the development of Practice Parameters for Speech-Language Pathology and Audiology Services. Using as a base the Preferred Practice Patterns developed by ASHA (ASHA, 1993), we expanded the therapeutic component of this document. We addressed each diagnostic grouping (e.g., voice, dysphagia, language 0–3) and constructed a flow chart of the process of care for that diagnosis. We submitted the draft practice patterns to the Agency for Health Care Administration for review.

As expected, the practice patterns were not sufficiently definitive. They were considered collectively as a "Best Practice" paper, the preceding step to development of a practice guideline or parameter. AHCA's three steps of developing a practice guideline are:

Scope of Practice Paper. At this level, information on who we are, how we are educated, where we practice, how we handle our clients, what makes us different, how we charge, how we are paid, and how we are licensed and/or certified is presented.

Best Practice Paper. How we most commonly do our work in a general sense; defining the steps to diagnosis, treatment, and discharge are explained in broad terms. Based on scientific data, these address the issues of our client needs. The ASHA Preferred Practice Patterns (ASHA, 1993) are an example of a best practice paper under this definition.

Practice Guideline. This is a medical algorithm. To describe, I will refer to elements of the *Clinical Practice Guideline for the Universe of Patients with Low Back Pain or Injury,* adopted by the Agency for Health Care Administration (1995). If you have low back pain, this document defines who can evaluate you, what options exist for the diagnosis, how long each activity should take (e.g., no more than 3 days of bed rest, no more than 7 days of medication), how many x-rays and what kind may be ordered, what information should be provided to you, when you may repeat an x-ray, how many sessions for therapeutic intervention are acceptable based on the scientific literature, and what interventions are not acceptable as there is no scientific literature to support it.

In order to develop a true practice guideline we needed to be more willing to assign numbers to much of what we do: How much time should an evaluation take? How many sessions are reasonable for rehabilitation? How many points, on average, should performance increase on an outcome scale?

A lesson learned in the development of guidelines related to the work done by the AHCA and its impact on physical therapy when the Low Back Pain guideline was endorsed. Despite the role physical therapists play in treatment of low back pain, the Agency did not include physical therapists among the consultants charged to write the document. The document was written by orthopedic surgeons, neurosurgeons, family physicians, and a psychiatrist. This guideline contains interventions which, as a result of outcomes studies, have known clinical and cost effectiveness. Listed as "ineffective options," because there are no published studies to support their effectiveness in the treatment of low back pain, are the following:

- massage
- ultrasound
- cutaneous laser treatment
- electrical stimulation
- spinal traction
- acupuncture
- biofeedback
- use of corsets

This practice guideline, designed for workers' compensation patients only, had been estimated to have the potential for saving Florida workers' compensation carriers approximately $100,000,000 in one year. Already, according to AHCA, the guideline has been endorsed by AETNA Insurance Company and is being published by the Joint Commission on Accreditation of Healthcare Organizations (JCAHO) as a reference for treatment of patients with low back pain.

Consequently, carriers paying for claims on back-injured patients may justifiably question payment for treatments listed as ineffective on this guideline. In the absence of outcomes research that can determine effectiveness, why should money be spent on these procedures? We as a profession, could easily find ourselves in the same dilemma without hard data to justify the effectiveness of our interventions. We have all witnessed clinical progress, but those observations alone are currently not sufficient justification for reimbursement.

THE CALIFORNIA EXPERIENCE

While not a statewide project, the Southern California Speech-Language and Audiology Director's Council, SCSLPADC (a consortium of Hospital/Rehabilitation facility-based directors) embarked on a treatment outcomes study in the early 1990s. Recognizing the need to answer the question "What are the results of our services for our patients?" these directors designed a study to do just that. They recognized the importance of documenting that our services are "reasonable and necessary" and that we do accomplish functional improvement in the lives of our clients.

The Outcome Task Force of SCSLPADC identified stroke patients as its study population. Their measurements were designed to focus on all parameters of treatment for speech, language, cognitive, and/or swallowing difficulties resulting from stroke. Questions on the data collection tool included identifying the stroke as right or left hemisphere, time post onset, therapy setting, and patient's age, educational level, and primary treatment goal. Duration of therapy and therapy type (individual vs. group) were detailed, as was reason for discharge.

The information gleaned from 200 patients revealed that goals were met 70 to 80% of the time for all subjects with treatment time averaging 45 minutes per session. Group treatment was rendered for less than 25% of all subjects.

Clinically significant differences were found from clinician to clinician in how and what goals are set, one of the problems identified in the Florida data collection effort. Variances in "realistic" goals may be quite large due to the experience of the treating clinician as may the pertinence of the goal to the identified communication disorder. These differences can make this "goal" a moving target, making uniform data collection problematic. In any of these state-initiated measures, the control of goal-setting, client demographics, and treatment-related variables are limited, if present at all. How do we assess if a disorder is mild, moderate, or severe? How do we consider comorbidities, compliance with treatment, and number of missed sessions as influences on the data we collect? These issues are recognized by both Florida and California as dilemmas in interpreting the data collected thus far.

THE GEORGIA EXPERIENCE

Building on the work of Florida, the Georgia Speech-Language-Hearing Association (GSHA) began its data collection efforts in November 1995. Its efforts were based on a GSHA resolution identifying the need for two work efforts:

1. Establishing a task force to study treatment outcomes in Speech-Language Pathology and Audiology
2. Establishing a data base that would identify outcome measures from all practice settings.

Initiated as part of a continuing education workshop, GSHA provided each participant with a comprehensive overview of health care initiatives leading to the need for data collection. It took the existing FLASHA form and expanded the number of diagnostic codes from 22 to 39. Examples of a completed form, client satisfaction measures, and discharge forms were included in its training packet. The discharge information was expanded to include billing information and level of functioning at time of discharge.

The most interesting part of this project was GSHA's determination to obtain a large number of forms in quick order. To encourage participation, members were offered free continuing education hours for participating in the study. GSHA hopes to have enough information to support efforts to reopen its licensure law to broaden its scope of practice. It also would like to use the data to lobby payers. The challenge is having sufficient data accumulated in a short period of time to accomplish the desired objectives.

OUTCOMES INITIATIVES OF THE COUNCIL OF STATE ASSOCIATIONS PRESIDENTS

As the need for outcomes research intensifies, the need for state-level activities becomes paramount. In response, the Council of State Association Presidents (CSAP) began regional projects in the Spring of 1996 to encourage greater outcomes measurement activities at the state level. At the same time, ASHA prepared a publication titled *Treatment Outcomes and Efficacy: A State Resource Guide* (ASHA, 1996).

This guide was presented to each state association president as a resource for potential short-term or long-term projects in order to help strengthen the strategic positioning of the professions in the context of service delivery information (Table 23–1). Nine regions throughout the United States were identified for this project with each region specifying what project would be accomplished.

The nine regions represented at this meeting, comprising 43 states and the Overseas Association, committed to a number of activities, as detailed in Table 23–2. For the first time, states are taking a regional approach to outcomes measurement. Perhaps a driving force is the pending quandary presented by the increased political movement

Table 23–1. ASHA Recommended Projects for State-level Outcomes Measurement Activities

SHORT-TERM PROJECTS

1. Member Education	a) Prepare articles to be published in state newsletter. b) Recruit a small number of people who would be willing to attend and speak at smaller meetings on the regional and local levels. c) Plan a presentation to be delivered at the annual conventions in each state. **Topics for consideration:** a) Importance of outcome information. b) Differences in outcome and efficacy. c) How professionals must advocate for their services utilizing outcomes information. d) Effect of managed care on the audiology and speech-language pathology professions.
2. Student Education	Arrange meetings with faculty of training programs to encourage inclusion of outcomes and efficacy in student courses.
3. Efficacy	a) Facilitate meetings of researchers and clinicians to discuss methods for improvement of working relationships. b) Identify and select a specific disorder-based topic and review the literature in order to identify gaps in efficacy research for a particular area. c) Identify and assemble a group to explore funding sources for clinically relevant efficacy research.
4. Payers	Arrange a payer meeting with local managed care companies and state agencies.

LONG-TERM PROJECTS

1. Outcomes Data Collection	a) Utilize an existing outcomes tool , i.e., ASHA's NOMS to collect data in each state. b) For a specified period of time, initiate data collection for a particular site of service or patient population.
2. Efficacy	Form a regional coalition with surrounding states for the purpose of discussing ways to conduct and fund efficacy research.

Table 23–2. 1996 CSAP Regional Projects

STATES INVOLVED	PROJECT CHOSEN
1. WI, IL, IN, MI, OH	Utilize the ASHA Treatment Outcomes forms in order to collect multistate (regional) information.
2. ND, NE, IA, MN	"Educate to Motivate" our members on the advocacy process 1. To present information to membership through state-selected vehicle. 2. Develop fact sheets. 3. Educate and obtain feedback from consumers. 4. Explore information about how to organize all information as a resource that can be accessed by membership.
3. RI, VT, NH, NJ, MA, ME, and Europe	1. Get electronically connected. 2. Consumer Advocacy presentation through Trialliance 3. Continuing Education-Taping seminars for CEUs videotape library. 4. Share lecturers.
4. CA, NV, NM, UT	From the ASHA model, select 5 strategies to develop grassroots advocacy in each of our states.
5. FL, LA, AL, GA, MS	1. Begin data collection 2. Newsletter article in all involved states
6. WV, PA, MD, DC	Outcome Data Collection Form. Revising the Maryland form to add schools and audiology settings and make changes for other professional settings.
7. OR, WA, ID, MT, WY	Educate members on the importance of outcome information.
8. NC, SC, KY, TN, VA	**Long term:** Ask member-at-large to identify home health sites in each state, and ask clinicians in those settings to collect treatment outcome data. **Short term:** Educate the members in each state by: 1. Writing articles (each state will pursue different topics) and sending these articles to each other for dissemination to our members. 2. Educating our Executive Board and Council through in-services/workshops. 3. Having states send each other information to disseminate to members regarding CEU workshops/conference events on managed care, outcomes and efficacy. **Note:** Another short-term goal is to speak to university researchers about ongoing studies.
9. CO, KS, TX, MO, AR	Develop educational tools to advocate speech, language, and audiological services.

toward block grants. These are large blocks of money targeted for a particular need and divided among the states based on previous spending history. The disbursement of the granted funds is left to the discretion of the individual states. These grants would create a shift from federal autocracy to state decision making, creating the potential for practitioner battles at the state level for the right to provide services through what are now federally funded, federally regulated programs. When in *each state* professionals must justify why they should get the money instead of some other medical or rehabilitative service, data to support the argument or consumer advocacy testimonials will need to be used in the fight for these dollars. The establishment of regional, cooperative efforts can assist in providing consistent outcomes data particular to similar demographic areas and establish a framework for supportive relationships as funding battles within the states escalate.

CONCLUSION

One of my favorite quotes comes from a meeting of the PEW Health Professions Commission Project on the Future of Allied Health (Dunn, 1994):

> Allied health professionals have relied on folklore to develop the culture of their professions. We have been slow to make a commitment to collecting and documenting evidence to advance our knowledge. When the beliefs of a profession are not documented and tested, educators rely more heavily on folklore as the basis of their course content, and the folklore continues to form the basis of student competencies. The risk of this strategy is that we pass along beliefs that are erroneous, benign, or potentially harmful to persons needing our services. [p. 163].

While we have made strides in projecting what is "best practice" for our clients, we have not laid the groundwork for accountability in terms meaningful to state legislators:

How many times should someone with dysphagia be seen?

On average, how long should a child with a language disorder continue in therapy?

How many treatment hours provide optimal effectiveness for a cognitively impaired adult, and at what point does the return in functioning no longer justify the expenditure in health care dollars?

Our answer to these and other questions has historically been, "It depends on the client." That answer today would be grossly insufficient, even irresponsible. Tightly controlled and studied techniques should begin to yield answers to commonly asked questions. We should be able to uncover trends.

There is a pessimist that battles inside all of us that prevents a unified effort of outcomes data collection. As a result, however, our clients may not fare well in the current system. There is comfort in pointing to factual information pertaining to the efforts of our interventions. There is security in being supported by a rich professional literature that secures our place in the lives of those whom we serve. There is little if any benefit in skirting the fair questions being asked repeatedly. If we do not do any documentable good, payers will not be obligated to pay us. Money spent for speech-language pathology could also be spent on care for asthma, heart disease, cancer, or prenatal care. If, however, we do improve clients' lives and our clinical science proves it, we do indeed deserve to be compensated for our skill. It is no more complicated than that.

REFERENCES

American Speech-Language-Hearing Association (1992). Omnibus Survey. Rockville, MD: Author.

American Speech-Language-Hearing Association (1993). *Preferred Practice Patterns for the Professions of Speech-Language Pathology and Audiology.* Supplement to March 1993 *Asha, 35,* 3.

Dunn, W. (1994). *Issues and Challenges for Allied Health Educators in the Future of the Allied Health Workforce.* Pew Health Professions Commission and U.S. Public Health Services Bureau of Health Professions.

Florida Association of Speech-Language Pathologists and Audiologists (1994). *Patient Tracking Study,* FLASHA Practice Parameters Task Force. Tallahassee, FL: Author.

Georgia Speech-Language-Hearing Association (1995). *Data Collection Instrument,* Task Force on Treatment Efficacy. Atlanta, GA: Author.

Lux, C., Foldivary, S., Santo, D., & Davis, G. (1994). Taskforce on Outcomes: Southern California Speech-Language Pathology and Audiology Director's Council Collaborative Research Project. Miniseminar at ASHA Annual Convention, New Orleans, LA.

State of Florida (1995). Medical Practice Guideline: the Universe of Patients with Acute/Chronic low Back Pain or Injury. Agency for Health Care Administration. Tallahassee, FL: Author.

Individual Patient Data Sheet

FLASHA Patient Tracking Study

Site Name: _____ Pt. I.D. _____ Site Code: _____

Sex: (circle) M F DOB: _____ Ethnicity Code: _____ Diagnosis Code: _____ Date of Onset: _____

Onset of Treatment date: _____ Date of Discharge: _____ Reason Code: _____ Previous Treatment: Y N

Diagnosis codes: (please see definitions)

01 aphasia	11 speech articulation delay	**Reason Code:**
02 apraxia	12 speech articulation disorder	1. met goals
03 dysarthria	13 voice-functional	2. funding
04 dysphagia-neurogenic	14 voice-organic	3. expired
05 dysphagia-structural	15 alaryngeal-TEP	4. d/c to diff. therapy site
06 dysphagia other	16 alaryngeal-traditional	5. other (patient preference,
07 cognitive-communication disorder	17 alaryngeal: device	etc.) Define _____
08 language disorder-socioemotional	18 fluency-prosody	
09 language disorder - specific	19 fluency-neurogenic	**Ethnicity Code:**
10 language delay	20 craniofacial / cleft palate	1 - white 4 - asian
	21 hearing loss-acquired	2 - african american 5 - other (specify
	22 hearing loss-congenital	3 - hispanic _____)

SITE CODE: 1-Outpatient Clinic (any type) • 2-SNF • 3-Inpatient Rehab. Hospital
4-Inpatient Acute Care Hospital • 5-Home Health

Month	1	2	3	4	5	6	7	8	9	10	11	12	13	14	15	16	17	18	19	20	21	22	23	24	25	26	27	28	29	30	31	Totals

Write units of service (15 minute blocks of direct time) in boxes that correlate with dates of service. When frequency of treatment changes, please circle this date. _Units of service recorded should be only those spent on the primary diagnosis identified for this patient._ If group sessions are used, please put a "g" after the units of service for that date. Use this data to complete the information below at time of discharge.

Additional clinically relevant information: _____

Summary DATA: Your estimate of Units of Service needed (prior to initiating therapy): _____

Actual Units Individual Therapy: _____ Actual Units Group Therapy: _____ Total Treatment Units: _____

Missed Units: _____   Length of time in treatment (days) _____

Ask your patient: Do you feel you benefited from this therapy?   Yes   No

Were you satisfied with the outcome of this therapy?   Yes   No

(continued)

Definitions - to be utilized for the purposed of FLASHA data collection only.

01 **aphasia** - an impairment, due to acquired and recent damage of the central nervous system, of the ability to comprehend and formulate language. Includes a variety of impairments in auditory comprehension, reading, oral-expressive language, and writing. May be influenced by physiological inefficiency or impaired cognition, but cannot be explained by dementia, sensory loss, or motor dysfunction.

02 **apraxia** - a neurogenic phonologic disorder resulting from sensorimotor impairment of the capacity to select, program, and/or execute, in coordinated and normally timed sequences, the positioning of the speech musculature for the volitional production of speech sounds.

03 **dysarthria** - a group of speech disorders resulting from disturbances of muscular control, weakness, slowness, or incoordination of the speech mechanism due to damage to the central or peripheral nervous system or both. The term encompasses coexisting neurogenic disorders of several or all the basic processes of speech: respiration, phonation, resonance, articulation, and prosody.

04 **dysphagia: neurogenic** - Developmental or acquired neuromuscular dysfunction resulting in disturbed motility patterns in any of the three stages of deglutition (oral, pharyngeal, esophageal) which may cause pulmonary aspiration, airway obstruction, or inadequate nutrition and/or hydration.

05 **dysphagia: structural** - Acquired/surgical or developmental abnormalities in anatomy resulting in disturbed motility patterns in any of the stages of deglutition which may result in pulmonary aspiration, airway obstruction or alterations in adequate nutrition and/or hydration.

06 **dysphagia: other** - The presence of dysphagia symptomology in the absence of a known or documented neurogenic or structural disorder.

07 **cognitive-communication disorder** - Any cognitive-communication problem that is the result of central or peripheral nervous system insult or dysfunction excluding language disorders associated with aphasia and hearing loss.

08 **language disorder: socioemotional** - any communication-language problem that is considered to be the result of a mental (DSM-III/IV) disorder (e.g., pervasive developmental disorder, mutism, substance abuse, etc.).

09 **language disorder: specific** - Any communication-language problem that is modality-specific and/or linguistic specific (e.g., specific language impairment, semantic deficit, syntactic deficit, dyslexia, dysgraphia, etc.) that is NOT classifiable as an aphasia, a cognitive-communication disorder, a language disorder-socioemotional, or a communication-language problem secondary to hearing loss.

10 **language delay** - any communication-language problem that is characterized by a significant difference between receptive / expressive language status and the individual's mental age and can not be classified as a cognitive-communication or a language disorder-specific.

11 **speech articulation delay** - speech characterized by delayed development, in childhood, of phonemic and / or prosodic features.

12 **speech articulation disorder** - speech characterized by abnormal production of phonemic and / or prosodic features not considered to be due to an apraxia, dysarthria, or fluency disorder.

13 **voice: functional** - any dysphonia secondary to vocal misuse-abuse / hyperfunction / muscle tension, hearing impairment, reduced vocal fold closure, psychogenic, or psychological trauma-based origin.

14 **voice: organic** - any dysphonia secondary to neurological insult, a progressive neuromuscular disease process, or other pathology unrelated to vocal misuse/abuse.

Alaryngeal - any communication disorder as a result of total laryngectomy. Post-surgical communication will be subsequent to tracheoesophageal puncture (TEP), acquisition of traditional esophageal speech, and / or through use of an artificial device. Please code appropriately.

15 **alaryngeal: TEP** (please specify type in space provided)

16 **alaryngeal: traditional** (please specify details in space provided)

17 **alaryngeal: device** (please specify type in space provided)

18 **fluency: prosody** - speech disrupted by atypical repetitions and prolongations (both silent and audible), altered prosodic features and/or negative emotions

19 **fluency: neurogenic** - speech disrupted by atypical repetitions and prolongations (both silent and audible), altered prosodic features and/or negative emotions resulting from a know neurological event

20 **cleft palate / craniofacial** - congenital or acquired differences in structure or function that result in disorders of speech and/or language

21 **hearing loss: congenital** - an impairment of auditory sensitivity existing at or dating from birth.

22 **hearing loss: acquired** - an impairment of auditory sensitivity which appears after birth. Not congenital.

CHAPTER 24

National Initiatives in Outcomes Measurement

Tanya M. Gallagher

INTRODUCTION

Outcomes measurement is becoming increasingly recognized as a distinct research methodology that has evolved at least partially from the fields of clinical epidemiology and information technology, and encompasses a broad range of data collection technologies, data treatment techniques, and interpretive assumptions. Among major factors accelerating interest in this work were national agency initiatives that underscored the potential value of and need for treatment outcomes information in health care and education service delivery organization and management. Attention within agencies responsible for service provision standards setting and monitoring, the financing of health care service delivery, health care policy and research, and education has shifted steadily from a primary emphasis on the structure and process characteristics of service providers and service facilities to an emphasis on service delivery outcomes. Information is being sought about the consequences and cost-effectiveness of the care provided and about the consumers' (by that is meant all interested parties) satisfaction with that care. The national debate on health care reform and concerns about spiralling health care costs have both supported and intensified these trends. For example, the Agency for Health Care Policy and Research (AHCPR), the primary federal agency responsible for supporting research on key health care delivery and treatment effectiveness issues through grants and contracts, developing outcomes research methodologies, analyzing health care policy issues, and evaluating the risks and effects of specific health technologies, was established by Congress in 1989, only 7 years ago.

The comprehensiveness of the agendas of national agencies regarding the incorporation of outcomes information into their decision making processes and their aggressive time-frames for implementation have placed considerable demands on service providers to collect outcomes data quickly and efficiently, and to learn how to use outcomes information effectively in program management, advocacy for services, and in the evolution of the knowledge base of health related professions (e.g., in the development and dissemination of practice guidelines, critical paths of care). This chapter reviews and summarizes:

1. the priorities of each of the major federal and private national agencies regarding outcomes data and their proposed or current use in meeting agency mandates;

2. the American Speech-Language-Hearing Association (ASHA's) efforts to meet the needs of speech-language pathologists (SLPs) and audiologists for national outcomes data information and for outcomes data collection instruments; and,

3. the ASHA national outcomes data on speech-language pathology services that have been collected to date.

HEALTH CARE AGENCY INITIATIVES

The influence of government on health care service delivery increased dramatically in the 1960s with the introduction of Medicare and Medicaid. After these programs were established, the government became a large-scale purchaser of health services, expanding what had been primarily controlled by local communities and independent health care professionals to include greater governmental involvement. Over time, the role of the federal government had been changed from that of being a limited provider of health care services to very restricted populations and a protector of the public's health, to that of being a major financial underwriter of health care. The agencies, policies and procedures that followed were an outgrowth of that expanded role (Kovner, 1990).

Major federal agencies that affect speech-language pathology service delivery can be categorized into two broad groups: those that establish and monitor standards, and those that finance or pay for services. All of these agencies can affect accessibility to service and patterns of service delivery through the exercise of their regulatory functions.

National not-for-profit agencies and associations also are involved in standards setting and monitoring and their evolution has followed a similar path to that of federal agencies. There has been a parallel shift of emphasis from structure and process quality indicators to outcomes assessment and monitoring.

STANDARDS SETTING AND OUTCOMES ASSESSMENT: HEALTH CARE

Several public and private agencies are involved in standards setting and monitoring health care services in speech-language pathology. Among the major agencies are the AHCPR, JCAHO, CARF, the NCQA, the HCFA's Office of Managed Care, and ASHA.

Agency for Health Care Policy and Research (AHCPR)

The U.S. Public Health Service, the first health care agency to be formed by the federal government, was established in 1789 to provide care for merchant seaman and members of the armed forces. Now a division of the U.S. Department of Health and Human

Services, subsequent legislation has continued to expand the scope of the Public Health Service (PHS) to encompass its current broad mission of protecting and advancing the nation's health.

Consistent with that mission, the Omnibus Budget Reconciliation Act of 1989 established the AHCPR as an agency of the PHS. AHCPR succeeded the National Center for Health Services Research and Health Care Technology Assessment and is the primary federal agency charged with producing and disseminating objective, policy-relevant information about the quality, effectiveness, and cost of health care (Calkins, Fernandopulle, & Marino, 1995).

AHCPR fulfills its mandate by supporting and conducting health services and health care policy research, assessing technologies used in health care, developing clinical practice guidelines, and disseminating treatment research and clinical practice guidelines to health care providers, policymakers, and consumers. Primary components of the agency are the Center for Medical Effectiveness Research, which awards grants and contracts on treatment outcomes, practice variations, and outcomes research methodologies; the Center for General Health Services Extramural Research, which awards grants and contracts on the organization, delivery, and financing of health care; the Center for Research Dissemination and Liaison, which publishes AHCPR reports; and the Office of the Forum for Quality and Effectiveness in Health Care, which develops, periodically reviews, and updates clinical practice guidelines (Ankrapp & DiLima, 1995).

The largest AHCPR-funded outcomes studies have been the Patient Outcomes Research Team (PORT) projects. These are 5-year, multimethod, multisite studies that bring together experts from various clinical fields and scientific disciplines to examine "alternative methods for diagnosing, treating, managing, or preventing a particular condition to determine which methods work best" (AHCPR, 1993, p. 2). Each of the initial 14 PORT projects received 5 to 6 million dollars in funding and addressed health conditions such as heart failure, urinary incontinence, cardiac rehabilitation, low back pain, and secondary and tertiary prevention of stroke. These projects included meta-analyses of published treatment effectiveness studies, decision analyses, analyses of available secondary data bases, and primary outcomes data collection (Johnston & Granger, 1994). The original PORT projects, unlike traditional clinical trials or efficacy research, focused on treatment outcomes for typical patients, in typical settings, receiving treatment from typical providers. Emphasis was placed upon treatment outcomes as patients experienced them, understood them, and cared about them, including quality of life and functional status. Six Inter-PORT Work Groups were formed to share information across projects and have focused on advancing methodologies relevant to the conduct of outcomes research (See Maklan, Greene, & Cummings, 1994 for review). The work of ASHA's Task Force on Treatment Outcome and Cost Effectiveness, which will be summarized below, followed general PORT methodologies and protocols.

The success of the PORT projects led to increased funding and a second round of PORTS, PORT II, which were begun in 1994. PORT-II's methodologies include experimental research designs such as randomized clinical trials.

A major goal of PORT activities is to develop meaningful clinical practice guidelines. As this information is being collected through various projects, AHCPR pursued its mandate to provide clinical guidelines by assembling panels of providers from a wide range of health care disciplines and consumers of health care services. AHCPR asked each panel to review available scientific information on a particular health condition or procedure, consider the expert testimony presented, and reach a consensus on recommendations for clinical practice. Recommendations were intended to help providers "make better medical care decisions and reduce the use of ineffective or inappropriate services" (AHCPR, 1992, p. 1). The Office of the Forum for Quality and Effectiveness in Health Care extensively peer reviewed and disseminated these guidelines.

Of particular concern to SLPs is the Post-Stroke Rehabilitation Guideline developed by AHCPR and disseminated in 1995 (AHCPR, 1995a). A multidisciplinary panel of 18 professionals in post-stroke rehabilitation and one consumer were invited to write the guideline. Despite the participation of speech-language pathologists on the panel, the opportunity to provide written and oral testimony, and to participate in the peer review process, ASHA has communicated its serious concerns about the guideline that was developed and disseminated (ASHA, 1995a). These concerns were:

1. that physical aspects are emphasized and communication is not sufficiently recognized (e.g., "Persistent motor deficits are often the primary indication for rehabilitation because of their influence on the performance of daily activities." (AHCPR Guideline, 1995a, p. 39);

2. that several statements are misleading (e.g., "Communication disorders occur in as many as 40% of patients with strokes . . . frequently they resolve spontaneously." (AHCPR Guideline, 1995a, p. 24); and, "Aspiration is silent in as many as 40% of patients who aspirate. Fortunately spontaneous improvement is frequent." (AHCPR Guideline, 1995a, p. 59); and,

3. that there are several errors of omission. For example, the roles and responsibilities of members of the rehabilitation team, except for physicians and nurses are not defined adequately and information regarding Augmentative and Alternative Communication devices/resources is omitted. (AHCPR Guideline, 1995a, p. 120).

The potential impact of practice guidelines such as these on the provision of speech-language pathology services to patients is clear and underscores that need for objective treatment outcomes information.

None of the PORT teams is collecting speech-language pathology outcomes data since condition or procedure priorities to date have reflected high-frequency, high-cost medical interventions. One of the motivations for creating the ASHA Task Force, discussed below, was to meet the need for speech-language pathology and audiology outcomes data.

AHCPR's commitment to consumer involvement was reflected in a recently announced major initiative. A 5-year, $10 million project entitled "Consumer Assessments of Health Plans Study" was recently awarded to a consortia led by the Research Triangle Institute, the RAND Corporation, and Harvard University to develop the best methods for measuring and communicating consumer satisfaction information about health plans. A variety of health plans and service delivery settings will be studied, including HMOs, fee-for-service plans, and public health clinics. Items will probe patient access, reasons for using and not using services, quality of care, and outcomes from the patient perspective (AHCPR, 1996).

In a related effort, AHCPR has combined efforts with the Health Insurance Association of America, a private organization, to help consumers make informed decisions about available health plans. This partnership will develop a managed care guide for public distribution (AHCPR, 1995b).

National Center for Medical Rehabilitation Research (NCMRR)

A federal partner to AHCPR in the support of outcomes data collection is the National Center for Medical Rehabilitation Research (NCMRR). NCMRR, a component of the National Institute of Child Health and Human Development of the National Institutes of Health, was established in 1990 to further the scientific knowledge base needed to promote the health, productivity, independence and quality of life of individuals with disabilities (Ankrapp & DiLima, 1995). Supporting outcomes research is one of the seven priorities outlined in the Center's Research Plan, published in 1993.

In 1994, NCMRR and AHCPR jointly sponsored a conference entitled "An Agenda for Medical Rehabilitation Outcome Research." Participants included professionals from a variety of disciplines including speech-language pathology, and representatives from federal agencies, relevant professional organizations, and consumer advocacy groups. The conference concluded that despite the inherent difficulties in designing and conducting outcomes studies, these efforts must and will continue because nothing less will adequately meet the information needs of the consumers, purchasers, providers, and researchers working to advance the knowledge base of rehabilitation professionals. Although not directly involved in standards setting, the outcomes research supported by the Center serves to inform efforts in this direction.

Joint Commission on Accreditation of Healthcare Organizations (JCAHO)

JCAHO is one of the major private, nonprofit, health care-standards-setting organizations. Voluntary self-regulation has been a long tradition within health care and JCAHO is perhaps the oldest and best known of the institutional accrediting bodies (Weitzman, 1990) (see Chapter 2). Originally formed in 1951 as the Joint Commission on Accreditation of Hospitals by the American College of Physicians, the American Medical Association, the Canadian Medical Association, and the American Hospital Association, JCAHO, renamed in 1987, sets standards and conducts voluntary accreditation and follow-up consultation programs for a range of health care institutions.

JCAHO accreditation is widely respected and qualifies hospitals for participation in Medicare and Medicaid. As of 1995, approximately 5000 of the nation's 6500 hospitals and 2800 other health care institutions were accredited by JCAHO (Ramsay, 1995). Many of its accreditation requirements also have been incorporated into state licensure laws.

JCAHO has been an active proponent of incorporating procedures for measuring quality of care and treatment outcomes into the accreditation process. Several sections of its accreditation manuals not only require that outcomes be continuously monitored, but that external reference data bases be used for comparative purposes. JCAHO also has been influential in advancing these issues in public policy arenas through its frequent interactions with the Health Care Financing Administration, AHCPR, and various Congressional bodies, conferences it has sponsored, and publications it disseminates. Examples of the latter include the *Joint Commission Perspectives* and the *Joint Commission Journal on Quality Improvement.*

Although indicators specific to rehabilitation are not yet required, the length of time that it takes to develop such indicators and their inevitability have accelerated efforts by related health care professionals (Hall & Johnston, 1994) and by SLPs and audiologists. In April, 1996, JCAHO asked various organizations and individuals who have developed performance measures, including ASHA, to submit them for potential inclusion in the Joint Commission's *National Library of Healthcare Indicators*. Dr. Loeb described this initiative as an effort "to meet the need for ongoing measurement and monitoring of relevant processes and outcomes as part of the accreditation process" (Loeb, personal correspondence, April 5, 1996). The outcomes instruments developed by the ASHA Task Force on Treatment Outcome and Cost Effectiveness, discussed below, were submitted for inclusion.

Rehabilitation Accreditation Commission (CARF)

Another major national, nonprofit standards setting and voluntary accreditation organization is the Rehabilitation Accreditation Commission (formerly the Commission on Accreditation of Rehabilitation Facilities—CARF). As has been the case with JCAHO, CARF has placed increasing emphasis on outcomes-based program evaluation, outcome measures, and evidence of client involvement in treatment planning. Its standards require the use of outcomes data and their links to input and process data in decision making at all levels of the organization (See Chapter 2).

National Committee for Quality Assurance (NCQA)

NCQA was recently established to set standards and accredit managed care plans. This nonprofit group, which was formed approximately 5 years ago with the help of HMOs, examines, rates, and compares managed care plans. NCQA has placed considerable emphasis upon continuous quality review and the collection of outcomes data in order to achieve its highest rating. Although accreditation by this group is voluntary, receipt of the industry's highest rating should provide an increasingly recognized competitive advantage to those HMOs so designated.

To facilitate the health care purchasers' ability to make meaningful comparisons among health plans, NCQA has developed the HEDIS employer scorecard. HEDIS includes five dimensions: quality of care, member access and satisfaction, membership utilization, finance, and descriptive information on health plan management and activities.

Office of Managed Care

The HCFA's Office of Managed Care is a federal partner to NCQA. One of the priorities of this office is to improve the quality of managed care by increasing competition on the basis of quality. The Office of Managed Care is working to provide comparative information on managed care plans to Medicare beneficiaries to help them make informed choices among available plans (Serafini, 1996).

American Speech-Language-Hearing Association (ASHA)

ASHA has established a standard-setting body and one of its operating boards to address specifically the quality of service in speech-language pathology and audiology. The Council on Professional Standards, a semiautonomous body, establishes standards in speech-language pathology and audiology, and the Professional Services Board monitors and accredits service facilities on a voluntary basis. In concert with CARF and JCAHO, ASHA's Professional Services Board has prioritized collection of data on the effects of treatment and evidence of mechanisms for continuous quality improvement within its review processes.

PAYMENT FOR SERVICES: HEALTH CARE

Several public and private agencies are involved in financing health care services. AHCPR recently released two reports that examined expenses and sources of payment for adult and child health care services based upon the 1987 National Medical Expenditure Survey (AHCPR, 1994a; AHCPR, 1994b). Medicare, the largest of the publicly funded programs, accounted for nearly 1 out of 5 of all expenditures. Medicaid and other public sources accounted for approximately 24% of the child health care costs. ASHA has recently estimated that 45% of its members receive Medicaid or Medicare reimbursement either directly or indirectly (ASHA, 1996). In both the public and private health care sectors information about treatment outcomes is becoming a central feature of major provider payment systems.

Health Care Financing Administration (HCFA)

The HCFA, a division of the U.S. Department of Health and Human Services, is the primary federal agency administering health care financing. Created by the Secretary of Health and Human Services in 1977, it has administrative responsibility for the Medicare program, and the federal portion of the Medicaid program. Medicare, a social insurance program, provides health benefits for individuals 65 years of age or older, those who are receiving Social Security disability benefits, and those who are undergoing dialysis treatment or kidney transplantation for end-stage renal disease. Medicaid is a jointly financed federal-state medical assistance program for eligible low-income individuals, including recipients of Aid to Families with Dependent Children, and in most states needy elderly, blind, and disabled individuals who receive support under the Supplemental Security Income program, low income pregnant women and infants, and those whose medical bills qualify them as needing assistance (Calkins, Fernandopulle, & Marino, 1995). As a part of its mandate, HCFA monitors quality assurance for the Medicare and Medicaid programs, and develops and implements standards for providers in federally funded health programs.

Providers are reimbursed for the Medicare-covered services they provide through intermediaries or carriers that contract with HCFA. Under the original legislation, providers were reimbursed on a "reasonable cost" fee-for-service basis. In 1983, as a cost containment measure, Congress changed the basis for hospital reimbursement from reasonable cost to a Prospective Payment System (PPS). Under this system the hospital is reimbursed a flat rate on a predetermined basis depending upon the patient's DRG category. A new payment system for Part B physician services was adopted in 1989 to be phased in from 1992 to 1996. This new fee schedule reflects resource-based relative value scales (RBRVS) and assigns relative values for services provided including adjustments for geographic variations in cost (Calkins et al., 1995). This shift and the increasing participation of Medicare in managed care arrangements will impact on the funds available for provision of speech-language pathology services in the outpatient environment and correspondingly intensify the need for outcomes data.

The method for reimbursing providers for Medicaid-covered services is determined by the states as long as they conform to general federal guidelines. States use prospective payment systems similar to Medicare and Medicare's DRG system, directly negotiated rates, or contractual arrangements with managed care organizations.

Free-standing rehabilitation hospitals and rehabilitation units within hospitals, as well as other specialty hospitals such as children's, long-term care, and psychiatric hospitals, are currently exempt from Medicare's PPS. Under the Tax Equity and Fiscal Responsibility Act of 1982 (TEFRA) rehabilitation facilities are reimbursed for reasonable costs up to a set amount. Dissatisfaction with the TEFRA reimbursement system has been widespread, and in the 1990 Omnibus Budget Reconciliation Act, Congress mandated that the Department of Health and Human Services propose a modification of the system or an alternative payment system for rehabilitation services. In its 1987 Report to Congress, HCFA indicated that among its goals would be the development of a prospective payment system for rehabilitation (Wilkerson, Batavia, & DeJong, 1992).

Several studies have concluded that diagnosis-based payment systems are not reliable predictors of rehabilitation resource utilization and that a functional status-based system would be preferable (Batavia, 1988; Hosek, Kane, Carney, Hartman, Reboussin, Serrato et al., 1986; McGinnis, Osberg, DeJong, Mae, Seward, & Branch, 1987; National Association of Rehabilitation Facilities, 1985). What the features of that system should be are still being discussed. One prospective payment system proposal, the FIM-FRGs, was developed to estimate length of stay for rehabilitation inpatient groups based upon FIM score estimates of functional status at admission, rehabilitation impairment category, and patient age (Stineman, Hamilton, Granger, Goin, Escarce, & Williams, 1994; Stineman, Escarce, Goin, Hamilton, Granger, & Williams, 1994). Formative work to design a PPS for rehabilitative services is still continuing. Other investigators have suggested that change in functional status is a better predictor of rehabilitation resource utilization than functional status at admission alone. Information on functional status change was considered to be particularly informative when used in combination with condition-specific activities of daily living (Harada, Sofaer, & Kominski, 1993).

Although a prospective payment system for rehabilitation has not yet been adopted, functional status measurement will be a key feature of any such plan. Efforts to develop a prospective payment system will continue to underscore the need for effective outcomes measurement of speech-language pathology services.

Private Insurers

The private insurance industry is undergoing dramatic change. Prior to 1980, Blue Cross, Blue Shield or commercial insurance companies provided health insurance plans to employers. Premiums were paid on an annual basis and providers were reimbursed on a fee-for-service basis for covered services up to set amounts. However, in 1980, a range of new options and alternatives were introduced under managed care (Kovner, 1990), and their roles in the health care industry continue to grow. Although the specific forms of managed care vary, a common feature is that the system of providers agrees to meet the specified health care needs of a predetermined population of enrollees for a predetermined budget amount.

Outcomes information is critical to determining appropriate levels of remuneration for speech-language pathology services given that financial risk in a managed care environment is shifted to the provider. Accurate prediction of potential resource use required by the enrollees covered under the plan becomes the responsibility of service providers and is essential for the viability and effectiveness of the service.

FEDERAL INITIATIVES REGARDING OUTCOMES ASSESSMENT IN EDUCATION

For the past 2 decades, business leaders and elected officials at all levels of government have been expressing deep concerns about public education. In the 1970s and 1980s these concerns focused on curricular content issues, and a movement sometimes referred to as "Back to Basics" advocated the establishment of minimum competency tests in reading and mathematics as a condition of high school graduation. Despite these efforts, concerns have persisted. Consequently, landmark national legislation has been enacted setting voluntary national educational standards specifying the expected outcomes of public education for the nation's children. This legislation, the *Goals 2000: Educate America Act,* which was signed into law in 1994, was the culmination of efforts begun in 1989 by President Bush at a summit conference with the nation's governors (Jennings, 1995).

Goals 2000 set voluntary content, performance, and opportunity-to-learn standards, and provided funds to states for "systemic reform" of their educational systems (O'Day, 1995). Eight National Education Goals to be achieved by the year 2000 were framed (See Table 24–1). These included the six national goals originally adopted at the governors' conference and two additional goals.

The Act established the National Education Standards and Improvement Council to provide models and support states in the development process. The Council has representation from education, business, parents, and the public. The Act also gave broad authority to the Department of Education to waive federal regulations restricting a state's educational reform efforts (Riley, 1995).

Subsequent to passage of the Goals 2000 Act, a panel that had been formed in 1990, the National Education Goals Panel became an executive branch agency responsible for monitoring and facilitating achievement of the National Education Goals. Members included eight Governors, four members of Congress, four state legislators, the U.S. Secretary of Education, and the President's domestic policy advisor. In a recent report, the Panel has described progress toward meeting the goals as "modest" (National Education Goals Panel, 1996).

Many of the changes occurring in health care are occurring also in education. The same questions regarding the cost-effectiveness of service and the functional outcomes of that service in education terms are being raised. For example, if speech-language pathology services are provided to young language-impaired children, will that mean that they will learn to read? Will fewer other support services be required such as resource teacher? Will children be able to attain grade level skills in other academic areas? How is overall academic achievement affected by the provision of speech-language pathology services? Does it matter if these services are provided when children are young, or is it more effective in terms of functional outcomes and cost to delay direct service provision until the children are older and can take more responsibility for

---

Table 24–1. National Education Goals

Goal 1:	"By the year 2000, all children in America will start school ready to learn."
Goal 2:	"By the year 2000, the high school graduation rate will increase to at least 90 percent."
Goal 3:	"By the year 2000, all children will leave grade 4, 8, and 12 having demonstrated competency over challenging subject matter including English, Mathematics, Science, Foreign Languages, Civics and Government, Economics, Arts, History, and Geography, and every school in America will ensure that all students learn to use their minds well, so that they may be prepared for responsible citizenship, further learning, and productive employment in our nation's modern economy."
Goal 4:	"By the year 2000, the nations teaching force will have access to programs for the continued improvement of their precessional skills and the opportunity to acquire the knowledge and skills needed to instruct and prepare all American students for the next century."
Goal 5:	"By the year 2000, United States students will be first in the world in Mathematics and Science Achievement."
Goal 6:	"By the year 2000, every adult American will be literate and will possess the knowledge and skills necessary to compete in a global economy and exercise the rights and responsibilities of citizenship."
Goal 7:	"By the year 2000, every school in the United States will be free of drugs, violence, and the unauthorized presence of firearms and alcohol and will offer a disciplined environment conducive to learning."
Goal 8:	"By the year 2000, every school will promote partnerships that will increase parental involvement and participation in promoting the social, emotional, and academic growth of children."

SOURCE: National Education Goals Panel, 1996(b).

---

guiding own their own learning? Does speech-language pathology intervention require the direct service delivery of speech-language pathologists, or can other care providers be used and service provided indirectly as effectively by teachers, parents, and aides?

Educational reform has echoed the same shift from structure and process indicators of quality to a greater emphasis on demonstrable, measurable outcomes. Some of the same challenges as those observed in the health care sector are also evident in educational settings. Reliable indicators and processes supporting routine inclusion of outcomes measurement in service delivery need to be developed for use within these settings as well as within health care settings. Educational professional practice patterns also need to be reviewed in the context of outcomes information, and this information used to enrich service provision. Organizational issues (e.g., the number of SLPs needed to service a school district; the types of service provision models used; the types of communication problems that will be addressed, at what ages, with what intensity) are similar to those raised in managed care. Further, since some speech-language pathology services within school settings are receiving reimbursement from Medicaid, the need to understand the importance of outcomes information is made even more acute.

School-based SLPs were among the first to deal with what have become important parameters of speech-language pathology service delivery in a managed care environment. They have had the longest history with managing case load from a population perspective. School-based SLPs were responsible for the population of children attending the school(s) to which they were assigned. Their roles, therefore, were defined on a population basis and their challenge was to provide services to those children within that population that evidenced communication problems. If risk factors within that population were great or changed over time, management of services required that service delivery models be adjusted to meet those shifts in demand. This is parallel to the type responsibility assumed by SLPs in a managed care environment when service provision is contracted with an insurer on a fixed cost per-member per-month basis. Similarly, school-based SLPs have had an extended history of using "care extenders" in the provision of service. These have included classroom teachers, other special service personnel, and parents and models of service delivery that are organized around these care providers, such as classroom inclusion, consultative models, and so on. As we face the challenges affecting practice in all settings, much could be learned by facilitating information sharing across employment settings.

ASHA: NATIONAL TREATMENT OUTCOMES INITIATIVES IN SPEECH-LANGUAGE PATHOLOGY AND AUDIOLOGY

ASHA has supported treatment outcomes assessment of speech-language pathology and audiology services for many years through its standards, quality improvement, and advocacy programs. These efforts were intensified in the early 1990s, however, in response to member needs to provide more information about the effectiveness of their services to policymakers, payers, and consumers. This was due partly to ongoing public interest in health care reform and the rapid growth of managed care models in the health care sector. In response to these pressures, ASHA's Executive Board in the Fall of 1993 authorized the formation of a task force to gather outcomes information on speech-language pathology and audiology services and explore the feasibility of establishing a national data base of outcomes data on these services. Early in 1994, ASHA's Task Force on Treatment Outcome and Cost Effectiveness (TOCE) was formed.

The Task Force began its work with two treatment outcome projects that predated its formation. One of these projects was to ask respected researchers in the field to review the published treatment efficacy literature and author summary papers in ten treatment areas. These technical reports were completed and published as supplements to the *Journal of Speech and Hearing Research* in 1996. They also were summarized into one-page briefs by ASHA staff for use with legislators, payers, and consumers and are available upon request from the ASHA National Office. (See Appendix 24–A for excerpts from these summaries).

In addition, a 3-year project was being completed to refine, pilot, and field test a functional communication measure of adults with speech, language, and cognitive communication disorders. Funding to support this work was provided in part through a grant from the U.S. Department of Education's National Institute on Disability and Rehabilitation Research. The instrument that was developed, the *Functional Assessment of Communication Skills for Adults (ASHA FACS),* was found to be a reliable and valid measure of functional communication across the domains of social communication; communication of basic needs; reading, writing, and number concepts; and daily planning for adults with aphasia resulting from left-hemisphere stroke and adults with cognitive communication disorders resulting from traumatic brain injury. The instrument was completed and marketed in 1995. The Task Force is currently collecting data from a group of users to add these outcomes data to other data being collected.

The Task Force next concentrated its efforts on retrieving and assembling utilization and outcomes data on speech-language pathology and audiology from existing national databases, evaluating data collection systems being used to obtain rehabilitation outcomes data, and providing information to members about managed care. Cost figures for speech-language pathology and audiology services were assembled by an actuarial firm, Milliman & Roberts, Inc., using HMO data. A subsequent report, *Managed Care Contracting: An Actuarial Analysis,* was prepared and published (Roberts, 1994).

Three outcomes data collection instruments being used in rehabilitation environments also were examined: the FIM (State University of New York at Buffalo, 1993), the LORS-III (Formations in Health Care Inc., 1991), and *RESTORE* (Formations in Health Care Inc., 1993). The first two instruments were designed for adults in inpatient rehabilitation settings, and the latter was intended for rehabilitation patients in outpatient settings.

The UDSMR encompasses the *Functional Independence Measure* and is one of the largest nationally aggregated rehabilitation data bases available. The UDS system is administered by the Center for Functional Assessment Research at the State University of New York at Buffalo, School of Medicine and Biomedical Sciences. The instrument was developed by a task force sponsored by the American Congress of Rehabilitation Medicine and the American Academy of Physical Medicine and Rehabilitation and was later endorsed by 11 national organizations concerned with medical rehabilitation. Data on patients became available to participating facilities in 1990 (Granger & Hamilton, 1992). As of June 1993, over 300,000 patient records from 470 inpatient medical facilities in 49 states have been entered into the UDS data base. The FIM assesses self-care, sphincter control, transfers (e.g., from bed to wheelchair), locomotion, communication, and social cognition using a 7-point scale (1 = total dependence; 7 = complete independence). Items of particular relevance to SLPs are those assessing eating, auditory comprehension, visual comprehension, vocal expression, nonvocal expression, social interaction, problem solving, and memory. There is limited applicability of items to audiology.

Upon close study, the Task Force concluded that several factors limited the FIM's ability to adequately measure treatment outcomes in speech-language pathology. Limitations were that: items were not specific enough to adequately characterize the communication processes being assessed; any member of the health care team could code communication items despite wide differences in their professional training to do so; ratings were entered for all scales regardless of their appropriateness to certain patient groups (e.g., patients with hip replacement); ratings were entered independent of whether intervention was provided or how often it was provided; and, the measure lacked sufficient sensitivity for capturing change in communication. Due to these limitations, the Task Force concluded that treatment outcomes of speech-language pathology services could not be reliably related to changes in FIM scores.

There were similar concerns about using LORS-III to represent functional status changes in communication. LORS-III, the smaller of the two nationally aggregated data bases, assesses activities of daily living (e.g., dressing, grooming), mobility, and verbal communication (i.e. auditory comprehension and oral expression). Reading comprehension, written expression, and alternative communication are coded only at discharge. The LORS-III uses a 5-point scale (0 = unable to perform task, 4 = independence). Each item is dually scored, usually by a nurse and the designated health care professional for the skills being evaluated (e.g., speech-language pathologist, physical therapist).

The Task Force contracted with Formations in Health Care, Inc. to analyze an exemplary data set on treatment outcomes for those LORS-III items in the database relating to speech-language pathology services. Data on 4419 stroke and head injury patients from 49 facilities were analyzed. Analyses indicated that patients' oral motor skills, communication skills, cognitive skills, and pragmatic skills, on average, improved from 20 to 35% across these skill domains. Although these data were not nationally representative, they did indicate the type of information that could be obtained from this type of data base. Because the items on the LORS-III are dually scored, comparisons also were made between the ratings made by speech-language pathologists and those made by other raters, most often nurses. This analysis indicated that ratings by SLPs were significantly lower than those made by other raters. Although it is not clear why raters differed, it does underscore the importance of discipline-designated raters in the reliability of change scores. As was the case with the FIM, the LORS-III does not provide information on the frequency and intensity of services delivered. Similar concerns to those noted for the FIM regarding item sensitivity, comprehensiveness, and possible ceiling effects unduly suppressing change scores also were expressed.

The third instrument examined was RESTORE. It was the only national outpatient rehabilitation data base available at the time. RESTORE uses the same rating scales as LORS-III but includes a data entry field for number of treatment units. Many of the concerns reviewed above applied to this instrument as well since the rating scales were the same as those for LORS-III. Analyses similar to those performed with the LORS-III database was not warranted, however, since the number of cases contained in the RESTORE database was too small (See Pietranton & Baum, 1995 for summary).

Following these efforts it became clear that in order to provide the types of utilization and outcomes information that SLPs and audiologists required, data could not simply be retrieved from the rehabilitation outcomes instruments already in use. Instruments more specific to the needs of these professionals would be needed.

The Task Force also identified treatment outcomes instruments developed and being used in the field. These were reviewed and the strengths of each noted. Five sites whose databases were sufficiently large and varied relative to their patient populations were studied further. Data across facilities were integrated and analyzed by Evaluation Systems International, Inc. Again, although not nationally representative, the data provided a great deal of information regarding the types of analyses that could be applied to automated systems. Three of the facilities that were maintaining outcomes data bases also were visited to explore coding and use issues that would be helpful in the design and maintenance of a speech-language pathology and audiology national outcomes database.

All of this information was used to design treatment outcomes instruments for speech-language pathology and audiology services and explore the development of an ongoing national data base. Four instruments have been completed to date: *The National Treatment Outcomes Measurement System for Speech-Language Pathology and Audiology: Speech-Language Pathology Services for Adults* (19 years of age and older);

The National Treatment Outcomes Measurement System for Speech-Language Pathology and Audiology: Speech-Language Pathology Services for Children Aged 5–18 Years in Health Care Settings (TOCE, 1995a); *The National Treatment Outcomes Measurement System for Speech-Language Pathology and Audiology: Speech-Language Pathology Services for Children aged 5–18 years in Educational Settings* (TOCE, 1995b); *The National Treatment Outcomes Measurement System for Speech-Language Pathology and Audiology: Speech-Language Pathology Services for Children Birth to Kindergarten* (TOCE, 1996a). One instrument is still under development, *The National Treatment Outcomes Measurement System for Speech-Language Pathology and Audiology: Audiology Services.*

The instruments were made available to selected field test sites on scannable forms. Each instrument includes four forms: Admission, Discharge, Patient Satisfaction, and Financial Information forms. Forms for the speech-language pathology service for adults instrument are attached (See Appendix 24–B). The Admission form includes information such as employment status, date of admission which is used to calculate LOS, admitted from, referral source, ICD–9 code, and functional communication measures. The Discharge form includes information such as date of discharge, the type of facility the individual was discharged to, the units of treatment provided (coded in 15-minute units), functional communication measures, and whether goals were met or continued treatment was recommended. The Patient Satisfaction form includes information such as the appropriateness of length and frequency of services, and patients' perceptions of their communication at an independent level (using a 5-point scale from strongly agree to strongly disagree). The Financial Information form includes information such as funding source, DRG code, and charges.

Functional communication status is coded at admission and discharge using a 7-point rating scale. The Manual provides a description of functional performance characteristics corresponding to each point on the scale for each type of primary communication disorder. These descriptions were based upon earlier work that ASHA had done in developing the *Program Evaluation System* (PES) (ASHA, 1987) and subsequent input from members who had used PES or its components. The points on the scale were designed to represent successive characteristics of communicative improvement that are typical given a particular primary communication disorder. FCMs are coded only for those communication disorders to be treated. In addition, on the school-based instrument, teachers are also asked to rate children on educationally relevant functional status measures at admission and discharge (see Appendix 21–C).

All of the instruments will be field tested for 6 months. The first instrument for which field testing was completed was the measure for adults. Ten health care systems, which included 100 programs providing speech-language pathology services along the continuum of health care settings, participated in the data collection. The sites were considered representative across program types and geographic regions although not in a statistical sense since they were not randomly selected from among all possible treatment settings.

Data from 1638 adult patients were obtained and analyzed in this initial data collection and data tables became available in June, 1996 (TOCE, 1996b). Statistical reliability and validity tests of the instruments are ongoing and until completed the data obtained should be considered to be preliminary and interpreted as exemplary.

Table 24–2 presents the mean FCM scores for primary communication disorders

Table 24–2. Mean FCM Admission Scores from Preliminary Test of National Outcome Measurement System: Speech-Language Pathology Services for Adults

PRIMARY COMMUNICATION DISORDER	SERVICE DELIVERY SETTINGS				
	Acute Inpatient	*Acute Rehab Unit*	*Rehab Inpatient*	*Skilled Nursing*	*Outpatient*
Speech Production	5.0	5.7	4.9	4.8	5.4
Voice	5.1	-	4.7	5.0	5.2
Ability to Swallow	4.8	6.9	6.2	4.5	-
Comprehension of Spoken Language	4.8	5.0	5.4	4.7	6.8
Production of Spoken Language	4.6	4.9	5.0	4.6	5.5
Comprehension of Written Language	-	5.1	4.9	4.3	5.5
Production of Written Language	-	4.7	4.3	3.7	5.2
Cognitive Communication	4.3	4.7	4.7	4.3	5.3

SOURCE: Task Force on Treatment Outcome and Cost Effectiveness, 1996. Missing data cells indicate that the number of responses received was not large enough to meaningfully compute a mean score.

across rehabilitation program settings, Table 24–3 presents the mean FCM change scores from admission to discharge across program settings, and Table 24–4 presents the mean FCM scores at discharge across program settings. These are averages of the data obtained within the designated settings and do not represent individual patients who have moved along a continuum of care from one type of setting to another.

Preliminary data within these tables indicate, for example, that patients with swallowing disorders within acute care inpatient settings are admitted, on average, at approximately FCM Level 3, ("Swallowing disorder prevents eating for a portion of nutritional needs and one-to-one supervision is required for eating."), and are discharged at approximately FCM Level 5, ("Swallowing is functional to meet nutritional needs, although self-monitoring and compensatory techniques are used."). In another example, preliminary data from patients within rehabilitation inpatient settings whose primary communication disorder is the comprehension of spoken language indicate that they are admitted, on average, at approximately FCM Level 4, ("Comprehension of spoken language is limited to the primary activities of daily living needs and simple ideas and frequently requires repetition and/or rephrasing."), and are discharged at approximately FCM Level 5, ("Comprehension of spoken language is normal for activities of daily living, but limited in complexity of form, content, or use; self-monitoring is inconsistent.") Data trends overall indicate that across primary communication disorders and program settings mean FCM changes from admission to discharge were approximately one FCM level. These improvements in communicative functioning lead to greater functional independence overall, which can be realized as economies throughout the health service delivery system (e.g., reduced levels of nursing care required, shortened LOSs).

Patient satisfaction data also were examined within this data set. On average, across

Table 24–3. Mean FCM Score Changes at Discharge Compared to Admission from Preliminary Test of National Outcome Measurement System: Speech-Language Pathology Services for Adults

FUNCTIONAL COMMUNICATION MEASURES	SERVICE DELIVERY SYSTEM				
	Acute Inpatient	Acute Unit Rehab	Rehab Inpatient	Skilled Nursing	Outpatient
Speech Production	0.9	1.0	1.2	0.7	0.8
Voice	1.1	-	0.9	0.8	1.1
Ability to Swallow	1.4	1.9	1.5	1.1	-
Comprehension of Spoken Language	0.9	1.1	1.0	0.6	0.8
Production of Spoken Language	1.0	1.1	1.2	0.7	0.7
Comprehension of Written Language	-	1.1	0.9	0.5	0.7
Production of Written Language	-	1.0	0.8	0.4	0.6
Cognitive Communication	0.9	1.1	1.1	0.5	0.7

SOURCE: Task Force on Treatment Outcome and Cost Effectiveness, 1996. Missing data cells indicate that the number of responses received was not large enough to meaningfully compute a mean score.

program settings, most adult patients' indicated that they judged their communication to be "better" following speech-language pathology services (range = 76–93%) and that their overall satisfaction with those services was high (range = 89–100%).

All of the data collected to date have been incorporated into ten illustrative "National Report Cards" that facilities using the ASHA instrument for adults in health

Table 24–4. Mean FCM Discharge Scores from Preliminary Test of National Outcome Measurement System: Speech-Language Pathology Services for Adults

PRIMARY COMMUNICATION DISORDER	SERVICE DELIVERY SETTING				
	Acute Inpatient	Acute Rehab Unit	Rehab Inpatient	Skilled Nursing	Outpatient
Speech Production	4.0	4.7	3.7	4.1	4.6
Voice	3.9	4.3	-	4.2	4.1
Ability to Swallow	3.3	4.0	3.7	3.4	-
Comprehension of Spoken Language	3.9	3.9	4.4	4.1	5.0
Production of Spoken Language	3.6	3.8	3.8	3.9	4.8
Comprehension of Written Language	-	4.0	4.0	3.7	4.8
Production of Written Language	-	3.6	3.5	3.3	4.6
Cognitive Communication	3.4	3.7	3.6	3.8	4.6

SOURCE: Task Force on Treatment Outcome and Cost Effectiveness, 1996. Missing data cells indicate that the number of responses received was not large enough to meaningfully compute a mean score.

care settings can refer to in a preliminary benchmarking of their service delivery patterns. Examples were provided in the recent Task Force report (TOCE, 1996).

Future work of the Task Force will focus on concluding the development and field testing of the five instruments described; reliability and validity studies of these instruments through independent, competitive grant awards administered through the American Speech-Language-Hearing Foundation; revision of the instruments as needed; and the establishment of an ongoing national treatment outcomes data base for speech-language pathology and audiology services.

CONCLUSION

Treatment outcomes information will become an increasingly important feature of rehabilitation service delivery. Public and private agency trends suggest that outcomes information will play a major role in accreditation, reimbursement, and the development of professional practice guidelines and critical paths (See Appendix 24–D for a listing of agencies). The quality, credibility, and comprehensiveness of the treatment outcomes information on speech-language pathology and audiology services will be critical to the healthy evolution of the professions.

It is clear that we will need to make a commitment to educating ourselves and students in training about how to collect and interpret outcomes data and how to most effectively incorporate outcomes data collection within standard service delivery practice. National trends also suggest that credible, national benchmarking of services will be required in the future. It is, therefore, imperative that we develop a speech-language pathology national data base that can be used in this fashion, and that that system reliably and validly reflect the impact of speech-language pathology services. Lastly, it is clear that we will have to proceed quickly. We must have the data when we are challenged to provide it. The timelines that national agencies are suggesting indicate that the need is fast approaching.

ACKNOWLEDGMENTS

The members of the Task Force on Treatment Outcome and Cost Effectiveness include Nancy B. Swigert (Co-project Officer), Herbert M. Baum (Project Staff Director), Robert M. Augustine, Audrey L. Holland, Raymond D. Kent, Roberta A. Kreb, Susan S. Russell, and Kenneth E. Wolf.

REFERENCES

Agency for Health Care Policy and Research (1996). AHCPR Announces Faculty of a New Initiative to Assist Consumers in Selecting High-Quality Health Plans. *AHCPR Release,* February 21, 1–5.

Agency for Health Care Policy and Research (1995a). *Clinical Practice Guideline Number 16: Post-Stroke Rehabilitation.* Silver Spring, MD: AHCPR Publications Clearinghouse.

Agency for Health Care Policy and Research (1995b). HIAA and AHCPR Join Forces to Help Consumers Choose and Use Managed Care Plans. *AHCPR Release,* August 28, 1–4.

Agency for Health Care Policy and Research (1994a). Expenses and Sources of Payment for Health Care Services by Type of Service, 1987. *Intramural Research Highlights,* 33, April, 5–8.

Agency for Health Care Policy and Research (1994b). Expenditures and Sources of Payment for Children's Health Care, 1987. *Intramural Research Highlights,* 29, February, 1–4.

Agency for Health Care Policy and Research (1993). Agency for Health Care Policy and Research: A Profile. *AHCPR Publication No. 93,* January, 1–2.

Agency for Health Care Policy and Research (1992). *AHCPR Fact Sheet,* March, 1–3.

American Speech-Language-Hearing Association (1987). *Program Evaluation System.* Rockville, MD: Author.

American Speech-Language-Hearing Association (1995a). *ASHA's Concerns with the Post-Stroke Rehabilitation Guideline.* Rockville, MD: ASHA Press Release.

American Speech-Language-Hearing Association (1995b). *Summaries of Treatment Efficacy Technical Papers.* Rockville, MD: Author.

American Speech-Language-Hearing Association (1996). *ASHA Legislative Agenda Mid-Year Report.* Rockville, MD: Author.

Ankrapp, B., & DeLima, S. (1995). *National Health Directory.* Gaithersburg, MD: Aspen Publishers.

Batavia, A. (1988). *The Payment of Medical Rehabilitation Services: Current Mechanisms and Potential Models.* Chicago, IL: American Hospital Association.

Calkins, D., Ferandopulle, R., & Marino, B. (1995). *Health Care Policy.* Cambridge, MA: Blackwell Science.

Formations in Health Care, Inc. (1991). *Level of Rehabilitation Scale-III.* Chicago, IL: Author.

Formations in Health Care, Inc. (1993). *RESTORE.* Chicago, IL: Author.

Granger, C., & Hamilton, B. (1992). The Uniform Data System for Medical Rehabilitation report of first admissions for 1990. *American Journal of Physical Medicine, 71*(2), 106–113.

Harada, N., Sofaer, S., & Kominski, G. (1993). Functional status outcomes in rehabilitation. *Medical Care, 31*(4), 345–57.

Hosek, S., Kane, R., Carney, M., Hartman, J., Reboussin, C., Serrato, C., et al. (1986). *Charges and Outcomes for Rehabilitative Care: Implications for the Prospective Payment System* (R-3424-HCFA). Santa Monica, CA: The RAND Corp.

Jennings, J. (1995). *National Issues in Education: Goals 2000 and School-To-Work.* Washington, DC: Institute for Educational Leadership.

Kovner, A. (1990). *Health Care Delivery in the United States.* New York: Springer Publishing Co.

McGinnis, G., Osberg, J., DeJong, G., Mae, M., Seward, L., & Branch, L. (1987). Predicting charges for inpatient medical rehabilitation using severity, DRG, age, and function. *American Journal of Public Health, 77,* 826–829.

National Association of Rehabilitation Facilities (1985). *NARF position article on a prospective payment system for inpatient medical rehabilitation services and a study regarding a prospective payment system for inpatient medical rehabilitation services: Final report.* Washington, DC: Author.

National Education Goals Panel (1996). *The National Education Goals Report.* Washington, DC.

O'Day, J. (1995). Systemic reform and Goals 2000. In J. Jennings (Ed.), *National Issues in Education: Goals 2000 and School-To-Work.* Washington, DC: Institute for Educational Leadership, 99–115.

Pietranton, A., & Baum, H. (1995). Collecting outcome data: Existing tools, preliminary data, future directions. *Asha,* 36–38.

Ramsay, C. (1995). *U.S. Health Policy Groups.* Westport, CT: Greenwood Press.

Riley, R. (1995). The Goals 2000: Educate America Act. Providing a World-Class Education for Every Child. In J. Jennings (Ed.) *National Issues in Education: Goals 2000 and School-To-Work.* Washington, DC: Institute for Educational Leadership, 3–25.

Roberts, S. (1994). *Managed Care Contracting: An Actuarial Analysis.* Rockville, MD: ASHA.

Serafini, M. (1996). He's high on managed health care. *National Journal, 9,* 2, 435.

State University of New York at Buffalo (1993). *Guide for Use of the Uniform Data Set for Medical Rehabilitation: Functional Independence Measure.* Buffalo: Research Foundation.

Stineman, M., Escarce, J., Goin, J., Hamilton, B., Granger, C., & Williams, S. (1994). A case-mix classification system for medical rehabilitation. *Medical Care, 32*(4), 366–379.

Stineman, M., Hamilton, B., Granger, C. Goin, J., Escarce, J. & Williams, S. (1994). Four methods for characterizing disability in the formation of function related groups. *Archives of Physical Medicine & Rehab, 75,* 1277–1283.

Task Force on Treatment Outcome and Cost Effectiveness (1994). *The National Treatment Outcomes Measurement System for Speech-Language Pathology and Audiology: Speech-Language Pathology Services for Adults.* Rockville, MD: ASHA.

Task Force on Treatment Outcome and Cost Effectiveness (1995a). *The National Treatment Outcomes Measurement System for Speech-Language Pathology and Audiology: Speech-Language Pathology Services for Children Aged 5–18 years in Health Care Settings.* Rockville, MD: ASHA.

Task Force on Treatment Outcome and Cost Effectiveness (1995b). *The National Treatment Outcomes Measurement System for Speech-Language Pathology and Audiology: Speech-Language Pathology Services for Children Aged 5–18 years in Educational Settings.* Rockville, MD: ASHA.

Task Force on Treatment Outcome and Cost Effectiveness (1996a). *The National Treatment Outcomes Measurement System for Speech-Language Pathology and Audiology: Speech-Language Pathology Services for Children Birth to Kindergarten.* Rockville, MD: ASHA.

Task Force on Treatment Outcome and Cost Effectiveness (1996). *ASHA's Treatment Outcomes Data Collection In Adult Health Care Settings: National Report Cards #1–10.* Rockville, MD: ASHA.

Weitzman, B. (1990). The quality of care: Assessment and Assurance. In A. Kovner (Ed.), *Health Care Delivery in the United States,* pp. 353–380. New York: Springer Publishing Co.

Excerpts from Summaries of ASHA
Treatment Efficacy Technical Papers

CHILD LANGUAGE DISORDERS

"There are over 200 studies regarding the effectiveness of language intervention. (. . .) Child langauge intervention studies indicate that the language treatment improves functional communication skills, thereby enhancing the quality of life and the social, academic, and vocational opportunities of the child."

DYSARTHRIA

"Effectiveness of speech treatment for individuals with dysarthia has been documented via group treatment studies, single-subject studies, and case reports."

COGNITIVE-COMMUNICATION DISORDERS
RESULTING FROM TRAUMATIC BRAIN INJURY

"Traumatic brain injury (TBI) patients receiving early intervention services were discharged at higher levels of cognitive functioning and had higher percentages of discharges to home versus long-term care facilities"

STUTTERING

"Treatment for stuttering results in improvement for approximately 70% of all cases. Studies on treatment effectiveness of school-age children indicate an average of 61% improvement in stuttering frequency. Over 100 studies with adults concluded that significant improvement typically occurs as a result of treatment in 60–80% of cases. A longer history of stuttering decreases the speed and degree of recovery."

"Studies have shown voice treatment to be a significant factor in improving the characteristics of voice and in reducing recurrence of laryngeal pathology"

PHONOLOGICAL DISORDERS IN CHILDREN

"The benefits of phonological treatment are overwhelming and widely documented in clinical and experimental studies dating back to the 1960s. Children who receive phonological treatment exhibit improved intelligibility and communicative functioning."

OROPHARYNGEAL DYSPHAGIA
(DIFFICULTY IN SWALLOWING)

"Efficacy studies indicate improvements in swallowing safety (reduced aspiration), improved nutrition, and efficiency as a result of both compensatory and direct treatment procedures. (. . .) Exercise programs for the active strengthening of muscle function and coordination of oropharyngeal muscle movements for swallowing have been found effective in returning patients to efficient oral intake."

Source: ASHA, 1995b. Reprinted with permission.

Admission, Discharge, Consumer Satisfaction, and Financial Information Forms from the National Treatment Outcomes Measurement System: Speech-Language Pathology Services for Adults *(TOCE, 1994).*

AMERICAN SPEECH-LANGUAGE HEARING ASSOCIATION

Treatment Outcomes Data Form
Admission

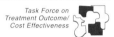
Task Force on Treatment Outcome/ Cost Effectiveness

MARKING INSTRUCTIONS

- Use No. 2 pencil or blue or black pen only.
- Do not use pens with ink that soaks through the paper.
- Make solid marks that fill the oval completely.
- Make no stray marks on this form.

WRONG MARKS   RIGHT MARKS

CORE ITEMS

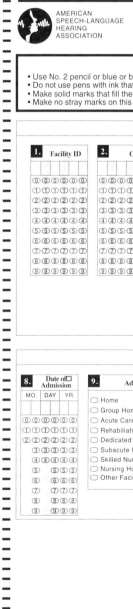

1. Facility ID

2. Client's ID

3. Client's Date of Birth
MO.   DAY   YR.

4. Client's Gender
○ Male   ○ Female

5. Client's Race/Ethnicity
○ Black (not of Hispanic origin)
○ Native American
○ Asian/Pacific Islander
○ Hispanic
○ White (not of Hispanic origin)
○ Other

6. Marital Status
○ Never Married
○ Married
○ Widowed
○ Separated
○ Divorced

6. Employment Status
○ Employed, Full-time   ○ Employed, Part-time
○ Unemployed   ○ Student
○ Homemaker   ○ Retired, Age
○ Retired, Disability   ○ Other

ADMISSION INFORMATION

8. Date of Admission
MO.   DAY   YR.

9. Admitted From
○ Home
○ Group Home
○ Acute Care Hospital
○ Rehabiliation Hospital
○ Dedicated Acute Rehab Unit
○ Subacute Unit
○ Skilled Nursing Unit/Facility
○ Nursing Home
○ Other Facility

9. Referral Source
○ Acute Care Hospital
○ Audiologist
○ Home Health Care
○ Managed Care/Utilization Review
○ Primary Care Physician
○ Rehabilitation Facility
○ Self-Referred
○ Specialty Physician
○ Speech-Language Pathologist
○ Other Health Professional (e.g., PT, OT)
○ Other (_____)

Continue on reverse side

548

11. Primary ICD-9-CM☐ Diagnosis

```
⓪⓪⓪⓪    ⓪⓪
①①①①    ①①
②②②②    ②②
③③③③    ③③
④④④④    ④④
⑤⑤⑤⑤    ⑤⑤
⑥⑥⑥⑥    ⑥⑥
⑦⑦⑦⑦    ⑦⑦
⑧⑧⑧⑧    ⑧⑧
⑨⑨⑨⑨    ⑨⑨
```

12. Was the client previously seen for treatment at this or any other facility for the same primary ICD-9-CM diagnosis?

○ Yes   ○ No

○ Unknown

13. Secondary ICD-9-CM☐ Diagnosis

```
⓪⓪⓪⓪    ⓪⓪
①①①①    ①①
②②②②    ②②
③③③③    ③③
④④④④    ④④
⑤⑤⑤⑤    ⑤⑤
⑥⑥⑥⑥    ⑥⑥
⑦⑦⑦⑦    ⑦⑦
⑧⑧⑧⑧    ⑧⑧
⑨⑨⑨⑨    ⑨⑨
```

13. Primary ☐ Communication☐ Disorder

```
⓪⓪⓪    ⓪⓪
①①①    ①①
②②②    ②②
③③③    ③③
④④④    ④④
⑤⑤⑤    ⑤⑤
⑥⑥⑥    ⑥⑥
⑦⑦⑦    ⑦⑦
⑧⑧⑧    ⑧⑧
⑨⑨⑨    ⑨⑨
```

11. Date of Onset/Identification☐ of Primary Communication☐ Disorder

MO.	DAY	YE.

```
①  ⓪⓪  ⓪⓪
①  ①①①  ①①
   ②②②  ②②
   ③③③  ③③
④  ④④④
⑤  ⑤⑤⑤
⑥  ⑥⑥⑥
⑦  ⑦⑦⑦
⑧  ⑧⑧⑧
⑨  ⑨⑨⑨
```

16. Was this☐ primary☐ communication☐ disorder☐ congenital?

○ Yes

○ No

○ Unknown

17. Was the client previously seen☐ for treatment at this or any☐ other facility for the primary☐ communication disorder?

○ Yes   ○ No

○ Unknown

18. Other☐ Communication☐ Disorder

```
⓪⓪⓪    ⓪⓪
①①①    ①①
②②②    ②②
③③③    ③③
④④④    ④④
⑤⑤⑤    ⑤⑤
⑥⑥⑥    ⑥⑥
⑦⑦⑦    ⑦⑦
⑧⑧⑧    ⑧⑧
⑨⑨⑨    ⑨⑨
```

19. FUNCTIONAL COMMUNICATION MEASURES

	CNT	Profound	Severe	Mod-Sex	Moderate	Mild-Mod	Mild	WANLY
Speech Production Disorder	⓪	①	②	③	④	⑤	⑥	⑦
Voice Disorder	⓪	①	②	③	④	⑤	⑥	⑦
Disorder of Rate, Rhythm, or Fluency	⓪	①	②	③	④	⑤	⑥	⑦
Ability to Swallow Function	⓪	①	②	③	④	⑤	⑥	⑦
Comprehension of Spoken Language	⓪	①	②	③	④	⑤	⑥	⑦
Production of Spoken Language	⓪	①	②	③	④	⑤	⑥	⑦
Recognition of Non-Spoken Language	⓪	①	②	③	④	⑤	⑥	⑦
Production of Non-Spoken Language	⓪	①	②	③	④	⑤	⑥	⑦
Comprehension of Written Language	⓪	①	②	③	④	⑤	⑥	⑦
Production of Written Language	⓪	①	②	③	④	⑤	⑥	⑦
Cognitive Communication	⓪	①	②	③	④	⑤	⑥	⑦
Hearing Sensitivity	⓪	①	②	③	④	⑤	⑥	⑦
Central Auditory Processing	⓪	①	②	③	④	⑤	⑥	⑦
No FCM (_ _ _ _ _ _ _ _ _ _ _ _)	⓪	①	②	③	④	⑤	⑥	⑦
Other Functional Indicator	⓪	①	②	③	④	⑤	⑥	⑦
Other Functional Indicator	⓪	①	②	③	④	⑤	⑥	⑦

20. Were the FCMs determined☐ by an audiologist or speech-☐ language pathologist?

○ Yes   ○ No

21. Were a set of treatment☐ goals established?

○ Yes, 30 days or less
○ Yes, 60 day
○ Yes, 90 day
○ No

22. Is English the primary☐ language spoken in the☐ household?

○ Yes   ○ No

23. Does the client use an☐ augmentative and☐ alternative communi-☐ cation device?

○ Yes   ○ No

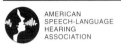

AMERICAN
SPEECH-LANGUAGE
HEARING
ASSOCIATION

Treatment Outcomes Data Form

Discharge

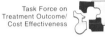

Task Force on
Treatment Outcome/
Cost Effectiveness

**MARKING☐
DIRECTIONS**

- Use No. 2 pencil or blue or black ink pen only.
- Do not use red ink or felt tip pens.
- Make solid marks that fill the oval completely.

WRONG MARKS   RIGHT MARK

---

1. Facility ID

⓪⓪⓪⓪⓪⓪
①①①①①①
②②②②②②
③③③③③③
④④④④④④
⑤⑤⑤⑤⑤⑤
⑥⑥⑥⑥⑥⑥
⑦⑦⑦⑦⑦⑦
⑧⑧⑧⑧⑧⑧
⑨⑨⑨⑨⑨⑨

2. Client's ID

⓪⓪⓪⓪⓪⓪⓪⓪
①①①①①①①①
②②②②②②②②
③③③③③③③③
④④④④④④④④
⑤⑤⑤⑤⑤⑤⑤⑤
⑥⑥⑥⑥⑥⑥⑥⑥
⑦⑦⑦⑦⑦⑦⑦⑦
⑧⑧⑧⑧⑧⑧⑧⑧
⑨⑨⑨⑨⑨⑨⑨⑨

3. Date of ☐ Discharge

MO.	DAY	YR.
⓪⓪	⓪⓪	⓪⓪
①①	①①	①①
②	②②	②②
③	③③	③③
④	④④	④
⑤	⑤⑤	⑤
⑥	⑥⑥	⑥
⑦	⑦⑦	⑦
⑧	⑧⑧	⑧
⑨	⑨⑨	⑨

☐

4. Discharged to:

- ○ Home
- ○ Group Home
- ○ Acute Care Hospital
- ○ Rehabilitation Hospital
- ○ Dedicated Acute Rehab Unit
- ○ Subacute Unit
- ○ Skilled Nursing Unit/Facility
- ○ Nursing Home
- ○ Other Facility
- ○ Other Pre-event Environment

5. Was the course and duration of treatment ☐ adequate to meet goals?

○ Yes   ○ No

If no, why? _____

If no, percentage of the treatment goals met:

○ 0%   ○ 20%   ○ 40%   ○ 60%   ○ 80%
○ 10%   ○ 30%   ○ 50%   ○ 70%   ○ 90%

Were the treatment goals limited by insurance☐ authorization or utilization review?

○ Yes   ○ No

6. Was the treatment program discontinued (i.e., the ideal ☐ course outlined)?

○ Yes   ○ No

If discontinued, please indicate why:

- ○ Client refused treatment
- ○ Client discharged from program before treatment was completed
- ○ Medical Complications/ Contraindications
- ○ Client plateaued
- ○ Insurance would not pay for continued treatment
- ○ Client would not play
- ○ Client expired
- ○ Other

7. Was the course of treatment interrupted?

○ Yes   ○ No

☐

8.

FUNCTIONAL COMMUNICATION MEASURES

	CNT	Profound	Severe	Mod-Sev	Moderate	Mild-Mod	Mild	WNL
Speech Production Disorder	⓪	①	②	③	④	⑤	⑥	⑦
Voice Disorder	⓪	①	②	③	④	⑤	⑥	⑦
Disorder of Rate, Rhythm, or Fluency	⓪	①	②	③	④	⑤	⑥	⑦
Ability to Swallow Function	⓪	①	②	③	④	⑤	⑥	⑦
Comprehension of Spoken Language	⓪	①	②	③	④	⑤	⑥	⑦
Production of Spoken Language	⓪	①	②	③	④	⑤	⑥	⑦
Recognition of Non-Spoken Language	⓪	①	②	③	④	⑤	⑥	⑦
Production of Non-Spoken Language	⓪	①	②	③	④	⑤	⑥	⑦
Comprehension of Written Language	⓪	①	②	③	④	⑤	⑥	⑦
Production of Written Language	⓪	①	②	③	④	⑤	⑥	⑦
Cognitive Communication	⓪	①	②	③	④	⑤	⑥	⑦
Hearing Sensitivity	⓪	①	②	③	④	⑤	⑥	⑦
Central Auditory Processing	⓪	①	②	③	④	⑤	⑥	⑦
No FCM (_ _ _ _ _ _ _ _ _ _ _ _)	⓪							
Other Functional Indicator	⓪	①	②	③	④	⑤	⑥	⑦
Other Functional Indicator	⓪	①	②	③	④	⑤	⑥	⑦

9. Were the FCMs determined by an audiologist or speech-language pathologist?   ○ Yes   ○ No

Continue on reverse side ⟩

☐

550

10. Was the client treated by an audiologist? ○ Yes ○ No

If yes, was a hearing aid fitted? ○ Yes ⟶ ○ Monaural ○ Binaural

○ No ○ Linear ○ Non-linear

11. Was the client treated by a speech-language pathologist? ○ Yes ○ No

12. Was the client treated by any support personnel? ○ Yes ○ No

13. If English is not the primary language, were treatment services provided in the primary language?

○ Yes ○ No

If yes, were treatment services provided by:

○ Speech-Language Pathologist/Audiologist
○ An interpreter
○ Family member as interpreter
○ Other _____

14. How many 15 minute units of treatment was the client provided as an individual and/or as part of a group?

Speech-Language Pathologist				Audiologist				Support Personnel		
Individual		**Group**		**Individual**		**Group**		**Individual**		**Group**

(each of the six columns contains bubble grids numbered 0 through 9)

15. Did the client acheive a higher level of functional communication ability than at admission? ○ Yes ○ No

16. Was the client able to resume their pre-event activites?

○ Yes, complete return
○ Yes, 75-90% return
○ Yes, 50-74% return
○ Less than 50% return

17. Was continued SLP/A treatment recommended at another level of care? ○ Yes ○ No

If yes,

○ Acute Care Hospital   ○ Nursing Home
○ Rehabilitation Hospital   ○ Home Health
○ Dedicated Acute Rehab Unit   ○ Outpatient Services
○ Subacute Unit   ○ Other _____
○ Skilled Nursing Unit/Facility

Treatment Outcomes Data Form

— PATIENT SATISFACTION —

AMERICAN SPEECH-LANGUAGE HEARING ASSOCIATION

Task Force on Treatment Outcome/ Cost Effectiveness

Marking Directions
- Use No. 2 pencil or blue or black pen only.
- Do not use red ink or felt tip pens.
- Make solid marks that fill the oval completely.

WRONG MARKS   RIGHT MARKS

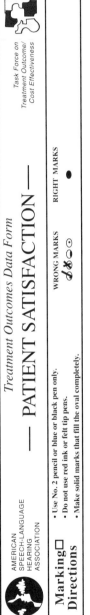

1. Facility ID

2. Client's ID

3. Form was completed by   ○ Client   ○ Family Member   ○ Caregiver

For each statement, please check the response which best indicates your experience or that of the client's with the speech-language pathology group and/or audiology group at this program.

4.

	Strongly Agree	Agree	Neutral	Disagree	Strongly Disagree	Not Applicable
My communication is better because I received these services.	○	○	○	○	○	○
I could not have improved without these services.	○	○	○	○	○	○
I feel that the length and frequency of my service program was appropriate.	○	○	○	○	○	○
My clinician was experienced and knowledgeable.	○	○	○	○	○	○
I feel the value of these services was so beneficial that I would have paid for them myself, even if they were not covered by my insurance.	○	○	○	○	○	○
I believe that I am communicating at an independent level.	○	○	○	○	○	○
I would recommend this program to others.	○	○	○	○	○	○
Overall, the program services were satisfactory.	○	○	○	○	○	○

552

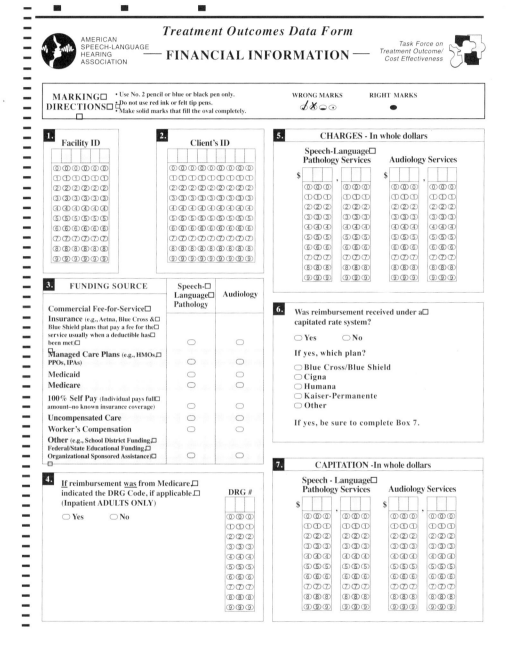

Reprinted with permission of the American Speech-Language-Hearing Association.

Functional Status Measures from the National Treatment Outcomes Measurement System: Speech-Language Pathology Services for Children in Educational Settings *(TOCE, 1994).*

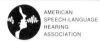

AMERICAN
SPEECH-LANGUAGE
HEARING
ASSOCIATION

Pediatric Treatment Outcomes Form
FUNCTIONAL STATUS MEASURES
(Educational Settings Only)

Task Force on Treatment Outcome/ Cost Effectiveness

Marking Directions

- Use a No. 2 pencil or black or blue pen.
- Do not use red ink or felt tip pens.
- Fill in the oval completely.
- Erase cleanly if you wish to change an answer, or "X" out if in pen.

Correct   Incorrect

1. Facility ID

2. Child's ID

3. Date of Completion

Entrance		
MO.	DAY	YR.

Dismissal		
MO.	DAY	YR.

4. STATUS MEASURES:

For each statement, please mark the response that indicates how well the student functions in each of these areas within the educational environment.

Does
Does with minimal assistance
Does with minimal to moderate assistance
Does with moderate assistance
Does with moderate to maximal assistance
Does with maximal assistance
Does not do
No basis for rating

a. The student's speech is understood. . . . . ⓪ ① ② ③ ④ ⑤ ⑥ ⑦

b. The student responds to questions regarding everyday and classroom activities. . . . . ⓪ ① ② ③ ④ ⑤ ⑥ ⑦

c. The student produces appropriate phrases and sentences in response to classroom activities. . . . . ⓪ ① ② ③ ④ ⑤ ⑥ ⑦

d. The student communicates wants, needs, ideas, and concepts to others either verbally
or by use of an augmentative/alternative communication system. . . . . ⓪ ① ② ③ ④ ⑤ ⑥ ⑦

e. The student uses appropriate vocabulary to function within the classroom. . . . . ⓪ ① ② ③ ④ ⑤ ⑥ ⑦

f. The student describes familiar objects and events. . . . . ⓪ ① ② ③ ④ ⑤ ⑥ ⑦

g. The student knows and uses age-appropriate interactions with peers and staff. . . . . ⓪ ① ② ③ ④ ⑤ ⑥ ⑦

h. The student initiates, maintains, and concludes conversations with peers and staff within
classroom environments. . . . . ⓪ ① ② ③ ④ ⑤ ⑥ ⑦

i. The student initiates, maintains, and concludes conversations with peers and staff in non-
classroon setttings. . . . . ⓪ ① ② ③ ④ ⑤ ⑥ ⑦

Continue on reverse side ⟶

```
                                                                    Does
                                                  Does with minimal assistance
                                           Does with minimal to moderate assistance
                                                 Does with moderate assistance
                                          Does with moderate to maximal assistance
                                                 Does with maximal assistance
                                                        Does not do
                                                    No basis for rating
```

j. The student indicates when messages are not understood. . . . . ⓪ ① ② ③ ④ ⑤ ⑥ ⑦

k. The student completes oral presentations. . . . . ⓪ ① ② ③ ④ ⑤ ⑥ ⑦

l. The student demonstrates the ability to give directions. . . . . ⓪ ① ② ③ ④ ⑤ ⑥ ⑦

m. The student demonstrates the ability to follow directions. . . . . ⓪ ① ② ③ ④ ⑤ ⑥ ⑦

n. The student demonstrates the ability to recall written information presented in the educational
   environment. . . . . ⓪ ① ② ③ ④ ⑤ ⑥ ⑦

o. The student demonstrates the ability to recall auditory information presented in the educational
   environment. . . . . ⓪ ① ② ③ ④ ⑤ ⑥ ⑦

p. The student demonstrates the ability to use verbal language to solve problems. . . . . ⓪ ① ② ③ ④ ⑤ ⑥ ⑦

q. The student demonstrates appropriate listening skills within the educational environment. . . . . ⓪ ① ② ③ ④ ⑤ ⑥ ⑦

r. The student recognizes and demonstrates comprehension of nonverbal communication. . . . . . . ⓪ ① ② ③ ④ ⑤ ⑥ ⑦

5. OTHER MEASURES:

Please respond to the following items using the scale rating from Strongly Agree to Strongly Disagree, or Not Applicable.

```
                                                                   Not applicable
                                                                Strongly disagree
                                                                     Disagree
                                                                     Neutral
                                                                      Agree
                                                               Strongly agree
```

a. The student speaks easily without apparent frustration. . . . . ① ② ③ ④ ⑤ ⑥

b. The student's speech does not call attention to itself. . . . . ① ② ③ ④ ⑤ ⑥

c. The student speaks loudly enough for small group and cooperative learning. . . . . ① ② ③ ④ ⑤ ⑥

d. The student demonstrates improved social and educational skills due to intervention by the
   audiologist. . . . . ① ② ③ ④ ⑤ ⑥

e. The student demonstrates improved social and educational skills due to intervention by the
   speech-language pathologist . . . . ① ② ③ ④ ⑤ ⑥

f. The student's successful progression through the educational process was positively affected by
   speech-language pathology and/or audiology intervention . . . . ① ② ③ ④ ⑤ ⑥

National Agency Addresses

AGENCY FOR HEALTH CARE POLICY AND RESEARCH

2101 East Jefferson Street, Room 501
Rockville, MD 20852
(301) 594–6662

AMERICAN SPEECH-LANGUAGE-HEARING ASSOCIATION

10801 Rockville Pike
Rockville, MD 20852
(301) 897–5700

CENTER FOR GENERAL HEALTH SERVICES
EXTRAMURAL RESEARCH

Agency for Health Care Policy and Research
2101 East Jefferson Street
Rockville, MD 20852
(301) 594–1349

CENTER FOR MEDICAL EFFECTIVENESS RESEARCH

Agency for Health Care Policy and Research
2101 East Jefferson Street
Rockville, MD 20852
(301) 594–1485

CENTER FOR RESEARCH DISSEMINATION AND LIAISON

Agency for Health Care Policy and Research
2101 East Jefferson Street
Rockville, MD 20852
(301) 594–1360

CARF . . . THE REHABILITATION ACCREDITATION COMMISSION

4891 E. Grant Rd.
Tucson, AZ 85712
(520) 325–1044

HEALTH CARE FINANCING ADMINISTRATION

330 Independence Ave. SW
Washington, DC 20201–0001
(202) 690–6726

JOINT COMMISSION ON ACCREDITATION
 OF HEALTHCARE ORGANIZATIONS

One Renaissance Boulevard
Oakbrook Terrace, IL 60181
(708) 916–5600

NATIONAL CENTER FOR MEDICAL REHABILITATION RESEARCH

National Institute of Child Health and Human Development
6100 Executive Building/Room 2A03
6100 Executive Blvd MSC 7510
Bethesda, MD 20892–7510
(301) 295–5800

NATIONAL COMMITTEE FOR QUALITY HEALTH CARE

1500 K Street NW
Suite 360
Washington, DC 20005
(202) 628–5788

NATIONAL EDUCATION GOALS PANEL

1255 22nd Street NW Suite 502
Washington, DC 20037
(202) 632–0952

OFFICE OF MANAGED CARE

Health Care Financing Administration
4360 Cohen Building
330 Independence Ave SW
Washington. DC 20201–0001
(202) 619–0815

OFFICE OF THE FORUM FOR QUALITY
AND EFFECTIVENESS IN HEALTH CARE

Agency for Health Care Policy and Research
Wilco Building
Room 310, 6000 Executive Boulevard
Rockville, MD 20852
(301) 594–1360

International Initiatives in Outcomes Measurement: A Perspective from the United Kingdom

SALLY BYNG, ANNA VAN DER GAAG,
AND SUSIE PARR

INTRODUCTION

In the United Kingdom in recent years, as in North America, the attention of health care professionals has been focused ever more sharply on the need to assess and evaluate the impact of intervention. In this chapter we provide a broad picture of the main initiatives in outcomes measurement in the United Kingdom, accompanied by a perspective on the influences shaping new developments and future trends. The first half of the chapter is therefore concerned with describing current activity in the development of a culture of evaluation, while the second half considers some of the dilemmas in outcomes measurement. The chapter concludes with a discussion of some of the principles which must underlie any new framework for developing outcomes.

THE CONTEXT OF CHANGE
IN THE NATIONAL HEALTH SERVICE

The National Health Service (NHS) has been the cornerstone of health care provision for the vast majority of the population in the United Kingdom. Historically the NHS has not operated under a fee-for-service system and all health care services have been provided through central government funding. The major difference between the U.K. and U.S. health care systems is that in the United States, consumer choices drive the market (Newman, 1995). The last six years have witnessed the most profound change to health care provision in the U.K. since the introduction of the NHS in 1946. The NHS still ensures that health care is free at the point of delivery to all who require its services, but since 1989 service providers have been separated organizationally from the commissioners (purchasers) of services. Commissioners decide, on behalf of a community or area of population, which health care services should be provided for that population and then purchase those services on behalf of that population. This has resulted in the introduction of managed competition between provider units for contracts with purchasers. It has also focused the minds of purchasers on the quality and effectiveness of services that they are purchasing (St. Leger, Schnieden, & Walsworth-Bell, 1992). As is happening in health care in most developed economies, these changes are highlighting the need for outcome measures that reflect the effects of the interventions provided.

When the profound changes to the organization of the NHS were introduced at the start of this decade, the government signaled the importance that evaluation of effectiveness would have in the development of health services in its strategy document "Health of the Nation" (1991):

> The development of better understanding of the effectiveness—and cost effectiveness—of interventions is essential. It is fundamental not only to setting strategic objectives; it is fundamental to all health planning and to each individual decision about how to use resources, from choice of treatment for individual patient to legislation on environmental protection. [p. 43]

This document goes on to define how outcomes measurement is to be interpreted: "Outcome measurement—that is measurement of the success of particular actions or sets of actions in improving health—shows not only change, but relates that change to identifiable actions, resources, or events. It enables specification and quantification of objectives increasingly to be not in terms of process, but of improvements to health. It allows the effectiveness of policies to be evaluated" (p. 43). Significantly, the crucial importance of the utilization of outcomes measurement for the maintenance and retention of services within the NHS is signaled. "In the long-term it will increasingly be developed as a way of holding the NHS and others to account for the success of their activities" (p. 43).

In order to underpin the better understanding of effectiveness and to achieve the objective of an "evidence-based health service" (Fahey et al., 1995), the government put in place a wide-ranging Research and Development Strategy (Department of Health,1993), one of whose key objectives was to facilitate the development of a knowledge-based NHS and encourage an evaluative culture within it. Within the Research and Development (R&D) Program, a number of initiatives has been established through which the development of outcome measures is promoted. Perhaps the most explicit is the Health Technology Assessment program, which refers to "the assessments of the effectiveness, costs and broader impact of all procedures used by health care professionals to promote health and to prevent and treat illness" (p. 8). This is an ambitious program which is commissioning a substantial amount of research to promote evaluation of comparison, cost-effectiveness, and outcomes across a wide spectrum of interventions (Department of Health, 1995).

The U.K. government has also demonstrated its commitment to the R&D Program's objectives by supporting a number of national information and dissemination centers. These centers are important to clinicians and managers alike, as they act as a nerve center for the exchange of information on many aspects of health care intervention including outcomes measurement. Each center has a specific role, which is briefly described below.

NATIONAL INITIATIVES IN OUTCOMES MEASUREMENT

The U.K. Clearing House on Health Outcomes

The U.K. Clearing House on Health Outcomes aims to develop and promote approaches to the assessment of health outcomes within routine health care practice. Its remit includes raising awareness among health care professionals, purchasers, and policymakers about key issues in health outcomes measurement, and to promote the role of health outcomes within decision making in health care commissioning and provision. The results of its early surveys suggested that process measurement was the predominant measurement in a majority of health care settings (UKCH, 1993). Consequently, the Center has focused its efforts on encouraging a shift from process to outcome measurement and the use of client-centered and clinically relevant outcomes criteria, notably health status questionnaires and quality-of-life measures.

The Clearing House provides an information and enquiry service. Its Outcomes Activities Database allows users to examine outcome measures currently in use, access a range of published and unpublished material on outcomes measurement, and exchange ideas and information on specific topics. In addition, a data base of Structured Abstracts (Outcomes Structured Activities Database [OSAD] allows users to make specific searches of the literature relating to the development and validation of outcome measures. Each submission to the data base is critically appraised and a commentary on the work is given. These data bases are available on CD ROM and can be accessed via the Internet.

Aside from this central activity, the Clearing House provides access to a range of publications and bibliographies. It also contributes to training and development for health care practitioners. It has links with other organizations concerned with outcomes measurement worldwide, such as the European Clearing House on Health Outcomes and the Australian Health Outcomes Clearing House, which fulfill similar functions.

The U.K. Cochrane Centre

The U.K. Cochrane Centre is part of an international collaboration established to evaluate all available evidence generated by randomized, controlled clinical trials. The collaboration evolved in response to Cochrane's incisive comment on the lack of a coordinated forum for the review and dissemination of information from such trials. Without regular systematic reviews, how could clinicians incorporate new knowledge into their practice? (Cochrane, 1979). The aim of the Centre is therefore to register all completed and continuing randomized controlled trials, to combine the results of trials, and to produce regularly updated systematic reviews or meta analyses. There are currently eight centers worldwide, covering 30 clinical areas. Those relevant to speech and language therapy include stroke, neonatal conditions, dementia and cognitive disorders, acute respiratory infections, and effective professional practice.

The Cochrane Centre disseminates information via CD ROM, the Internet and academic press, and through international conferences.

NHS Centre for Reviews and Dissemination

The NHS Centre for Reviews and Dissemination (CRD) was established in 1994 to provide the NHS with information on the effectiveness of health care interventions and to promote research-based practice. It is a sibling organization of the U.K. Cochrane Centre. The CRD's activities include regular reviews of research on the effectiveness of health care interventions, health promotion, and service delivery. Many of these reviews are undertaken by experts commissioned by the CRD. The most recent review relevant to speech and language therapy is focusing on the efficacy of preschool language intervention programs.

The Centre provides users with information on two data bases, one of which concentrates on abstracts of reviews of effectiveness (known as Database of Abstracts of Reviews on Effectiveness [DARE]) and the other on economic evaluations of health care. It has recently established a facility aimed specifically at disseminating information to nurses and therapists, known as the Practice and Service Development Initiative.

The U.K. Centre for Evidence-Based Medicine

"Evidence-based medicine" is a relatively new term for describing a well-established principle of good professional practice. It has been defined as the conscientious, explicit, judicious use of current best evidence in making decisions about the care of individual clients. It is an integral part of professional development.

The Centre for Evidence-Based Medicine, or Evidence-Based Health Care, was established in 1995 to promote and support the practice of evidence-based medicine among all U.K. health professionals. It aims to achieve this by critically appraising research evidence where it is available and disseminating this information to clinicians. It also provides training workshops in how to apply the principles of evidence-based medicine, and has plans to assist in the establishment of a graduate program to train researchers in the application of randomized controlled trial methodologies and systematic reviews.

The Centre publishes a journal that presents structured abstracts of key clinical articles, each accompanied by a commentary from a clinical expert. This follows a similar format to the American College of Physicians "Journal Club," a highly successful journal edited by Brian Haynes of McMaster University.

The Centre plans to conduct its own research into the application of evidence-based health care, including implementing randomized controlled trials, evaluations of clinically useful measures of the "economics" of diagnosis and therapy, and surveys and observational studies into clinical competence and clinical information needs of U.K. clinicians.

The National Centre for Clinical Audit

The National Centre for Clinical Audit (NCCA) was established in 1995 to provide a national focus for new developments in clinical audit. Unlike other national centers described above, the NCCA is a partnership of health care organizations that have chosen to work together to promote audit as a collaborative activity. As such it is committed to promoting multidisciplinary audits and to disseminating information on clinical audit activities across the health care disciplines.

The Centre has developed criteria for excellence in clinical audit and has used this to establish a data base of clinical audits featuring examples of good practice. Users can access this database via CD ROM and the Internet.

In addition to its function as an information center, the NCCA offers training in clinical audit methodologies and organizes conferences on clinical audit. Like other information and dissemination centers, it is dependent on clinicians to contribute to and make use of the data base. Figure 25–1 summarizes the functions of the various resource centers in the United Kingdom.

The Clinical Outcomes Group

In addition to these national centers, the U.K. Department of Health has established a Clinical Outcomes Group, a multiprofessional body with responsibility for the development, dissemination, and monitoring of clinical guidelines. Clinical guidelines are a recent development in the U.K., and they follow much the same format as the guidelines proposed and implemented through the Agency for Health Care Policy and Research in the United States (AHCPR, 1992). Clinical guidelines are systematically developed statements that assist the individual clinician and patient in making decisions about appropriate health care for a particular condition. The principles underlying the strategy for clinical guidelines in the U.K. stipulate that guidelines should, wherever possible, contain a systematic review of the literature. If such evidence is not available, then the statements should be based on expert opinions agreed by means of

	U.K. Clearing House on Health Outcomes	Cochrane Centre	Centre for Reviews and Dissemination	Evidence-Based Medicine	National Centre for Clinical Audit
Focus:	outcome measures	clinical effectiveness	systematic reviews	evidence - based health care	multi-disciplinary clinical audit
Audience:	health care practitioners, purchasers, policymakers	health care practitioners, purchasers, policymakers	health care practitioners, purchasers, policymakers	health care practitioners, purchasers, policymakers	health care practitioners, purchasers, policymakers
Access:	CD ROM Web site	CD ROM Web site Conferences	CD ROM Web site	Journals Web site	CD ROM Web site
Design Criteria:	quasi-experimental	randomized controlled trials (rct)	randomized controlled trials (rct)	rcts & quasi-experimental	quasi-experimental

Figure 25–1. U.K. resource centers relating to outcomes measurement and clinical effectiveness

consensus. The guidelines should be widely disseminated to clinicians and clients. In the United States, this process is achieved through three guidelines documents, one detailed document, and two accessible documents for use by clinicians and clients. As yet, the United Kingdom has not adopted this model for disseminating information, but it may well do so in the future.

Resource allocation and decisions about client care must be informed by clinical guidelines as well as by outcomes data, information from reviews, and clinical trials (Mechanic, 1995; Ham, 1995). What is becoming increasingly clear is the need to integrate information in order to avert the potential avalanche of financial and clinical decision making based on incomplete evidence.

WHAT NATIONAL ARE THE IMPLICATIONS OF THESE INITIATIVES FOR SPEECH AND LANGUAGE THERAPISTS?

Speech and language therapists in the United Kingdom, like their medical colleagues, have welcomed the development of these national centers, which provide them with efficient access to information. It is obvious that the value of such centers is, however, largely dependent upon the volume and quality of information provided by clinicians and researchers. Much of the data currently available to speech and language therapists are derived from medical and nursing research. There is no doubt that access to this information informs the debate within speech and language therapy and widens the picture on outcomes measurement, efficacy, and the methodological obstacles shared by many health care researchers. However, there is a dearth of U.K.-based research on outcome measures and treatment efficacy, and at present many of the studies submitted to the centers have originated in the United States, Canada, and Australia.

Speech and language therapy has, up to now, had a relatively low profile among the larger research funding agencies in the United Kingdom. In addition, multidisciplinary research is now more likely to obtain funding from such agencies than ever before. This development is possibly an advantage to the larger professions like nursing and medicine, who have already undertaken a substantial body of unidisciplinary research, but it is in many ways a disadvantage to smaller health care professions like speech and language therapy who need to procure more speech and language therapy-focused research before, or at least in addition to, embarking on research of a multidisciplinary nature. Moreover, speech and language therapists in the United Kingdom have not had the research infrastructure or indeed the public profile required to support many large-scale studies.

The other area of difficulty, shared by all other health care professions, is the increasing emphasis on randomized controlled clinical trials as the "gold standard" (Fahey et al., 1995) in establishing clinical effectiveness. There are two major implications of this gold standard in terms of information exchange, both of which relate to the problem of selectivity. First, valuable data from good quality nonrandomized studies are excluded altogether.

Randomized controlled trials may provide valuable information on whether or not an intervention will reliably produce the desired effect under controlled circumstances. They may not tell the clinician very much about how effective such intervention is when it is used in everyday practice (Epstein, 1990). Data from nonrandomized research studies, which may make use of existing client data, allows the application of statistical techniques such as matching and stratification to compare intervention effects in more routine clinical settings. In the United Kingdom, the advent of sophisticated computerized information systems makes this kind of research more possible.

The other implication is that randomized controlled trials that are never published, often those with unfavorable results, may not be submitted for inclusion in data bases at all. This may occur in trials funded by industry in particular (Godlee, 1994). This "imbalance" is nothing new in the research field, but the fact that the information is now more available than ever to more clinicians and purchasers in an easily accessible, digestible form has considerable implications for its influence on practice and service provision. Critical appraisal of all the available evidence for and against a particular intervention depends upon access to that evidence.

There is another equally important limitation to these centers. They are not by and large "user friendly" to lay people, nor have they taken into account the views of lay people. They do not appear to be promoting public involvement in health care planning and policymaking, and perhaps through their emphasis on national and international perspectives they fail to nurture the importance of local needs and local perspectives on health care delivery (Annette & Rifkin, 1990). A recent government publication (Department of Health, 1996), entitled "Promoting Clinical Effectiveness," emphasized the importance of "patient partnership," including encouraging "ready access to meaningful and easily understood information on clinical effectiveness" (p. 7). As yet, there are few obvious ways in which this strategy is being implemented.

These issues are of particular relevance to the work of the Cochrane Collaboration and the NHS Centre for Reviews and Dissemination. The Outcomes Clearing House is not using the randomized controlled trial as a gold standard for inclusion as the majority of studies of outcomes in health care do not take place within the randomized controlled trial design. However, the influence of this gold standard is considered by many therapists to be restrictive rather than helpful in the search for valid and reliable clinical outcomes.

There is in effect a paradox generated by the growth of interest in outcomes and efficacy research in the United Kingdom. One the one hand, the U.K. government has recognized the need to disseminate information to practitioners on an ongoing basis. This initiative is to be warmly welcomed by clinicians and researchers alike. On the other hand, the criteria for inclusion is limiting the type of information being disseminated, and thereby its impact on working practices. Epstein (1990), in his discussion of the outcomes movement in the United States, cautioned against "carrying a good thing too fast and too far" (p. 269). We would argue that a similar caution applies to the explosion of information centers in the United Kingdom.

DILEMMAS IN SPEECH AND LANGUAGE THERAPY OUTCOMES MEASUREMENT IN THE UNITED KINGDOM

This growth in the importance of outcomes measurement and access to information about outcomes poses certain difficulties for all health care professionals. The political and clinical importance of these measures presupposes not only that satisfactory measures are available, but also that studies implementing those measures are available to provide the necessary evidence. Unfortunately this is not the case; neither are there adequate measures nor is there adequate evidence. In this section we go on to describe briefly some of the issues and difficulties in obtaining such evidence.

As Frattali points out in Chapter One, many of the issues surrounding treatment efficacy are inextricably linked to outcomes measurement. Reviews of the literature both in the United Kingdom and the United States reveal a dearth of treatment efficacy studies in the field of communication disorders. There is a similar lack of valid and reliable outcome measures for assessing efficacy (Frattali, 1986; Olswang, 1990; McReynolds, 1990; Clark & Elliot, 1992).

Issues in Treatment Efficacy Studies

Speech and language therapy services in the United Kingdom have little information on variations in practice across the country. This is an issue for all health care professions, and it has been at the center of the outcomes debate for many years (Epstein, 1990). Variation in medical practice has been well documented in the United States (Wennberg, 1990; Wennberg et al., 1987). In the United Kingdom, staffing ratios can vary enormously from one service to another (e.g., Mackenzie et al., 1993), and recruitment and retention of staff affects patterns of service delivery on all levels. Other influences on variations in practice include undergraduate and post-graduate educational experience, individual preferences, and local management directives. There is a need for more systematic analysis of these variables and their impact on speech and language therapy services.

Few studies have taken into consideration the importance of contextual influences on outcome. The few U.K. treatment efficacy studies which do exist have concentrated on clinic-based evaluations of intervention and have frequently failed to examine the impact of the therapeutic intervention on the clients' everyday life (e.g., Lincoln et al., 1984; David et al., 1982). They have not taken into account the views of carers or indeed the clients themselves in determining the impact of intervention.

To date, there has been a lack of specificity in the therapy being described. Speech and language therapy in the United Kingdom does not have competing alternative therapy techniques for any one specific communication disorder which would lend themselves to critical evaluation. Instead, it typically uses a portfolio of therapeutic techniques integrated into one therapeutic program. For example, clients with an acquired language disorder may require a combination of language therapy, literacy work, and counseling, both for themselves and for their "carers," among other procedures. The therapist, in other words, is delivering a therapeutic package consisting of different types of therapy, which are determined by the needs and wishes of the individual client. It is these "typical packages" of treatment that require evaluation, rather than the various types of treatment which make up the package.

There is, therefore, a need for rigorous and detailed investigation of treatment packages. The majority of such studies carried out in the aphasia field to date (Lincoln et al., 1984; David et al., 1982) have tended to be large group studies and randomized controlled trials, which made little or no investigation of the relationship between the type of language problem and the type of therapy used or indeed the amount of therapy given (Howard, 1986; Pring, 1986). For example, in the Lincoln study, which involved 32 therapists, "no specific type of speech therapy was advocated" (p. 1198). In addition, although it was recommended that clients should receive 48 hours of treatment, 75% of the sample received less than 18 hours of treatment altogether. These studies uncover important methodological problems and shortcomings (for a detailed review of issues in evaluating the efficacy of aphasia therapy, see Wertz, 1995).

Randomized controlled trials continue to represent the "gold standard" in the assessment of health care interventions in the United Kingdom (Fahey et al., 1995). This poses problems for clinicians who find quasi-experimental designs and case studies to be more appropriate methods of enquiry. As Frattali points out in Chapter 1, this frustration is shared by colleagues in the United States. The combination of inductive and deductive methodologies would seem more suitable to the complexities of evaluation in this field.

There is now widespread agreement among therapists in the United Kingdom that current standardized tests are too narrow in that they do not attempt to assess the effect of intervention on the client's communication skills in different settings. The views of communication impaired people and their relatives are rarely taken into account in the measurement of outcome of therapy, as Worrall (1992) has argued that they should be. In addition, existing rating scales tend to be global scales, which cannot provide the detail required to measure subtle changes in communication over time with any degree of accuracy. There is also a problem with their reliability in that global rating scales are frequently open to a large number of interpretations (Clarke & Elliott, 1992). These concerns are reinforcing the belief that the range of methodologies used in outcomes measurement needs to be extended, which we will go on to discuss later.

Issues in Outcomes Measurement

Outcomes measurement is a relatively recent preoccupation in the United Kingdom, as it is in the United States. A review of the literature on outcome measures for the rehabilitative professions in the United Kingdom revealed a paucity of research and very little in the way of guidelines for practitioners on appropriate and reliable measures of outcome (Clarke & Elliott, 1992). These authors recommend that research into outcomes should concentrate on "getting inside" therapy and evaluating the service infrastructure, rather than adopting a "checklist mentality and focus on throughput." We would suggest that "getting inside therapy" will involve developing more appropriate methods of describing the therapy itself, the timing and intensity of therapy, and the precise nature of the therapist's skills.

Data collection in the United Kingdom has focused on measures such as admissions, discharges, and waiting times, the number of times a client has been in contact with a service, and so on. Outcomes measurement has therefore been limited to information on the pattern of admissions and discharges, with little or no systematic collection of information on the pattern of recovery or even the amount of intervention a client with a particular condition might receive.

Newly developed information systems do provide rudimentary outcomes data. Speech and Language Audit Software (Reid & Linsey, 1993), for example, stores information on individual treatment goals and client and carer satisfaction measures. However, these satisfaction measures do not go far enough in involving consumers in service evaluation.

Increasing demand for speech and language therapy and diversification of roles has meant that therapists are working with many different disciplines, crossing the boundaries of health, education, and social service agencies. Like their colleagues in the United States, therapists need to manage their information differently for different agencies, and must tune themselves to local working practices and philosophy accordingly.

The other major issue for those involved in outcomes measurement is that of attribution. Changes in communication skills are determined by multiple causal factors, such as motivation, age, severity of the condition, level of support, personality, and associated skills such as literacy. It is therefore extremely difficult to isolate the contribution of the intervention itself. In addition, changes in speech and language therapy staffing levels, the amount and type of intervention delivered to clients by different therapists, and variations in support systems such as clerical, technical, and other multidisciplinary services need to be taken into account in any evaluation of the impact of therapy. These influences are increasingly difficult to measure in a health care service characterized by constant change. The importance of interdisciplinary collaboration in establishing the range of causal factors cannot be overstated.

QUALITATIVE METHODS: AN ADDITIONAL ROUTE TO OUTCOMES MEASUREMENT?

There is then a growing awareness that the means of investigating the client's perspective needs to move beyond the conventional procedures used by health care professionals. Worrall (1993) suggests that the disabling aspects and functional implications of a communication disorder such as aphasia can only be properly assessed through some form of consultation between "patient" and professional. This line of thinking opens the door for more *qualitative* studies of communication disorders. The goal of qualitative research is "the development of concepts which help us to understand social phenomena in natural (rather than experimental) settings, giving due emphasis to the meanings, experiences and views of all the participants" (p. 43) (Pope & Mays, 1995). It investigates the social world, and perspectives on that world, in terms of the concepts, perceptions, and accounts of the people it is about, a departure and contrast from the process of testing out constructs developed by professional experts.

Qualitative data can be gathered in a number of ways. These include interview, observation, analysis of documents, and focus group discussion. The data can also be analysed in a variety of ways. For example, it may yield a *narrative* account, that is, one which conveys the sense of the individual's progress (or "career") through the changing phases of a chronic illness (Phillips, 1990). In contrast, *categorized* data is coded by theme or category to create a conceptual analysis of the social situation. One of the strengths of qualitative investigation is the way in which it can be designed to achieve crisply conceptual analysis while retaining a sense of the individual account (Conrad, 1990).

Qualitative research also offers the opportunity to examine the distinction between *insider* and *outsider* knowledge of a condition, that is the understanding of the ill or disabled person compared with that of the professional offering medical or social intervention. The full understanding of the insider perspective is a complex and delicate pursuit. It can be approached through questioning which addresses peoples' views of symptoms, conceptualizations of the condition, explanations and theories of the cause and nature of the problem, what they expect and achieve from medical intervention, their health beliefs, strategies for coping, and their integration of the illness and its management into their everyday lives and relationships (Conrad, 1990). The focus on interviews could be seen to exclude the communication disordered population from contributing, but recent research suggests that the experience and opinions of people even with severe expressive forms of communication difficulty can be probed qualitatively (Parr, Byng, & Gilpin, 1997).

Clearly, this kind of investigation, the pursuit of insider knowledge, is directly relevant to issues of efficacy and outcome. As yet, these implications remain largely unexplored. Indeed, it is acknowledged that the pure science orientation of much medical and rehabilitation research has meant that qualitative investigation is regarded with some suspicion. In a recent account of approaches to the analysis of qualitative data, Bryman and Burgess (1994) point out that the roots of medical unease lie in the vague and inexplicit accounts of the research process which characterize traditional ethnographic studies.

However, major developments in qualitative methodology have taken place in the last decade. These range from the development of software systems, which undertake categorized data analysis, to the consolidation of explicit, specific (and therefore replicable), and highly focused research procedures. Explicit methodology is crucial in demonstrating the potential rigor of qualitative research. Replicability of the study is ensured if the raw data is retained and the methods of analysis and interpretation detailed. Triangulated studies can ensure validity of data analysis. In essence, this process involves approaching a research issue from a number of different viewpoints and through a number of different studies. Again, explicit and rigorous methodology is both appropriate and essential (West, 1990).

Alongside this newfound explicitness concerning methodology, there is at present a concern to articulate the relative contributions of qualitative and other approaches in research, which has been addressed by a number of writers (Mason, 1994; Marshall & Rossman, 1989; Pope & Mays, 1995). Qualitative research may be used as a precursor to, alongside, and after, quantitative research. As a precursor, it can be used to develop hypotheses, explore and elaborate concepts, and define terminologies. Alongside quantitative research, it can explain, illuminate, qualify, or illustrate aspects of the findings. Used after quantitative research, it can follow up subgroups of interest, explore unexplained relationships, and illuminate decision processes. It can also be used to generate ideas, theories, and strategies and as a way of testing hypotheses against case histories.

An integrated use of qualitative and quantitative research may consolidate generalization of findings: the theories and issues emerging in a small-scale study may form the basis of large-scale studies. However, findings from small-scale qualitative studies may be generalizable if they are drawn from a soundly-selected sample. Purposive sampling involves designing the sample to include a full range of relevant experience, rather than trying to find homogeneous groups.

Qualitative investigations can therefore meet conventional demands for validity and replicability through specified methodology and focused discussion. However, it can be argued that the paradigms of pure science are inappropriate in the domains of applied science, and that these constructs need to be replaced with equally specific and rigorous demands, say for *credibility, transferability, dependability,* and *confirmability* (Lincoln & Guba, 1985). The potential of qualitative research has been recognized by many commissioning bodies, including those in the health and social services. Qualitative studies, properly designed and rigorously implemented, have effected changes in policy and practice within many professions (e.g, Finch, 1988). Qualitative methods can no longer be considered the "soft," easy option in treatment efficacy studies.

Qualitative methods are currently being used predominantly in research, but also have the potential to be incorporated into clinical procedures such as audit and outcomes assessment. The time required for both the interview and its transcription, analysis, and interpretation, might be thought to be prohibitive, but as Long (1994) points out, "In-depth qualitative interviews have a higher unit cost per interview, but even a very small sample may provide a wide range of information and highlight key problems more effectively than a similarly priced large-sample survey" (p. 178).

The use of qualitative methods in both efficacy and outcomes studies has clear potential, but as yet, few exemplars. There is a sense in which the development of outcomes measurement in the United Kingdom is following a twin track approach: one which is responding to the immediate demands on services, and the other which is responding to the call for more research and ultimately more carefully crafted measurements. The pressure felt by practitioners to have available the required data is often in conflict with the desire to be using more appropriate measures. The necessity for urgent research and development action in this arena is underlined.

British speech and language therapists, like their colleagues in the United States, are striving for a range of outcome measures which accurately reflect their practice. There is widespread agreement on the need for a multidimensional approach to measurement. Kane (1987) suggests that what is needed is "the clinical equivalent of a Swiss army knife, something small and easily taken into the field, with enough blades and attachments to fit any number of circumstances that may arise" (p. 99).

In the next section we describe some of the current initiatives being taken in the development of outcomes measurement in speech and language therapy in the United Kingdom, although, generally, even these developments do not address the dilemmas previously discussed. In turn, consideration of these initiatives highlights a further area for attention in outcomes measurement, which we go on to consider.

SPEECH AND LANGUAGE THERAPY INITIATIVES IN OUTCOMES MEASUREMENT

The Role of the Royal College of Speech and Language Therapists

The Royal College of Speech and Language Therapists (RCSLT), the U.K. professional organization, has been actively involved in disseminating information on outcomes measurement through its various publications. "Communicating Quality: Professional Standards for Speech and Language Therapists" (CSLT, 1991; RCSLT, 1996) recommends the use of a combination of consumer outcome measures (for example, consumer satisfaction surveys, consumer forums) and clinical outcome measures (measures completed by therapists). The College has produced a series of consumer satisfaction questionnaires, each one tailored to the concerns of a particular client group. These questionnaires are used widely in the United Kingdom to provide client and carer feedback to therapists and their employers.

The need to record the views of clients is reinforced by Long (1994) who defines an outcome of health and social care as "more than an end-point; it involves a valuation of that end-point, and in particular a benefit to the patient/consumer. In measuring outcomes, it is thus necessary to take account of the multiple perspectives of health and social outcome; this must be reflected in the measures used" (p. 165). This perception is increasingly a focus of attention by health care providers, and the means of measuring or assessing that perception is generally through the implementation of questionnaires and surveys. However, these, in their own turn, have limitations, as Kleinman (1988) vividly (if wordily) explains:

> Symptom scales and survey questionnaires and behavioural checklists quantify functional impairment and disability, rendering quality of life fungible. Yet about suffering they are silent. The thinned-out image of patients and families that perforce must emerge from such research is scientifically replicable but ontologically invalid; it has statistical, not epistemological, significance; it is a dangerous distortion. [p. 28]

This concern about the oversimplification of complex and changing experience has led to questions about the meaning and validity of data gathered through surveys, checklists, and so on, which have often been constructed from a professional perspective and rarely generated predominantly by service user groups. Qualitative interviews may well prove a more satisfactory alternative.

The RCSLT Audit Manual (RCSLT, 1993) suggests that the choice of clinical outcome measure must be determined by the type of condition and the nature of the intervention. Acknowledging that outcomes measurement is still in its infancy, the Manual advocates the use of a combination of clinical outcomes which can assess the direction of the client's progress over a period of time. These include standardized and nonstandardized communication assessments, individual goal setting techniques, rating scales, and checklists of communication behavior. This is seen as an interim solution rather than an wholly adequate answer to the problem of outcomes assessment.

This interim solution was generated as a result of a pilot investigation of audit procedures for speech and language therapists (van der Gaag, Glass & Reid, 1993). This study looked at a range of process and outcome measures used by therapists in different parts of the United Kingdom. Therapists were asked to select the clinical communication assessments most suited to their clients' condition and intervention. Initial and final scores on these assessments for the duration of the study were recorded. At the end of the study period, the percentage of clients who showed positive, negative, or no change in score was calculated, giving a global outcome statistic on the direction of change over time.

A number of difficulties emerged. The first was the large number of assessments used—23 adult communication assessments and 24 child assessments in total. The second was the variability in clinical diagnosis, which presumably accounted for the large number of assessments used. This limited the extent of cross comparison that could be made. Third, some clients were assessed on several different outcome measures, and showed improvement on one measure and deterioration on another. For example, clients with motor neurone disease showed a deterioration on the Dysphagia rating scale, but improvement on a rating scale measuring the use of a communication aid. A negative outcome on one scale did not necessarily mean that intervention had been unsuccessful.

Despite these difficulties, speech and language therapists in the United Kingdom are continuing to apply the technique as an interim measure. It satisfies their employers in that it provides a crude indication of the direction of change over time. It satisfies to some extent therapists' desire to use whatever measure is clinically appropriate, and translate a complex clinical picture into a simple clinical outcome.

The Enderby Outcomes Scale

The Enderby Outcomes Scale attempts this translation of a complex clinical picture into a simple clinical outcome (Enderby, 1992). This scale uses a series of 5-point rating scales, which are based on the WHO definitions of "Impairment, Disability, Handicap," with the additional category of "Well-being." Therapists define the impact of each of these on a severity rating scale. In addition, there is a rating scale for the overall outcome of therapy, which measures the degree of change in the client. Where possible, the client/carer are involved in rating progress during the intervention period.

Clinical Guidelines for the Management of Speech and Language Impairments (Department of Health, 1994; RCSLT 1997)

This publication complements "Communicating Quality: Professional Standards for Speech and Language Therapists" (RCSLT, 1991, 1996). It provides existing research evidence of effectiveness as well as professional consensus on what constitutes good practice in specific clinical areas. These clinical guidelines are to be used in conjunction with data from outcomes research and systematic reviews. They will require regular updating as new evidence comes to light and new technology changes practice.

Software Initiatives

Computerized information systems have only recently begun to have an impact on speech and language therapy services in the United Kingdom. There is an increasing recognition that such systems can provide therapists and their employers with a range of clinical and financial information not previously recorded on a routine basis. As health budgets become devolved to general practitioners and the shift from hospital to community-based care becomes more evident in the United Kingdom, therapists require information on costs and clinical outcomes for a variety of agencies purchasing their services. The implementation of managed care and the approach of explicit rationing makes such data collection essential to survival.

There is an increasing number of generic health care information systems in use in the United Kingdom. In some areas therapists are being asked to implement such systems with little or no consultation as to their relevance to speech and language therapy. Inevitably, this has led to difficulties in managing data and obtaining useful information.

The most acceptable and indeed successful information systems are those which have been customized for speech and language therapy services. Speech and Language Audit Software (SiLAS; Reid, Linsey, & van der Gaag, 1993) is the most recent and the most comprehensive such system now in widespread use in the United Kingdom. It is a client-based system, which follows the logical progression of a client from referral to assessment, identifying needs, setting intervention goals, and recording outcomes.

SiLAS allows therapists to record treatment goals for each client contact, and record to what extent goals have been met. The system can then generate reports showing to what extent goals have been met over a particular time period by diagnosis, age, time since onset, and so on. In addition to these treatment goals, SiLAS incorporates consumer questionnaires developed by the RCSLT Audit Research Team, which record client and care perceptions of and satisfaction with the service being received. Client and therapist data on outcome can then be correlated.

Systems like SiLAS are user-friendly, flexible, and are designed to give users maximum opportunity to manipulate data to suit their local requirements. By giving therapists control over their own data, and in particular the ability to generate their own customized reports, these systems encourage a culture of careful data collection, which previous generations of information technology have not. This has important implications for the future of outcomes measurement, as it adds to the baseline of accurate data on prevalence, mean length of intervention, and so on, from which further research can be launched. It also paves the way towards identifying variations in outcome in different geographical areas and differences in procedures or interventions that may be associated with differences in outcome.

However, such systems do not go far enough in examining variability between individuals with the same impairment, or outcome in terms of functional status (Fitzpatrick, 1994). This may well be possible from a technological point of view, but it cannot be achieved until researchers turn their attention to ways of understanding and measuring the "illness experience" (Fitzpatrick, 1994) and describing the recovery process from the client's perspective. In other words, conventional descriptive epidemiological data collection, while vital to our understanding of the value of speech and language therapy, cannot go far enough. It is becoming increasingly clear that qualitative studies offer ways of addressing effectiveness of service which are not mechanistic and reductionist but which acknowledge and encompass the diversity of patient experience and understanding. In the next section we describe some changes to the definition of disability being proposed by disability activists in the United Kingdom, which have fundamental implications both for how the role of the speech and language therapist is construed and, therefore, for the nature and content of outcome measures.

WHAT NEXT? BEYOND CLIENT SATISFACTION QUESTIONNAIRES AND STANDARDIZED ASSESSMENTS: A NEW FRAMEWORK FOR OUTCOMES MEASUREMENT

The increasing use of qualitative methods, especially in research into chronic impairment and disability (with which speech and language therapists are much concerned), has revealed how much the difficulties encountered by people with disabilities arise not so much as a result of the impairment, but also from barriers and limitations constructed by society. This has led to a redefinition by activists within the disability movement in the United Kingdom of the familiar World Health Organization (WHO) (1980) definitions of impairment, disability, and handicap. These represent a construction of disability familiar to members of medical and rehabilitation professions and within speech and language therapy. These WHO definitions are being used as the basis for classification of communication disorders (Raaijmakers & Dekker, 1993) and are forming the framework for the development of outcome measures (Enderby, 1992).

The WHO definitions represent the medical model of disability. They are developed by professional and expert "outsiders," not by people with impairments. They focus on the *inabilities* of the impaired individual, and on the assumed goal of cure or improvement, while the disability is seen to stem directly from the impairment, and is itself the focus for treatment or cure. *Disability* is therefore defined as "any restriction or lack (resulting from impairment) of ability to perform an activity in the manner or within the range considered normal for a human being." *Handicap* is defined as "the disadvantage for a given individual resulting from the impairment or disability, that limits or prevents fulfillment of a role that is normal (depending on age, sex, social and cultural factors) for that individual."

A more radical definition of disability (and one which is challenging to professional groups concerned with rehabilitation) has been developed by members of the disability movement in the United Kingdom. Thus, Finkelstein and French (1993) collapse the notions associated with disability and handicap into one concept. According to their definition, disability arises not from the impaired individual's inability to perform normal activities, but from the barriers and restrictions imposed by society upon the impaired person. Disability therefore becomes "the loss or limitation of opportunities that prevents people who have impairments from taking part in the normal life of the community on an equal level with others due to physical and social barriers" (p. 28). Defined in this way, disability becomes something which can be mitigated, not by treatment or cure, but by recognition and removal of the barriers. The barriers may not always be external, in that they may take the form of prejudice and oppressive notions of disability which are internalized by the disabled person. Thus, in discussing the effects of acquired hearing loss, Woolley (1993) writes:

> While still a hearing person, the deafened person learned to have able-bodied attitudes towards disability which deaf and disabled movements now identify as key disabling factors in their oppression. But the newly deafened person continues to function from these oppressive attitudes and sees them daily reinforced by society now that she also has a disability. . . . The fundamental experience of loss and tragedy remains and the deafened person still struggles with despair, powerlessness, loss of self-confidence and positive self-image. The deafened person blames her deafness and hates being deaf, with self-contempt, therefore, lurking at the periphery of her consciousness. [p. 78]

The disability movement in the United Kingdom and beyond, therefore, is centrally concerned with the identification and removal of internal and external *barriers* and with the concurrent development of the positive *disabled identity*. Barriers for people with communication impairments specifically have begun to be identified (LeDorze & Brassard, 1995; Parr, Byng & Gilpin, 1997), although the limitations of the contribution of barriers alone to the disability experienced by communication disabled people, is also under investigation. These two concepts—barriers and disabled identity—are understood to be fundamental to the metamorphosis of disability from a negative to a positive state, a process which is seen to be remote from medical concepts of cure and treatment.

This perspective on impairment and disability has implications for outcomes measurement. Fitzpatrick (1994), reviewing health needs assessment in chronic disability concludes that "It is possible to focus too exclusively on the health status or quality-of-life deficits of the individual with chronic illness, thereby ignoring the impact that the social context has in shaping and determining handicaps" (p. 195). The new emphasis on outcomes measurement has "reinforced the tendency to look at ways in which the individual has health-related problems requiring personal adjustment and thereby to ignore changes in the broader context which may more readily improve quality of life" (p. 196) (Fitzpatrick, 1994).

All of these developments suggest that we are in the transitional phase of a change of culture. This change of culture is characterized by three elements: (1) the emergence of new qualitative methodologies for measurement, to ensure that "the data collected and the interpretations made are both useful and meaningful" (Frattali, this volume), (2) a new focus on developing interventions that include the person with the communication disability as a collaborative partner in the planning and execution of the therapy (French, 1994), and (3) the ongoing analysis of the components of packages of intervention provided by speech and language therapists to make more explicit what we are doing and what motivates our actions (Byng, 1995).

This culture change means that the role of the speech and language therapist needs to be confirmed and clarified, so that we can maintain some perspective on what we do and why. The goals of our intervention may change or take on a different character, and this has implications for how we evaluate outcome: "Outcome measures must relate directly to the expected changes as a consequence of an intervention. Thus, outcome of contact has to be related to stated goals, which have generally not been formulated with the precision necessary to permit evaluation. Often outcome measures have related to only one aspect of care, leading to false impressions of treatment and lack of credibility in the eyes of clinicians" (p. 61) (Enderby, 1992). It is therefore critical that we make explicit the range and extent of our role, encompassing the different components of intervention that we offer, since if our role is changing then so will our goals. It is imperative that the different components of the "package of intervention" provided by speech and language therapists are included in any framework for developing outcome measures.

Components of the Package of Intervention
Offered by the Speech and Language Therapist

The following list of components describes the full scope of the intervention by speech and language therapists, of which all the components can be measured to some extent:

- Assess the uses of language and communication required by the communication impaired person;
- Assess the nature and effects of the communication impairment with respect to the whole language and communication system;
- Facilitate coping with communication impairments or adjustment to changes in communication skills, for both the communication impaired person and his or her family, friends, and carers;
- Address therapy to the actual communication impairment;
- Increase the use of all other potential means of communication to support, facilitate, and compensate for the impaired aspect of communication;
- Enhance the use of the remaining or existing communication skills;

- Provide opportunities to use newly acquired and emerging communication skills, not just in a clinical environment, but in more familiar communicative situations;

- Facilitate changes to the communication skills and awareness of those around the person with a communication impairment and in society at large to address the external barriers to communication.

(Adapted from Byng, 1993).

These components of the package of care are different in scope, with different goals and effects. They therefore require very different forms of evaluation. The type of outcome measure that would be used to establish the effects of attempting to change the communication skills of, for example, colleagues of a dysfluent person in the workplace would be very different from the kind of outcome measure required to establish how well the dysfluent person was coping with his or her dysfluency or was able to modify speech. Yet each of these areas could legitimately be the focus of the speech and language therapist's intervention.

CONCLUSION

Outcome measures not only need to be relevant to the goal of the intervention, but different types of outcome measure need to be available for different audiences. The third-party payer (or purchaser in U.K. terminology) will not need a detailed breakdown of the impact of different intervention programs or packages on specific aspects of communication or life skills. Rather, a more global measure providing a simple statistic or guide to the broad scope of change would probably be more useful. A therapist, on the other hand, needs much more detailed information about impact and outcome of specific procedures/interventions on specific areas of need/function. A client might require a different kind of knowledge about the impact of intervention, whereas a carer or parent will again want different information.

Measuring outcomes is not just a matter of data collection (Long, 1994). It requires careful consideration of why outcomes are to be assessed, the type of interventions for which outcome is to be evaluated, and for whom. This will in turn require a careful search for appropriate measures and study designs to do so, so that outcome can be attributed to the intervention. St. Leger, Schnieden, and Walsworth-Bell (1992) sound an important additional cautionary note: "An ideological stance is implicit in every attempt to evaluate health services and distribute health care resources. Investigators of service effectiveness should try to make plain the ideological assumptions which lead to the perception of need for a particular study and which inevitably will influence the choice of study aims and objectives" (p. 16).

This culture change needs to be reflected in the education of speech and language therapists. Educational establishments need to equip students with the necessary knowledge and skills to undertake both quantitative and qualitative studies. Experienced practitioners may also need to review their skills and expand their knowledge base to accommodate new methodologies, to make explicit the components of their practice, and to emphasize a client-centered, power-sharing, enabling approach to working with people with disabilities (Pound, 1996).

Schein (1996) suggests that "Culture is not a suit of clothes to be changed at will" (p. 39). If culture change occurs, it does so as a by-product of fixing the fundamental problems identified and the new strategies which emerge. The challenge for speech and language pathology is to ensure that, within the emerging culture, we can continue to provide interventions and services which are both relevant and accessible to clients, and which result in meaningful outcomes.

REFERENCES

Agency for Health Care Policy and Research (1992). U.S. Department of Health and Human Services. Agency for Health Care Policy and Research Publications. Rockville, M.D. ACHPR Publication 92/0038.

Annett, H., & Rifkin, S. (1990). *Improving Urban Health.* Geneva: WHO.

Bryman, A., & Burgess, R. (Eds.) (1994). *Analysing qualitative data.* London: Routledge.

Byng, S. (1993). Hypothesis testing and aphasia therapy. In A. Holland and M. Forbes (Eds.), *World Perspectives on Aphasia.* Singular Publishing Group Inc.

Byng, S. (1995). What is aphasia therapy? In C. Code & D. Muller (Eds.), *The Treatment of Aphasia: From Theory to Practice.* London: Whurr Publishers.

Clark, N., & Elliott, S. (1992). *Clinical Audit in the Nursing and Therapy Professions.* Maidstone Priority Care Group: Maidstone Hospital.

Cochrane, A. (1979). 1931–71; A critical review, with particular reference to the medical profession. In Teeling Smith, G. (Ed.), *Medicine for the Year 2000.* London: Office of Health Economics.

Conrad, P. (1990). Qualitative research on chronic illness: a commentary on method and conceptual development. *Social Science of Medicine, 30*(11), 1257–1263.

College of Speech and Language Therapists (1991). *Communicating Quality: Professional Standards for Speech and Language Therapists.* London: CSLT.

David, R., Enderby, P., & Bainton, D. (1982). Treatment of acquired aphasia: speech therapists and volunteers compared. *Journal of Neurology Neurosurgery and Psychiatry, 45,* 957–961.

Department of Health (1993). *Research for Health.* Department of Health.

Department of Health (1994). *Improving the effectiveness of the NHS: Clinical Guidelines.* Department of Health EL (94):74.

Department of Health (1995). *Report of the NHS Health Technology Assessment Programme.* Department of Health.

Department of Health (1996). *Promoting Clinical Effectiveness: A Framework for action in and through the NHS.* London: HMSO.

Enderby, P. (1992). Outcome measures in speech therapy: impairment, disability, handicap and distress. *Health Trends, 24*(2), 62–64.

Epstein, A. (1990). The outcomes movement: will it get us where we want to go? *New England Journal of Medicine, 323*(4), 266–269.

Fahey, T., Griffiths, S., & Peters, T. (1995). Evidence based purchasing: understanding results of clinical trails and systematic reviews. *British Medical Journal, 311,* 1056–1060.

Finch, H. (1988). *Barriers to the receipt of dental care.* Social Community Planning and Research, London.

Finkelstein, V., & French, S. (1993). Towards a psychology of disability. In: J. Swain, V. Finkelstein, S. French, & M. Oliver (Eds.), *Disabling barriers-enabling environments.* London: OU Publications and Sage.

Fitzpatrick, R. (1994). Health needs assessment, chronic illness and the social sciences. In J. Popay and G. Williams (Eds), *Researching the People's Health.* London & New York: Routledge.

Frattali, C. (1986). Are we reaching our goals? Developing outcome measures. In Larkins, P. (Ed.), *In Search of Quality Assurance: What Lies Ahead?* Rockville, MD: ASHA.

French, S. (1994). *On Equal Terms: Working with disabled people.* Butterworth: Heinemann.

Godlee, F. (1994). The Cochrane Collaboration. *British Medical Journal, 309,* 969–970.

Ham, C. (1995). Health care rationing *British Medical Journal, 310,* 1483–1484.

Hayward, J. (1996). Promoting clinical effectiveness. *British Medical Journal, 312,* 1491–1492.

Health of the Nation (1991). *A Consultative Document fo Health in England.* London: HMSO.

Howard, D. (1986). Beyond randomised controlled trials; the case for effective case studies of the effects of treatment in aphasia. *British Journal of Disorders of Communication 21,* 89–102.

Kane, R.L. (1987). Commentary: functional assessment questionnaire for geriatric patient—or the clinical Swiss army knife. *Medical Care Supplement,* S95–99.

Kleinman, A. (1988). *The Illness Narratives: Suffering, Healing and the Human Condition.* Basic Books.

Le Dorze, G., & Brassard C., (1995). A description of the consequences and significance of aphasia on aphasic persons and their relatives and friends, based on the WHO model of chronic diseases. *Aphasiology, 9*(3), 239–255.

Lincoln, N., McGuirk, E., Mulley, G., Jones, A., & Mitchell, J. (1984). Effectiveness of speech therapy fro aphasic stroke patients. A randomised controlled trial. *Lancet,* 1197–2000.

Long, A. (1994). Assessing health and social outcomes. In J. Popay and G. Williams (Eds.), *Researching the People's Health.* London & New York: Routledge.

Lincoln, Y., & Guba, E. (1985). *Naturalistic inquiry.* Beverly Hills: Sage.

Mackenzie, C., Le May, M., Lendrem, W., et al., (1993). A survey of aphasia services in the UK. *European Journal of Disorders of Communication, 28*(1), 43–61.

Marshall, C., & Rossman, G. (1989). *Designing qualitative research.* London: Sage.

Mason, J. (1994). Linking qualitative and quantitative data analysis. In A. Bryman and R. Burgess (Eds.), *Analysing qualitative data.* London: Routledge.

Mechanic, D. (1995). Dilemmas in rationing health care services; the case for implicit rationing. *British Medical Journal, 310,* 1655–1659.

McReynolds, L. (1990). Historical perspectives on treatment efficacy research. In Olswang, L., Thompson, C., Warren, S., & Minghetti, N., Eds. (1990), *Treatment Efficacy Research in Communication Disorders.* Rockville, MD: ASHA.

Newman, T. (1995). Is there convergence between Britain and the U.S. in the organisation of health services? *British Medical Journal, 310,* 1652–1655.

Oakley, K. (1996). What do we know about knowledge? *Demos, 6,* 15–17.

Olswang, L (1990, January). Treatment efficacy research; a path to quality assurance. *ASHA,* 45–47.

Parr, S., Byng, S., & Gilpin, S (1997). *Talking back: The experience of living with aphasia after stroke.* Milton Keynes: Open University Press.

Phillips, M. (1990). Damaged goods: oral narratives of the experience of disability in American culture. *Social Science of Medicine, 30*(8), 849–857.

Pope, C., & Mays, N. (1995). Reaching the parts other methods cannot reach: an introduction to qualitative methods in health and health services research. *British Medical Journal, 311,* 42–45.

Pound, C. (1996). *Bulletin of the Royal College of Speech and Language Therapists,* 532.

Pring, T. (1986). Evaluating the effects of speech therapy for aphasics; developing the single case methodology. *British Journal of Disorders of Communication, 21,* 103–115.

Raaijmakers, M., & Dekker, J. (1993). *Toepassing van de ICIDH in de logopedie.* NIVEL/NVLF, Gouda, Utrecht.

Reid, D., Linsey, M., & van der Gaag, A. (1993). *Speech and Language Audit Software* (SiLAS). Glasgow: Mosaic.

Royal College of Speech and Language Therapists (1993). RCSLT: London. *Audit: A Manual for Speech and Language Therapists.*

Royal College of Speech and Language Therapists (1996). *Communicating Quality: Professional Standards for Speech and Language Therapists* (2nd ed.). London: RCSLT.

Schein, E. (1996). Culture matters. *Demos, 8,* 38–39.

St. Leger, A.S., Schieden, H., & Walsworth-Bell, J.P. (1992). *Evaluating Health Services' Effectiveness.* Milton Keynes Open University Press.

Tyrrell, B. (1996). The shapers of things to come: the history of planning *Demos, 8,* 5–7.

UK Clearing House on Health Outcomes (1993). Activities of the Clearing House. *Outcomes Briefing Issue 1,* p. 3–8.

van der Gaag, A, Glass, K., & Reid, D. (1993). A Pilot investigation into Clinical Audit Procedures for Speech and Language Therapists. Report to the Department of Health.

West, P. (1990). The status and validity of accounts obtained at interview: a contrast between two families with a disabled child. *Social Science of Medicine, 30*(11), 1229–1239.

Wennberg, J.E., Freeman, J.L., & Culp, W.J. (1987). Are hospital services rationed in New Haven or over utilised in Boston? *Lancet, 1,* 1185–1189.

Wennberg, J.E. (1990). Better policy to promote the evaluative clinical sciences. *Quality Assurance in Health Care, 2*(1), 21–29.

Wertz, R.T. (1995). Efficacy. In C. Code & D. Muller (Eds.), *Treatment of Aphasia: From Theory to Practice.* London: Whurr Publishers Ltd.

Woolley, M. (1993). Acquired hearing loss: acquired oppression. In J. Swain, V. Finkelstein, S. French, & M. Oliver (Eds.), *Disabling barriers-enabling environments.* London: OU Publications and Sage.

Worrall, L. (1992). Functional communication assessment: an Australian perspective. *Aphasiology, 6*(1), 105–111.

World Health Organization (1980). *International classification of impairments, disabilities and handicaps.* Geneva: Author.

Index

References to figures are *italicized*. References to tables are followed by a *t*.

Accrediting agencies
  listing of, 50
    American Speech-Language-Hearing Association, 50
    Council on Healthcare Provider Accreditation, 50
    Joint Commission on Accreditation of Healthcare Organizations, 50
    Rehabilitation Accreditation Commission, 50
  requirements, 29–41
    American Speech-Language-Hearing Association, professional services board, 37–39
    Joint Commission on Accreditation of Healthcare Organizations, 37–39, 39–41
      agency, description of, 37, 39
      care of patients, 40–41
      implementation, 38–39
      patient function, assessment of, 39–40
      standard 3.0 quality improvement, program evaluation, 37–38
    Rehabilitation Accreditation Commission, 29–37, 30–37
      accreditation criteria, 30–32
      accreditation principle, 30
      agency, description of, 29–30
      information analysis, utilization, 34–35
      outcomes measurement, promotion of, 32
      program evaluation principle, 32–33
      program quality, 36–37
      quality of services, 33–34
Acute inpatient rehabilitation outcomes, 463
Administrators, automated outcomes management systems for, 191
African-American perspective, of impairment, 230–231
Agency for Health Care Policy and Research, 528–530, 556
AHCPR. *See* Agency for Health Care Policy and Research
ALS. *See* Amyotrophic lateral sclerosis
American Speech-Language-Hearing Association, 532–533, 556
  aphasia assessment, 256–257, 258t

Functional Assessment of Communication Skills for Adults, 74
national treatment outcomes initiatives, 537–543, 541–542t
Professional Services Board, 37–39
  outcomes measurement requirements, description of, 37–39
  agency, description, 37
  implementation, 38–39
  standard 3.0 quality improvement, program evaluation, 37–38
Amsterdam-Nijmegan Everyday Language Test, 73
  aphasia assessment and, 259
Amyotrophic lateral sclerosis, motor speech disorder with, 337
ANCC. *See* Assessment of Needs for Continuing Care
ANELT. *See* Amsterdam Nijmegan Everyday Language Test
Aphasia, 245–266
  American Speech-Language-Hearing Association, assessment, 256–257, 258t
  Amsterdam-Nijmegan Everyday Language Test, 259
  communication
    direct assessment, 257–259
    effectiveness index, 255t, 255–257
    measures, 253–254
      rating scales, 254–255
      profile, 254–255, 256
  daily living, communicative abilities in, 257
  level of outcomes measurement, 248–252, 249t, 251t
  psychosocial outcome, well-being measures, 259–260
  quality-of-life issues, 260–261
    depression scales, 260
    health-related quality-of-life measures, 260–261
    psychosocial outcome measures, 260
    well-being, measures of, 261
  rehabilitation measures, 251t, 252–253
  research, 248
  value change, in therapy, *57*
ASHA. *See* American Speech-Language-Hearing Association

Asian/Pacific Islander perspective, of impairment, 231–233
Assessment of Needs for Continuing Care, 69
Automated outcomes management system design, 186–208
  for administrators, 191
  case example, 199–205
  for clients, 191
  for clinicians, 191
  design team, 192–193
    purpose, composition, 192–193
  features of system, 193–199
    commercially available systems, 197–199, 200–201t
    diagnostic categories, 195
    hardware, 197
    percent improvement by diagnostic category, 196
    report generation features, 189t, 194–196, 195–196
    software, 196–197
  framework, 187–192, 189t
  for general public, 191
  for managed care organizations, 191
  report format, 192
  for researchers, 192
  stakeholders, identifying, 190–192
  uses of system, 189–190

Behavioral cognitive outcome measures, in stuttering, shift from, 394–395
Benchmarking, financial outcome data, 119–120
Brain injury
  right-hemisphere, 281–292
    clinical research, 283t, 288–291, 289–290t
    outcome measurement, 282–288, 283–287t
      needs, 291–292
    traumatic, 268–281
      clinical research, 274–281
        disability, 277–279
        handicap, 279–281
        impairment, 274–277
          attention, 276–277
          memory, 276–277
        outcomes measurement needs, 2812
      disabilities, 269–273
      handicaps, 273–274
    motor speech disorder with, 345
    outcome measures, 268–269
      impairment, 268–269, 270–271t

CADL. See Communicative Abilities in Daily Living; Communicative abilities in daily living
California initiative, outcomes measurement, 519–520
CARF. See Rehabilitation Accreditation Commission
Cause-and-effect diagrams, 180–181
Center for General Health Services Extramural Research, 556
Center for Medical Effectiveness Research, 556

Center for Research Dissemination and Liaison, 556
Cerebral palsy, motor speech disorder with, 345
CETI. See Communicative Effectiveness Index
Charges, vs. cost, in financial outcome data, 115–116
Child language disorders, 406–437, 407
CHPA. See Council on Healthcare Provider Accreditation
Class I methods, outcomes measurement, 19–20
Class II methods, outcomes measurement, 20–22
Class III methods, outcomes measurement, 22
Classification of outcomes
  Nagi classification, 13, 14
    active pathology, 13
    disability, 13, 14
    functional limitation, 13
    impairment, 13
  Wilson, Cleary conceptual model, 13–16, 15
    biological variables, 14
    functional status, 15
    general health perceptions, 15
    overall quality of life, 15–16
    physiological variables, 14
    symptom status, 15
  World Health Organization classification, 11–13, 12
    disability, 12
    handicap, 11–13, 12
    impairment, 12
Clearing House on Health Outcomes, United Kingdom, 560
Cleary, P.D., 15
Clinicians, automated outcomes management systems for, 191
Cochrane Centre, United Kingdom, 560
Codman, Ernest A., 2–3
Cognitive communication disorders, 267–320
  dementia, 292–305
    clinical research, 299–303
      disabilities, 301–303
      handicaps, 303
      impairments, 300–301
    outcome measures, 294–299
      disabilities, 296–298
      handicaps, 298–299
      impairments, 294–296
  right-hemisphere brain damage, 281–292
    clinical research, 283t, 288–291, 289–290t
    outcome measures, 282–288, 283–287t
  traumatic brain injury, 268–281
    clinical research, 274–281
      disability, 277–279
      handicap, 279–281
      impairment, 274–277
        attention, 276–277
        memory, 276–277
    disabilities, 269–273
    handicaps, 273–274
    outcome measures, 268–269
      impairment, 268–269, 270–271t
Communication Profile: Functional Skills Survey, 73
Communicative Abilities in Daily Living, 72

Communicative Effectiveness Index, 72
Computerized systems, finanical outcome analysis, 122t
Consequences of disorder, World Health Organization classification, *12*
Consumer satisfaction measurement, 89–112
  methods, 95
    focus groups, 101–106, *102*
      public school setting, 104–106, 105t, 107t
      university setting, 102–104
    interviews
      face-to-face, 100t, 100–101
      telephone, 100t, 100–101
    surveys, 91–108, 95–108
      following acute rehabilitation stay, 100t
      health care setting, 95–100, 96–97t, 99t
  overview, 90–91
  quality, consumer-oriented dimensions of, 91–94
  service factors, importance-performance matrix, *102*
Continuum of care outcome measures, source of resources, 474
Control charts, 181
Cost. *See also* Economic outcome data
  in financial outcome analysis
    charges, distinguished, 115–116
    conformity, 130, 131t
    effectiveness, 129–130, 130t
    per client, *124*
Council of State Associations Presidents, 520–523, 521–522t
Council on Healthcare Provider Accreditation, 50
Critical pathways, financial outcome and, 118
Cultural diversity, 225–241
  clinical practice and, 234
  disability, differing views of, 227–234
  impairment, cultural interpretation of, 227–234
    African-American perspective, 230–231
    Asian/Pacific Islander perspective, 231–233
    Hispanic perspective, 227–230, 228–229t
    Native American perspective, 233–234
  research, 237–238
    paradigm shift, 237–238
  standardized instruments, 234–237, 235t
    adapting, 235–236
    interpreters, 236–237
    translating, 235–236
Curriculum alignment, in schools, outcomes measurement and, *442*

Daily living, communicative abilities in, aphasia and, 257
Dementia, 292–305
  clinical research, 299–303
    disabilities, 301–303
    handicaps, 303
    impairments, 300–301
  outcome measures, 294–299
    disabilities, 296–298
    handicaps, 298–299
    impairments, 294–296

Deming, W. Edward, 3–5
Depression scales, aphasia and, 260
Design, automated outcomes management system, 186–208
  for administrators, 191
  case example, 199–205
  for clients, 191
  for clinicians, 191
  design team, 192–193
    purpose, composition, 192–193
  features of system, 193–199
    commercially available systems, 197–199, 200–201t
    diagnostic categories, *195*
    hardware, 197
    percent improvement by diagnostic category, *196*
    report generation features, 189t, 194–196, *195–196*
    software, 196–197
  framework, 187–192, 189t
  for general public, 191
  for managed care organizations, 191
  report format, 192
  for researchers, 192
  stakeholders, identifying, 190–192
  uses of system, 189–190
Disablement process, quality of life, relationship, *77*
Disability, World Health Orgainzation Classification, *12*
Disease, consequences of, World Health Organization classification, *12*
Dismissal criteria, in schools, 447–448
Diversity, cultural, 225–241
  clinical practice and, 234
  disability, differing views of, 227–234
  impairment, cultural interpretation, 227–234
    African-American perspective, 230–231
    Asian/Pacific Islander perspective, 231–233
    Hispanic perspective, 227–230, 228–229t
    Native American perspective, 233–234
  research, 237–238
    paradigm shift, 237–238
  standardized instruments, 234–237, 235t
    adapting, 235–236
    interpreters, 236–237
    translating, 235–236
Donabedian, Avedis, 3–4
Duke-UNC Health Profile, 79
Dysphagia, 321–333
  historical overview, 322–323
  negative outcomes, 323–324
  positive outcomes, 323–324
  study types, 324–328
    quality-of-life instruments, 328
    randomized studies, 326–328
    single case studies, 325
    videofluorographic assessment, intervention completed at time of, 325–326

Economic outcome data, 113–132
  analysis, 125–128, 126–129t
  benchmarking, 119–120
  computerized systems, 122t
  cost
    vs. charges, 115–116
    conformity, 130, 131t
    effectiveness, 129–130, 130t
    per client, 124
  critical pathways, financial outcome and, 118
  data collection mechanisms, 120
  differentiating outcomes data, 114–115
  formulae, financial, generation of, 128–131
  integrated financial outcome analysis, 123–125, 124
  measurement systems, 120–123, 122t
  outlier analysis, 116–117
  overview, 131
  uses of, 118–119
  value analysis, 117–118
Efficacy, vs. effectiveness, in outcome measurement,
    16–18, 17t
Enderby outcomes scale, 571
Experimental methods, outcome measurement, 18,
    19–20

Face-to-face interviews, consumer satisfaction, 100t,
    100–101
FCP. See Functional Communication Profile
FIM. See Functional Independence Measure
Financial outcome data, 113–132
  analysis, 125–128, 126–129t
  benchmarking, 119–120
  computerized systems, 122t
  cost
    vs. charges, 115–116
    conformity, 130, 131t
    effectiveness, 129–130, 130t
    per client, 124
  critical pathways, financial outcome and, 118
  data collection mechanisms, 120
  differentiating outcomes data, 114–115
  formulae, financial, generation of, 128–131
  integrated financial outcome analysis, 123–125, 124
  measurement systems, 120–123, 122t
  outlier analysis, 116–117
  overview, 131
  uses of, 118–119
  value analysis, 117–118
Florida initiative, outcomes measurement, 515–517
Flow charts, 180
Fluency disorders, 387–405
  behavioral cognitive outcome measures, shift from,
    394–395
  effectiveness, defined, 390
  efficacy, defined, 389–390
  models, for outcomes research in, 388–389t,
    396–400
  outcomes, defined, 389
  process, defined, 388
  World Health Organization model, 395–396

  expansion of, with Wilson, Cleary model,
    396–400, 398t
Focus groups, consumer satisfaction, 101–106, 102
  public school setting, 104–106, 105t, 107t
  university setting, 102–104
Focus on Therapeutic Outcomes, Inc., 475
Formations in Health Care, Inc., 475
Formulae, financial, generation of, 128–131
FOTO. See Focus on Therapeutic Outcomes, Inc.
FSQ. See Functional Status Questionnaire
Functional, defined, 64
Functional abilities, measurement of, 62–75
  differentiating features, 64–75, 66–69t
  functional, defined, 64
  global measures, 65–70, 66–70t
  Minimum Data Set, Nursing Home Resident
    Assessment and Care Screening, 69
  Pediatric Evaluation of Disability Inventory, 68
  purposes, 63–64
  rehabilitation, general, 65–70, 66–70t
  WeeFIM, 68
Functional communication measures, 70–75, 72–74t
  American Speech-Language-Hearing Association
    Functional Assessment of Communica-
    tion Skills for Adults, 74
  Amsterdam Nijmegan Everyday Language Test, 73
  Communication Profile: Functional Skills Survey,
    73
  Communicative Abilities in Daily Living, 72
  Communicative Effectiveness Index, 72
  Functional Communication Profile, 72
  Functional Linguistic Communication Inventory,
    74
  Performance Status Scale for Head and Neck Can-
    cer Patients, 73
  Revised Edinburgh Functional Communication
    Profile, 72
Functional Communication Profile, 72
Functional Independence Measure, Version 4.0, 67
Functional Linguistic Communication Inventory, 74
Functional status, modality-specific behaviors, quali-
    ty of life, interrelationships, 57–61, 59t
Functional Status Questionnaire, 81

Georgia initiative, outcomes measurement, 520
Graphical tools, 182

Handicap
  usage of term, 154–155
  World Health Organization classification, 11–13, 12
HCFA. See Health Care Financing Administration
Health Care Financing Administration, 533–534, 556
  700 Form, 51
  701 Form, 53
  Office of Survey and Certification, 474
Health care settings, outcomes measurement in,
    453–476
  acute inpatient rehabilitation outcomes, 463
  continuum of care outcome measures, source of
    resources, 474

description, health care outcomes, 454–462, 455t, 457–461t

Focus on Therapeutic Outcomes, Inc., 475

Formations in Health Care, Inc., 475

health care continuum, outcomes, 462–467

Health Care Financing Administration Office of Survey & Certification, 474

home care, 465–466
  source of resources, 476

Joint Commission on Accreditation of Healthcare Organizations, 475

long-term care
  outcomes, 463–465
  source of resources, 474

managed care, 466–467
  network accreditation, source of resources, 475

Marianjoy Rehabilitation Hospital & Clinics, 475

Medirisk Corp. Headquarters, 475

National Association for Home Care, 476

National Committee for Quality Assurance, 475

outcome-oriented rehabilitation principles methods, source of resources, 476

outcomes management, 467–470, 469t

outpatient services, 465–466

Rehabilitation Accreditation Commission, 476

Rehabilitation Outcome Reporting System, 475

rehabilitation services accreditation, source of resources, 476

risk adjustment, 456–462

Santa Clara Valley Medical Center, 474

subacute care center, 463–465

Health-related quality-of-life measures, aphasia and, 260–261

Hearing Handicap Inventory for Elderly, 81

Hispanic perspective, of impairment, 227–230, 228–229t

Histograms, use of, 181

History of outcomes measurement, 2–8

Home care services outcomes, 465–466, 476

HQL. *See* Health-related quality-of-life measures

Huntington's disease, motor speech disorder with, 338–339

IEP. *See* Individualized education program

Impairment, World Health Organization classification, 121

Individualized education program, outcomes measurement and, 447

Initiatives, outcomes measurement
  national, 527–545
    American Speech-Language-Hearing Association, national treatment outcomes initiatives, 537–543, 541–542t
    health care, 528–533
      Agency for Health Care Policy and Research, 528–530
      American Speech-Language-Hearing Association, 532–533
      Joint Commission on Accreditation of Healthcare Organizations, 531–532

National Center for Medical Rehabilitation Research, 531

National Committee for Quality Assurance, 532

Office of Managed Care, 532

payment for services, 533–535
  Health Care Financing Administration, 533–534
  private insurers, 534–535

Rehabilitation Accreditation Commission, 532

health care agency initiatives, 528

outcomes assessment education, federal initiatives, 535–537, 536t

state, 514–524
  California, 519–520
  Council of State Associations Presidents, 520–523, 521–522t
  Florida, 515–517
  Georgia, 520
  practice guidelines, 517–519
    practice parameters, 517–519

Inpatient rehabilitation outcomes, acute, 463

Integrated financial outcome analysis, 123–125, *124*

International initiatives, outcomes measurement, United Kingdom, 558–578

JCAHO. *See* Joint Commission on Accreditation of Healthcare Organizations

Joint Commission on Accreditation of Healthcare Organizations, 39–41, 475, 531–532, 557
  care of patients, 40–41
  description of, 39
  outcomes measurement requirements, 39–41
  patient function, assessment of, 39–40

Leaders in outcomes movement, 2–5

Legislative requirements, 47–48
  Omnibus Budget Reconciliation Act, 47
  Social Security Act, Part 484, Resident Assessment, 47–48

Life, quality of
  with aphasia, 260–261
    depression scales, 260
    health-related quality-of-life measures, 260–261
    psychosocial outcome measures, 260
    well-being, measures of, 261
  disablement process, relationship, *77*
  functional status, modality-specific behaviors, interrelationships, 57–61, 59t
  instruments, dysphagia, 328
  measurement of, 75–82
  COOP charts, 79
    differentiating features, *77*, 77–82, 79–81t
    disablement process, quality of life, relationship, *77*
    Duke-UNC Health Profile, 79
    Functional Status Questionnaire, 81
    Hearing Handicap Inventory for Elderly, 81
    McMaster Health Index Questionnaire, 80

Life, quality of (*continued*)
    Medical Outcome Study Health Status Question-
        naire (SF-36), 79
    Nottingham Health Profile, 80
    purposes, 76–77
    Quality of Well-Being Scale, 81
    Sickness Impact Profile, 79
    tool selection, 82–83, 84t
    Voice Handicap Index, 81
Linguistic diversity, 225–241
    clinical practice, 234
    impairment, cultural interpretation, 227–234
        African-American perspective, 230–231
        Asian/Pacific Islander perspective, 231–233
        Hispanic perspective, 227–230, 228–229t
        Native American perspective, 233–234
    research, 237–238
        paradigm shift, 237–238
    standardized instruments, 234–237, 235t
        interpreters, 236–237
        translating, 235–236
Long-term care outcomes, 463–465, 474

Managed care organizations, 45–46
    automated outocmes management systems for, 191
    description, 45–46
    outcomes, 466–467
Marianjoy Rehabilitation Hospital & Clinics, 475
McMaster Health Index Questionnaire, 80
MCOs. *See* Managed care organizations
MDS. *See* Minimum Data Set, Nursing Home Resi-
        dent Assessment and Care Screening
Measurement of outcomes, 16–22
    classification of methods, 17t, 18–19
        experimental, 18
        nonexperimental, 19
        quasi-experimental, 18
    efficacy *vs.* effectiveness, 16–18, 17t
    experimental methods, 19–20
    multiple-attacks approach, 23
    nonexperimental methods, 22
    outcomes research *vs.* efficacy research, 16
    quasi-experimental methods, 20–22
        program evaluation, 20–21
        quality improvement methods, 20–21
    requirements, 28–54
    synthetic analysis, 22
Medicaid program, 44–45
Medical Outcome Study Health Status Questionnaire
    (SF-36), 79
Medicare program, 42–44, 45
    3705.2 assessment, 43
    3905.3 plan of treatment, 43
    3905.4 progress reports, 43–44
    description of, 44–45
    program, description of, 42
Medirisk Corp. Headquarters, 475
MHIQ. *See* McMaster Health Index Questionnaire
Minimum Data Set, Nursing Home Resident Assess-
        ment and Care Screening, 69

Modality-specific behaviors
    functional status, quality of life, interrelationships,
        57–61, 59t
    measurement of, 61–62
        differentiating features, 62
        purposes, 62
MOS. *See* Medical Outcome Study
Motor speech disorders, 334–353
    chronic disability model, 335–336
    nonprogressive, 343–348
        diseases, 344–345
            cerebral palsy, 345
            stroke, 344–345
            traumatic brain injury, 345
        intervention effectiveness analysis, 345–346
            improving pathologies, 345–346
            stable pathologies, 345
        rationale for measurement, 346–348
            intervention
                documenting effectiveness of, 346–347
                effectiveness value, 348
            recovery, extent, pattern of, 346
    progressive, 336–343
        diseases, 337–339
            amyotrophic lateral sclerosis, 337
            Huntington's disease, 338–339
            multiple sclerosis, 337–338
            Parkinson's disease, 338
        impairment-level intervention efficacy, docu-
            mention, 339–343
            augmentative communication systems, 343,
                344
            speech treatment, 342–343
            staging of treatment, 340–341t, 340–342
        intervention effectiveness analysis, 339
        rationale for measurement, 339
MS. *See* Multiple sclerosis
Multiple-attacks approach, outcome measurement,
    23
Multiple sclerosis, motor speech disorder with,
    337–338

Nagi classification of outcomes, 13, *14*
    active pathology, 13
    disability, 13, *14*
    functional limitation, 13
    impairment, 13
National Association for Home Care, 476
National Center for Medical Rehabilitation Research,
    531, 557
National Center on Educational Outcomes Model,
    443–446, *444,* 445–446t
National Centre for Clinical Audit, United Kingdom,
    561–562, *562*
National Committee for Quality Assurance, 475, 532
National Committee for Quality Health Care, 557
National Education Goals Panel, 557
National initiatives, outcomes measurement, 527–545
    Agency for Health Care Policy and Research,
        528–530

American Speech-Language-Hearing Association, 532–533
   national treatment outcomes initiatives, 537–543, 541–542t
  health care, 528–533
  Joint Commission on Accreditation of Healthcare Organizations, 531–532
  National Center for Medical Rehabilitation Research, 531
  National Committee for Quality Assurance, 532
  Office of Managed Care, 532
  outcomes assessment education, federal initiatives, 535–537, 536t
  payment for services, 533–535
    Health Care Financing Administration, 533–534
    private insurers, 534–535
  Rehabilitation Accreditation Commission, 532
Native American perspective, of impairment, 233–234
NCMRR. *See* National Center for Medical Rehabilitation Research
NCQA. *See* National Committee for Quality Assurance
Neurological Outcome Scale, Evaluation System for Outpatient Rehabilitation Programs, 67
NHP. *See* Nottingham Health Profile
Nightingale, Florence, contribution of, 2
Nonexperimental methods, outcome measurement, 19, 22
Nottingham Health Profile, 80

OBRA. *See* Omnibus Budget Reconciliation Act
Office of Forum for Quality And Effectiveness in Health Care, 557
Office of Managed Care, 532, 557
Office of Survey and Certification, Health Care Financing Administration, 474
Omnibus Budget Reconciliation Act, 47
Outcome
  defined, 10–16
  occurance of, 9–10
  overview of, 8–9
Outcome classification
  Nagi classification, 13, *14*
    active pathology, 13
    disability, 13, *14*
    functional limitation, 13
    impairment, 13
  Wilson, Cleary conceptual model, 13–16, *15*
    biological variables, 14
    functional status, 15
    general health perceptions, 15
    overall quality of life, 15–16
    symptom status, 15
  World Health Organization classification, 11–13, *12*
    handicap, 11–13, *12*
    impairment, 121
Outcome measurement
  overview, 16–22
    classification of methods, 17t, 18–19
      experimental, 18

      nonexperimental, 19
      quasi-experimental, 18
    efficacy *vs.* effectiveness, 16–18, 17t
    experimental methods, 19–20
    multiple-attacks approach, 23
    nonexperimental methods, 22
    outcomes research *vs.* efficacy research, 16
    quasi-experimental methods, 20–22
      program evaluation and quality improvement methods, 20–21
    synthetic analysis, 22
  requirements, 28–54, 46–47
    accrediting agencies, requirements of, 29–41
      American Speech-Language-Hearing Association
      Joint Commission on Accreditation of Healthcare Organizations, 39–41
      agency, description of, 39
      patient function, assessment of, 39–40
      professional services board, standard 3.0
        quality improvement, program evaluation, 37–38
      American Speech-Language-Hearing Association professional services board, 37–39
      description of, 37–39
      agency, description of, 37
      implementation, 38–39
      Joint Commission on Accreditation of Healthcare Organizations, care of patients, 40–41
      Rehabilitation Accreditation Commission, 29–37
      agency, description of, 29–30
      description of, 30–37
        accreditation criteria, 30–32
        accreditation principle, 30
        information analysis, utilization, 34–35
        management principle, 32
        outcomes measurement, promotion of, 32
        program evaluation principle, 32–33
        program quality, 36–37
        quality of services, 33–34
    accrediting organizations, 50
    Health Care Financing Administration
      700 Form, 51
      701 Form, 53
    legislative requirements, 47–48
    managed care organizations, 45–46
      description, 45–46
    Omnibus Budget Reconciliation Act, 47
    payer requirements, 41–47
      Medicaid program, 44–45
      Medicare program, 42–44, 45
        3705.2 assessment, 43
        3905.3 plan of treatment, 43
        3905.4 progress reports, 43–44
        program, description of, 42, 44–45
    regulatory requirements, 47–48
    Social Security Act, Part 484, Resident Assessment, 47–48

Outcomes research, *vs.* efficacy research, in outcome measurement, 16
Outlier analysis, financial outcome, 116–117
Outpatient services outcomes, 465–466

Pacific Islander perspective, of impairment, 231–233
Pareto charts, 181
Parkinson's disease, motor speech disorder with, 338
Payer requirements, 41–47
  Medicaid program, 44–45
  Medicare program, 42–44, 45
    3705.2 assessment, 43
    3905.3 plan of treatment, 43
    3905.4 progress reports, 43–44
    program, description of, 42, 44–45
PDSA. *See* Plan-do-study-act cycle
Pediatric Evaluation of Disability Inventory, 68
Pediatric language disorders. *See* Child language disorders
Performance Status Scale for Head and Neck Cancer Patients, 73
Phonological disorders, 406–437, 408–409
Plan-do-study-act cycle, *181*
Practice guidelines, state initiatives, 517–519
Private insurers, initiatives, 534–535
Private practice, outcomes measurement in, 503–515
  case example, 507, 509–510
  cost effectiveness, 509
  functional outcomes
    emergence of, 507–508
    reporting, 508–509
  practice patterns, measuring, 506–507
  three-party service delivery system, 503–506
    payer, 505–506
Professional services board, American Speech-Language-Hearing Association, 37–39
Program evaluation, 151–171
  aggregation, levels of, *152*
  comparative data, 160–163, 162
  components, 163–168, 164–165t
    baseline data, 166
    comparative information, 166–167
    data collection, 167
    framework for program goals, 163
    indicators of performance, 166
    interpretation of data, 168
    measurement points, 166
    model, 167
    performance index, 167–168
    population for analysis, 166
    program goals, 163
    report of data, 167
  consumer satisfaction, as indicator of value, 159
  data elements for, example, 155t
  defined, 152–153
  disablement framework, 154–155
  goal attainment, 158-
  handicap, usage of term, 154–155
  improvement, 160
    integration, evaluative functions, 153
    level of function, 157t
    management report, sample, 164t-165t
    methods, quality improvement methods, outcome measurement, 20–21
    report cards, 162–163
    reporting process, 168–169
      accuracy, 169
      tailoring to audience, 168–169
      timely reports, 169
    systems approach, 155–157t, 155–158
    value, 159
PSB. *See* Professional services board
Psychosocial outcome, well-being measures, aphasia and, 259–260
Public school setting, consumer satisfaction focus groups, 104–106, 105t, 107t

Quality improvement, 172–185
  analysis tolls, 180–182, *182*
  cause-and-effect diagrams, 180–181
  clinical example, 182–183
  clinical outcomes, optimizing, 176–179, 177t
    critical paths, 178–179
    practice guidelines, 178
    preferred practice patterns, 177–178
  control charts, 181
  data collection tools, 180–182, *182*
  defined, 173
  flow charts, 180
  graphical tools, *182*
  histograms, 181
  methods, 20–21
  model, 179–183, *180, 180–181*
  overview, 173–176
  Pareto charts, 181
  plan-do-study-act cycle, *181*
  problem solving tools, 180–182, *182*
  run charts, 181
  scatter diagrams, 181
Quality of life
  with aphasia, 260–261
    depression scales, 260
    health-related quality-of-life measures, 260–261
    psychosocial outcome measures, 260
    well-being, measures of, 261
  disablement process, relationship, *77*
  functional status, modality-specific behaviors, interrelationships, 57–61, 59t
  instruments, dysphagia and, 328
  measurement of, 75–82
    COOP charts, 79
    differentiating features, *77*, 77–82, 79–81t
    disablement process, quality of life, relationship, *77*
    Duke-UNC Health Profile, 79
    Functional Status Questionnaire, 81
    Hearing Handicap Inventory for Elderly, 81
    McMaster Health Index Questionnaire, 80

Medical Outcome Study Health Status Questionnaire (SF-36), 79
Nottingham Health Profile, 80
purposes, 76–77
Quality of Well-Being Scale, 81
Sickness Impact Profile, 79
tool selection, 82–83, 84t
Voice Handicap Index, 81
Quality of Well-Being Scale, 81
Quasi-experimental methods
outcome measurement, 18, 20–22
program evaluation, quality improvement, 20–21
QWB. *See* Quality of Well-Being Scale

Rehabilitation Accreditation Commission, 29–37, 50, 476, 532, 556
agency, description of, 29–30
outcomes measurement requirements, description of, 30–37
accreditation
criteria, 30–32
principle, 30
information analysis, utilization, 34–35
outcomes measurement, promotion of, 32
program evaluation principle, 32–33
program quality, 36–37
quality of services, 33–34
Rehabilitation Institute of Chicago Functional Assessment Scale, 67
Rehabilitation Outcome Reporting System, 475
Rehabilitation services accreditation, source of resources, 476
Researchers, automated outocmes management systems for, 192
Revised Edinburgh Functional Communication Profile, 72
RIC-FAS. *See* Rehabilitation Institute of Chicago Functional Assessment Scale
Right-hemisphere brain damage, 281–292
clinical research, 283t, 288–291, 289–290t
outcome measures, 282–288, 283–287t
Risk adjustment, principles of, 456–462
Royal College of Speech and Language Therapists, in United Kingdom, role of, 569–571
Run charts, use of, 181

Santa Clara Valley Medical Center, 474
Satisfaction of consumer, measurement, 89–112
methods, 95
focus groups, 101–106, *102*
public school setting, 104–106, 105t, 107t
university setting, 102–104
interviews
face to face, 100t, 100–101
telephone, 100t, 100–101
surveys, 95–100
following acute rehabilitation stay, 100t
health care setting, 95–100, 96–97t, 99t
overview, 90–91

quality, consumer-oriented dimensions of, 91–94
service factors, importance-performance matrix, *102*
Scatter diagrams, 181
Schools, outcomes measurement in, 438–452
curriculum alignment, *442*
dismissal criteria, 447–448
history of, 439–443, 441t, *442*
individualized education program, 447
National Center on Educational Outcomes Model, 443–446, *444,* 445–446t
service delivery model effectiveness, 448–450
speech, language services, students enrolled in, outcome indicators, 447–450
students with disabilities, outcomes for, 443–446
Senility, 292–305
clinical research, 299–303
disabilities, 301–303
handicaps, 303
impairments, 300–301
outcome measures, 294–299
disabilities, 296–298
handicaps, 298–299
impairments, 294–296
Sickness Impact Profile, 79
SIP. *See* Sickness Impact Profile
Social Security Act, Part 484, Resident Assessment, 47–48
State initiatives, outcomes measurement, 514–524
California, 519–520
Council of State Associations Presidents, 520–523, 521–522t
Florida, 515–517
Georgia, 520
practice guidelines, 517–519
practice parameters, 517–519
Stroke, motor speech disorder with, 344–345
Stuttering, 387–405
behavioral cognitive outcome measures, shift from, 394–395
effectiveness, defined, 390
efficacy, defined, 389–390
models, for outcomes research in, stuttering, 388–389t, 396–400
outcomes, defined, 389
process, defined, 388
stuttering, 390–393
World Health Organization model, 395–396
expansion of, with Wilson, Cleary model, 396–400, 398t
Subacute care center outcomes, 463–465
Survey, consumer satisfaction tool, 91–108, 95–100
following acute rehabilitation stay, 100t
health care setting, 95–100, 96–97t, 99t
Synthetic analysis, outcome measurement, 22

TBI. *See* Traumatic brain injury
Team, for automated outcomes management systems design, 192–193
purpose, composition, 192–193

Telephone interviews, consumer satisfaction, 100t, 100–101
Three-party service delivery system, private practice, outcomes measurement in, 503–506
    payer, 505–506
Traumatic brain injury, 268–281
    clinical research, 274–281
        disability, 277–279
        handicap, 279–281
        impairment, 274–277
            attention, 276–277
            memory, 276–277
    disabilities, 269–273
    handicaps, 273–274
    motor speech disorder with, 345
    outcome measures, 268–269
        impairment, 268–269, 270–271t
Treatment efficacy research, 134–150
    clinical research, 134–135
    components of, 136
    data analysis, interpretation, 145–147
    defined, 134–147
    dependent variables, 140–145
    designs, 138–139
    efficacy, *vs.* outcome research, 135–136
    independent variables, 139–140
    research questions, 136–138

United Kingdom
    Centre for Evidence-Based Medicine, 561
    Clearing House on Health Outcomes, 560
    Cochrane Centre, 560
    outcomes measurement initiatives, 558–578
    Royal College of Speech and Language Therapists, 569–571
Universities, outcome measurement in, 477–502
    classroom measurement goals, 481
    clinical practicum measurement goals, 481
    consumer satisfaction focus groups in, 102–104
    goals, 479–482
    institutional goals, 479–480, 480t
    laboratory measurement goals, 481–482
    programmatic measurement goals, 479–480, 480t
    sample, 483–491, *485–492*
    types, 482–483
        classroom assessment, 496–497
        commonly used approaches, 482–483, 483–484t
        variation types, 482

Value, outcome measurement and, 209–224
    audit, 216–222
    client/family, 222
    clinicians, 219–222, *220–222*
    corporate environments, 211–212
    financial outcome, 117–118
    implementation, 2156–216
        testing system, 215–216
    integrity procedures, 216–222
    outcomes information, use of, 219
    payer, 222
    rehabilitation managers, 219–222, *220–222*
    report structure, 217
    reporting of outcomes data, 216–219
    training, 214–215
        barrier, 214, 215
        overview, 214
        reliability testing, 215
        solution, 214, 215
Videofluorographic assessment, dysphagia intervention completed at time of, studies, 325–326
Voice disorders, outcome measurement, historical perspective, 354–386
    in 1940s, 355–357
    in 1950s, 357–358
    in 1960s, 358–360
    in 1970s, 360–364
    in 1980s, 364–371
    in 1990s, 371–379
Voice Handicap Index, 81

WeeFIM, 68
Wennberg, John, 5
WHO. *See* World Health Organization
Wilson
    Cleary conceptual model, outcomes, 13–16, *15*
        biological variables, 14
        functional status, 15
        general health perceptions, 15
        overall quality of life, 15–16
        symptom status, 15
    I. B., 15
World Health Organization
    classification of outcomes, 11–13, *12*
        handicap, 11–13, *12*
        impairment, 121
    stuttering, outcomes model, 395–396